J. Cale Johnson, Krisztián Simkó

Gastrointestinal Disease and Its Treatment in Ancient Mesopotamia

Die babylonisch-assyrische Medizin in Texten und Untersuchungen

Begründet von Franz Köcher

Herausgegeben von
Nils P. Heeßel und Marten Stol

Band 11

J. Cale Johnson, Krisztián Simkó

Gastrointestinal Disease and Its Treatment in Ancient Mesopotamia

The Nineveh Treatise

DE GRUYTER

The work on this volume as part of the project BabMed – Babylonian Medicine has been funded by the European Research Council (ERC) under the European Union's Seventh Framework Programme (FP7/2007–2013; Project No. 323596).

European Research Council
Established by the European Commission

ISBN 978-1-5015-1526-2
e-ISBN (PDF) 978-1-5015-0657-4
e-ISBN (EPUB) 978-1-5015-0645-1
DOI https://doi.org/10.1515/9781501506574

Library of Congress Control Number 2024933235

Bibliographic information published by the Deutsche Nationalbibliothek
The Deutsche Nationalbibliothek lists this publication in the Deutsche Nationalbibliografie; detailed bibliographic data are available in the Internet at http://dnb.dnb.de.

Cover image: Line art of Manuscript C (K 2386+) from the fourth chapter of the Stomach Treatise, copied by Krisztián Simkó
Typesetting: Michael Peschke, Berlin

www.degruyter.com

Table of Contents

Acknowledgements

First and foremost, we would like to express our sincere and unending thanks to Markham J. Geller, who has continually supported our work on the edition published here in almost every way imaginable. This work began with a joint edition of STO that Geller and Johnson worked on for a number of years during the BabMed Project (2013–2018). During that time, the entire text, in as far as it had been recovered at that point, was read in weekly meetings for several months by the BabMed team in Berlin, and then again as part of the online reading group for medical texts that Mark led at that time. We would like to express our sincere and heartful thanks to everyone who participated in the BabMed Project and the online reading group. When Cale Johnson moved to Leiden in 2016 and then again to Birmingham between 2018 and 2020, Mark agreed that Cale should finish the edition on his own, particularly with the access to the British Museum that, it was hoped, the position in Birmingham would make possible. As it happened, Cale was only able to visit the British Museum a handful of times before the Covid pandemic struck, and he was called back to Berlin as Professor für Wissensgeschichte des Altertums in 2020; the still fundamental need for a careful reassessment of all the fragments in the British Museum remained unfulfilled.

In 2020, Krisztián Simkó, who had also played a key role in the BabMed Project, took up a three-year postdoc at the British Museum as part of the NinMed Project (2020–2023) under the leadership of Jon Taylor and in collaboration with Mark Geller and Irving Finkel. This was a great opportunity to complete the work on the primary sources in the British Museum, so Johnson and Simkó agreed to jointly edit the entire work again from scratch. Now including numerous textual improvements based on first-hand examination of the tablets and fragments (as well as a dozen new joins), this new edition, which has led to the edition that we publish here, was again read over a number of months by the online reading group associated with the NinMed Project. Often, in the course of these reading sessions, numerous contradictory and usually strongly held points of view on a given philological problem were presented, but only rarely was there a clear consensus. Thus, although these online reading sessions have been incredibly helpful and instructive, we have sought to arrive at our own view of each philological problem, as justified briefly in our footnotes. Needless to say, the authors are jointly responsible for the readings and interpretations of the text presented here and no one else should be held responsible for any errors or poorly made philological decisions that remain in the volume. Although the membership of these online readings groups continually shifted over time, we would like to single out a few people who have been at nearly every session and from whose suggestions we have greatly benefitted again and again: Mark Geller, Irving Finkel, Jon Taylor, Strahil Panayotov, Sona Eypper, Gilles Buisson, Annie Attia, and Antoine Cavigneaux.

We would especially like to thank our reviewers for the series *Die babylonisch-assyrische Medizin in Texten und Untersuchungen*, Marten Stol and Nils Heeßel, who went amazingly beyond the call of duty and sent us literally hundreds of questions and suggestions over the course of six months. Even though we did not always accept their suggestions, the volume has been massively improved by the intense critical rigour of this review process, and we are truly thankful for the huge amount of effort that they expended as part of this process. We also want to extend our sincere thanks to Albrecht Doehnert, the editorial director responsible for BAM at De Gruyter, who has continually supported the project, including the somewhat innovative format that we make use of in this volume. Thanks to Kristin Kleber for making available to us the GoviB-Projekt RTI scanning dome in the VAM and Georg Neumann for scanning several recalcitrant tablets. We would like to thank Stefan Maul for sending detailed images of the tablets edited in *Bannlösung (nam-érim-búr-ru-da): Die Therapie eines auf eidlichen Falschaussage zurückgeführten Leidens* (KAL 10, as well as for the numerous suggestions for our text that he included in that volume); special thanks to Enrique Jiménez for giving us early access to the eBL portal as well as sponsoring the creation of the eBL join-finding algorithms, which have delivered numerous little gifts to us over the past three years. And, of course, we would like to thank the management, curators and staff at the British Museum and Vorderasiatisches Museum for helping us both to access and make sense of the tablets over the years.

Cale Johnson would like to thank his wife, Grace, and his daughter, Abigail, for their never-ending love and support over the last decade while elements of this volume were being prepared and reworked.

https://doi.org/10.1515/9781501506574-201

Abbreviations

AbB F.R. Kraus (ed.), *Altbabylonische Briefe in Umschrift und Übersetzung* (1964–)

ABRT J.A. Craig, *Assyrian and Babylonian Religious Texts*, 2 vols. (1895–1897)

AHw W. von Soden, *Akkadisches Handwörterbuch*, 3 vols. (1965–1981)

AMC Assur Medical Catalogue

AMT R. Campbell Thompson, *Assyrian Medical Texts from the Originals in the British Museum* (1923)

ARET 5 D.O. Edzard, *Hymnen, Beschwörungen und Verwandtes aus dem Archiv L.2769*, Archivi reali di Ebla Testi, vol. 5 (1984)

ASKT P. Haupt, *Akkadische und sumerische Keilschrifttexte* (1881–1882)

BAK H. Hunger, *Babylonische und assyrische Kolophone* (1968)

BAM F. Köcher, *Die babylonisch-assyrische Medizin in Texten und Untersuchungen*, 6 vols. (1963–1980)

BAM 7 M.J. Geller, *Renal and Rectal Disease Texts*, Die babylonisch-assyrische Medizin in Texten und Untersuchungen, vol. 7 (2005)

BAM 8 M.J. Geller, *Healing Magic and Evil Demons: Canonical Udug-hul Incantations*, Die babylonisch-assyrische Medizin in Texten und Untersuchungen, vol. 8 (2016)

BAM 9 U. Steinert (ed.), *Assyrian and Babylonian Scholarly Text Catalogues: Medicine, Magic and Divination*, Die babylonisch-assyrische Medizin in Texten und Untersuchungen, vol. 9 (2018)

BAM 10 M.J. Geller and S.V. Panayotov, *Mesopotamian Eye Disease Texts: The Nineveh Treatise*, Die babylonisch-assyrische Medizin in Texten und Untersuchungen, vol. 10 (2020)

BAM 13 E. Schmidtchen, *Mesopotamische Diagnostik. Untersuchungen zu Rekonstruktion, Terminologie und Systematik des babylonisch-assyrischen Diagnosehandbuches und eine Neubearbeitung der Tafeln 3–14*, Die babylonisch-assyrische Medizin in Texten und Untersuchungen, vol. 13 (2021)

BRM 4 A.T. Clay, *Epics, Hymns, Omens and Other Texts*, Babylonian Records in the Library of J. Pierpont Morgan, vol. 4 (1923)

BRON BRONCHIA (the seventh treatise of the Nineveh Medical Encyclopaedia)

CAD A.L. Oppenheim et al. (ed.), *The Assyrian Dictionary of the University of Chicago*, 20 vols. (1956–2010)

CDA J. Black, A. George, and N. Postgate, *A Concise Dictionary of Akkadian*, 2nd (corrected) printing (2000)

CRAN CRANIUM (the first treatise in the Nineveh Medical Encyclopaedia)

CT Cuneiform Texts from Babylonian Tablets in the British Museum

CTMMA 2 I. Spar and W.G. Lambert (ed.), *Literary and Scholastic Texts of the First Millennium B.C.*, Cuneiform Texts in the Metropolitan Museum of Art, vol. 2 (2005)

CTN 4 D.J. Wiseman and J.A. Black, *Literary Texts from the Temple of Nabû*, Cuneiform Texts from Nimrud, vol. 4 (1996)

CUSAS 12 M. Civil, *The Lexical Texts in the Schøyen Collection*, Cornell University Studies in Assyriology and Sumerology, vol. 12 (2010)

CUSAS 18 A.R. George, *Babylonian Divinatory Texts Chiefly in the Schøyen Collection*, Cornell University Studies in Assyriology and Sumerology, vol. 18 (2013)

CUSAS 32 A.R. George, *Mesopotamian Incantations and Related Texts in the Schøyen Collection*, Cornell University Studies in Assyriology and Sumerology, vol. 32 (2016)

Emar VI/4 D. Arnaud, *Recherches au pays d'Aštata, Emar VI/4, Textes de la bibliothèque: Transcriptions et traductions* (1987)

IAS R.D. Biggs, *Inscriptions from Tell Abū Ṣalābīkh*, Oriental Institute Publications, vol. 99 (1974)

KADP F. Köcher, *Keilschrifttexte zur assyrisch-babylonischen Drogen- und Pflanzenkunde* (1955)

KAR E. Ebeling, *Keilschrifttexte aus Assur religiösen Inhalts*, 2 vols. (1919–1923)

KUB Keilschrifturkunden aus Boghazköi

LTBA 2 W. von Soden, *Die akkadischen Synonymenlisten*, Die lexikalischen Tafelserien der Babylonier und Assyrer in den Berliner Museen, vol. 2 (1933)

MARV H. Freydank et al. (ed.), *Mittelassyrische Rechtsurkunden und Verwaltungstexte*, 10 vols. (1976–2010)

MDP Mémoires de la Délégation en Perse

MSL B. Landsberger et al. (ed.), *Materialien zum sumerischen Lexikon / Materials for the Sumerian Lexicon* (1937–)

MSL SS 1 M. Civil et al., *The Sag-Tablet, Lexical Texts in the Ashmolean Museum, Middle Babylonian Grammatical Texts, Miscellaneous Texts*, Materials for the Sumerian Lexicon Supplementary Series, vol. 1 (1986)

PBS Publications of the Babylonian Section, University of Pennsylvania

RIAA L. Speleers, *Recueil des inscriptions de l'Asie antérieure des Musées Royaux du Cinquantenaire à Bruxelles: Textes sumériens, babyloniens et assyriens* (1925)

SAA 7 F.M. Fales and J.N. Postgate, *Imperial Administrative Records, Part 1: Palace and Temple Administration*, State Archives of Assyria, Vol. 7 (1992)

SAA 10 S. Parpola, *Letters from Assyrian and Babylonian Scholars*, State Archives of Assyria, vol. 10 (1993)

SAD M.P. Streck, *Supplement to the Akkadian Dictionaries* (2018–)

SBH G. Reisner, *Sumerisch-babylonische Hymnen nach Thontafeln griechischer Zeit* (1896)

SEAL Sources of Early Akkadian Literature (http://www.seal.uni-leipzig.de)

SF A. Deimel, *Schultexte aus Fara* (1923)

SpTU 1 H. Hunger, *Spätbabylonische Texte aus Uruk*, vol. 1 (1976)

SpTU 4 E. von Weiher, *Uruk. Spätbabylonische Texte aus dem Planquadrat U 18*, vol. 4 (1993)

https://doi.org/10.1515/9781501506574-202

STO	STOMACH (the eighth treatise in The Nineveh Medical Encyclopaedia)
STT	O.R. Gurney et al., *The Sultantepe Tablets*, 2 vols. (1957–1964)
STVC	E. Chiera, *Sumerian Texts of Varied Contents*, Oriental Institute Publications, vol. 16 (1934)
TCL	Textes cunéiformes, Musées du Louvre
UET	Ur Excavations, Texts
VS	Vorderasiatische Schriftdenkmäler der Königlichen Museen zu Berlin
YOS	Yale Oriental Series, Babylonian Texts

Chapter 1
Introduction

Without anatomical textbooks and the disciplines built up around them, we moderns might assume that ancient peoples, including the authors and transmitters of the Mesopotamian medical treatise edited here, had no accurate conception of the gastrointestinal tract. Maybe it is easier to imagine this kind of knowledge if we think of the gastrointestinal tract merely as the tube that runs from mouth to anus. Given the regular movement of food through it and the corresponding generation of excrement and other effluvia, not to mention the connection of eating and drinking with a host of internal states from inebriation to the agony of food poisoning, the gastrointestinal tube is a deeply cultural entity. The Mesopotamian physicians who first wrote down their diagnoses and prescriptions in the 2nd millennium BCE were well aware of this tube running through the body, and as we will see throughout this volume, their treatments were often aimed at introducing drugs into it, either through medicines to be drunk or medicines introduced through the anus in the form of enemas or suppositories. Before we turn to some of the specifics of how Mesopotamian physicians treated gastrointestinal problems, let us take a moment to reflect on this gastrointestinal pathway and its *longue durée* prehistory as a cultural entity and domain.

Already with the Neanderthals but also with our *Homo sapien* ancestors, fire was one of the first domesticated and domesticating technologies. James C. Scott's rewrite of the millennia leading up to the early Mesopotamian states, *Against the Grain*, frames fire in environmental terms as an early way of manipulating the distribution of naturally occurring foodstuffs prior to their domestication, but foremost as the basis for the cooking of food.[1] Human beings are able to make do with a relatively small digestive tract because we use culturally transmitted techniques—including recipes handed down through the generations—to predigest our food before we eat it:

> The application of fire to raw food externalizes the digestive process; it gelatinizes starch and denatures protein. The chemical disassembly of raw food, which in a chimpanzee requires a gut roughly three times the size of ours, allows *Homo sapiens* to eat far less food and expend far fewer calories extracting nutrition from it.[2]

Of course, the larger argument that Scott and others have been making over the years is that the earliest Near Eastern states really emerged, as states, largely through their efforts to control the planting and harvesting of staple crops like barley and wheat and, likewise, through their management of huge herds of domesticated animals.[3] To a great degree, the elaboration of the proto-cuneiform and cuneiform writing systems resulted from the need to manage and audit vast amounts of grain, livestock, and the labour involved in producing both. At the same time that urbanism in southern Mesopotamia was producing a new kind of food security (or perhaps a different kind of insecurity), mediated through state-level organizations and their newly invented bookkeeping methods, it was also producing a new kind of disease, namely contagious diseases that are spread through closely packed urban populations.[4] It was in the midst of these infrastructures of food production and consumption, human waste and disease that the earliest forms of technical medicine probably came into being.

Even if the prehistorical phases of Mesopotamian thought about the digestive tract were not written down and are certainly lost, perhaps we can use a recent, popular description of the embryology and development of the gastrointestinal tract to think about the accessibility of the gastrointestinal tract to ancient Mesopotamians.[5] Here is Giulia Enders's description of the earliest states in the development of the cardiovascular, nervous and digestive tracts in a human foetus:[6]

1 Scott 2017: 37–43.

2 Scott 2017: 40–41

3 See Paulette 2016 for a nice survey of staple crop economies in Mesopotamia; for an interesting comparative meditation on state-managed herding, see Corcoran-Todd, Price and Caramanica 2022.

4 See the broad-brush overview in the opening chapters of Barrett and Armelagos 2013 as well as Algaze's discussion of McNeill's Paradox in the context of Mesopotamia (2018: 23–26).

5 Overviews of the history of the gastrointestinal tract or digestion often skip ancient Mesopotamia. In the recent collection of papers in Collard and Samama 2021, for example, the only reference to Mesopotamia is a citation of Stol 2006 in Pietrobelli's paper on theories of digestion in Greco-Roman antiquity (Pietrobelli 2021: 36 n. 24)

6 Enders 2015; translation from the German original published in 2014.

https://doi.org/10.1515/9781501506574-001

> If we could see more than meets the eye, we could watch as a clump of cells grows into a human being in a woman's belly. We would suddenly see how we develop, roughly speaking, from three tubes. The first tube runs right the way through us, with a knot in the middle. This is our cardiovascular system, and the central knot is what develops into our heart. The second tube develops more or less parallel to the first along our back. Then it forms a bubble that migrates to the top end of our body, where it stays put. This tube is our nervous system, with the spinal cord, including the brain, at the top and myriad nerves branching out into every part of the body. The third tube runs through us from end to end. This is our intestinal tube—the gut.
>
> The intestinal tube provides many of the furnishings of our interior. It grows buds that bulge out farther and farther to the left and right. These buds will later develop into our lungs. A little bit lower down, the intestinal tube bulges again and our liver has begun to develop. It also forms our gall bladder and pancreas. But, most importantly, the tube itself begins to grow increasingly clever. It is involved in the complex construction of our mouth, creates our esophagus, with its ability to move like a break dancer, and develops a little pouch so we can store food for a couple of hours. And, last but not least, the intestinal tube completes its masterpiece—the eponymous intestine or gut.[7]

Crucially for us, as historians and philologists of the ancient Near East, the only one of these three tubes that was readily accessible to ancient healers and physicians in Mesopotamia, or at least indirectly observable through its intake of food and output of wastes, was the gastrointestinal tube. The cardiovascular and nervous systems would remain very poorly understood until the emergence of internal anatomy in the work of Herophilus in Alexandria.[8] In contrast, the gastrointestinal tube was an ever-present object of interaction and investigation through the foods, drinks, and drugs that were introduced into it and the various different kinds of wastes, gases, and effluvia that passed out of it. Moreover, as human experiencers of these intakes and outputs, eaters, drinkers, and excreters like us were also well aware of the sensations and internal states that could be brought about by the ingestion of a drug, contaminated food or the odd malfeasant microbe.

Even so, for ancient Mesopotamians, the digestive system was still a 'black box': certain things could be added to the system, producing various responses and effluvia, but its internal structure and processes were largely unknown. To fill in this gap in their knowledge, ancient Mesopotamian healers postulated a number of different models for processes within the gut, and many of these black-box hypotheses were modelled on processes observable in the social or natural environments in which they lived. Two dominant models are visible in later textual traditions: (i) waterways and canals, which carried all manner of goods and people, not to mention waste and trash, and (ii) ceramic vessels, such as the fermentation vat.[9] Each of these models had its advantages: waterways and canals, at a much larger scale than the human digestive tract, allowed for the imagination of many different types and intensities of gastrointestinal dysfunction, not to mention processes such as the accumulation of silt or putrefaction of non-flowing water. In contrast, vessels such as the fermentation vat were analogous to the internal organs in size and often served as containers for processes of fermentation, especially of alcohol.

The chief metaphors in the Stomach Treatise (hereafter STO), for example, describe the gastrointestinal tract either in terms of waterways and canals with minute creatures shovelling out an intestinal blockage—sometimes as a waterway or a well with still, unflowing water—or alternatively in terms of containers of one kind or another, such as a fermentation vat whose mouth is covered (*kīma kakkulli pīšu katim*), a waterskin (*nādu*) or leather bag (*luppu*), or a second kind of fermentation vat (*namzītu*). The metaphorical vehicles at work in these images or models range in scale from the weir of a canal, in which a team of human workers could remove a blockage (a common everyday scene in ancient Mesopotamia), down to a number of vessels no larger than the gastrointestinal organs themselves. Moreover, as George argues in his 2016 publication of the incantations from the Schøyen Collection, there seems to have been a tradition of compiling gastrointestinal models in the form of incantations; the purpose of the incantations about the *namzītu* vessel was, as George says:

> not cultic but medical. The brewing jar *namzītum* was a tall pot with a pointed bottom that rested on a stand. Liquids and solids were put in at the top, and the end product collected from a hole in the bottom. The hole could be closed with a stopper or plug (*purussu*). One of the Sumerian terms for it is ^{dug}níg-dúr-bùru (Urra X 213), explicitly "the pot with a hole in the bottom." It is easy to see that such a vessel provides a functional analogue of the human digestive system, from mouth to anus.[10]

This sliding scale of 'functional analogies', from a massive weir controlling the flow of water through a canal to George's eloquently described and human-sized 'pot with a hole in the bottom', thus represents a set of models for the gastrointesti-

7 Enders 2015: 10.

8 See von Staden 1989 in conjunction with the review in Hankinson 1990 for the key sources and an overview of the issues.

9 For the ancient Mesopotamian models of the gastrointestinal tract in terms of waterways, see Steinert 2013 and the papers collected in Wee 2017. A brief discussion of the food canal imagery can also be found in Simkó 2018: 538–540.

10 George 2016: 135–136. See also the discussion of the Akkadian equivalent of *nazzītu*, viz. *namzītu*, in Gaspa 2014: 135–138.

nal tract. Indeed, in line with the Mesopotamian penchant for using sliding scales like this as theoretical models,[11] it is best, in our view, to speak of these metaphors as theoretical models for the Stomach Treatise edited in this volume.

Regardless of the metaphorical model in use, healthy digestion—where food enters the body through the mouth, moves downward in the food tube until it reaches the end of the tube and exits the body in the form of waste, all without discomfort and at a reasonable speed—served as a norm, against which abnormal behaviour of the tube could be judged. Gastrointestinal disease could be observed if the system became blocked up and the food did not proceed normally or if the nourishment did not produce the expected levels of satisfaction, fullness, energy, or inebriation.

Early Incantations against Gastrointestinal Illness in Mesopotamia

While food production and storage were already being documented in the earliest proto-cuneiform records (ca. 3300 BCE), the treatment of human disease would not begin to emerge in written form until the middle of the third millennium BCE, seven or eight centuries after the first written documents. As it happens, these earliest treatments were incantations written down in the Early Dynastic III period (ca. 2600–2500 BCE), occasionally including short ritual instructions, such as having the patient drink water from the Tigris and the Euphrates (see below). Although some examples of Early Dynastic incantations were already surveyed in Krebernik's pathbreaking *Die Beschwörungen aus Fara und Ebla*,[12] two recent publications are particularly important for making sense of this early group of treatments employed for gastrointestinal illness: Andrew George's publication of incantations from the Schøyen Collection[13] and the recent synthesis of belly incantations published by Ulrike Steinert and Luděk Vacín.[14] Let us first look briefly at a few examples of Early Dynastic, Ur III and Old Babylonian incantations before turning to more traditional medical sources.

Early Dynastic incantations are often difficult to interpret, but it is clear that terms like 'sick belly' (Sum. ša$_3$ gig) or 'sick innards' (Sum. lipiš gig) occur frequently in the attested incantations. More importantly, for our purposes here, two of the central themes in the Stomach Treatise, namely the gastrointestinal tract (usually represented by Sum. ša$_3$ 'belly') and the deleterious effects associated with 'bile' (Sum. ze$_2$)[15] are obliquely connected in an incantation found in Ebla (see below), but let us turn first to a topos that occurs in several Early Dynastic incantations: the juxtaposition of 'sick belly' (ša$_3$ gig) with 'tree' (ĝiš) and 'reed' (gi) in two passages from Fara:

$^{\text{viii 5}}$TUR EDEN ša$_3$ UD mu-na-ak / $^{\text{viii 6}}$**ša$_3$-da ĝiš an-TAG$_4$.TAG$_4$+SAG-da** / $^{\text{viii 7}}$**gi TAG$_4$.TAG$_4$+SAG-da** / . . . / $^{\text{viii 12}}$ša$_3$ gig / $^{\text{ix 1}}$ZUM ḫe$_2$-DU[16]
$^{\text{iii' 4}}$**ša$_3$ gig-da** / $^{\text{iii' 5}}$**ĝiš an da TAG$_4$+SAG** / $^{\text{iii' 6}}$**gi da TAG$_4$+SAG**[17]

In both passages, the main verb (viz. an-TAG$_4$.TAG$_4$+SAG-da and TAG$_4$+SAG respectively) describes an event that is 'with the (sick) belly' (ša$_3$ gig.da) but takes first the 'tree' (ĝiš) and thereafter the 'reed' (gi) as its direct object; unfortunately, there is no consensus on the translation of either an-TAG$_4$.TAG$_4$+SAG-da or TAG$_4$+SAG.[18] We translate a largely parallel version of the same incantation below, but the importance of these two excerpts is that the same topos reappears in a syllabically written version of much the same incantation in Ebla,[19] in western Syria, and in the syllabic version from Ebla, the Sumer-

11 Besides the perspectival elements in the Etana and Adapa tales, see also the role of scale in the matrilineal genealogy in Johnson 2014a.

12 Krebernik 1984. See also Cunningham 1997, as well as Rudik's (2011) dissertation for surveys of the Early Dynastic incantation tradition.

13 George 2016.

14 Steinert and Vacín 2018, see in particular pp. 701–702 and comparable Old Babylonian materials; see also Peterson 2019.

15 In present-day usage, bile and gall are largely interchangeable (strictly speaking, bile is secreted in the liver, stored in the gallbladder and used to break down fats in the small intestine), but Assyriologists generally translate Sum. ze$_2$ as 'gall' rather than 'bile' in order to stress its connection to the gallbladder. In extispicy texts, for example, the logogram ZE$_2$ (also generally read as Akk. *martu*) refers to the gallbladder rather than gall or bile. With one possible exception, see the commentary to STO 3: 30, *martu* always seems to refer to gall or bile in our treatise and we consistently translate it with 'bile'. For a fascinating discussion of the Early Dynastic orthography AB$_2$.ŠA$_3$.GE as a writing of /ze/, see Balke 2015 and the response in Keetman 2021.

16 VAT 12597 viii 5–7 and viii 12–ix 1, corresponding to Krebernik 1984: no. 7, sections a–b and f, pp. 48–52.

17 VAT 12524 iii' 4–6, corresponding to Krebernik 1984: no. 11, section g (see also section b), pp. 76–80.

18 Rudik (2011: 115–116) reviews a couple of possible interpretations of KID$_2$+SAG, also rendered as TAG$_4$+SAG, but neither of these suggestions seems to fit the context of gastrointestinal illness, bile or jaundice. For a discussion of the parallel expression UD+DUL$_3$, see below.

19 In the syllabically written version from Ebla ša$_3$ gig corresponds to ša gi and lipiš gig to li-bi$_2$-iš gi; see Krebernik 1984: no. 9 i 6 and ii 1–2, Cunningham 1997: 36 and Rudik 2011: 123–128.

ian phrase lu$_2$ ze$_2$ 'someone (suffering from) bile' is used as a rubric, presumably in order to classify the type of illness described in the tablet. Thus, in one of the first intercultural moments in the third-millennium tradition, the recipients of this Mesopotamian incantation tradition, in Semitic-language speaking Ebla, felt the need to label 'sick belly' (ša$_3$ gig) as a bile-related illness.

Alongside these well-known, if still cryptic, Early Dynastic incantations, Andrew George's publication of incantations from the Schøyen Collection includes several Early Dynastic compendia of incantations that are particularly important for the early history of the treatment of gastrointestinal disease. Interestingly enough, one of these Early Dynastic compendia also includes a version of the Fara incantations above:

> [vii 5] en$_2$.e$_2$.nu.ru / [vii 6] ša$_3$ gig mu.ak ša$_3$ gig libiš gig mu.ak / [vii 7] **ša$_3$ gig.da ĝiš UD+DUL$_3$** / [vii 8] **gi.da UD+DUL$_3$** / [vii 9] šeg$_9$.bar nu ma AN.AN.AN a.da.ša$_3$.ša$_3$
>
> (*Description of medical condition*) *Incantation: 'The sick belly was at work. The sick belly and sick insides were at work. With the sick belly, the trees are . . . . The reeds are . . . . (Like) a wild ram . . . .*
>
> [viii 1] a.ni ^{d}en.lil$_2$.še$_x$(GAN$_2$) / [viii 2] lu$_2$ nin.da.ra.še$_3$.gi$_4$ / [viii 3] a.ĝu$_{10}$.ra a.ba.du$_{11}$.ga / [viii 4] ba.ra.MUNSUB / [viii 5] a.ne a.na nu.zu / [viii 6] ĝa$_2$ a.na.pad$_3$
>
> (*Marduk-Ea formula*) *He sent a messenger to his father: 'Please say to my father: 'I cannot . . . .' (Enlil answered:) 'What does he not know? What can I show him?'*
>
> [viii 7] a idigna a buranun u$_3$.ma.de$_2$ / [viii 8] lu$_2$ ša$_3$ gig mu.ni.naĝ / [viii 9] *šu*.si ĝiri$_3$.si.na[20] / [ix 1] ḫa.mu.ta.sar / [ix 2] KAS (×5)[21]
>
> (*Treatment*) *You might try pouring (together) water from the Tigris (and) water from the Euphrates. Have the person with the sick belly drink it, and then it (= the illness) will flee from his fingers and toes.'*

As George emphasises, the parts of this incantation that line up with the earlier Fara incantations allow us to make some sense of this very early tradition of treating gastrointestinal problems. Both the key terms (ša$_3$ gig and lipiš gig) and the idiom that combines 'tree' (ĝiš) and 'reed' (gi) with the verbal logogram TAG$_4$+SAG seem to be replicated here but with a different orthography for the verb, namely UD+DUL$_3$. Although we leave these verbs untranslated above, George suggests the following translation: 'it sheltered among the trees, it sheltered among the reeds' (perhaps describing a reservoir or source for the illness that caused the intestinal distress described as 'sick belly' and 'sick innards').[22] Be that as it may, it is clear that there was a relatively widespread tradition for treating gastrointestinal illness in the middle of the third millennium BCE. Moreover, there may even be an oblique trace of this tradition preserved in the Stomach Treatise: in the last line of the incantation, it is said that 'it (presumably the ailment affecting the patient) will flee from his fingers and toes'; two millennia later we find a similar, although decidedly odd, expression in our compendium: *ina* ŠU.SI GIR$_3$-*ka* GAL-*ti ša$_2$* 2,30 EN$_2$ ŠUB-*di* 'with the big toe of your left foot, you cast the incantation' (STO 1: 185).

The incantation just presented also includes a treatment encoded, within the incantation, in the form of a Marduk-Ea formula. This is a common way of offering treatments at this early stage of the tradition, where distinctions between *dicenda* and *agenda* have not yet been indicated; these short embedded treatments of the Early Dynastic period were only explicitly labelled as 'rituals' (written kid$_3$.kid$_3$.bi, du$_3$.du$_3$.bi, or *kikkiṭaša*) in the Old Babylonian period. Through the example of an Old Babylonian text, in which an existing instruction within the incantation is paired with an explicitly marked ritual that describes much the same procedure, George suggests that *dicenda* and *agenda* can operate independently:

> [This] confirms Irving Finkel's thesis, that incantations of the Asalluḫe-Enki type were vehicles "for the preservation and transmission of medical praxis" (Finkel 1980: 51), and gives a glimpse of the process which resulted in the splitting of this transmission into two sets of instructions: "incantation" and "ritual."[23]

---

20 George (2016: 121) follows Krebernik (1984: 67) in suggesting that Sumerian na here means 'spell' but it is a very common sign that plays many different roles in different contexts. We take it as the animate third person possessive followed by a locative or genitive.

21 MS 4549/1 obv vii 5–ix 2, corresponding to George 2016: 120–121 with plates 1–2.

22 George (2016: 120) notes that UD+DUL$_3$ corresponds, partly via an UD.GAL.NUN equivalency (UD = AN), to an.dul$_3$ 'shade, shadow', but it remains unclear how this fits into the context.

23 See the tables of 'appended rituals' in George 2016: 5–6.

It is noteworthy that where these *agenda* are specified in the richer Old Babylonian corpus, they nearly always represent broadly defined pharmaceutical treatments of one kind or another,[24] but also here in our Early Dynastic incantation with the Marduk-Ea formula, a pharmaceutically oriented treatment seems to be prescribed with water taken from the Tigris and Euphrates rivers and consumed by the patient as a healing potion.[25]

The second Early Dynastic incantation that we present here follows right after the one described above in the new compendium published by George, but in this case, interestingly enough, a duplicate was also found in a lavatory drain in Abu Salabikh (near the ancient city of Nippur).

> [ix 3] en$_2$.e$_2$.nu.ru / [ix 4] ša$_3$ gig ša$_3$.ga.ni an.na.e.e / [ix 5] libiš <gig> e$_2$:baḫar.nun.za.ku / [ix 6] ur.gin$_7$ mu.da.BAD.BAD
>
> *Incantation: 'The sick belly was coming forth against his belly. Baḫar-enunzaku . . . the sick innards as if it were a dog.*
>
> [ix 7] ša$_3$ gig libiš gig utu.AN.še$_3$ a.ĝa$_2$.la šim.gin$_7$ / [ix 8] ma.ni.keš$_2$ / [ix 9] ^{d}nin.girim$_x$(A.BU.ḪA.DU) / [ix 10] ki.a bi$_2$.du$_8$
>
> *He bound the sick belly and the sick innards to the sun as if it were a sack of aromatics. Ningirim released them in the netherworld.*
>
> [x 1] ša$_3$ gig libiš gig / [x 2] izi ZI.ZA.A-gin$_7$ / [x 3] ni$_2$.bi ḫe$_2$.te.PI / [x 4] KAS (×5)[26]
>
> *The sick belly and the sick innards will die down on their own, like a fire in the rushes.'*

Here again we largely follow George's interpretation, but there are interesting contrasts with the first incantation: no Marduk-Ea formula and, indeed, no real *agenda* or *dicenda*. Instead, we get a brief historiola explaining that Bahar-enunzaku will attach these illnesses to the sun-god Utu, who will, in turn, carry them back to the netherworld, where they will be released by Ningirim. Even if Ningirim is the primary deity found in connection with the incantations in the third millennium, no incantation (in the strict sense of *dicenda*) is at work here. As George also points out, it is particularly intriguing that a duplicate of this so-called 'incantation' was found in a lavatory in Abu Salabikh,[27] perhaps suggesting 'a belief that stomach disorders could be brought on by the lavatory demon'.[28] The key takeaway from these two incantations, however, is that the category of 'incantation' is quite elastic, stretching from actually performative *dicenda* to historiolas that explain the underlying logic for removing the illness, and even a kind of prognosis: 'it will die down like a fire in the rushes' (viz. a self-limiting illness for which no clear treatment was presumably available).

In his publication of the incantations from the Schøyen Collection, George goes on to edit a number of later Old Babylonian incantations that are also relevant to our central themes (and we will look at one further Old Babylonian incantation from this volume below), but at this point we turn to an even more recent survey of 'sick belly' incantations in the Ur III and Old Babylonian periods: the contribution of Ulrike Steinert and Luděk Vacín to the Mark Geller Festschrift published in 2018.[29] Although many important themes of the 'sick belly' incantations are discussed by Steinert and Vacín, two general features of the Old Babylonian texts are particularly important: (i) the expressions 'invocation for sick belly' (ka.inim.ma ša$_3$ gig.ga.kam) and 'invocation for bile' (ka.inim.ma ze$_2$.kam) often serve as rubrics for incantations describing ordinary gastrointestinal pain (ša$_3$ gig) and the various conditions associated with bile (ze$_2$), and (ii) incantations labelled in this way often occur in close proximity, as a thematic group, within a single compendium. Evidence for the latter can be found in Old Babylonian incantation collections published by George as texts no. 7 and 8 below, where the gastrointestinal (ša$_3$ gig) and bile (ze$_2$) incantations as well as the related condition known as 'wasting disease' (*šu-ḫu-ḫu-um*) regularly co-occur.[30]

---

24 Only two of the appended rituals in George 2016: 5–6 are of significance to us here: a 'potion of chopped leeks and oil' for jaundice in YOS 11 14c and 'purging with salt solution' for bloat in MS 3085 obv. ii 10′–16′ (George 2016: 133–134).

25 For the same treatment, see the snake-bite incantation in MS 4549/1 vi 7–vii 4 (George 2016: 100–101). As George argues, the source of water may not have necessarily been the two rivers, but they may have been converted from mundane into holy water through a ritual or simply obtained from holy temple wells.

26 MS 4549/1 obv ix 3–x 4, corresponding to George 2016: 121–122 with plates 1–2.

27 The text was published as IAS 549.

28 George 2016: 121 with n. 1, citing George 2015: 86–90.

29 It should be stressed that Steinert and Vacín 2018 is primarily an edition of BM 92518 and is substantially indebted to Böck 2014a and 2014b, but it does represent an up-to-date summary of all relevant Old Babylonian materials.

30 See also Steinert and Vacín 2018: 710. For terms that are etymologically related to this 'wasting disease', see STO 3: 147, STO 4: o (unplaced line from a parallel from Assur), and STO 5: 226′.

Table 1: Thematic arrangement of gastrointestinal and bile-induced ailments in Old Babylonian incantation collections and STO

Sections in texts 7 and 8[31]		Corresponding Rubric	Parallel between texts (or in STO)	
7h	(iv 1′–19′)	ka.inim.ma ze$_2$.[kam]		
7i	(iv 20′–v 11)	[ka.inim.ma] ⸢ze$_2$⸣		(STO 3: 99–107)
7j	(v 12–25)	ka.inim.ma [ze$_2^?$].⸢kam⸣	8l	
7k	(v 26–33)	ka.inim.ma [. . .]		
7l	(v 34–37)	ka.inim.ma ša$_3$ gig.ga *ša-pa-ru-um*	8e	
7m	(v 38–48)	[ka.inim.ma ša$_3$ gig *pa-ša*]-⸢*ru-um*⸣	8f	
7n	(vi 1–3)	(missing)		
7o	(vi 9–44)	(missing)	8i	(STO 1: 153–161; STO 1: 164–169)
7p	(vii 1–7)	⸢ka⸣.inim.ma ša$_3$ [gig.ga]	8j	
7q	(vii 8–36)	[ka].⸢inim⸣.ma [. . .]	8k	
8d	(i 45′–ii 16′)	(missing)		
8e	(ii 17′–20′)	ka.inim.ma ša$_3$ gig.ga	7l	
8f	(ii 21′–29′)	(missing)	7m	
8g	(ii 30′–32′)	[ka.inim].ma ša$_3$ [gig.ga]		
8h	(ii 33′–39′)	ka.inim.ma ša$_3$ [gig-ga]		
8i	(ii 40′–iii 37)	[ka.inim].⸢ma ša$_3$⸣ [gig.ga]	7o	(STO 1: 153–161; STO 1: 164–169)
8j	(iii 39–47)	(missing)	7p	
8k	(iv 1–19)	ka.inim.ma *šu-ḫu-ḫu-um*	7q	
8l	(iv 20–31)	[ka.in]im.[ma x x]	7j	

The tenuous connections between these two domains, viz. ša$_3$ gig and ze$_2$, which we identified in the Early Dynastic materials from Fara and Ebla above, are fully demonstrated in the labelling of Old Babylonian incantations and their configuration in larger compendia. Moreover, the specific Old Babylonian (and occasionally Old Assyrian) incantations that are best attested and apparently central to each of these two traditions also anchor the blocks of incantations that appear in the first and third tablets of the Stomach Treatise, namely the two different versions of the 'Belly Plant' (also known as 'Heart Grass') incantation in STO 1: 153–161 and 164–169 and the well-known bile incantation in STO 3: 99–107.[32] The fact that no other blocks of incantations occur in our treatise is probably a good indication that the gastrointestinal tract (the theme of the block in STO 1: 86–93 and 111–235) and bile (the theme of the block in STO 3: 94–126) were the two main organizing themes within the first three tablets of the treatise,[33] whereas the rest of the treatise seems to be concerned with a rather different family of illnesses centred on fever.

One of the curious features of the Old Babylonian and Old Assyrian incantations that reappear in and anchor the blocks of incantations in the Stomach Treatise is that they represent examples of what Niek Veldhuis has called 'chain incantations', viz. an incantation in which a repeated turn of phrase is used to represent a chain of transmission. Here, for example, is an incantation against sty in translation:[34]

31 For text no. 7 (MS 3097) and no. 8 (MS 3085), see the discussions and partial editions in George 2016: 34–38 and 122–127 with plates 21–30.

32 For the key bibliography and further discussions, see the relevant sections of STO 1 and 3.

33 For a discussion of these blocks of incantations in medical treatises, see Johnson 2018. Steinert and Vacín (2018: 710, citing Stol 1993: 27–32 and Böck 2014b: 111–118) suggest a 'recurring link between bile and belly in Akkadian/Sumerian expressions referring both to bodily complaints as well as to emotional trouble', but we should be extremely cautious about importing this line of thought into the medical treatises. The mixture of gastrointestinal symptoms and emotional upset that Böck describes in literary sources and lexical lists (centred on the use of Sum. ša$_3$ = Akk. *libbu* in both domains) is extremely rare in the Stomach Treatise and only consists of the occasional symptom (STO 1: 94 and STO 2: 151, for example), never an emotional or psychological diagnosis like *ḫīp libbi*.

34 Goetze 1955; Veldhuis 1993.

Table 2: Chain of transmission in an incantation against sty

1–2	The earth, they say, the earth bore the mud,
3–4	The mud bore the stalk,
5–6	The stalk bore the ear,
7–8	The ear bore the sty,
9–11	In, they say, the field of Enlil, the seven bur field,
12–13	Sîn reaped, Šamaš gathered,
14–16	Into, they say, the eye of the young man the sty entered.

The distinguishing feature of a chain incantation like this, for our purposes here, is that, although it includes divinities—here Sîn reaping and Šamaš gathering—it does not posit supernatural intermediaries between the deities and the affected person. It almost seems as if the stray barley grain that causes the sty is accidental.[35] In contrast to the widely used Marduk-Ea formula, the absence of supernatural intermediaries is surprising. Even where a somewhat distorted version of the Marduk-Ea formula appears, as in STO 1: 86–92, the mediating supernatural being, typically played by an exorcist in the actual ritual, is left out. Here, for example, are the stage directions in the last three lines of the incantation in STO 1: 86–92.

> [90] Gula, the provider of good health for mankind, saw this and brought the young man into the temple of Asalluhi (= Marduk),
> [91] merciful Marduk looked upon him, and then (said): 'Belch and feel better, young man!'
> [92] If there is flatulence (lit. wind), may it go out through the anus! If there is a belch, may he let it out through the throat! (End of incantation)

Whether in the form of a direct conversation between a patient and his belly, chain incantations that omit any supernatural mediators between god and human beings, or, as here, a transformation of the Marduk-Ea formula so that the deity addresses his instructions directly to the patient, these august incantations largely avoid—at least in the Stomach Treatise—the characteristic use of the Marduk-Ea formula for the framing of knowledge deriving from the gods.

A Brief History of Pharmaceutically Oriented Compendia for Gastrointestinal Illness

Although brief pharmaceutical instructions had long been a part of incantations, chiefly involving salt and/or thyme in connection with gastrointestinal illness, it would only be in the Ur III period (ca. 2100–2000 BCE) that specific instructions for making drugs were collected into a large compendium,[36] detached here, for the first time, from an incantatory matrix. Much of the text is unreadable, but as Civil admirably demonstrates in his *editio princeps*, these sequences of ingredients and step-by-step instructions are organised in terms of how the drugs were to be administered to patients, for example, via poultice (niĝ$_2$ ab.la$_2$.e), drinking (lu$_2$ al.naĝ.naĝ) or perhaps an enema (an.ku$_4$.ku$_4$).[37] Without even a hint of diagnostic categories, it is actually quite difficult to link any specific recipe to our gastrointestinal corpus, but certain ingredients, such as salt (mun) together with *kasû*-plant (gazi) seem to transcend the linguistic barrier between Sumerian and Akkadian, along with the few centuries between this last of the Sumerian compendia and the first of the Akkadian ones.

In the subsequent Old Babylonian period, new discursive forms were transferred from the legal domain in order to tie the individual pharmaceutical recipes in older compendia to symptoms and, in part, diagnoses. Already in *legal* compendia from the Ur III period, fully casuistic 'if . . . then' formulations (Sum. tukum.bi) were in use, and this pattern was now extended to pharmaceutical recipes (Akk. *šumma*), with symptoms and, eventually, diagnoses included as well.[38] At the same time, we also see the stereotypical ending of later medical recipes used for the first time: the ever-optimistic 'he will recover' (Akk. *iballuṭ*) or alternatively 'he will get well' (Akk. *inêš*), with both terms originally meaning simply 'he will

35 See Veldhuis 1993: 57 and, more recently, Panayotov 2017: 214–215.

36 See Civil 1960 for the publication of the multi-column tablet CBS 14221 from Nippur; another much smaller tablet with a single prescription dating to the Ur III period was published in Civil 1961.

37 The so-called Ebla pharmaceutical text, dating to the end of the Early Dynastic period, clearly represents a rather different tradition: it is essentially an herbal, listing drugs and their uses. For our purposes here only the third drug may be relevant, namely MU U$_2$ *mar-tum*, which is analogous to the list of drugs for treating bile (U$_2$ ZE$_2$) in STO 3: 20–26 (see Fronzaroli 1998: 232).

38 Johnson 2015: 295–300.

live'. These two discursive elements—symptomatology in the protasis and one of the optimistic prognostic statements at the end of the apodosis—would remain the nearly omnipresent frame for pharmaceutical recipes throughout the rest of the Mesopotamian medical tradition. Although relatively few of the Old Babylonian medical texts have been published, here are a few short passages from the most accessible Old Babylonian compendium (BAM 393):[39]

> obv. 4 6,40[40] *a-wi-lum a-u*$_2$*-ri-qa*$_2$*-nam ma-ru-uṣ* / obv. 5 *i-ši-id šu-ši-im i-na ši-iz-bi-im ta-ra-sa*$_3$*-an-ma* / obv. 6 *i-na ka-ka-bi-im tu-uš-ba-at-ma i-na hi-il-ṣi*$_2$*-im* / obv. 7 *tu-uš-te-te-ma ta-ša-qi*$_2$*-šu-ma i-ne*$_2$*-a-aš*
> obv. 23 6,40 *a-wi-lum ṣe-e-tam ḫa-mi-iṭ ti-la-q[u-ur-da-am]*[41] / obv. 24 *ṭi-gi-ma-am iz-qu*$_2$*-qa*$_3$*-am am-ma-aš-ta-⸢ka⸣-[al]* / obv. 25 *li-bi-tam la-bi-ir-tam i-na e-⸢li⸣-[im]* / obv. 26 *tu-uš-te-te-ma ⸢i⸣-[ša-ti-ma i-ne*$_2$*-a-aš]*[42]
> rev. 11 ⸢6⸣,40 *a-wi-lum li-ba-šu na-pi-iḫ zi-bi-bi-a-n[am]* / rev. 12 *⸢i⸣-na ru-uš-tim i-ša-ti-ma i-ne*$_2$*-a-[aš]*
> rev. 26 6,40 *a-wi-lum li-ib-ba-šu i-ta-na-an-pa-aḫ* / rev. 27 *ni-na-a-am i-na ši-ka-ri-im i-ša-ti-ma i-ne*$_2$*-a-aš*[43]

> (obv. 4–7) If someone[44] suffers from jaundice (*amurriqānu*): you soak root from *šūšu* ('liquorice') in milk and you leave (the mixture) out overnight under the stars, then you combine it in pressed oil and you make him drink it; then he will get well.
> (obv. 23–26) If someone suffers from burning fever (*ḫimiṭ ṣēti*): you combine *tillaqurdu* (a plant), ash, *isqūqu* (a type of groats), *maštakal* ('soapwort'), old brick in *el(l)u* (a fine quality oil) and he drinks it; then he will get well.
> (rev. 11–12) If someone's belly (*libbu*) is swollen: he drinks *zibibânu* ('black cumin') in *rūštu* (a fine quality oil); then he will get well.
> (rev. 26–27) If someone's belly (*libbu*) is constantly swollen: he drinks *nīnû* ('mint') in beer; then he will get well.

Jaundice, especially the kind called *amurriqānu*, is one of the central preoccupations of the third tablet of the Stomach Treatise, with numerous recipes mentioning either the root of the plant *šūšu* or milk, but these two ingredients are not actually found in combination in our corpus. Likewise, the condition *ḫimiṭ ṣēti*, presumably a type of strong fever, is dealt with extensively in the fourth tablet of our treatise, yet the set of ingredients listed for this condition in the Old Babylonian recipe are not found together in our corpus; in fact, only *isqūqu* and *maštakal*, as well as oil,[45] occur. The next two prescriptions include swollen belly, a condition otherwise not known from the Stomach Treatise; however, swollen internal organs (Akk. *qerbū*) occur several times in the texts, with the verb usually spelt as MU$_2$.MU$_2$(-*ḫu*) or MU$_2$.MEŠ.[46] Of the two drugs used here in BAM 393 for treating swollen belly, black cumin co-occurs with garlic in a series of remedies for swollen and cramped internal organs (STO 2: 87–88 and 90–91), whereas *nīnû* is attested as a simplicium against a complex set of symptoms, including swollen internal organs (STO 4: 62).

While many technical compendia in the Old Babylonian period strike the modern reader as *ad hoc* and largely incoherent,[47] this is certainly not the case for pharmaceutical recipe collections and contemporary incantation compendia. These two types of compendia—pharmaceutical and incantatory—are quite carefully distinguished and never intermingled,

---

39 Although Finkel (1999: 213 n. 3) questioned the Old Babylonian dating of BAM 393, suggesting it might be a later copy of an Old Babylonian original (personal communication in Schwemer 2007: 27 n. 23), based on renewed collations, Schwemer maintains it is actually Old Babylonian.

40 Based on its position in the text, we take 6,40, in line with Abusch and Schwemer 2011: 65, as standing for Akkadian *šumma* 'if'. A recent discussion of this difficult orthography is found in BAM 10 p. 255, with the reading *aš*$_3$*-šar*$_2$, which Geller and Panayotov take as a forerunner to their reconstructed first millennium form *ana ašri* (*šanîmma*). For a discussion of this first millennium form, see our comments to STO 1: 8.

41 For the restoration of this passage, see Haussperger 1997: 144 n. 2 and, more recently, Mayer 2009: 434 and SAD D/T/Ṭ 91.

42 We restore the end of this line based on the frequent co-occurrence of the verbs *išattī-ma inêš* as in BAM 393 rev. 12 and 27.

43 For an edition of BAM 393, see Haussperger 1997 and Geller 2006. George has recently published another large pharmaceutical compendium (CUSAS 32 73) and Irving Finkel is currently preparing several others for publication.

44 Our use of gender-neutral 'someone' here and throughout the volume is admittedly anachronistic, but it should be kept in mind that Akk. *awīlum* referred not simply to males but to elite males, presumably as a prototype. Perhaps the use of the logogram NA, if it derives from the third person animate possessive pronoun in Sumerian, is already an early sign of this neutrality.

45 The specific types of oil mentioned in BAM 393, viz. *el(l)u* and *rūštu*, do not occur in the Stomach Treatise. For a discussion of *el(l)u*, see Stol 1985a: 122.

46 For our rendering of MU$_2$.MU$_2$(-*ḫu*) and MU$_2$.MEŠ as standing for Akkadian *napḫū*, instead of the Ntn-form *ittananpaḫū*, see the comments to STO 1: 21.

47 See, for example, CUSAS 18 16, which combines omens that would be carefully separated into physiognomic, medical and *šumma ālu*-type omens in later traditions.

at least if we limit ourselves to large compendia.[48] Throughout the rest of the second millennium, the compendial tradition is further refined, and, at some point that is not really clear to present-day researchers, specific compendia become associated with learned professions or disciplines such as *āšipūtu* 'exorcistic practice' or *asûtu* 'medicine'. The apparently single-minded focus of compendia in the Old Babylonian period on either pharmaceutical recipes or incantations, but never both, seems to be the first hint, in the historical record, of a clear distinction between *āšipūtu* and *asûtu*, but the evidence in the Old Babylonian period is still circumstantial. It is really only in the seventh century BCE, in the rather unusual context of Assurbanipal's Library and the Nineveh Medical Encyclopaedia, that we can be relatively sure that a pharmaceutical compendium belongs to 'medicine' (*asûtu*), while a collection of incantations probably belongs to the competing discipline of 'exorcism' (*āšipūtu*).[49]

The lengthy period of time between these Old Babylonian compendia and the Neo-Assyrian treatise edited in this volume—the Middle Babylonian and Middle Assyrian periods—is poorly understood, at least in terms of recipe-based pharmaceutical treatments.[50] Several recent publications, including Zomer's survey of the incantations from this period[51] as well as Sibbing-Plantholt's work on the Kassite medical letters along with her description of the spread of Gula's cult in Assyria and Babylonia,[52] now provide us with a relatively broad framework for looking at the history of medicine in the Middle Babylonian and Middle Assyrian periods. Still, a survey of the specifically therapeutic sources from these periods is certainly a desideratum for a better understanding of the processes through which Mesopotamian medical knowledge was transmitted to the first millennium BCE. The case of the Babylonian physician Rabâ-ša-Marduk illustrates the conundrum here well: a Babylonian-born physician, Rabâ-ša-Marduk rose to the top of his profession in southern Mesopotamia and was dispatched to Hattusha on behalf of the crown, yet there is only a single therapeutic text known to identify itself in its colophon as 'from the house of Rabâ-ša-Marduk' (BAM 11).[53] At the same time, distant loci of peripheral Akkadian such as Hattusha, Emar and Ugarit produced occasional therapeutic texts[54] along with a number of incantation collections, some of which include incantations also found in the treatise edited in this volume.[55]

By far, the most important source for the Stomach Treatise between the Old Babylonian and the Neo-Assyrian periods is the Middle Assyrian text BAM 66. It combines a forerunner to Diagnostic Handbook 31 (obverse and the first three lines of the reverse) with a forerunner to the first 22 lines of the fourth tablet of our treatise (the remainder of the reverse), carefully separated by a double ruling.[56] This juxtaposition is not fortuitous: both Diagnostic Handbook 31 and STO 4 are focused on burning fever (*himiṭ ṣēti*) and related types of fever, with the forerunner text BAM 66 possibly representing a kind of Vademecum for the *ṣētu* type of fevers in its original *Sitz im Leben*. While STO 4, as we might expect of a therapeutic text, carefully works its way through different types of fevers,[57] Diagnostic Handbook 31 is organised in terms of the number of days that the patient will suffer from *himiṭ ṣēti* fever, ranging from three days to a full month. As Finkel first recognised, BAM 66 seems to represent a somewhat distinctive prognostic tradition, in which defining the length of illness ('that man will be sick for n days') and avoiding its prolongation ('to avoid prolonging his sickness') were the central goals.[58] More recently, as part of a broader argument about the possible links between Mesopotamian sources and Greco-Roman fever theory, Maddalena Rumor has suggested that the time periods found in Diagnostic Handbook 31 can

---

48 Note, however, that smaller Old Babylonian tablets with one or only a few medical recipes sometimes make mention of incantations to be recited as part of healing procedures: the instruction *šiptam tanaddī-ma* 'you recite the incantation, and then' occurs, for instance, in H 170 Side A ln. 6′, which is a small landscape format tablet from Meturan (Cavigneaux and Al-Rawi 1993: 104–105), and in the Old Babylonian medical text UET 6/3 895 rev. 14 from Ur.

49 Geller 2018: 33–34.

50 See Lambert 1969 for an edition of a Middle Assyrian medical text.

51 Zomer 2018.

52 For the Kassite medical letters, see Sibbing-Plantholt 2014, whereas Gula's cult in Assyria and Babylonia in the second half of the second millennium BCE is discussed extensively in Sibbing-Plantholt 2022: 63–105.

53 For Rabâ-ša-Marduk, see Heeßel 2009, as well as Devecchi and Sibbing-Plantholt 2020.

54 See, for example, Burde 1974, Tsukimoto 1999 and Klinger 2010.

55 See, in particular, Emar VI/4 737: 4–7, which runs parallel with STO 1: 135–136, and also a couple of other distant parallels in the same text that correspond to the opening line of the incantation in STO 1: 213–218 and perhaps STO 1: 232. Although Emar VI/4 737 does not include therapeutic prescriptions, Arnaud (1987: 345–346) already recognised in his *editio princeps* that this text is clearly oriented to gastrointestinal disease. For a new edition of the text, see Zomer 2018: 261–263.

56 See Finkel 1994 and Heeßel 2000: 348 for the key observations, summarised in Johnson 2014b.

57 For a survey of fever texts, see Bácskay 2018; the classic study of fever in Mesopotamia is Stol 2007.

58 Finkel 1994: 88.

be associated, via the lunar models that underlie the *Kalendertext* tradition, with the Hippocratic doctrine of critical days.[59] Be that as it may, her observations certainly open up a new perspective on fever theory in ancient Mesopotamia.

Assurbanipal's Library and the Nineveh Medical Encyclopaedia

Even if it is often described as a massive universal library put in place by the Neo-Assyrian king Assurbanipal (669–631 BCE), there are two rather distinct entities that we might describe as Assurbanipal's Library: the sum-total of official archival materials recovered from a series of archives from seventh-century Nineveh, now largely held in the British Museum (this is the usual sense of the term),[60] or we might ask for more specific evidence and attempt to define a consistent and explicitly delimited official archive belonging to Assurbanipal.[61] Indeed, the relatively small group of tablets that form the medical corpus in Nineveh, and in particular the tablets belonging to the Nineveh Medical Encyclopaedia, exhibit both a distinctive standard Assurbanipal colophon as well as a series of shared layout features, namely the well-known two-column 'library' format. The particular Assurbanipal colophon found on tablets belonging to the Nineveh Medical Encyclopaedia (hereafter NME) is known as colophon q and reads as follows:[62]

> Palace of Assurbanipal, ruler of the World, king of the land of Assur, on whom Nabû and Tašmētu have bestowed wisdom (lit. wide ears),
> He acquired for himself shining eyes, the pinnacle of scholarship,
> Of the kings who came before me, none were able to comprehend this task.
> Prescriptions (organised) from head to foot, gleanings from extraneous materials, technical lore
> (And) whatever pertains to the great medical expertise of Ninurta and Gula,
> I have written on tablets, checked and double-checked, and
> I deposited them in my palace for my reading and recitation.[63]

Thus, regardless of how the broader notion of Assurbanipal's Library eventually comes to be seen, with our much narrower concept, we can be quite sure that the Nineveh Medical Encyclopaedia, in which the corpus edited here constitutes one of the twelve interconnected treatises, was explicitly and self-consciously conceptualised as a distinct royal editorial project in the seventh century BCE.

Within the NME, this colophon is normally preceded by two crucial pieces of metadata: first, a so-called catchline, which is the first line of the following tablet in the treatise, and, second, a reference to the tablet number (viz. tablet designation)—in the sequence of tablets forming the treatise—of the text that has reached its conclusion just before the colophon. The beginning of the colophon of the first tablet of the Stomach Treatise reads as follows (STO 1: 247–249):

> (Catchline) 'If someone's belly is sick: he drinks pure cow milk (and) ghee for two days' (corresponding to the first line of the following tablet, viz. STO 2: 1)
>
> (Tablet designation) First tablet of 'If someone suffers from phlegm, which has turned into gastric constriction' (corresponding to the first line of the tablet that this colophon is attached to, and, incidentally, the incipit or title of the treatise as a whole, viz. STO 1: 1)
>
> (Colophon) Palace of Assurbanipal . . . (see above)

As it happens, the precise configuration of these three pieces of metadata in the colophon (catchline, tablet designation and colophon) only appears or is fully preserved in three of the five tablets in the Stomach Treatise: STO 3 omits the enu-

59 Rumor 2021, especially pp. 65–70.

60 For an overview, see Reade 1998–2000; the excavation history is surveyed in Turner 2021.

61 This second approach, which we adopt here, is at the heart of Jon Taylor's project on library colophons in the British Museum, entitled 'Reading the Library of Assurbanipal: A Multi-sectional Analysis of Assyriology's Foundational Corpus'.

62 Corresponding to BAK 329. There are a couple of medical tablets from Nineveh that include, perhaps accidentally, a different colophon, viz. colophon b (BAK 318): see BAM 548 iv 14′–22′ (BRON 5) and BAM 7 23 iv 29′–35′ (ANUS 3), but the reasons for this remain unclear (see Panayotov 2018: 110).

63 For colophon q in the Stomach Treatise, see STO 1: 249–255, STO 2: 264–270, STO 3: 255–261, STO 4: 260′–264′ (partially preserved) and STO 5: 238′–244′.

meration, and we only have the end of the colophon in STO 4. This type of chaining or linkage between catchlines and incipits is one of the most important pieces of evidence for the internal structure of our treatise and the NME as a whole: the catchline named in STO 1: 247 is, in fact, the first line in STO 2; the catchline in STO 2: 262 is the first line of STO 3 and so on, up until the final tablet where, as the pattern would predict, the catchline seemingly corresponds to the incipit of the treatise that follows STO in the Nineveh Medical Encyclopaedia, namely the EPIGASTRIUM/ABDOMEN treatise.[64]

If, as we tentatively assume here, the NME was an editorial project that took place under the auspices of Assurbanipal himself, as the colophon suggests, it is somewhat surprising that no catalogue of the NME is known from Nineveh itself. What we do have is a catalogue from Assur, which outlines the therapeutic text material in first-millennium Mesopotamia by listing the incipits of the extant treatises. Since this catalogue, known as the Assur Medical Catalogue (hereafter AMC), and its relationship to the NME have already been studied extensively in the secondary literature,[65] we do not need to go into the matter here except to note that, where the AMC is preserved, it agrees with the attested incipits of the Stomach Treatise. The relevant section of the AMC (ll. 29–35) reads as follows:

29 [DIŠ NA *su-a-lam* GIG *ana ki-is* ŠA$_3$ GUR-*š*]*u*$_2$: DIŠ NA ŠA$_3$-*šu*$_2$ ⸢GIG⸣
30 [DIŠ NA SAG ŠA$_3$-*šu*$_2$ GU$_7$-*šu*$_2$: DIŠ NA UD.DA KUR-*i*]*d* : DIŠ NA ŠA$_3$-*šu*$_2$ KUM$_2$ DAB-*it*

---

31 [NIGIN$_2$ 5 DUB.MEŠ DIŠ NA *su-a-lam* GIG *ana ki-is* Š]A$_3$ GUR-*šu*$_2$ EN IM *iš-biṭ-su-*⸢*ma*⸣
32 [. . .] x U$_2$ NAG-*ma* ⸢*la*⸣ *i-ar*$_2$-⸢*ru*⸣
33 [*ṣe-me-er* (?) . . . KA]Š NAG-*ma* SUḪUŠ.MEŠ-*šu*$_2$ *pa-al-qa*
34 [*di-ig-la ma-a-ṭi* (?) . . . GI]G *ki-ṣir* ŠA$_3$ GIG *ki-is* ŠA$_3$
35 [GIG . . . DIR]I *u*$_3$ *nik-mat* IM *u* UD.DA

29 'If someone suffers from phlegm, which has turned into gastric constriction' (STO 1: 1); 'If someone's belly is sick' (STO 2: 1);
30 'If someone's epigastrium causes him pain' (STO 3: 1); 'If someone is overwhelmed by fever' (STO 4: 1); 'If someone's belly has been seized by heat' (STO 5: 1)

---

31 Total of five tablets (of the treatise) 'If someone suffers from phlegm, which has turned into gastric constriction', including (prescriptions for the case that) wind has bloated him,
32 . . . someone took (lit. drank) a drug, and subsequently, he does not throw up
33 (and) he is distended (STO 2: 177) . . . someone drinks high-quality beer, and then his lower extremities are impaired.[66]
34 (and his) vision is diminished (STO 2: 184) . . . someone suffers from . . . someone suffers from a knotted-up belly (STO 2: 245 or 251), someone suffers from gastric constriction (STO 1: 4 and *passim*)
35 . . . someone is full of . . . and someone has an accumulation of flatulence (lit. 'wind') and heat

The first thing that should be reiterated here is that this catalogue of medical incipits derives from Assur rather than Nineveh and is largely reconstructed. Nonetheless, where the fragments of the text exist, in a text that is quite consistent in its layout and proportions, the placement and length of the incipits in lines 29–30 do line up with our reconstruction of a five-tablet edition of the Stomach Treatise.[67] The next catchline, which is not included here because it presumably corresponds to the incipit of the following EPIGASTRIUM/ABDOMEN treatise (see above), only occurs in line 36; the inter-

64 The catchline of STO 5 reads 'If someone's epigastrium heaves, his hips and his limbs constantly cause him pain'; this catchline corresponds to the first line of AMT 43/6, which may thus be a manuscript of the first tablet of the EPIGASTRIUM/ABDOMEN treatise. As Steinert (2018a: 232–233) and Panayotov (2018: 103–104) showed, however, the precise arrangement of the three treatises following STO (VIII) in the Nineveh Medical Encyclopaedia, namely EPIGASTRIUM (IXa), ABDOMEN (IXb) and KIDNEY (X), remains unclear.

65 See, in particular, Scurlock 2014: 295–306 and Heeßel 2018a: 314–315, as well as the papers published in BAM 9, especially Steinert 2018a and 2018b, and Panayotov 2018.

66 For the verb *palāqu*, see our comment to STO 2: 184

67 *Pace* Köcher 1978: 19–20 and Scurlock 2014: 299; see also Panayotov 2018: 102.

mediate section in line 31–35 does not list tablet incipits but seems to present, instead, highlights from different parts of the Stomach Treatise. Although the function of this thematic appendix, also known as an '*adi*-section' after the first word that introduces it, viz. EN for Akk. *adi* 'including', is decidedly unclear,[68] the references that are identifiable mostly point to the second tablet, which is the least innovative part of our treatise and focuses exclusively on pharmaceutical measures. These sections may be highlighted because they point to an exception in pharmaceutical practice, as in the case when someone takes an apparently emetic drug but does not vomit (STO 2: 177) or when someone produces seemingly exceptional symptoms (i.e., drunkenness) due to the overconsumption of one of the most common medical ingredients in Mesopotamian pharmaceutical practice, viz. beer (STO 2: 184). At the same time, more conventional medical problems such as knotted-up belly (STO 2: 245 or 251) and gastric constriction (STO 1: 4 and *passim*) are also included among the thematic highlights in lines 31–35, which makes it very difficult to determine what the overall purpose of the *adi*-sections in AMC was.

What we learn from both the metadata included in the colophons at the end of each tablet and the traces of compendial structure recorded in the Assur Medical Catalogue is that the treatise edited in this volume, viz. the Stomach Treatise, was carefully situated within the overall architecture of the Nineveh Medical Encyclopaedia. It forms the eighth of twelve interconnected treatises, each of which offers an extensive collection of treatments for ailments that affect a specific part of the body. The sequence of the twelve treatises in the NME follows human anatomy, proceeding from the head, the first treatise, to the feet and toes, the ailments of which are dealt with extensively in the twelfth and final treatise.

CRANIUM (I)
EYES (II)
EARS (III)
NECK (IV)
NOSEBLEED (V)
TEETH (VI)
BRONCHIA (VII)
STOMACH (VIII)
EPIGASTRIUM/ABDOMEN (IX)
KIDNEY (X)
ANUS (XI)
HAMSTRING (XII)

It needs to be emphasised at this point that this compendial structure, also known as the 'from-head-to-toe' sequence, is not a specific characteristic of the Nineveh Medical Encyclopaedia but a common feature of most first-millennium technical compendia, and, as such, it is also employed by other cornerstone texts of the Mesopotamian healing professions.[69] In fact, the basic principle of organising knowledge in terms of human anatomy can already be detected approximately a millennium earlier in the context of Old Babylonian anatomical word lists: the twelve-sided prism MS 2888 allots a bilingual Sumerian-Akkadian list of terms for the parts of the human body to its twelve columns.[70] The sections do not line up precisely with the NME, as the following parallel makes clear, but the structural principles are much the same:

NME (7th century BCE)	MS 2888 (1800–1600 BCE)
CRANIUM (I)	Cranium (I)
EYES (II)	Hair (II)
EARS (III)	Face (III)
NECK (IV)	Eye (IV)
NOSEBLEED (V)	Mouth (V)
TEETH (VI)	Neck (VI)
BRONCHIA (VII)	Hand (VII)
STOMACH (VIII)	Chest (VIII)
EPIGASTRIUM/ABDOMEN (IX)	Guts (IX)
KIDNEY (X)	Anus (X)
ANUS (XI)	Feet (XI)
HAMSTRING (XII)	Whole body (XII)

68 For the *adi*-sections in AMC, see generally Steinert 2018a: 231–232. Up to now, nothing in our text supports Panayotov's (2018: 94) contention that these are non-canonical *aḫû* materials.

69 See, for example, the second chapter of the Diagnostic Handbook with its twelve tablets (Tablet 3–14) that record symptoms in connection with specific parts of the body: the first seven tablets (Tablet 3–9) are concerned with the head area, including the eyes, the nose, the tongue and so on, whereas the remaining five tablets (Tablet 10–14) focus on the rest of the body (Heeßel 2000: 24–30 and Schmidtchen 2021: 17–24).

70 CUSAS 12: 154–158.

The different genres of the two texts and the impressionistic nature of the labels—all modern impositions rather than ancient rubrics—might raise doubts, but nonetheless, the overall similarity of the two structures is relatively clear: both proceed from head to foot, both devote approximately half their length to the organs and orifices of the head, and both distinguish—when it comes to the internal organs—between the respiratory tract (BRONCHIA / Chest), the gastrointestinal tract (STOMACH / Guts) and the rectal area (ANUS / Anus). One might say that the uncertainties about the existence of an EPIGASTRIUM/ABDOMEN treatise in the NME and the AMC (see above) are already a part of the tradition since the Old Babylonian text assigns the twelfth face of the prism to whole-body conditions, while a thousand years later the AMC treats non-anatomical conditions in a separate section, which is, strictly speaking, not part of the NME.[71]

The Stomach Treatise (STO): The Nineveh Treatise on Gastrointestinal Illness

Situated between the upper trunk of the body and the renal-rectal region, the internal organs of the gastrointestinal tract are dealt with extensively in the eighth treatise of the Nineveh Medical Encyclopaedia. This treatise, now called the Stomach Treatise (abbreviated as STO) but often cited in the secondary literature using the first word of its incipit, viz. *Suālu*, offers an extensive and multifaceted collection of treatments for ailments that were seen by Mesopotamian healers as resulting from the malfunctioning of the digestive tract.

Consisting of five tablets and approximately 1300 lines of text (ca. 260 to 270 lines per tablet), in its original state in Ashurbanipal's Library, STO was one of the longest treatises in the Nineveh Medical Encyclopaedia; only the treatise on respiratory illness (BRON) and the one concerned with the neck (NECK) exceed STO in length, both consisting of six tablets rather than the five tablets in STO.[72] These longer treatises are still very fragmentary, however, and will require a great deal more reconstruction and editorial work before we can understand their contents and structure. STO, on the other hand, represents the most intact part of the entire Encyclopaedia, and the core fragments of its first three tablets have long served as anchors for the study of Babylonian medicine (see the research history below). A large part of the fifth chapter can also be recovered with the help of the somewhat damaged manuscript BAM 579, which, though broken in half along its vertical axis, still has very well-preserved sections of text in its first and fourth columns and also some fragmentary lines in its second and third columns. Three individual manuscripts represent the fourth tablet of STO, but all three manuscripts are in a very fragmentary state and allow the reconstruction of no more than seventy lines of text, which makes the fourth tablet the least understood part of our treatise on gastrointestinal illness. Nonetheless, despite all the missing parts in the fourth and fifth tablets, STO is the longest treatise in the Nineveh Medical Encyclopaedia that is currently available to us, with approximately 950 to 1000 preserved lines of text.

STO 1

The first tablet of STO is preserved in the manuscript K 191+, an almost intact tablet that Franz Köcher copied as BAM 574. Since Köcher's publication, several new joins to the tablet have been identified, and a corner fragment possibly belonging to a second manuscript of STO 1 has also come to light. The progress made in recent years in reconstructing the textual basis for STO 1 has considerably improved our understanding of its overall layout and thematic structure; we will return to the details of this progress in the second chapter.

As it now stands, STO 1 can be divided thematically into three larger units. The first unit is pharmaceutical in nature and contains a long series of prescriptions for various forms of gastric constriction or colic. Most often, the text refers to

71 Another apparent inheritance from the Old Babylonian anatomical tradition is the bipartite structure of these compendia: in MS 2888, the twelfth face is assigned to whole-body terms such as 'stature' or 'shadow', while in later compendia such as Esagil-kīn-apli's edition of the Diagnostic Handbook and the Physiognomic Corpus, or the two major sections of the Assur Medical Catalogue, this bipartite structure seems to signify something other than a simple opposition between parts and wholes.

72 The treatise EPIGASTRIUM/ABDOMEN may have had an even higher number of tablets, perhaps eight, but this treatise is in an extremely fragmentary state, and given also the contradictory nature of evidence gleaned from the few related fragments from Nineveh in comparison to what is said about EPIGASTRIUM/ABDOMEN in the Assur Medical Catalogue, it is difficult to be certain about the exact length and structural outline of this treatise. For EPIGASTRIUM/ABDOMEN, see Abusch and Schwemer 2011: 126–128, Scurlock 2014: 304–305, Panayotov 2018: 103 and Steinert 2018a: 232–236.

this condition with the Akkadian term *kīs libbi* or another conjugated form of the verb *kasû* 'to bind', which is the basis of the word *kīs* 'constriction' as in STO 1: 80: *libbašu iktanassūšu* 'his belly constantly binds him'. Other symptoms such as swollen internal organs, indigestion, vomiting and flatulence frequently co-occur with *kīs libbi*, and drug-based remedies administered through healing potions and enemas are the most characteristic treatments. Incantations are not a major component in the first thematic unit of STO 1: only two incantations occur in this part of the text, a poorly understood opening incantation in STO 1: 5–7 and a single Akkadian incantation (STO 1: 86–93) situated between two large blocks of therapeutic prescriptions. The passage dealing with gastric constriction is the second longest thematic unit in STO 1 and extends over the first two columns of the tablet BAM 574, which correspond to lines 1–110 of the composite text.

The second thematic unit starts at the bottom of the second column of BAM 574, in line 111 of the composite text, extends over the entire third column of the tablet and ends in line 238, in the middle of the fourth column. This is the longest unit in STO 1 and consists of an extended series of incantations that are occasionally accompanied by concise ritual descriptions. The incantations are geared toward internal problems, addressing conditions such as blocked-up intestines, stomach aches or flatulence. The core of this block of incantations is made up of three different versions of the well-known 'Belly Plant' incantation, often known as the Heart Grass incantation in earlier work. In these versions of the Belly Plant incantation, the internal disease is depicted in somewhat abstract terms as a plant that, after being picked, transmits the ailment through a whole chain of hosts, while other incantations, as we saw above, portray the stomach as a disturbed fermenting vat, an inflated waterskin, a blown-up leather bag or even as a dark windowless building filled with terror. The tone of the individual incantations also varies greatly: sometimes statements of fact are reported in an unemotional way, while in other cases, the incantations speak of begging and pleading, as in begging the belly not to inflict pain on its owner or pleading with the flatulence to leave the body. Only two invocation or incantation rubrics occur in this unit, but both point to internal problems: the somewhat obscure 'belly that pursues him' in STO 1: 146 and the more straightforward 'flatus (lit. wind) that the belly holds' in STO 1: 237.

The last thematic unit is found in STO 1: 239–246, and here, the text returns to pharmaceutical praxis, recording treatments for a loose or collapsed navel. The medicines are taken internally as healing potions except for one instance where it is administered in the form of a localised treatment: a mixture dripped directly into the navel.

STO 2

The second tablet of STO is known from the tablet K 71B+, which represents the best-preserved manuscript in the Stomach Treatise; the manuscript was copied by Franz Köcher as BAM 575. This tablet is almost entirely pharmaceutical in content, containing a long list of prescriptions for a mixed set of medical problems. It proceeds from a general statement about an internal ailment, viz. 'if someone's belly is sick' (STO 2: 1–14), to more specific symptomatologies affecting the patient (STO 2: 15–86). Accordingly, as we move through this section, additional symptoms were added to the basic condition of having a sick belly, including throbbing sensations (STO 2: 15), yellow bruises and lesions (STO 2: 21) and piercing pain accompanied by the inability to hold one's urine and other effluvia (STO 2: 25). These specific additional symptoms are followed by a more general or comprehensive statement about the patient, viz. 'if someone's belly is sick, and in addition, he has any (other) illness' (STO 2: 51), after which the text becomes somewhat fragmentary.

Up through line 86, STO 2 offers a number of different treatments, presumably for the same kinds of illness, but then in line 87, a new topic is introduced with a new group of symptoms, including swollen and cramped internal organs, flatulence and the feeling of having to vomit. The main focus here seems to be on swollen (*napāḫu*), cramped-up (*ebēṭu*) and bloated (*emēru*) internal organs; these are the diagnostic symptoms that feature prominently in the next long section of the text (STO 2: 87–135), alongside occasional symptoms like flatulence (STO 2: 90, 124 and 130), fever in various parts of the abdomen (STO 2: 101, 108 and 130), regurgitation (STO 2: 105, 127, 130 and 133), diminished appetite (STO 2: 108 and 113), the build-up of phlegm (STO 2: 108, 113 and 115) and coughing (STO 2: 113). At the end of the section, mention is made, in a rather surprising way, of the patient's temples: 'his temples are splitting apart' (STO 2: 133). However unexpected, in a gastrointestinal context, this seems to represent a turning point in our text since it is followed in the next entry by another reference to the head, but this time in connection with constipation (STO 2: 136). Interestingly, this unusual symptom description is not accompanied by a pharmaceutical treatment but instead a short magical spell, together with a rubric that describes its use for constipation and a ritual that is to be recited over the patient's belly (STO 2: 137–138).

Loss of appetite (STO 2: 139–152), built-up mucus in the digestive system (STO 2: 153–159) and flatulence (STO 2: 160–171) are leading symptoms in the next part of our text, occurring alongside twisted internal organs and fits of coughing (STO 2: 147), an upset stomach (STO 2: 151) as well as a combination of paralysis with stinging pain and the wasting away of bad-smelling flesh (STO 2: 165–167). The first use of a disease name in STO 2 also occurs at this point of our text, with a reference to the disease *bibiktu*, which manifests itself in overindulgence—because the patient is unable to satisfy their appetite—and leads to swollen internal organs and a complete loss of appetite (STO 2: 172). Other named diagnoses appear later on in STO 2: *zēzēnu* appears in line 179 (a condition in which patients are unable to pass waste even after taking the prescribed drugs) and *tašnīqu* in line 242 (a disease that is characterised by a patient who spits up blood along with their phlegm).

Two prescriptions merit further attention since they, uniquely in our corpus, deal with drunkenness: several symptoms are associated with consuming beer in these prescriptions, such as impaired use of the lower extremities, diminished vision, the inability of a patient to speak or form a thought and the feeling of having one's head seized; in one instance, the condition indicated by these symptoms is labelled as 'constantly starring eyes' (STO 2: 184–189).

Finally, in the last part of our tablet, treatments are collected for someone who has 'particles in the throat', also framed in terms of having 'stuff in the belly' (STO 2: 190–218), as well as for the medical conditions described with the verb *kaṣāru* 'to tie, to knot, to cluster' such as *kiṣirti libbi* 'clots in the belly' (STO 2: 219–241) and *kiṣir libbi* 'knotted-up belly' (STO 2: 245–255).

STO 3

The third tablet of the Stomach Treatise is also based on a single manuscript, namely K 61+, which was copied by Franz Köcher as BAM 578. The tablet is in a relatively good state of preservation, with only thirty lines or so missing from the bottom half of its third column. In terms of content, STO 3 can also be divided into three thematic units. Unlike the first tablet of our treatise, however, the division here is not based on an opposition between pharmaceutical treatments and incantations but instead according to different topics in each section: the first unit is concerned with bile (Akk. *martu* = Sum. ze$_2$) and related diseases (STO 3: 1–143), and it is followed by two further units with treatments for the two main types of jaundice, namely *amurriqānu* (STO 3: 144–232) and *aḫḫāzu* (STO 3: 233–253). The Akkadian term *martu* is etymologically related to the infinitive *marāru* 'to be(come) bitter' and the universal experience of vomiting and/or acid reflux, where digestive acids in the small intestine enter the stomach, undoubtedly served to define qualities (yellow, acidic, connected to excessive eating and drinking) that were associated with bile. Of these qualities, the colour yellow seems to be the most prominent feature, as codified in the block of incantations in STO 3, linking 'bile disease' to the two types of jaundice dealt with later on in this tablet. As such, this block of incantations may have served as a thematic centre of gravity for the tablet as a whole.

The first condition treated in STO 3 is described as resulting from bile moving through and affecting different parts of the body. The focus of this unit is naturally on the gastrointestinal tract, but sometimes the illness of 'bile disease' manifests itself without any apparent connection to the patient's stomach or gastrointestinal tract, as in STO 3: 50, which lists warm sensations in the chest and heels, bleeding gums and difficulties with speaking as the signs of the disease. This may suggest that bile here is conceived as a somewhat abstract entity that can leave the gastrointestinal tract and affect other parts of the body. Most symptoms are still related to the digestive system and include, for instance, pain in the epigastrium together with bile being belched up (STO 3: 1), retching (STO 3: 27), swollen internal organs (STO 3: 28), loss of appetite (STO 3: 29), being blocked up (STO 3: 38) as well as nausea and dizziness (STO 3: 47). In the next part of the section, bile appears in the company of other conditions: firstly, in line 70, it is mentioned alongside *amurriqānu* and *aḫḫāzu*, even if these two types of jaundice are separately dealt with later on in the same tablet. The text then turns to treatments for *ašû*, *lubāṭu*, *qidḫu*, *pašittu* and *tuganû* (STO 3: 77–92), followed by the first block of incantations (STO 3: 94–126) and another set of bile treatments (STO 3: 127–143). It is, therefore, the variety of different illness classifications, often placed alongside corresponding incantations, that sets STO 3 apart from the first tablet of the treatise. Although it never says so explicitly, the configuration of elements in STO 3 seems to suggest that 'bile disease' may have served as the overarching category. If so, this would align with the rubrics in the older phases of the incantation tradition that we looked at earlier.

At the beginning of the second thematic unit, the diagnoses focus on *amurriqānu*-jaundice: according to one of the symptomatologies, patients were said to suffer from *amurriqānu* if their body and face were yellow and had a condition called 'wasting away of the flesh' (STO 3: 147). As the other symptom descriptions in this section suggest, this type of jaundice could often lead to a lethal outcome (STO 3: 145–146), but still, the text goes on to offer a number of different treatments for this condition. Moreover, a specific case of *amurriqānu* is recorded towards the end of the unit, when the focus shifts from the gastrointestinal tract to the eyes, which could also be affected by the type of jaundice known as *amurriqānu*. Not surprisingly, yellow eyes signalling *amurriqānu*-jaundice is also a key topic in the second tablet of the Eye Treatise.

In its last thematic unit, STO 3 turns to another type of jaundice called *aḫḫāzu*: the condition is described here at the beginning of the section as an illness that causes a yellowing of the body, a yellow and black face and a black tongue (STO 3: 233). Treatments for *aḫḫāzu*-jaundice follow this diagnostic entry, but some evidence gleaned from the closing statements (STO 3: 250–253) might suggest that this form of jaundice may have been considered more serious than *amurriqānu* or perhaps even untreatable.

STO 4

Unlike the previous tablets of our treatise, STO 4 is not represented by a single well-preserved manuscript but instead is known from three fragments that once belonged to two-column library tablets. Around seventy lines of text, mostly from the first column, can be recovered with the help of these fragments: AMT 14/7+ and AMT 44/6+ preserve the top of the first column, whereas AMT 23/5+ contains text from the bottom half of the first column of STO 4. Short sections are known from the second and fourth columns as well, together with the remains of the standard Ashurbanipal q colophon. Due to the fragmentary nature of the material, new copies were drawn of all three manuscripts, and these have been included in the second chapter.

Based on what has been preserved of the text, it is likely that the fourth tablet of the Stomach Treatise partly centred on fever and its effects on the gastrointestinal tract, with two feverish conditions carefully separated from one another in the first column: treatments for *ṣēta kašid* are collected in the top half of the first column, corresponding STO 4: 1–22, whereas *ṣēta* $SA_2.SA_2$ is the focus in the bottom half of the first column and the first few lines of the second column, corresponding to STO 4: 39′–69′. This second type of *ṣētu* fever also seems to be the topic of the unplaced lines a–h, recovered with the help of the Neo-Assyrian excerpt tablet BAM 174, but then the text turns to a different condition, namely constipation, with little obvious connection to fever (STO 4: i–o). The rest of the tablet is in a very fragmentary state, with only small sections containing a few medical incipits preserved in the fourth column, one of which mentions grief that constantly afflicts the patient along with the absence of phlegm (STO 4: 222′–223′).

STO 5

The tablet K 5834+ is the only known manuscript of the fifth tablet of STO; it was copied by Franz Köcher as BAM 579. The manuscript broke in half along its vertical axis but still preserves the format of a standard two-column library tablet with intact sections of text in the first and fourth columns and several more fragmentary lines in its second and third columns. Even with all its losses, however, enough of BAM 579 is preserved so that we can make sense of the fifth and final tablet of the Stomach Treatise.

Fever in the gastrointestinal tract is one of the central topics in the fourth tablet of our treatise, and it also reappears here at the beginning of the fifth tablet, although it quickly shifts to other types of fevers, such as the presence of heat (Akk. *ummu*) in the belly (STO 5: 1–71); treatments for a more serious form of fever known as 'burning heat' or 'burning fever' (STO 5: 34–44) are also recorded in this part of our text.

Pharmaceutic treatments for an ailment resulting from the breaking of an oath (*māmītu*) are also included in STO 5. This condition is first mentioned in a fever prescription at the beginning of the text (STO 5: 44) and occurs later on in a long list of ailments, such as 'blast of wind' disease, burning fever, paralysis, stiffness, numbness and 'hand-of-ghost' disease (STO 5: 119′–148′). The procedures recorded at this point in our text are unique in that they contain exceedingly long lists of ingredients, supply exact measurements for each ingredient, and describe complex forms of dosing. Measuring ingredients seems to be a characteristic feature of STO 5, with similarly unique prescriptions found at the end of the tablet. The four long prescriptions that are recorded at the end of the treatise do not generally provide any reference to a specific medical context, yet in most cases they replace the straightforward medical incipits with a label stating that the potions were a 'royal secret' (193′–235′). In line with this remarkable label, the last four prescriptions in STO showcase aspects of the drug-making process that were otherwise rarely, if ever, recorded in writing in the therapeutic literature.

Research History

The first publication of elements from our treatise, which was aware of its medical character, seems to be Sayce's paper 'An Ancient Babylonian Work on Medicine' from 1885. In this paper, Sayce states that 'some two years ago [ca. 1882 or 1883]' he had copied 'a great medical work which must have been to the Babylonians what the Papyrus Ebers was to the Egyptians'.[73] The two fragments that had captured Sayce's attention were K 191+, mistakenly transcribed as K 161 in Sayce's paper, and K 61+: K 191+ now forms the core of STO 1, the first tablet of the Stomach Treatise, while K 61+ is the core of STO 3, the third tablet. Drawing on the equally fragmentary and still very poorly understood lexical materials, Sayce had identified a few key terms, primarily *asû* 'physician' and the logogram U_2, rendered by him as Akk. *akalu* 'food', which he correctly surmised was probably 'medical food' or, as we might say, 'ingredient'. More likely, however, if we read between the lines, Sayce had likely recognised the similarities between the cuneiform medical recipes in STO and the analogous lists of ingredients and instructions in Papyrus Ebers. Understandably enough, given the early date at which Sayce was writing, Sayce's transcriptions and translations of these deeply logographic recipes were basically incoherent. Only the occasional syllabically written lines from incantations were anywhere close to a correct rendering. Here is his edition of STO 1: 89:

> Sayce's transcription and translation
> itanapats kima nuni ittanakbir cima tsiri
> 'it spreads itself like the fish, it swells like a snake'
>
> Our transliteration, transcription and translation:
> *i-ta-na-pa-aṣ ki-ma* KU_6.MEŠ / *it-ta-nak-bir ki-ma* MUŠ
> *ittanappaṣ kīma nūnī ittanakbir kīma ṣēri*
> 'he keeps flopping around like fish (and) continually puffs himself up like a snake'

Thus, where non-technical syllabic writing was in use, Sayce could already correctly transcribe and understand the text; elsewhere in this pioneering effort, especially when confronted with logographic orthographies or technical terms, Sayce's translations are less comprehensible.

In the wake of Sayce's work and Bezold's cataloguing efforts, these two fragments were studied by Baron Felix Freiherr von Oefele and Friedrich Küchler, with Küchler producing the *editio princeps* of the first three tablets of the Stomach Treatise in 1904.[74] Oefele's work, in contrast to Küchler's editorial work, aimed at broader interpretation and comparison,[75] and while Oefele's early research history remains interesting,[76] his efforts to make sense of K 191+ (STO 1) are less so. Rather than focusing on advances in interpretation, which were largely tied to the development of Akkadian dictionaries in the twentieth century, it might be more useful here to look at the gradual reconstruction of the key texts themselves. If we look, for example, at the photo of the reverse of K 191+ (STO 1) published as the frontispiece in Oefele's *Keilschriftmedizin in Parallelen* from 1904,[77] it includes approximately 60 lines, many of which are partial or fragmentary.[78] In the hand-copies in Küchler's edition, which appeared in the same year (1904), no additional fragments had been joined to K 191+. Seventy-five years later, in 1980, Franz Köcher's hand-copy of the same tablet in the sixth volume of his *Die babylonisch-assyrische Medizin in Texten und Untersuchungen* (BAM) included two major joins and brought the line total for the reverse of K 191+ (STO 1) to 116 lines, nearly twice as many as Küchler. Today, four decades after Köcher's publication of BAM 6, thanks to a number of additional joins discussed in the second chapter of this volume, every line on the reverse of

73 Sayce 1885: 1.
74 See Stol 1985c for an overview of these early phases of the research history.
75 See, in particular, Oefele 1902 and ^{2}1904.
76 See especially Oefele 1902: 4–15.
77 This photo, along with a few others, were taken years earlier and had served as the basis for all of Oefele's work.
78 These lines now correspond to STO 1: 150–196 (BAM 574+ iii 19–65), altogether 47 lines, and STO 1: 243–255 (BAM 574+ iv 47–59), altogether 13 lines.

K 191+ (STO 1) is partly or entirely recovered: 65 lines in the third column and 59 lines in the fourth column, for a total of 124 lines on the reverse of the tablet.

While the reconstruction of the textual sources has been an ongoing concern for cuneiformists over the last 140 years or so, clear advances in our understanding of the content of the compendium can really be located in three major works: Küchler's 1904 *editio princeps*, the edition of the incantations concerned with gastrointestinal illness in Timothy Collins's University of Chicago dissertation from 1999 and, most importantly, Danielle Cadelli's 2000 Sorbonne / Université de Genève dissertation, which edited the entire treatise as far as it had been recovered in the twentieth century.[79] Alongside the numerous new joins and collations made over the last few years, the only major addition to the compendium, as reconstructed by Cadelli, was the recognition that Marten Stol's 'fever tablet' could be located in the bottom left corner of the obverse of STO 4,[80] including a further join made by M. Geller while inspecting these fragments. The massive and unprecedented amount of collaborative work on this text, as part of both the BabMed and NinMed projects over the last decade, is described in the acknowledgements at the beginning of the book.

Editorial Principles

Alongside the standard canons of philological work and translation, we advocate in this edition for a number of special layout and formatting conventions meant to make the Mesopotamian medical tradition more tractable and user-friendly. Two organizational principles are particularly important for the configuration of the edition in this volume: first, any and all textual elements that can, with substantial certainty, be demonstrated to be part of the Stomach Treatise of the NME should be included in this volume of BAM; second, all of the elements that are relevant to any given line should be visible on the same page of our edition. These two editorial principles are meant to emphasise the fundamentally compendial character of these texts, on the one hand, while on the other hand, producing an edition that is easily used both in the form of a printed book and as a PDF or other digital format, in which it is difficult to look at more than one page at a time. Let us first turn to the 'same-page' principle and only afterwards return to the notion of compendial context.

The same-page principle states that all elements relevant to a single line of the *Haupttext* should appear on the same page, including transliterations, translations and commentary. All commentary appears in footnotes tied to the most relevant word or phrase on the page; no separate commentary appears elsewhere in the volume. Thus, we maintain only two primary zones of attention on the page, namely transliteration and translation, with footnotes at the bottom of the page. These two primary zones (transliteration and translation) are enumerated using the same line numbers, which run the entire length of a tablet, but are separated from each other by the element ☨. Names of ingredients and logographically written verbs are systematically transcribed in the translation so as to avoid adding a third or fourth zone within the page and further dividing the attention of the reader. In our experience, the combination of three separate zones for transliteration, transcription and translation often yields a largely unreadable page layout, while efforts to spread these different zones across different pages usually lead to great confusion and are unusable in digital formats. Footnotes are meant above all to justify the transliteration and the translation of the main text.

We systematically distinguish between manuscripts of the Stomach Treatise in the Nineveh Medical Encyclopaedia and all other parallels. Manuscripts seek to reproduce the compendial structure of an entire section, tablet or other logical unit of the treatise in the specific version known from the NME, whereas parallels are, in principle, derived from a different compendial context, even where it is difficult to specify this other context. The only basis for adding a parallel to one of our lines is the similarity of expression within the context of one or more lines.[81] Manuscripts are assigned sigla and appear at the top of a given line entry, while parallels do not receive sigla and appear both indented and in a smaller font. As a rule, the commentary in the footnotes should not focus on the variants found only in the parallels, nor attempt to describe the distinct compendial context of parallels. We hope to edit large parts of this parallel material, such as the materials from Assur, in separate volumes in the BAM series in future, where the compendial structure of the Assur medical corpus will serve as the *Haupttext* rather than the compendial structure of the NME.

79 Parts of Cadelli's dissertation have since been published in Cadelli 2019 and 2021.

80 See Johnson 2014b.

81 See Johnson 2018 for further discussion.

The translations strive for consistency throughout the entire treatise, so the English translations themselves serve as a kind of virtual index alongside the traditional lexical index at the end of the volume. Above all, the translations seek to capture the logical sequence of actions described in the texts. This is represented, for example, through the use of full stops (periods) to mark logical 'stopping points' in a given procedure, such as the 'the patient will vomit' at the end of an emetic prescription. Individual steps within a procedure are separated from each other with commas. Symptomatologies are normally separated from treatment by a colon, while stereotypically final phrases like *iballuṭ* are separated from the rest of a prescription by a semicolon. Drug ingredient identifications are largely conventional: we have focused, above all, on correctly identifying the Akkadian lemma rather than arguing for or against specific translations or equivalencies.

The edition in this volume is based on both direct inspection of the original tablets in the British Museum as well as high-quality photos of the texts. When direct inspection shows that Köcher's hand copies, published in earlier volumes of the BAM series, are mistaken, this is indicated by the addition of an asterisk in the transliteration, or, for more complex divergencies from Köcher's hand copies, these differences are detailed in a footnote. The next chapter takes up the numerous collations, corrections, and new joins in detail.

Chapter 2
Joins and Collations

Tablets describing the diseases of the gastrointestinal tract from Assurbanipal's Library at Nineveh have been available in the form of hand-copies for more than a hundred years. These copies, especially the ones published by Franz Köcher as BAM 574, 575, 578 and 579 in his sixth and final volume in *Die babylonisch-assyrische Medizin in Texten und Untersuchungen* (1980), are still a reliable source of information, which makes recopying the whole set of tablets from Nineveh a time-consuming and needless task.[82] The copies that are made available in the present volume are limited to new joins to the already published text material as well as unplaced Kouyunjik fragments identified here, for the first time, as possibly representing parts of the Nineveh Medical Encyclopaedia. An exception was made with the fourth tablet of the Stomach Treatise: due to the fragmentary state of this tablet, it was necessary to make new hand-copies of all three manuscripts. Producing new copies that reflect the current state of research was also a desideratum since all three manuscripts of STO 4 include joined fragments that are still only recorded as separate stand-alone pieces in Reginald Campbell Thompson's *Assyrian Medical Texts* (1923).[83]

In the course of work on the Stomach Treatise in the British Museum, we had the opportunity to collate all relevant tablets and fragments from Nineveh. This work yielded, on the one hand, several new readings that considerably improved the interpretation of the more fragmentary passages in Köcher's hand-copies. On the other hand, the direct work on the corpus has led to the identification of several new joins, most of them direct joins included as hand-copies here for the first time.[84] In the following pages the new joins are discussed in detail, starting with the corner piece fragment AMT 30/6+, which is the only non-contiguous join that we propose here. It can be assigned with confidence to BAM 574+, the main manuscript of STO 1. This is followed by further Kouyunjik fragments that probably belong to our treatise but cannot yet be placed as part of any available manuscript. A list of collated passages, including copies of the collated signs, can be found at the end of this chapter.

BAM 574 (+) AMT 30/6 + K 14163 + K 20273 // AO 7765

AMT 30/6 is a fragment with seven lines written on the obverse and another eight lines on the reverse; two unpublished pieces, K 14163 and K 20273, were later joined to the fragment.[85] In a recently published paper, Steinert and Vacín offer a detailed discussion of AMT 30/6 + K 20273 along with AO 7765, which is a duplicate fragment from the collections of the Musée du Louvre.[86] Steinert and Vacín point out that AMT 30/6+ and AO 7765 contain a series of incantations, rubrics and short ritual instructions for diseases that affect the gastrointestinal tract: one spell is a first-millennium Sumerian version of a bilingual Old Babylonian incantation for the belly, while another seems to be a version of the so-called 'Belly Plant' incantation. Importantly, different versions of the 'Belly Plant' incantation are also included in the first tablet of the Stomach Treatise. In the absence of any duplicating passages and with only one seemingly parallel incantation, Steinert

---

82 As described in detail in the previous chapter, the first, second and third tablets of the Stomach Treatise are the key text witnesses in one of the earliest major studies on therapeutic medicine, viz. Friedrich Küchler's *Beiträge zur Kenntnis der Assyrisch-Babylonischen Medizin* (1904), with the publication of the first hand-copies along with transliterations, translations and philological commentary. The only earlier study discussing excerpts from the first tablet of STO is Archibald Henry Sayce's article 'An ancient Babylonian Work on Medicine I' from 1885: a masterful achievement for its time. Copies of several more pieces that later turned out to be part of our treatise appeared as unplaced fragments in Erich Ebeling's *Keilschrifttexte medicinischen Inhalts* (1922–1923) and Reginald Campbell Thompson's *Assyrian Medical Texts* (1923).

83 For an overview of the current state of research regarding the reconstruction of STO 4, see Johnson 2014b. Since this article was published, the most important development in the reconstruction of this tablet has been a new join made between AMT 14/7 and the unpublished Kouyunjik fragment K 17800 (see below).

84 It is important to mention that collaboration with the Electronic Babylonian Literature Project also yielded several possible joins. These joins were checked and, in most cases, confirmed by Krisztián Simkó while working in the collections of the British Museum. The new joins are always credited to the person who first suggested them, and this information is found in footnotes throughout the edition.

85 AMT 30/6 is a copy of the Kouyunjik fragment K 2510; for an early translation of this fragment, see Campbell Thompson 1926: 75–76.

86 Steinert and Vacín 2018: 732–737. For partial editions and discussions of the text, see also Campbell Thompson 1926: 75–76, Falkenstein 1931: 10, 44, 47 and 57, Collins 1999: 145–148 and 169–171, and Stol 2006: 114 with n. 103. A line art copy of the Louvre fragment AO 7765 appeared posthumously in Nougayrol 1979: 69.

https://doi.org/10.1515/9781501506574-002

and Vacín did not think that AMT 30/6+ and AO 7765 could be part of our treatise but rather described it as 'a varying compilation of material belonging to or overlapping with topics contained in the series Suālu [i.e., the Stomach Treatise]'.[87] As we suggest here, however, these fragments actually belong to STO 1.

Both AMT 30/6+ and AO 7765 are cornerpiece fragments from the lower right-hand corner of standardised two-column library tablets and include text that was written at the end of the second and the beginning of the third column. The corresponding passage has not been preserved in BAM 574+, viz., the main manuscript of STO 1. Except for a few fragmentary signs, this part of the manuscript is so damaged that it was impossible to reconstruct the missing text. This large gap can now be filled with the help of AMT 30/6+: the placement of this fragment as a non-contiguous join to BAM 574+ is supported by shared physical characteristics, including the same script size as well as ductus and similarities in the spacing of signs. Moreover, both BAM 574+ and AMT 30/6+ have a clay texture ranging from yellow to light orange in colour. These similarities in content, ductus and the fabric of the tablets themselves are also reinforced by another manuscript from the collections of the Musée du Louvre.

The Louvre fragment AO 7765 comes from a tablet with somewhat different physical characteristics. This fragment not only duplicates the non-contiguous join AMT 30/6+, but once this join breaks off in the third column, it continues on with the same text that is preserved by the main manuscript BAM 574+ (ll. 145–149). Therefore, it is very likely that AO 7765 comes from Assurbanipal's Library and represents a second manuscript of STO 1.[88]

Altogether thirty-nine lines of text can be retrieved with the help of the newly joined pieces, extending over the end of the second and the beginning of the third column of the standard two-column library tablets. This passage contains incantations, rubrics and short ritual instructions:

Table 3: Thematic layout of STO 1: 111–149

111–116	(BAM 574+ ii 46–51): Akkadian incantation for the belly
117–122	(BAM 574+ ii 52–57 // AO 7765 obv. 1′–2′): Akkadian incantation for the belly
123	(BAM 574+ ii 58 // AO 7765 obv. 3′): short ritual
124–130	(BAM 574+ ii 59–65 // AO 7765 obv. 4′–11′): Sumerian incantation for the belly
131–131a	(BAM 574+ ii 66 // AO 7765 obv. 12′–13′): short ritual and rubric
132–133	(BAM 574+ iii 1–2 // AO 7765 rev. 1–2): Sumerian incantation for the belly
134	(BAM 574+ iii 3 // AO 7765 rev. 3): short ritual
135–137	(BAM 574+ iii 4–6 // AO 7765 rev. 4–6): Akkadian incantation for the belly
138	(BAM 574+ iii 7 // AO 7765 rev. 7): short ritual
139–145	(BAM 574+ iii 8–14 // AO 7765 rev. 8–14): 'Belly Plant' incantation
146	(BAM 574+ iii 15 // AO 7765 rev. 15): rubric
147–149	(BAM 574+ iii 16–18 // AO 7765 rev. 16–18): ritual instructions

Lines 111–122: The first two sections in lines 111–122 include two Akkadian incantations for the belly. They are preserved, for the most part, by a fragment that Köcher published as BAM 577; this fragment was later joined to BAM 574+.[89] The last two legible lines of BAM 577 belong to the end of the second incantation and contain a standard closing formula that features Asalluḫi and Gula as the owners and authors of the spell (ln. 120). Then, in the last line of BAM 577, there are traces of the commonly used phrase *iqbûnim-ma anāku ušanni* (ln. 121). The same phrase seems to occur in the fragmentary first line of AO 7765, with traces of the first-person singular independent pronoun *anāku* and the beginning of the conjugated verb form *ušanni*. The second line of AO 7765 preserves the form TI-*e*, after which a horizontal ruling was drawn in the clay (ln. 122). BAM 577 is damaged at this point, but as it happens the form TI-*e* also occurs in the last line of the first

87 Steinert and Vacín 2018: 733.

88 See also Steinert and Vacín 2018: 733. Stray fragments from Assurbanipal's library are known from various collections: see, for instance, the Louvre fragment BAM 34 (= AO 7482), which most probably is a second manuscript of the Nineveh medical compilation represented by BAM 494+. Similarly, the fragment BAM 4 (= Div 158) in the collections of the Istanbul Archaeological Museums duplicates the Nineveh manuscript BAM 480+, which contains the first tablet of the medical treatise concerned with head diseases (viz. CRAN 1). Moreover, the cornerpiece fragment MFA 1981.156, housed in the Museum of Fine Arts, Boston, is a manuscript of the 16th tablet of Šumma ālu, with a relatively well-preserved Assurbanipal colophon (Type b); for an edition of this fragment, see Bácskay and Niederreiter 2021.

89 For BAM 577 as a possible join to BAM 574+, see already BAM 6 pp. xxviii-xxix; the physical contact between the pieces was confirmed by Geller in 2007. This join is also discussed in Johnson 2018: 56 n. 3 and Steinert 2018a: 230.

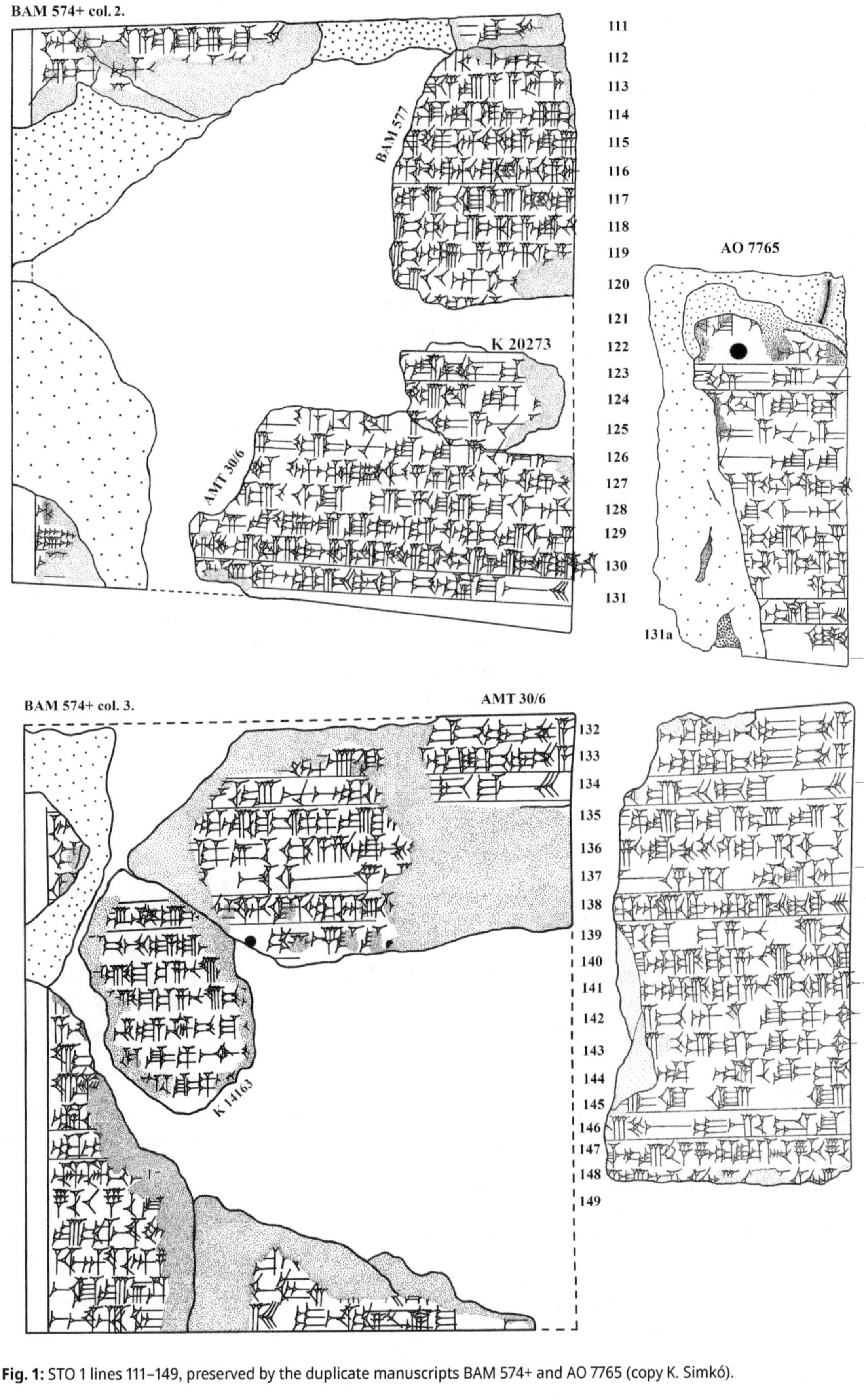

Fig. 1: STO 1 lines 111–149, preserved by the duplicate manuscripts BAM 574+ and AO 7765 (copy K. Simkó).

incantation (ln. 116). It is used there as part of a longer formula that instructs Gula to take her payment (TI-*e* = Akk. *leqê*) for healing the patient. Lines 120–122 can thus be reconstructed as follows:

> 120 [(. . .) *šipat Asa*]*lluḫi u Gu*[*la*]
> 121 [*šipat Ningirim bēlet šipti šunu iqb*]*ûnim*$^{?}$-*ma anāku u*[*šanni*]
> 122 [*Gula bulluṭī qīšta*] ***leqê***

Compare the standard closing formula of the first incantation in lines 115–116:

> 115 [(. . .)] *šiptu ul yattun*
> 116 [*šipat Asalluḫi āšip ilī iddī-ma anāku aššī*] *Gula bulluṭī qīšta* ***leqê***

Line 123: The next section contains the description of a short ritual that was performed in connection with the two Akkadian belly incantations. This is the first preserved line of AMT 30/6+ and the third line of the duplicating fragment AO 7765. Accordingly, BAM 574+ has a one-line break between the last legible line of its direct join BAM 577 (ln. 121) and the first legible line of its non-contiguous join AMT 30/6+ (ln. 123). This line is only known from AO 7765 and contains traces of the above-mentioned standard closing formula (ln. 122).

Lines 124–130: In the next section, the text continues with a Sumerian incantation for the belly; the same incantation is also known from an Old Babylonian bilingual version preserved by the tablet BM 92518 (CT 4 8).[90] Steinert and Vacín offer a new edition of the Old Babylonian text, with a full apparatus and detailed discussions, demonstrating beyond doubt its relationship to the first-millennium monolingual version.[91] In the Stomach Treatise, the right side of the column is preserved by the non-contiguous join AMT 30/6+ and the Louvre fragment AO 7765. BAM 574+ remains damaged up to the last two lines of the incantation, at which point traces of the signs NAM (ln. 129) and LU$_2$ DUMU (ln. 130) appear at the beginning, right next to the vertical ruling separating the columns. These readings find support in the formulaic and somewhat repetitive nature of the passage, as it contains an abbreviated version of the Marduk–Ea formula, with the depiction of Marduk (Asalluḫi in our text) as the one casting the spell (nam.šub). Then, the incantation instructs us that salt and thyme, viz., the drugs for curing the illness, are to be placed into the mouth of the patient. The patient is described as 'the man, son of his god' (lu$_2$.u$_{18}$.lu dumu dingir.ra.na)[92] in line 129, and the same formulation seems to reappear at the beginning of line 130 as well:

> 127 [.. n]e : ^{d}asal.lu$_2$.ḫi igi : nig$_2$ ge$_{26}$.e : gen.na dumu.gu$_{10}$
> 128 [.. n]e$^{?}$.ke$_4$: u$_3$ ^{u2}ḫa.šu.u$_2$ šu u.me.ti
> 129 na[m.šub eridu^{ki}.ga u.m]e.ni.si$_3$: **lu$_2$.u$_{18}$.lu dumu dingir.ra.na** ka.bi.ta u.me.ni.gar
> 130 **lu$_2$ du[mu dingir.ra.na** še$_{10}$.gen$_7$ ḫe$_2$.du]r$_2$.re bu.luḫ.gen$_7$ «ri» ḫe$_2$.en.si.il.e : im.ma gu.du.a.ni.ta ḫe$_2$.em.ma.ra.⸢e$_3$⸣

The formulaic passage in lines 129–130 is missing from the Old Babylonian version of the incantation, nor is it mentioned anywhere in the Old Babylonian version that salt and thyme were to be placed in the patient's mouth.[93] A very similar set of instructions is known from the Sumerian gall incantation, where it is clearly stated that the healer should place a lump of salt into the patient's mouth.[94] Then, a description of different bodily functions follows both in the gall incantation and STO 1. The verbs in this passage are usually translated intransitively, with the digestive complaint as the subject that should leave the body like excrement and flatulence or in the form of a burp.[95] As the reappearance of the phrase 'man, son of his god' in

---

90 See now also the unpublished fragment K 13368: 6′–9′, which runs parallel with our lines 124–127.

91 Steinert and Vacín 2018. See also Alster and van Dijk 1972: 354, S. Cohen 1980: 102–103, Sullivan 1980: 131–134 Text 17, Foster ^{2}1996, vol. 1: 124, Cunningham 1997: 148 no. 311, Wasserman 2003: 194 no. 57, George 2016: 7 and SEAL no. 7065. For AMT 30/6+ as a possible first-millennium parallel to the Old Babylonian bilingual belly incantation, see already Falkenstein 1931: 10, 44, 47 and 57.

92 The phrase 'man, son of his god' also occurs in a somewhat similar context in Utukkū lemnūtu Tablet 13–15: 131–133 (BAM 8 p. 472) and the anti-witchcraft text Abusch and Schwemer 2016: 120 ln. 95‴–96‴.

93 George (2016: 7) interprets the Old Babylonian passage as the description of a procedure, where 'a lump of salt and thyme is hurled into the distance, to disintegrate as it strikes the ground, so that by analogy the digestive complaint will follow the same trajectory and suffer the same fate'. For a revision of this thesis, based partly on the first-millennium variant, see Steinert and Vacín 2018: 726–727.

94 For the gall incantation, see Alster and van Dijk 1972, Michalowski 1981, Böck 2014a: 122–126, Böck 2014b: 105–107, as well as George 2016: 6–7 and 123–125. Another parallel is found in the ŠA$_3$.GIG.GA incantation OIP 16 11 obv. 6′–8′, for which see Michalowski 1981: 17, Michalowski 1992: 324 no. 1 and Peterson 2013: 1.

95 See, e.g., Cohen 1976: 103, Sullivan 1980: 134 and Steinert and Vacín 2018: 722.

line 130 of our text suggests, however, it may be possible to take this as a transitive construction, where the patient himself is doing all the necessary actions: after the digestion of salt and thyme, the patient may be able to free himself from the digestive complaint by voiding it like faeces, farting it out like flatulence and burping it up as if it were a belch.[96]

Lines 131–131a: The last line of the second column contains a set of ritual instructions that presumably starts with the word KID$_3$.KID$_3$.BI, for Akk. *kikkiṭṭašu* 'its ritual procedure': traces of this form, specifically of the first KID$_3$, seem to be preserved by the main manuscript BAM 574+. The rest of the line can be recovered with the help of the non-contiguous join AMT 30/6+ and the Louvre fragment AO 7765. The ritual in this line involves the patient sucking (*mazāqu*) on some kind of medical substance, which may be a small block of salt and a piece of thyme.[97] This rare procedure, recorded several times in our text, is otherwise only attested in a closely related collection of treatments meant to cure digestive diseases.[98] In STO 1, it first occurs in line 131 and reappears four other times later in the text:

> 131 *kikkiṭ*[*ṭašu* x x x x *ana muḫ*]*ḫi šipti tanaddi ina pîšu umazzaq-ma ina šikari tašattī-ma inâš*
> 134 [*kikkiṭṭašu* x x x x *šipta*] *sebēšu tamannu ina pîšu umazzaq-ma inâš*
> 138 [*kikkiṭṭašu*] *kirbān ṭābti nuḫurta teleqqe ana muḫḫi šipti tanaddi ina pîšu umazzaq-ma inâš*
> 170 *kikkiṭṭaš*[*u* x x x x *šipta sebēš*]*u tamannu ina pîšu u*[*mazzaq-ma*] *inâš*
> 212 *kikkiṭṭašu nuḫurta ṭābta teleqqe šipta šalāšīšu ana libbi tanaddī-ma imazzaq-ma iballuṭ*

The Louvre fragment AO 7765 does not end with this short ritual but carries on with what is most probably a rubric containing a reference to the corresponding therapeutic context (i.e., sick belly). Small differences between manuscripts like this are not uncommon in the Nineveh Medical Encyclopaedia: another example can be found in the treatise on eye diseases, first tablet line 153′, where one manuscript includes a similar rubric (BAM 510+ iii 29e′) but a second manuscript omits it (BAM 513+ iii 47k′–iv 1).[99]

Lines 132–134: The next two sections of STO 1 contain another Sumerian spell (ll. 132–133) followed by a short ritual (ln. 134) which is very similar to the one in line 131 in that it has the patient sucking on healing drugs. The incantation is addressed to Marduk (Asalluḫi in our text), who is being asked to loosen the constriction in the patient's stomach. The non-contiguous join AMT 30/6+ and the Louvre fragment AO 7765 preserve the second half of these lines, but there is no known parallel that would help us recover the rest of the text. A characteristic feature of this Sumerian spell is that it lacks the closing formula TU$_6$ EN$_2$ for Akk. *tē šipti* ('incantation-formula'): the text simply comes to an end after the last appeal is made to Marduk to loosen the constriction in the patient's stomach. An abrupt ending like this is also found in the second Akkadian belly incantation, the last line of which contains a request to Gula to accept the payment offered to her for curing the patient (ln. 122). As in our line here, this request is not followed by any closing formula.

Lines 135–138: This section includes an Akkadian incantation for the belly (ll. 135–137) and the same short ritual (ln. 138) that is cited in lines 131 and 134. The first signs that occur at the beginning of all three lines of the incantation are preserved by the main manuscript BAM 574+, whereas the non-contiguous join AMT 30/6+ and the Louvre fragment AO 77665 contain more than half of the remaining text. With the help of the available parallels, in particular ABRT 2 11+, the missing part can be recovered as well.[100]

> 135 ⸢EN$_2$⸣ [x x x x x x x] *ka-su-šu$_2$-ma* SAḪAR SIG$_3$.SIG$_3$*-ta ma-l*[*a-a rit*]-⸢*ta-šu$_2$*⸣
> EN$_2$ ^{d}ŠAKKAN$_2$ *ina* ED[IN Š]A$_3$*-ba-šu$_2$ ka-si-šu-ma* / SAḪAR.MEŠ *mu-ti* ⸢*ma*⸣*-la-a rit-ta-a-šu$_2$* (ABRT 2 11+ iii′ 27′–28′)
> 136 *ul* [*um-mu pe-ta-a*]*t pa-ni-šu$_2$ ul a-ḫa-tu mu-š*[*e-qa-at re-ši-šu$_2$*]
> *ul um-mu* ⸢*pe-ta*⸣*-at pa-ni-š*[*u$_2$*] / *ul a-ḫa-tu m*[*u-še-q*]*a-*⸢*a*⸣*-at re-ši-š*[*u$_2$*] (ABRT 2 11+ iii′ 29′–30′)
> 137 ⸢*ki*⸣-[*ma* DI GI] ⸢DA⸣ *na-ši pat-r*[*i* TU$_6$ EN$_2$]
> GIM DI G[I DA *na-ši pa*]*t-ri* TU$_6$ [EN$_2$] (ABRT 2 11+ iii′ 31′)

96 Compare also the translations offered by George (2016: 7) and SEAL (no. 7065).

97 In agreement with Steinert and Vacín 2018: 732, thyme and salt may have been the drugs used here, because they are the drugs mentioned in the preceding spell.

98 AMT 52/1: 16–17: [DU$_3$.DU$_3$].BI *ina* UGU LAG MUN EN$_2$ 3-*šu$_2$* ŠID-*nu* / [*ina* K]A-*šu$_2$ u$_2$-man-zaq-ma ina-eš* (see also CAD M/1 437, as well as Steinert and Vacín 2018: 731–732).

99 EYES 1: 153′ (BAM 10 p. 95).

100 Only the best-preserved parallel ABRT 2 11+ iii′ 27′–31′ is cited here; other parallels include AMT 52/1: 10–14, AMT 45/5+ ii 11′–14′ and Emar VI/4 737: 4–7. For this incantation, see Collins 1999: 169–171 and Stol in Loretz 2011: 398–399.

Lines 139–145: There are three versions of the so-called 'Belly Plant'[101] incantation embedded in STO 1: the shortest version appears here in lines 139–145 (Version 1), and it is followed by two longer versions in lines 153–161 (Version 2) and 164–169 (Version 3). Version 1 seems to be an abbreviated version of Version 3. The main difference between these two versions is that the shorter one (Version 1) does not use any comparative clauses but simply asks for the belly of a certain entity—affected by the Belly Plant—to be released (*libbi* X *lippašir*). The long version in lines 164–169 (Version 3), on the other hand, always compares the belly of one entity to the belly of some other entity, before asking for its release (*kīma libbi* X *ippaššaru libbi* Y *lippašir*). While these two versions mention the same entities, a longer list of creatures occurs in Version 2 of the 'Belly Plant' incantation, recorded in lines 153–161. One key difference between Version 2, in lines 153–161, and Versions 1 and 3, in lines 139–145 and 164–169, is that Version 2 also mentions the natural habitat of the creatures suffering from digestive disease but does not plead for the recovery of each individual creature separately. The Belly Plant is only asked at the very end of these lines to abandon all of the creatures it has affected.

Table 4: A summary of the entities mentioned in the different versions of the 'Belly Plant' incantation

Versions 1 and 3	Version 2
Me when I picked the Belly Plant	Šamaš when he picked the Belly Plant
Šamaš	Sîn in the clouds
Heaven and Earth	Ox in the stall
Beasts	Ram in the fold
Patient	Ass in the herd
	Dog at the door-bolt
	Hog in the pigsty
	Young man during play
	Young woman in the bedroom
	Patient

Line 146: Starting with the label *ka'inimma* in line 146, a rubric follows the short 'Belly Plant' incantation in lines 139–145. While this label is preserved in the main manuscript BAM 574+, AO 7765 also includes a description of the pertinent medical condition in the second half of the line; the non-contiguous join AMT 30/6+ is broken at this point. Accordingly, the incantation was used for patients who had a specific problem with their belly that was expressed by the verb *redû* 'to pursue'. Thus, the rubric in line 146 seems to signal a change in topic from gastric constriction (*kīs libbi*), dealt with earlier in the text, to the seemingly unique medical condition described as 'pursuing belly'.

Lines 147–149: The last section of our reconstructed passage corresponds to the beginning of a fragmentary ritual, which is preserved only by the main manuscript BAM 574+ and the Louvre fragment AO 7765. The non-contiguous join AMT 30/6+ ends in the second to last line of the first 'Belly Plant' incantation (ln. 144) and cannot be used anymore to connect AO 7765 to BAM 574+. In the same line, however, there is a shift in the way the text is arranged by the two extant manuscripts. Compared to BAM 574+, the Louvre fragment seems to have longer lines, since pieces of text preserved at the end of lines in the Louvre fragment only occur at the beginning of the following lines in BAM 574+. This has led to some overlaps between BAM 574+ and AO 7765, such as the phrase *sebīšu u sebīšu* that first occurs in AO 7765 rev. 16 and reappears again in BAM 574+ iii 17 (ln. 147). Similarly, the difficult form *ištu naḫbî* is attested in the same position in AO 7765 rev. 17 and BAM 574+ iii 18 (ln. 148). These overlaps suggest that AO 7765 is, in fact, a second manuscript of the first tablet of the Stomach Treatise since it not only duplicates the non-contiguous join AMT 30/6+, but after this join breaks off in line 144, it continues on with the same text that is written in BAM 574+.

101 For the corpus of these incantations, called 'Heart Grass' in earlier literature, see Reiner 1985: 94–100, Veldhuis 1990, Veldhuis 1993: 48–61, Collins 1999: 137–151, and George 2016: 129–132. See also Steinert and Vacín 2018: 704–707, who provide a detailed overview of the sources and suggest the more appropriate designation 'Belly Plant spell'.

BAM 574 + K 21858 + K 21905

K 21858 and K 21905 are unpublished Kouyunjik fragments that were joined by W.G. Lambert in 1991 and have now been placed as direct joins to the top of the second column of BAM 574+. With the help of these fragments, the beginning of a six-line long section can be recovered in lines 67–73, with four individual treatments for painful internal organs. The first two prescriptions include a series of simple drugs to be consumed in various carrier liquids, such as beer, wine and water (ll. 67 and 68–69). Then, a more complex prescription follows with measured ingredients boiled in three litres of beer and administered to the patient in the form of an enema (ll. 70–71). The last piece of text that can be recovered using the direct join K 21858+ corresponds to the first two lines of another complex prescription for painful internal organs (ll. 72–73). This prescription starts with the unexpected form UD-*ma* for Akkadian *enūma* 'when' and includes another set of instructions for making healing potions.

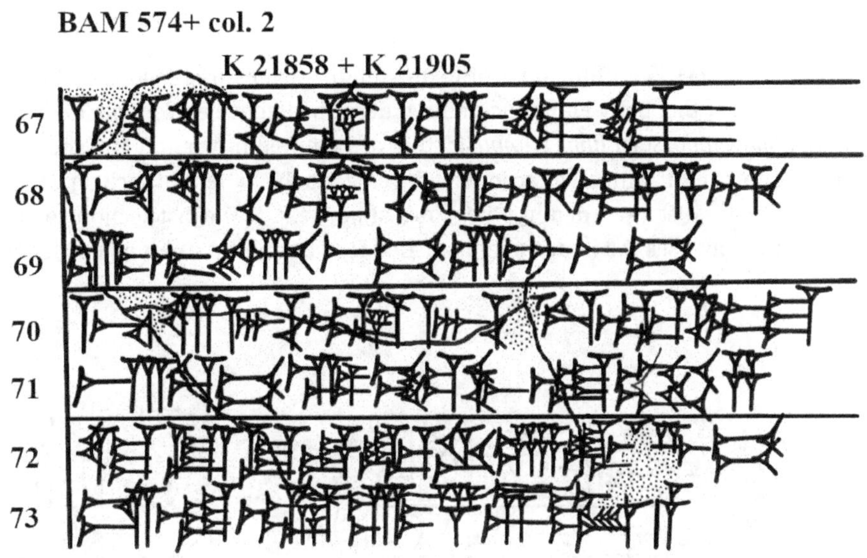

Fig. 2: BAM 574 + K 21858 + K 21905 (copy K. Simkó)

BAM 574 + K 22170

K 22170 is also an unpublished Kouyunjik fragment and is now a direct join to the second column of BAM 574+. This fragment preserves the beginning of lines 98–100, including an incipit that mentions the same medical condition treated earlier in our text, viz. *kīs libbi* 'gastric constriction'. There are two treatments recorded in this three-line section; both of them involve healing potions for patients suffering from gastric constriction. Line 98 also contains two subscript glosses, of which the second one is still well preserved and offers an alternative spelling for the drug name *tarmuš*. The first gloss shows signs of intentional erasure with some traces still legible. According to these remaining traces, some part of a plant, presumably its seed, may have originally been included in this gloss as a possible alternative to the main ingredient *imḫur-ešrā*.[102]

102 For these glosses, see now Bácskay 2021: 55–56, who does not see the first gloss as erased.

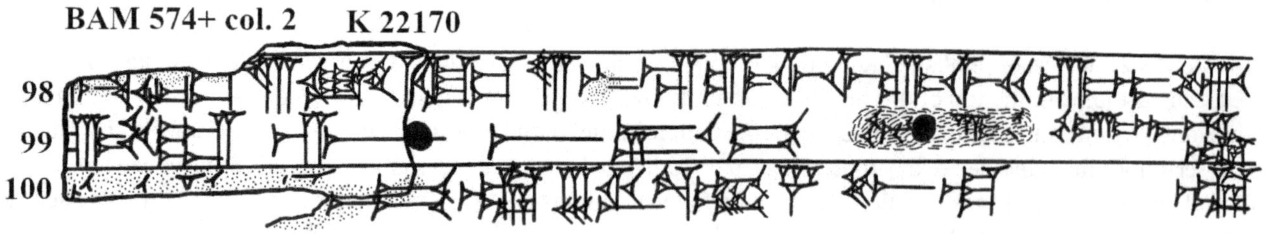

Fig. 3: BAM 574 + K 22170 (copy K. Simkó)

BAM 574 + K 22164

This small fragment joins the third column of BAM 574+, with four lines of text extending over three sections. The first section (ll. 168–169) belongs to the end of a version of the 'Belly Plant' incantation described above as Version 3 because it contains all the comparative clauses (*kīma libbi* X *ippaššaru libbi* Y *lippašir*) that are omitted in Version 1 of the same incantation.[103] This incantation is followed by a short ritual with an instruction addressed to the patient to suck on healing drugs (ln. 170); as mentioned above, the same ritual is also recorded in other lines of our text.[104] The last section consists of a two-line Akkadian incantation, which presumably uses the image of a disturbed fermenting vat as an object of comparison for an upset stomach (ll. 171–172).

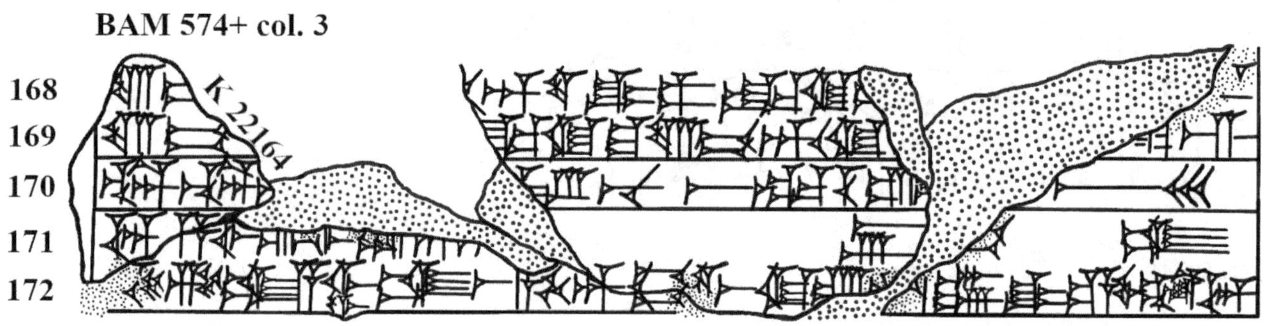

Fig. 4: BAM 574 + K 22164 (copy K. Simkó)

BAM 574 + K 22089

K 22089 is the last physical join to the first tablet of the Stomach Treatise. The fragment joins the third column of BAM 574+, in lines 173–178, and consists of an incantation as well as an appended ritual. The incantation depicts wind, i.e., flatulence, as a pure entity that comes down from the mountains to affect the belly of mankind. The belly is then described as having flesh and what appears to be some kind of liquid, perhaps oil, framed in terms suitable for a therapeutic context.[105] The incantation warns the wind about consuming the belly and then ends by saying that the wind should leave through the anus like a vineyard snake. The following healing ritual prescribes a potion made out of three healing drugs.

103 The short version of the 'Belly Plant' incantation, without the comparative clauses (viz. Version 1), occurs in lines 139–145, whereas another version containing a long list of creatures with their natural habitat (viz. Version 2) is recorded in lines 153–161.

104 See lines 131, 134, 138 and 212.

105 Based on our tentative reading of line 174, oil (Akk. *šammu*) co-occurs with the verb *pašāšu* ('to anoint') in the Gt-stem. Anointing with oil is one of the most common forms of external treatment in therapeutic texts.

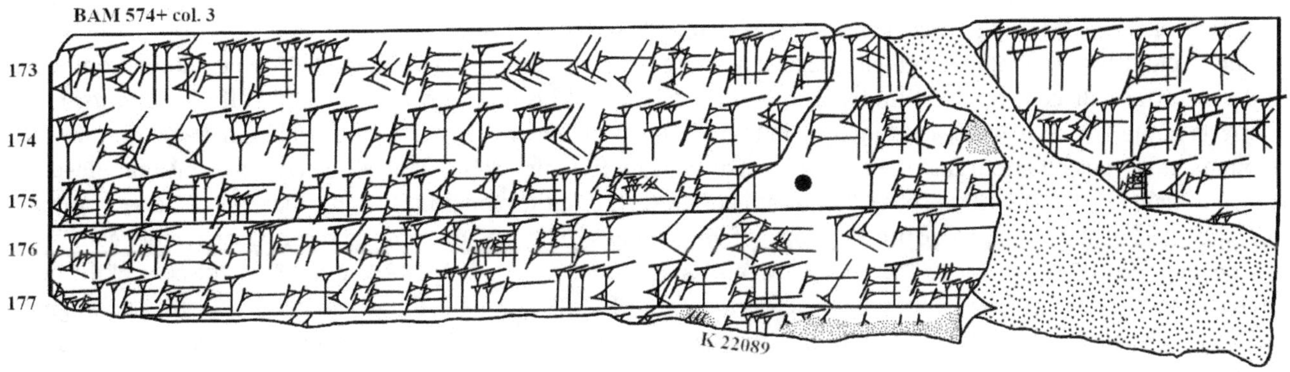

Fig. 5: BAM 574 + K 22089 (copy K. Simkó)

BAM 578 Column 1

Several fragments could be identified that join a sixteen-line section towards the end of the first column of BAM 578+, viz. the main manuscript of the third tablet of the Stomach Treatise. Some of the fragments are still unpublished such as the flake K 22008 from the edge of the tablet, which preserves the beginning of lines 47–53. In lines 47–49, the text contains prescriptions for a complex set of symptoms, including dizziness, nausea, as well as pain in the neck, hips, shins and feet;

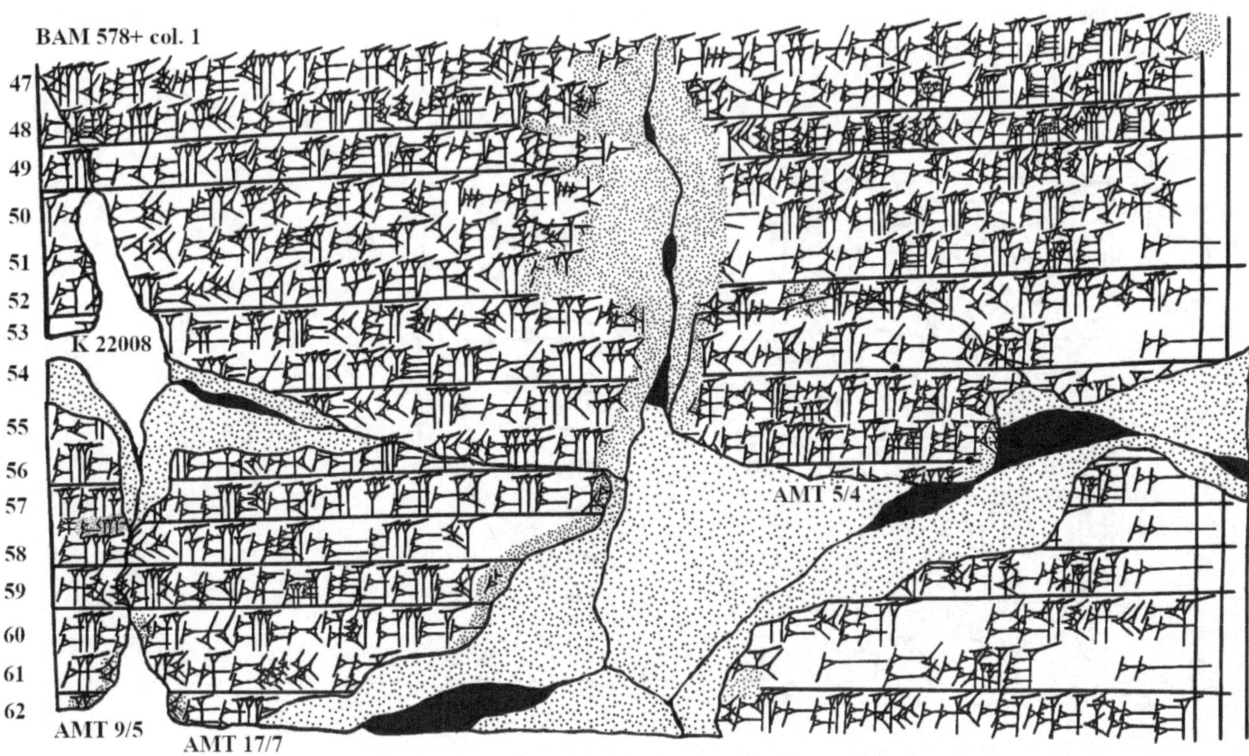

Fig. 6: BAM 578 + AMT 5/4 + AMT 9/5 + AMT 17/7 + K 22008 (copy K. Simkó)

according to the diagnosis in line 47, these symptoms represent a disease that is related to bile, which has 'seized' (*ṣabātu*) the patient. The text records two treatments for this condition. Both treatments consist of channelling the medicine into the rectum of the patient, the first time in the form of an enema (ln. 47–48) and the second time as a suppository (ln. 49) that is sprinkled with oil first to make it easier to insert into the patient's anus.

The unpublished Kouyunjik fragment K 22008 also preserves the beginning of lines 50–53, where another group of symptoms is traced back to the same underlying medical condition. This time, however, patients suffering (*marāṣu*) from the effects of the bile-related disease do not seem to have any problems with their digestive tract. Instead, they produce symptoms in various other parts of their body, such as warmth in their heels and chest, as well as gums that bleed and make it difficult for the patients to speak. The treatment for this condition consists of simply making the patient vomit.

One of the largest sets of emetic prescriptions is found in lines 50–64 and can now be reconstructed more completely with the help of K 22008 and a few other joined fragments. The small fragment AMT 9/5 comes from the edge of the tablet and joins AMT 17/7, which, in turn, can be attached to BAM 578+, filling in most of the gap in lines 55–62. The fragment AMT 5/4 also belongs to our tablet: it can be directly joined with the rest of the section, forming the recipe section in the second half of lines 53–57.

BAM 578 + AMT 58/8

AMT 58/8 is a direct join to the top of the second column of BAM 578+ and contains prescriptions for three different sets of diseases. The first set is found in the last line of the first column of BAM 578+ (ln. 70); the corresponding treatment also starts at this point, but then it continues in the first line of the second column of our tablet (ln. 71). The first line of the joining fragment, AMT 58/8, represents the closing section of this treatment, which was employed for someone suffering from bile or one of the two types of jaundice, *aḫḫāzu* and *amurriqānu*. The text records two more prescriptions for the same medical conditions (ll. 72–76) before it turns to another set of diseases that also includes bile, but now alongside less well-known medical conditions like *qidḫu* and *lubāṭu* (ll. 77–78). Unlike in the previous section of our text, there is only one treatment recorded in connection with this second set of diseases. Finally, *ašû*, *pāšittu* and *lubāṭu* constitute the third group of diseases in lines 79–80, which are to be treated using a single prescription.

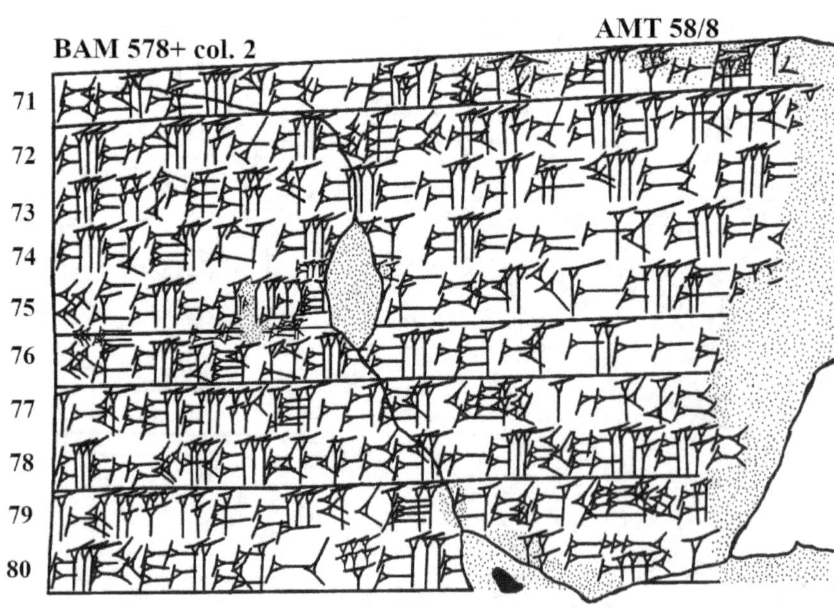

Fig. 7: BAM 578 + AMT 58/8 (copy K. Simkó)

BAM 578 + K 13344 + K 17699

Two unpublished fragments from the Kouyunjik collection of the British Museum, K 13344 and K 17699, are physical joins to the second column of BAM 578+, yielding a passage that includes two incantations (ll. 119 and 122–123), each accompanied by a ritual (ll. 120–121 and 124–125) and a rubric mentioning bile at the end (ln. 126). The new joins preserve the last line of the first incantation with the expected closing formula, attributing the spell to Ea and Asalluḫi as well as the healing deities Damu and Gula. The other incantation is in a fragmentary state of preservation, except for the last line, which contains an appeal for the patient's life. The healing potions that appear in the appended rituals were to be made from a mixture of plants, salt and aromatics and consumed on an empty stomach.

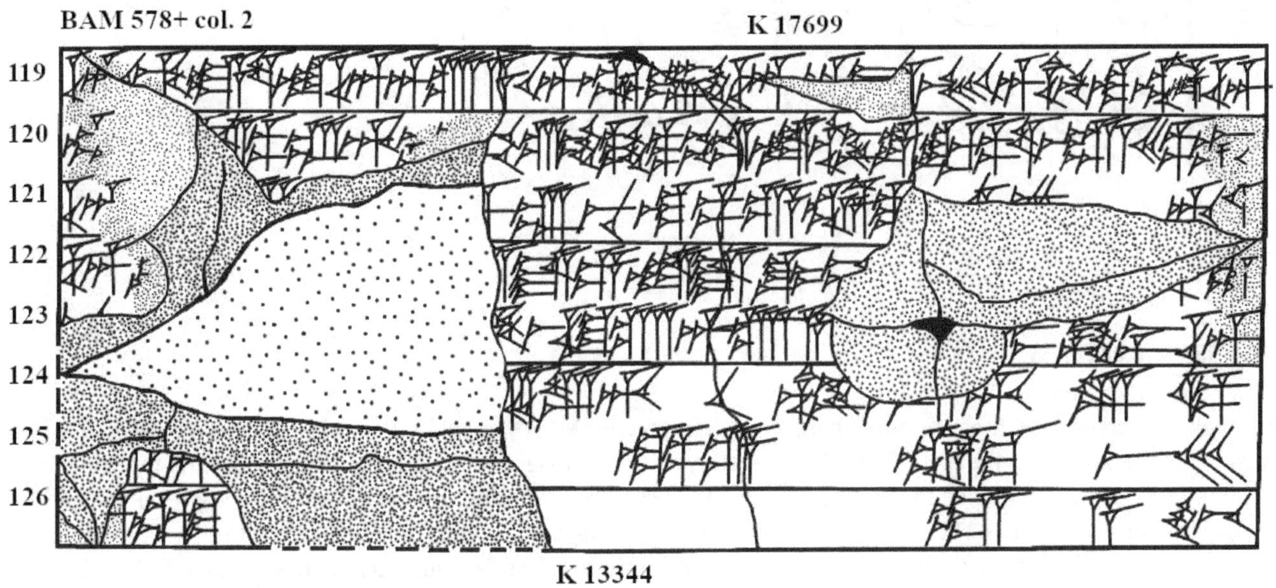

Fig. 8: BAM 578 + K 13344 + K 17699 (copy K. Simkó)

BAM 578 + K 5762

The unpublished Kouyunjik fragment K 5762 is a direct join to the third column of BAM 578+ and can now be used to fill the small gap at the beginning of ll. 155–161. The newly restored passage is part of a lengthy section that collects treatments for *amurriqānu*-jaundice. Nearly all of the treatments in this section are *simplicia*, consisting of a single healing drug for a single disease, and they include, for the most part, the same set of instructions for both the preparation of the drugs (pounding and mixing the ingredients with carrier substances) and their subsequent administration as healing potions.

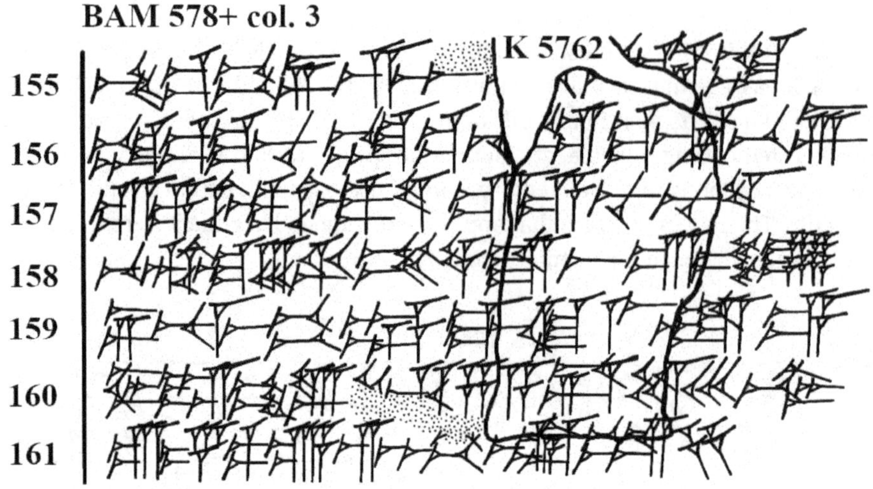

Fig. 9: BAM 578 + K 5762 (copy K. Simkó)

BAM 578 + AMT 9/6

Köcher already considered the possibility that the small fragment AMT 9/6 might belong to BAM 578+ and copied this piece as a non-contiguous join to the lower half of the reverse, where it preserves text both from the third and fourth columns of the tablet.[106] Köcher positioned the fragment so that the preserved four lines in its fourth column represent a continuation of a four-line section in BAM 578+, with two treatments for *aḫḫāzu*-jaundice (healing potions) and a diagnostic entry (ll. 248–251). This placement was recently reconfirmed through a first-hand examination of the pieces, which also yielded a point of contact between them, where AMT 9/6 can be physically attached to BAM 578+. This is partially due to the fact that BAM 578+ preserves just enough of its rough clay structure at this point, so AMT 9/6 can be physically joined to it. Collations provide further support for the placement of AMT 9/6 as a physical join to BAM 578+ because of sign traces still visible in line 250. These traces most likely belong to UD, used as the first syllable in the conjugated verbal form *ud-du-ḫa* '(his eyes) are covered (with yellow filaments)'. The sign is visible on the damaged surface of BAM 578+, but its head stretches out to the left, where it corresponds to the traces preserved by AMT 9/6.

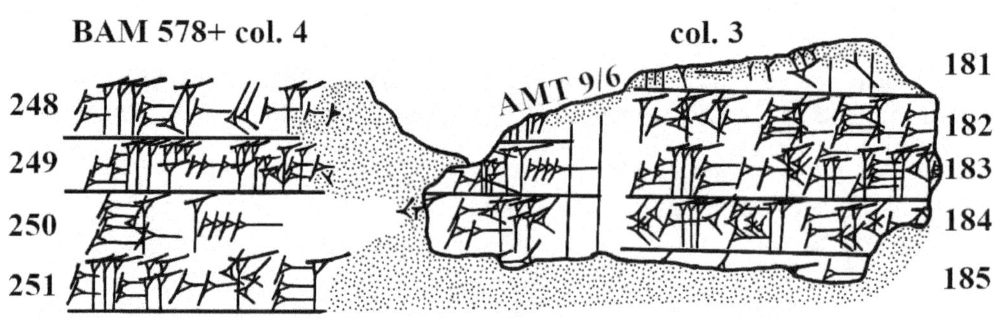

Fig. 10: BAM 578 + AMT 9/6 (copy K. Simkó)

106 Köcher 1980: xxix with plates 135 and 137.

BAM 579 + K 18594

K 18594 is an unpublished fragment from the Kouyunjik collection and the only direct join that can be assigned to the fifth tablet of the Stomach Treatise. It belongs to the third column of the corresponding manuscript, viz. BAM 579, joining the tablet at the end of an unusually long prescription (ll. 145′–148′), which lists more than a dozen healing drugs and instructs the healer to use these drugs together with beer, vinegar and *kasû*-plant juice as an enema. As it happens, the goal of the healing procedure is indicated—after the enumeration of all the technical details—at the very end of the prescription. Accordingly, this enema could be used to treat many different conditions, including the 'blast of wind' disease, burning fever, paralysis, stiffness and numbness, as well as further medical problems labelled as 'hand-of-ghost' and 'hand-of-oath'.

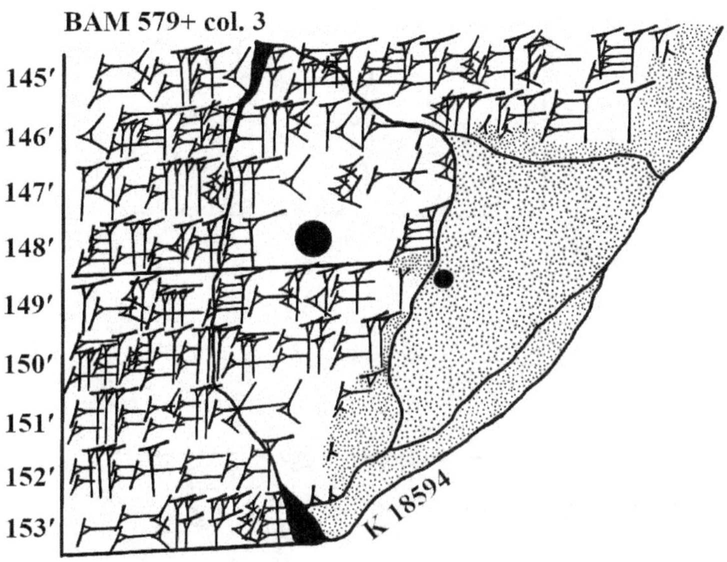

Fig. 11: BAM 579 + K 18594 (copy K. Simkó)

The newly joined piece K 18594 helps us restore parts of the following treatment (ll. 149′–153′). Here, the prescription starts with the usual discourse pattern *šumma amēlu* 'If someone', but then a difficult sign sequence follows which, although meant to describe the medical condition being treated, does not yet yield a clear meaning.

Addendum: After the completion of the manuscript, we received information from Zsombor Földi about the join BAM 578 + K 6941, corresponding to STO 3: 95-108. Unfortunately, this information arrived too late for us to include K 6941 in this volume.

Manuscripts of STO 4

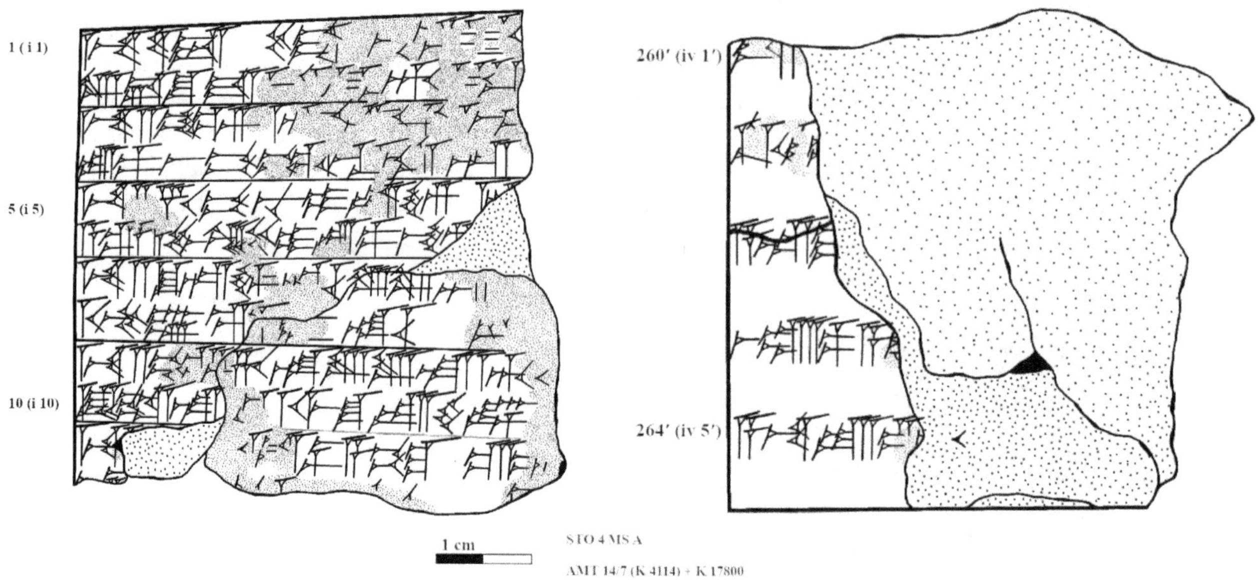

Fig. 12: STO 4 MS A (copy K. Simkó)

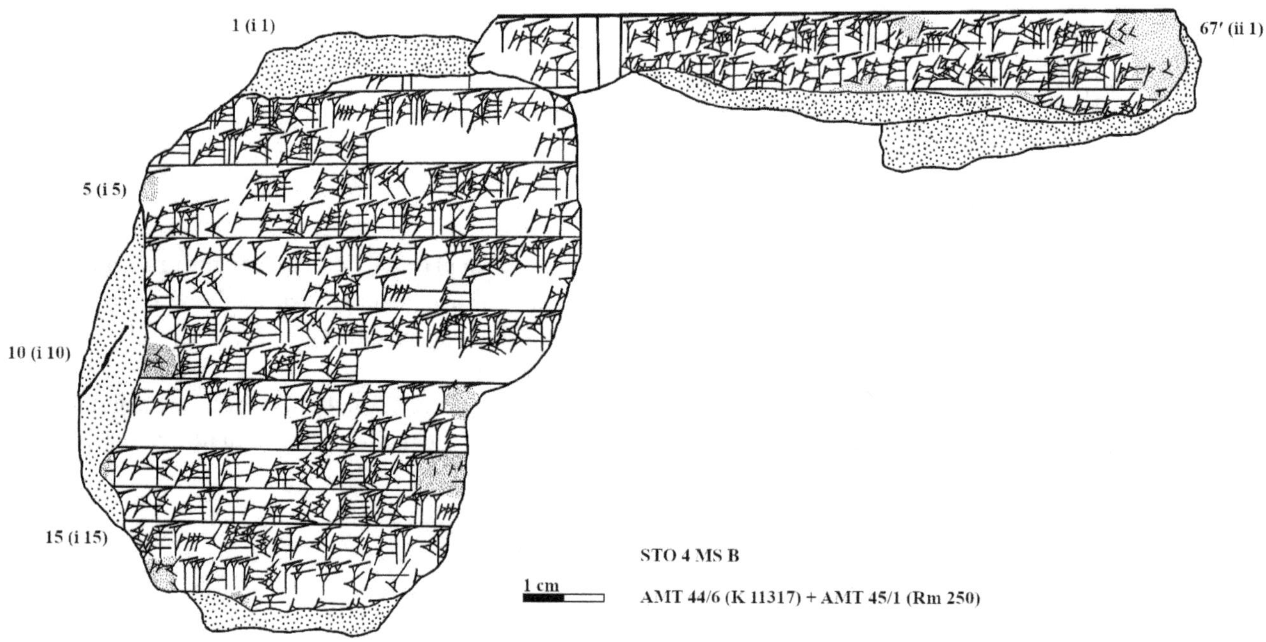

Fig. 13: STO 4 MS B (copy K. Simkó)

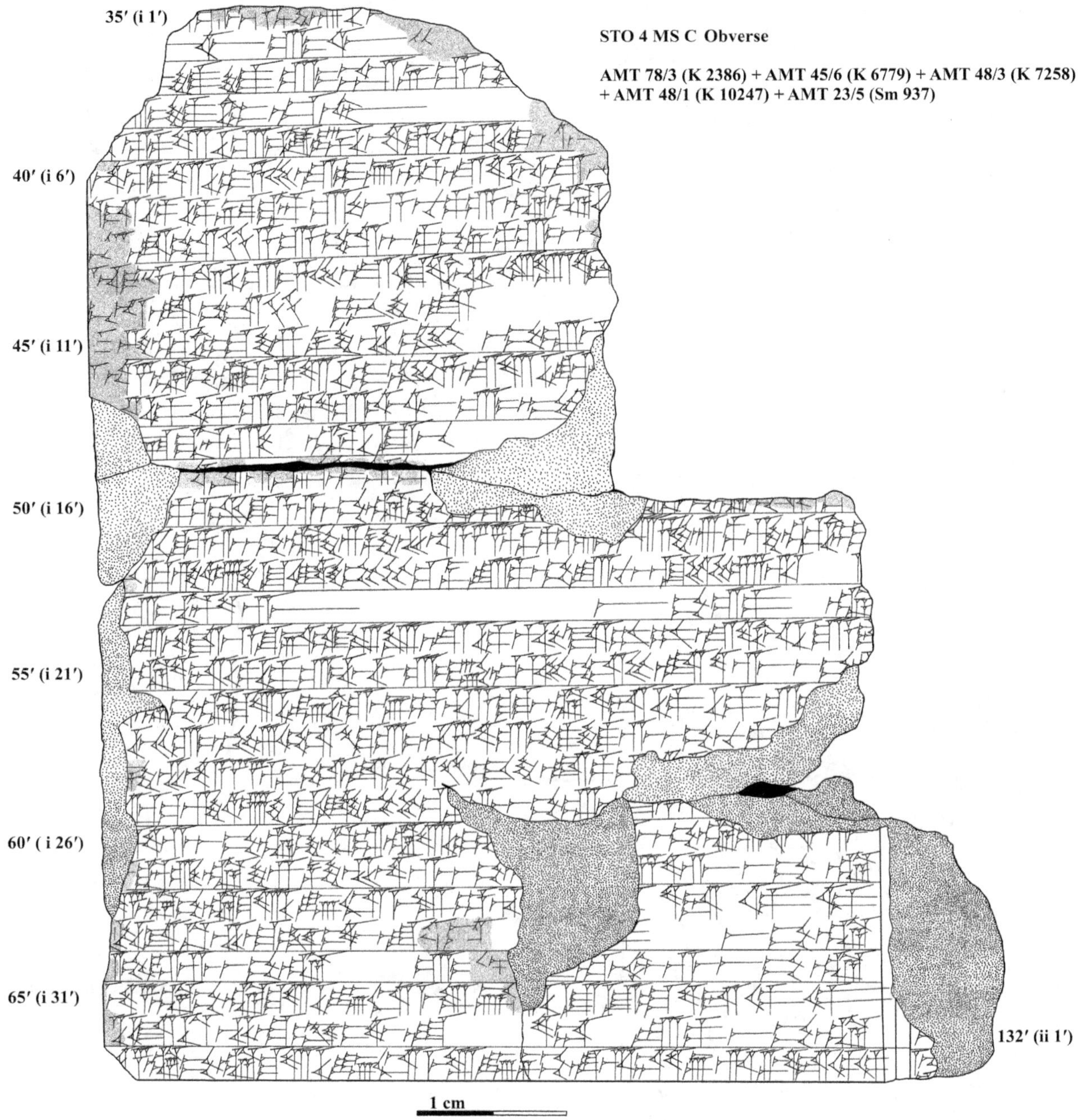

Fig. 14a: STO 4 MS C obverse (copy K. Simkó)

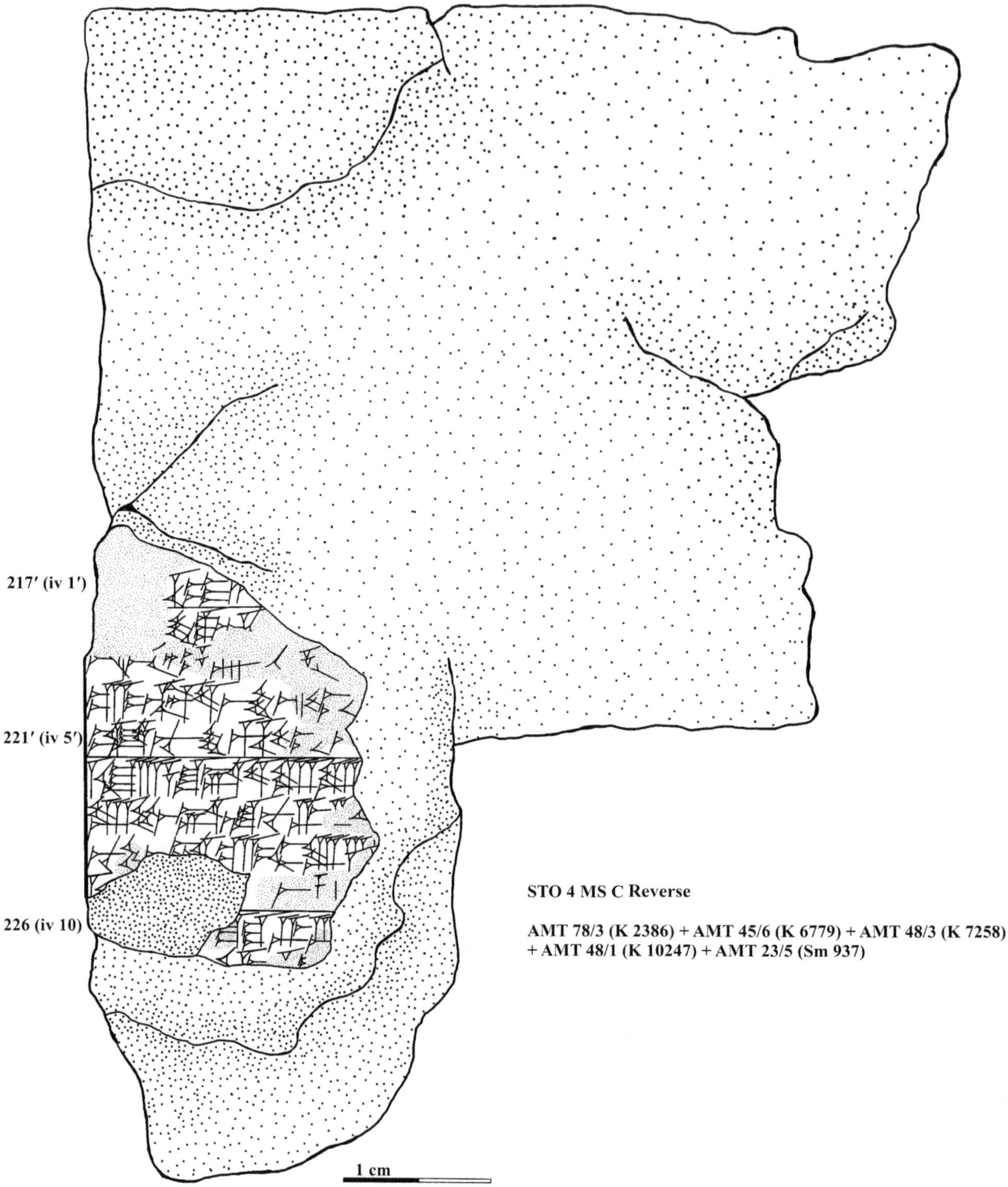

Fig. 14b: STO 4 MS C reverse (copy K. Simkó)

Unplaced Fragments

AMT 39/5 (K 14541)

AMT 39/5 is a fragment from the left-hand edge of a tablet.[107] This small fragment has a clear link to our treatise since it is concerned with *kīs libbi* 'gastric constriction', the same medical condition that is discussed at length in the first half of STO 1. However, compared to the main manuscript BAM 574+, AMT 39/5 has a slightly different handwriting, making it unlikely that it is an indirect join to this manuscript. If it is from a different manuscript, AMT 39/5 may represent a piece of text from the missing part of STO 1, most likely in the ten-line gap at the end of the first column of BAM 574+.

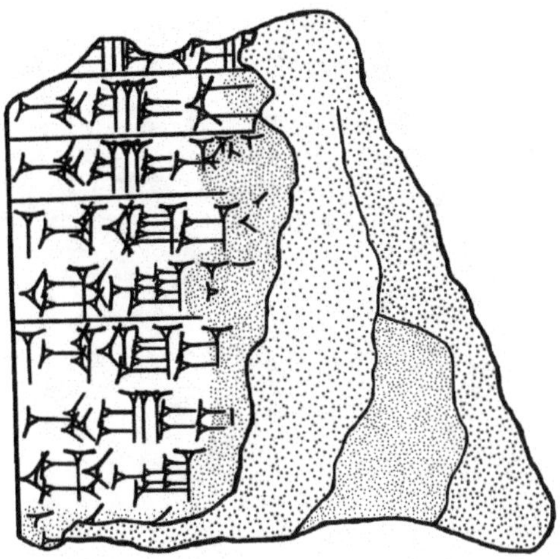

Fig. 15: AMT 39/5 (copy K. Simkó)

1′	[NUMUN] ⌜$^{u2}u_5$⌝-*r*[*a-nu* . . .]	Seed from *urânu* ('anise') . . .
2′	NUMUN ^{u2}AB$_2$.[DUḪ . . .]	Seed from *kamantu* (a plant) . . .
3′	NUMUN ^{u2}⌜u_5⌝-[*ra-nu* . . .]	Seed from *urânu* ('anise') . . .
4′	DIŠ NA *ki-is* Š[A$_3$ GIG . . .]	If someone suffers from gastric constriction . . .
5′	*ul-tu* x [. . .]	from . . .
6′	DIŠ NA *ki-*⌜*is*⌝ [ŠA$_3$ GIG . . .]	If someone suffers from gastric constriction . . .
7′	NUMUN ^{u2}x [. . .]	seed from . . .
8′	*ul-tu* [. . .]	from . . .
9′	x x x [. . .]	. . .

107 For a brief discussion of this fragment, mistakenly cited as K 15451, see Campbell Thompson 1929: 85.

K 18128

The unpublished Kouyunjik fragment K 18128 cannot be placed as a direct join to any of our manuscripts but seems to contain the same type of therapies that are collected in STO 2: a healing potion is administered first on an empty stomach, then afterwards, an enema (now missing from the fragment) and finally a bandage. BAM 575, the main manuscript of STO 2, has just enough room for this fragment in lines 36–41 of its first column, where K 18128 could be placed as a direct join. However, the depth of this fragment is far greater than what is missing from lines 36–41 of our tablet.[108]

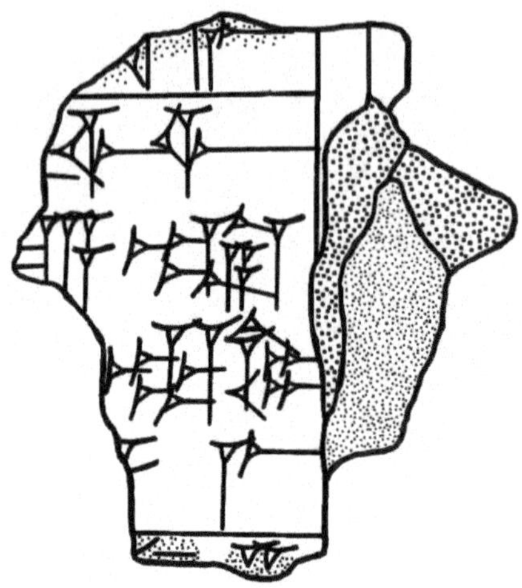

Fig. 16: K 18128 (copy K. Simkó)

1′	[. . . *te-ṭer*$_5$]-⌜*ri* LAL$_2$⌝	. . . you smear . . . (and) you bandage him.
2′	[. . .] ⌜^{u2}⌝IGI-*lim*	. . . *imḫur-līm* ('faces a thousand' plant)
3′	[. . . NU *pa*]-⌜*tan*⌝ NAG	. . . he drinks it on an empty stomach
4′	[. . .] ZU$_2$.LUM	. . . *suluppū* ('dates')
5′	[. . . SU]R LAL	. . . you smear . . . (and) you bandage him.
6′	[. . .] x x	. . .

AMT 29/3 (K 2408)

AMT 29/3 is a fragment from the left-hand edge of a tablet that cannot be joined directly to any known manuscript of the Stomach Treatise.[109] Nevertheless, the fragment may belong to our corpus since it contains prescriptions for the gastrointestinal tract. The condition mentioned in this context is *urbatu*, a parasitic infestation, presumably some kind of worm that lodges itself in the intestines and causes different gastrointestinal symptoms (e.g., swollen intestines, dry stool, flatulence and noisy intestines).[110] This condition is otherwise not attested in our corpus but occurs in connection with the belly in medical texts from Assur. One of the key text witnesses for *urbatu* is the three-column tablet BAM 159, where treatments

108 Personal communication J. Taylor, July 2021.

109 For this fragment, see Campbell Thompson 1929: 85, as well as Scurlock and Andersen 2005: 82–83 with n. 258.

110 For this intestinal parasite, see Kinnier Wilson 1968: 243–244 (discussed under the alternative Akkadian reading *išqippu*), Scurlock and Andersen 2005: 82–83, Böck 2014a: 109 and 179–180, as well as Parys 2014: 48

for this condition follow a series of prescriptions for bile (i 29–44) and afterwards for the two main types of jaundice, namely *amurriqānu* (i 45–ii 10) and *aḫḫāzu* (ii 11). BAM 159 then presents several treatments for swollen intestines and contorted legs (ii 12–19) before turning to *urbatu*, the discussion of which takes up a large part of the text (ii 20–48).[111] A similar arrangement seems to have been at work in our treatise as well: STO 3 collects prescriptions for bile and the two types of jaundice; this is followed in the first seventy lines of the fourth tablet by prescriptions that are concerned with fever. The rest of STO 4 has not been preserved, but based on the arrangement in BAM 159, one might reasonably assume that prescriptions for *urbatu* were recorded in the missing part of the text, after the fever recipes, which, like the swollen intestines and contorted legs in BAM 159, separate the last treatment for jaundice from the first *urbatu* recipe.

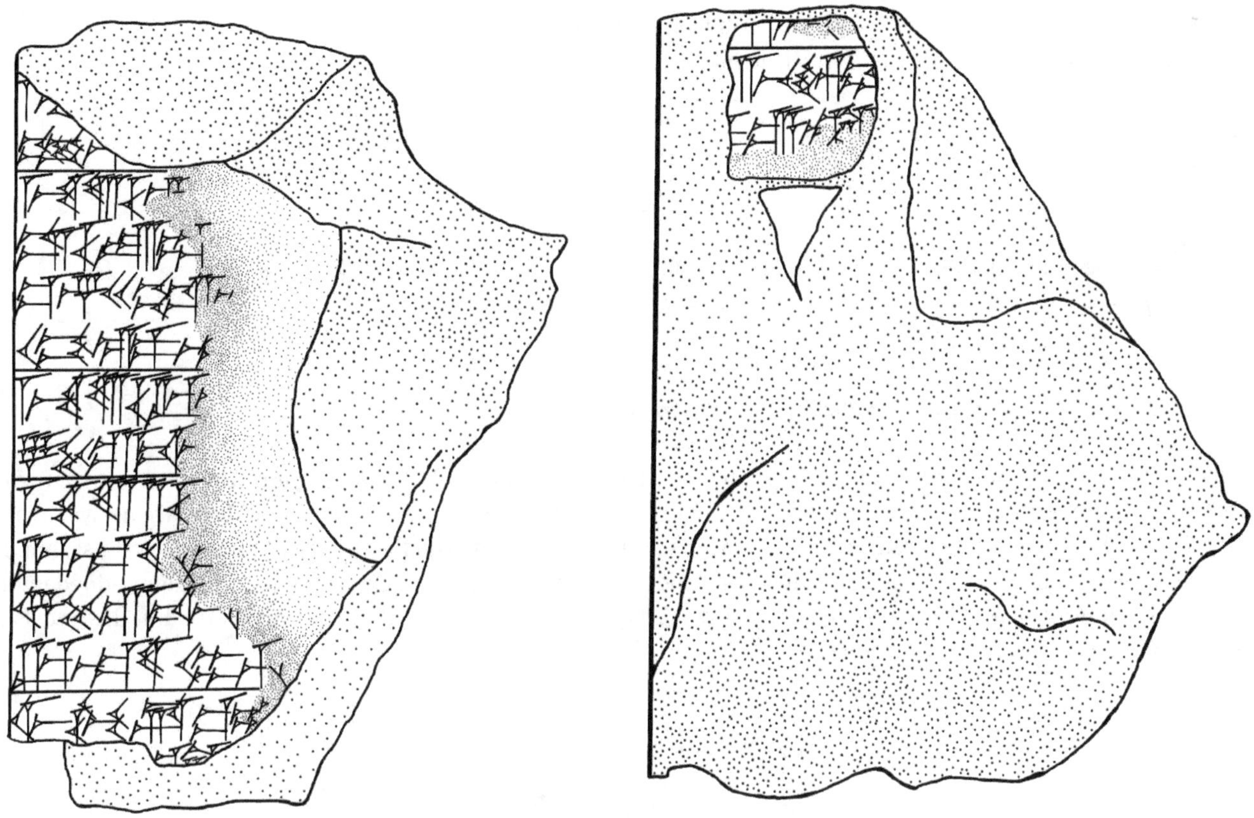

Fig. 17: AMT 29/3 (copy K. Simkó)

Obverse

1′	DIŠ N[A . . .]	If someone . . .
2′	GAZ S[IM . . .]	you crush (and) sift . . .
	________________	________________
3′	DIŠ NA ŠA$_3$-*šu*$_2$ ⸢e⸣ [. . .]	If someone's belly . . .
4′	SAḪAR-*šu*$_2$ ta ⸢ab⸣ [. . .]	you . . . its dust . . .
5′	^{giš}ŠUR.MIN$_3$ ^{šim}B[ULUḪ$^?$ . . .]	*šurmēnu* ('cypress'), *baluḫḫu* (an aromatic)$^?$ . . .
6′	*u* KAŠ SAG NA[G . . .]	he drinks it in . . . and high-quality beer . . .
	________________	________________

111 For an edition and in-depth analysis of BAM 159, see Parys 2014, who convincingly restores *amurriqānu* as the condition being treated in the fragmentary passage BAM 159 i 45–ii 10 (pp. 43–45).

7′	DIŠ NA ŠA$_3$-*šu*$_2$ *ur-b*[*a-ta*$_5$ . . .]	If someone's belly . . . by *urbatu* worms . . .
8′	7 ŠE ^{u2}⌜IGI⌝-[*lim*$^?$ . . .]	seven grains of *imḫur-līm* ('faces a thousand' plant)$^?$ . . .
9′	DIŠ NA ŠA$_3$.MIN-*šu*$_2$ [. . .]	If someone's internal organs . . .
10′	*ur-ba-ta*$_5$ G[IG . . .]	he suffers from *urbatu* worms: . . .
11′	15 ŠE ^{u2}IGI-⌜*lim*⌝ [. . .]	fifteen grains of *imḫur-līm* ('faces a thousand' plant) . . .
12′	*ur-ba-tu*$_2$ mi x [. . .]	*urbatu* disease . . .
13′	*ši-gu-uš* ^{giš}KI[RI$_6$ . . .]	*šigguštu* (a plant) from the garden . . .
14′	[x x x] ⌜NAG⌝ [. . .]	. . . he drinks it . . .
Reverse		
1′	[x x] x x x [. . .]	. . .
2′	[DIŠ NA] MIN bad im ⌜du⌝ [. . .]	If someone DITTO . . .
3′	[NU *p*]*a-tan* ⌜NAG⌝ x [. . .]	he drinks it on an empty stomach . . .

AMT 1/6 (K 16440), 9/4 (K 8557), 22/5 (K 15238) and 49/3 (K 16442)

The allocation of these remaining fragments to the Stomach Treatise is more tentative, taking into account the presence of internally administered treatments in these texts.[112] They are only partially similar, however, and there are no systematic overlaps between the step-by-step instructions that make up these treatments and the specific steps in our treatise, nor do they mention any specifically gastrointestinal medical conditions. Therefore, the placement of the fragments edited in the following pages must remain provisional, bearing in mind that the type of internal treatments recorded in these texts is not entirely limited to gastrointestinal illnesses.

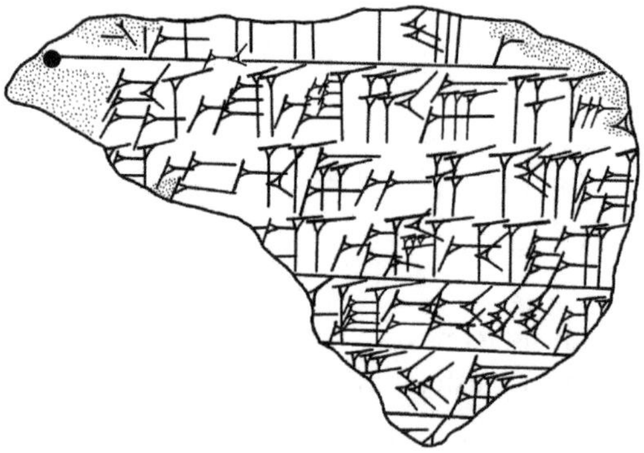

Fig. 18: AMT 1/6 (copy K. Simkó)

112 For the fragment AMT 1/6, see Herrero 1984: 64 and Stol 1998: 345. The fragment copied in Böck 2000: plate 15 under the acquisition number K 16440 (corresponding to AMT 1/6) is actually K 16640. A translation of AMT 49/3 is found in Campbell Thompson 1929: 80.

1′	[. . .] x x $_{\text{TIL}}$ x x ⸢*ana* ŠA$_3$⸣ D[UB . . .]	. . . (gloss: complete$^?$) . . . you pour . . . in (the mixture) . . .
2′	[. . .] SIG$_7$-*su tu-ḫa-sa* A.MEŠ-*š*[*u*$_2$ . . .]	. . . you mince . . . while it is fresh . . . its juice . . .
3′	[. . . GIM *ra-bi-k*]*i tara-bak* I$_3$ *ḫal-ṣa ana* ŠA$_3$ DU[B . . .]	. . . you stir them like a paste, you pour pressed oil in (the mixture) . . .
4′	[. . . *baḫ-r*]*a* GU$_7$ *baḫ-ra* [NAG . . .]	. . . he eats steaming hot (food), he drinks steaming hot (drinks) . . .
5′	[. . . ZI$_3$ MUN]U$_6$ ZI$_3$.KUM ḪI.ḪI x [. . .]	. . . you mix flour from *buqlu* ('malt') (and) *isqūqu* ('a type of groats') . . .
6′	[. . . ZI$_3$] NIG$_2$.ŠE.S[A.A . . .]	. . . flour from *labtu* ('roasted barley') . . .
7′	[. . .] x [. . .]	. . .

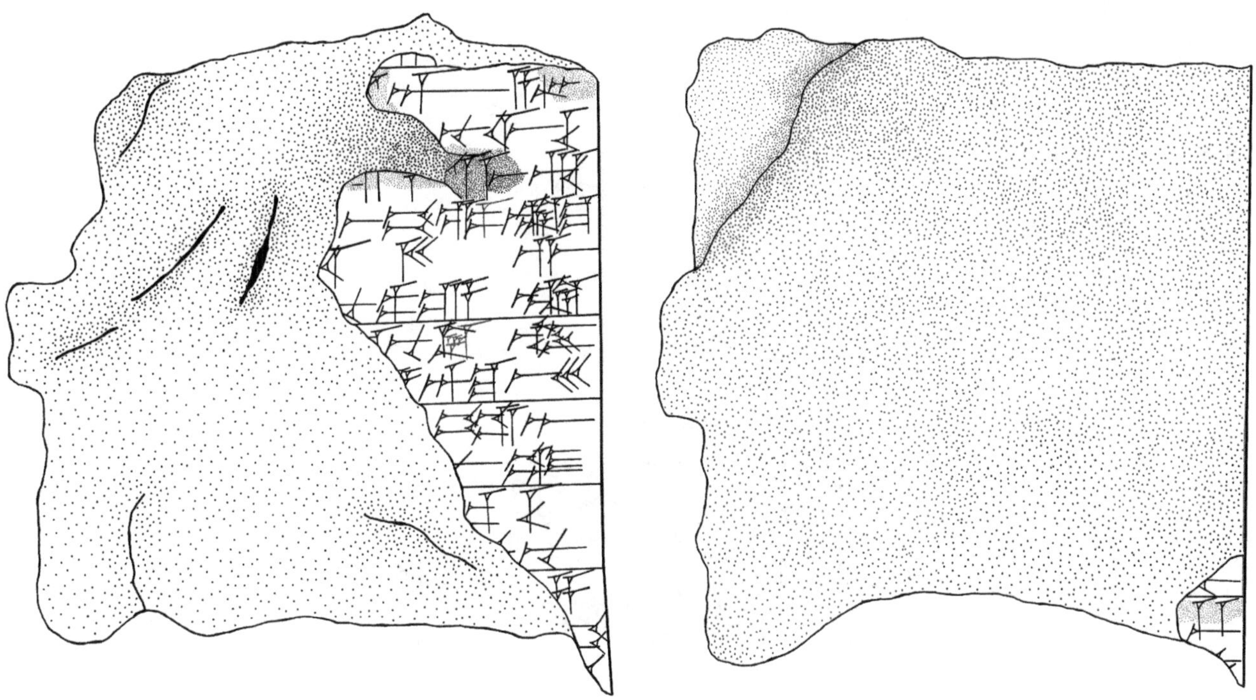

Fig. 19: AMT 9/4 (copy K. Simkó)

1′	[. . .] x [x x]	. . .
2′	[. . . U]Ḫ$_2^?$.^{d}ID$_2$	. . . *ru'tītu* (a kind of sulphur)$^?$
3′	[. . .] NU IGI-*šu*$_2$	. . . which has not yet seen it[113]
4′	[. . .] ⸢^{u_2}*a-na*⸣-*me-ri*	. . . *anameru* (a plant)

113 The reference here may be to the time of day for picking a plant, as in STO 2: 160, where the root of the 'dog's tongue' plant is gathered before it has seen the sun (*ša ina nasāḫīka Šamaš lā īmuru*). The passage here differs somewhat from other attestations of this instruction, since it has the third person object suffix appear on the verb; elsewhere a phonetic complement is attached to the verb to indicate its subordinate position in the sentence (viz. IGI-*ru* = Akk. *īmuru*), or longer Sumerian verb forms are used, such as IGI.DU$_8$.A or IGI.LA$_2$ (see Reiner 1995: 37 with n. 149 and 150).

5′	[. . .] *ina* KAŠ SAG NAG-*ma*	. . . he drinks it in high-quality beer and
6′	[. . .] x DIŠ-*niš* SUD$_2$	. . . you pound together
7′	[. . .] NU *pa-tan* NAG	. . . he drinks it on an empty stomach.
8′	[. . .] x nu NINDU MUN	. . . from an oven, salt
9′	[. . . GA]R-*an-ma ina-eš*	. . . you place it . . .; then he will get well.
10′	[. . .] ^{šim}BULUḪ	. . . *baluḫḫu* ('ferula gummosa')
11′	[. . . n]u$^?$ tum	. . .
12′	[. . . K]A$^?$-*šu*$_2$	. . . his mouth
13′	[. . .] x nu	. . .
14′	[. . .] ⸢za⸣	. . .
15′	[. . . b]i	. . .
16′	[. . . *ina-e*]*š*$^?$	. . . he will get well$^?$.

Reverse

1′	[. . .] x	*too fragmentary for translation*
2′	[. . .] ⸢ŠUB$^?$⸣	
3′	[. . .] x	

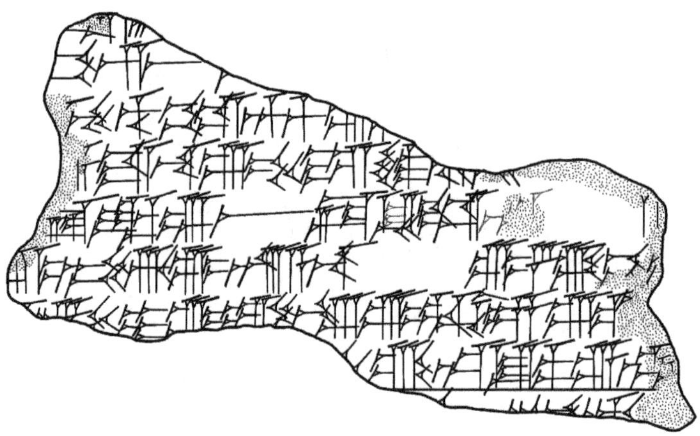

Fig. 20: AMT 22/5 (copy K. Simkó)

The form NU IGI-*šu*$_2$ otherwise appears in medical incipits as a symptom of the belly that does not let the patient accept (*lā ušamḫaršu*) bread and beer, but then one would expect a symptom to occur in the preceding line (line 2′) as well, instead of the common medical ingredient *ru'tītu*.

1′ [. . . NA]G.⸢MEŠ⸣ [. . .]

2′ [. . . *ina*] KAŠ SUD$_2$ x [. . .]

3′ [. . .] x NUMUN GADA $^{šim.d}$MAŠ ⸢^{u2}⸣GI[DRU SIPA . . .]

[KI MIN] NUMUN ^{u2}*qut-ri* NUMUN GADA / [*ni-k*]*ip-ta* GIDRU SIPA / [^{u2}M]A$_2$.ERI$_4$.IŠ.MA$_2$.LA$_2$ PA ^{giš}ḪA.LU.UB$_2$ (BAM 92 i′ 8′–10′)

4′ [. . . ^{u2}*ṣ*]*a-da-na* ^{u2}KUR.RA ARA$_3$-⸢*en* SIM⸣ [. . .]

[x x] x ^{u2}NIGIN ^{u2}*ṣa-*⸢*da*⸣*-na* / [^{u2}KUR.R]A ARA$_3$-*en* SIM / [x x] bi ^{u2}LUM.ḪA (BAM 92 i′ 11′–13′)

5′ [. . . *ina* A G]AZI^{sar} SILA$_{11}$-*aš* I$_3$.GIŠ ŠEŠ$_2$-⸢*su*⸣ L[AL$_2$-*ma* TI]

tu-sa-maḫ / [*ina* A GA]ZI^{sar} *ta-la$_2$-aš* / [x x] ŠEŠ$_2$-*su* LAL-*ma* TI (BAM 92 i′ 13′–15′)

6′ [. . .] ⸢^{u2}⸣*tar-muš* ^{u2}GIR$_2$*-a-na* ^{u2}*ša$_2$-ga-*⸢*bi*⸣*-g*[*al-zu*]

[^{u2}IGI-*li*]*m* ^{u2}IGI.NIŠ / [^{u2}*tar*]*-muš* ^{u2}GIR$_2$*-a-na* / [^{u2}*ša$_2$*]*-ga-*⸢*bi*⸣*-gal-zu* (BAM 92 i′ 16′–18′)

7′ [. . . U$_2$ SIG.ME]Š ⸢*ša$_2$*⸣ KUR-*i* ⸢^{u2}*ṣi-bu*⸣*-ru* ^{u2}*al-lum-za* ^{u2}Ḫ[AB x x x x]

^{u2}*ḫal-tap-a-na* / [U$_2$ SIG.MEŠ] *ša$_2$* ⸢KUR-*e*⸣ ^{u2}*ṣi-bu-ra* / [^{u2}*al*]*-lum-*[*za*] ^{u2}ḪAB / [x x š]a$^?$ ud [(x)] (BAM 92 i′ 19′–21′)

8′ [. . . GEŠTIN] ⸢DU$_{10}$⸣.GA *ba-lu pa-tan* ⸢NAG⸣.[MEŠ TI][114]

TEŠ$_2$.BI *ta-sak$_3$* / [*ina* GEŠT]IN DU$_{10}$.GA [(x)] NAG.MEŠ TI (BAM 92 i′ 21′–22′)

9′ [. . .] x x x ⸢ti⸣ [. . .]

1′ . . . he keeps drinking it . . .

2′ . . . you pound it in beer . . .

3′ (If) DITTO, you grind (and) sift seed from *qutru* (a plant), seed from *kitû* ('flax'), *nikiptu* ('spurge'), *ḫaṭṭi rēʾî* ('shepherd's staff' plant), *mirišmarû* (a plant), leaves from *ḫaluppu* (a tree)

4′ . . . *supālu* (a kind of juniper),[115] *ṣadānu* (a plant) (and) *nīnû* ('mint'), you mix them with . . . (and) *barīrātu* ('sagapenum'),

5′ you knead (the mixture) in juice from *kasû* ('tamarind'), you anoint him with oil (and) you bandage him; then he will recover.

6′ You pound *imḫur-līm* ('faces a thousand' plant), *imḫur-ešrā* ('faces twenty' plant), *tarmuš* ('lupin'), *patrānu* ('like a knife' plant), *šagabigalzu* (a plant),

7′ *ḫaltappānu* (a plant), *qatunu* ('thin' plant) from the mountains, *ṣibaru* ('aloe'), *alluzu* (a plant), *būšānu* ('smelly' plant) (and) . . .

8′ together (and) he keeps drinking them in sweet wine on an empty stomach; then he will recover.

9′ . . .

---

114 For lines 6′–8′, see also BAM 161 vii 20–25 but with considerable variations.

115 For the rare orthography ^{u2}NIGIN possibly corresponding to Akk. *supālu*, see the commentary to STO 2: 156.

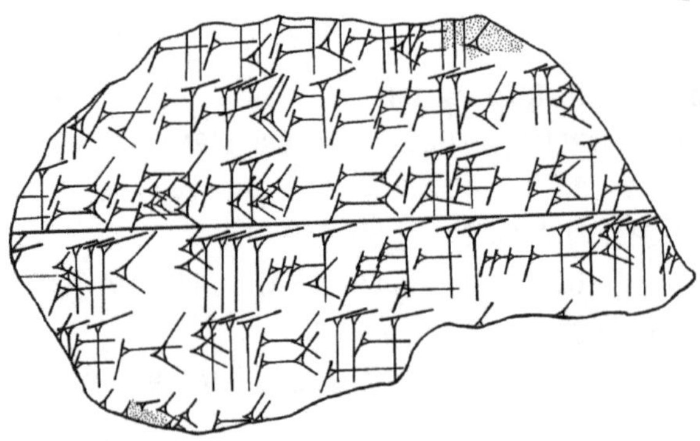

Fig. 21: AMT 49/3 (copy K. Simkó)

1′	[. . . ^{gi}]^{š}⌜*si-ḫu* ^{giš}*ar-ga*⌝-[*nu* . . .]	. . . *sīḫu* (‘wormwood’), *argannu* (a conifer) . . .
2′	[. . . ^{giš}*e-r*]*e-nu* ^{giš}ŠUR.MIN$_3$ ^{giš}*dap$_2$-ra-nu* GI [. . .]	. . . *erēnu* (‘cedar’), *šurmēnu* (‘cypress’), *daprānu* (a kind of juniper), reed . . .
3′	[. . . T]EŠ$_2$.BI GAZ SIM *ina* KAŠ SAG *ina* ^{urudu}Š[EN.TUR . . .]	. . . you crush (and) sift them together (and) . . . in high-quality beer using a small copper pot . . .
4′	[. . . *e*]*m-ru u* ŠA$_3$.MEŠ-*šu$_2$* MU$_2$.MEŠ-*ḫu* ŠA$_3$.M[EŠ . . .]	. . . are bloated and his internal organs are swollen, his internal organs . . .
5′	[. . . I$_3$.SA]G$^?$ SUMUN ŠA$_3$-*bi* TEŠ$_2$.B[I$^?$ GA]Z$^?$ [. . .]	you crush$^?$ . . . (and) old fine oil in it together$^?$ . . .
6′	[. . .] x x x [. . .]	. . .

Collations

1. STO 1: 1 = BAM 574+ i 1: *šu-ru-* 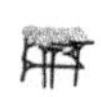 ^{giš}NAM.TAR

2. STO 1: 2 = BAM 574+ i 2: 7 U$_2$. 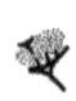 .A

3. STO 1: 5 = BAM 574+ i 5: dam 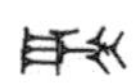 MIN

4. STO 1: 16 = BAM 574+ i 16: *ša* 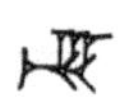 14-*šu$_2$*

5. STO 1: 18 = BAM 574+ i 18: *lu ina* A *lu in*[*a* 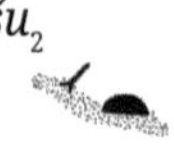

6. STO 1: 21 = BAM 574+ i 21: *mu-še-er-* 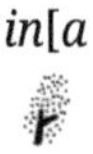

7. STO 1: 22 = BAM 574+ i 22: [*ina* ŠA$_3$] 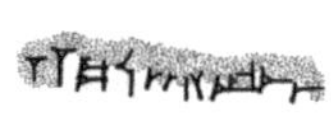

8. STO 1: 24 = BAM 574+ i 24–25: $^{\text{u2}}$*ur-*⌜*ba*⌝*-* 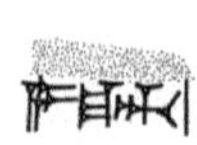

9. STO 1: 25 = BAM 574+ i 25: DIŠ-*niš* GAZ 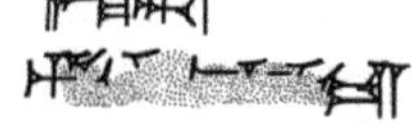 ḪAB

10. STO 1: 26 = BAM 574+ i 26: *ki-* 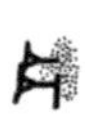 (. . .) 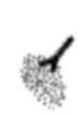

11. STO 1 32 = BAM 574+ i 32: TEŠ$_2$.BI 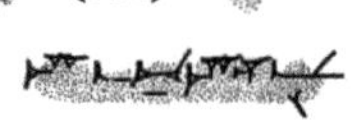 *pa-tan*

12. STO 1: 33 = BAM 574+ i 33: 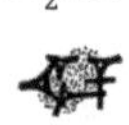 *-ik-ta*

13. STO 1: 34 = BAM 574+ i 34: [NAG.MEŠ 2] 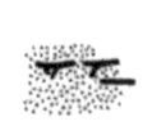 *ina*

14. STO 1: 34 = BAM 574+ i 34: ⸢*tu*⸣-  -*laḫ*$_2$-*ma*

15. STO 1: 35 = BAM 574+ i 35: ^{urudu}ŠEN. 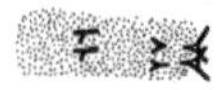

16. STO 1: 36 = BAM 574+ i 36: [^{u2}ḪAR.ḪAR] 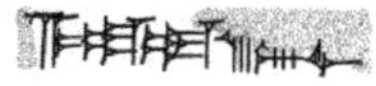

17. STO 1: 38 = BAM 574+ i 38: ⸢1/2 SILA$_3$ 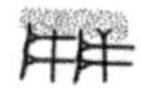 -*si*-^{d}ID$_2$⸣

18. STO 1: 39 = BAM 574+ i 39: ŠE$_{10}$ 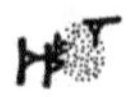 ^{mušen}

19. STO 1: 40 = BAM 574+ i 40: *an-nu*- 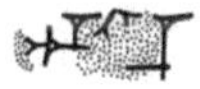 .BI

20. STO 1: 41 = BAM 574+ i 41: 3 UD- 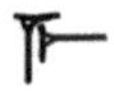

21. STO 1: 41 = BAM 574+ i 41: NINDA. 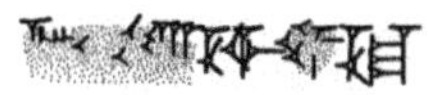

22. STO 1: 42 = BAM 574+ i 42: *ta-sak*$_3$ *ina* 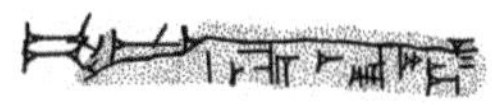

23. STO 1: 43 = BAM 574+ i 43: TI- 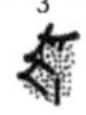

24. STO 1: 44 = BAM 574+ i 44: NU *pa-tan* 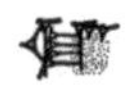

25. STO 1: 45 = BAM 574+ i 45: ⸢GU$_7$⸣.  -*ma* TI

26. STO 1: 46 = BAM 574+ i 46: *ina* KAŠ *u* 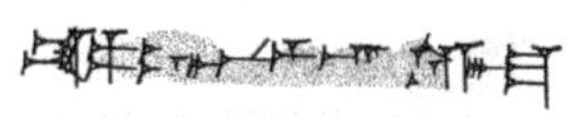

27. STO 1: 47 = BAM 574+ i 47: DIŠ KI MIN 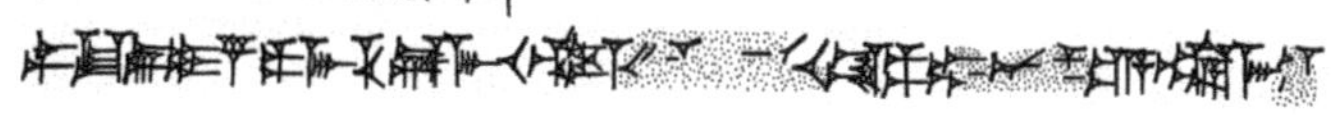

28. STO 1: 48 = BAM 574+ i 48: ⸢DIŠ⸣ 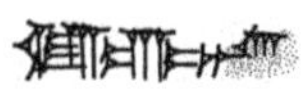 .ḪAB⸣

29. STO 1: 48 = BAM 574+ i 48: ⸢*ta*⸣-*sa-laq* 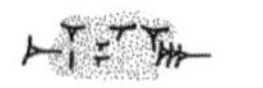 ⸢TI⸣

30. STO 1: 49 = BAM 574+ i 49: [DIŠ K]I ⸢MIN⸣ 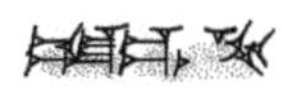

31. STO 1: 50 = BAM 574+ i 50: [DIŠ KI MIN x x x x 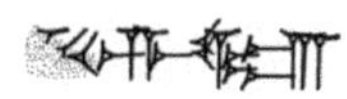

32. STO 1: 51 = BAM 574+ i 51: NU 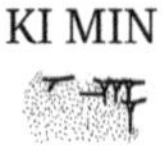

33. STO 1: 62–65 = BAM 574+ i 62′–65′ 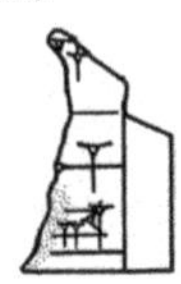

34. STO 1: 76 = BAM 574+ ii 11: *lu ina* I$_3$.ŠAḪ 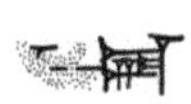 GU$_7$

35. STO 1: 78 = BAM 574+ ii 13: SUḪUŠ ^{giš} 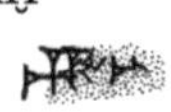

36. STO 1: 79 = BAM 574+ ii 14: *ba-lu pa*-⸢*tan*⸣ 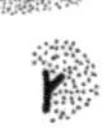

37. STO 1: 86 = BAM 574+ ii 21: *zi-ir kar*- 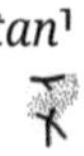

38. STO 1: 86 = BAM 574+ ii 21: *ku-uṣ*- 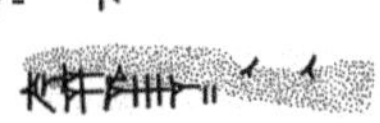

39. STO 1: 91 = BAM 574+ ii 26: 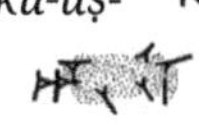 *re-me*$_2$-*nu*

40. STO 1: 92 = BAM 574+ ii 27: *šum*$_2$-*ma* 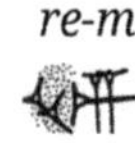

41. STO 1: 94 = BAMT 574+ ii 29: ⸢DIŠ⸣ [NA *e-t*]*a*- 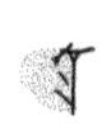 -*ša*$_2$-*aš*$_2$

42. STO 1: 97 = BAM 574+ ii 32: [DIŠ KI MIN x x x  .⸢SILA$_{11}$⸣.GA$_2$

43. STO 1: 105 = BAM 574+ ii 40: 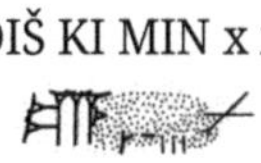 .UŠ

44. STO 1: 106 = BAM 574+ ii 41: *ik-ta*- 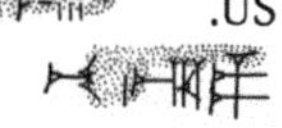 ^{giš}ŠINIG

45. STO 1: 107 = BAM 574+ ii 42: SUḪUŠ 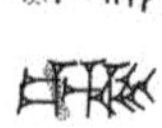 .TAR

46. STO 1: 109 = BAM 574+ ii 44: 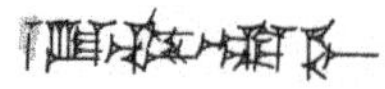 -*li*$_3$

47. STO 1: 163 = BAM 574+ iii 32 *ina* KA[Š 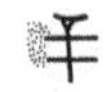

48. STO 1: 166 = BAM 574+ iii 35 *iṣ-ṣa-bat* 

49. STO 1: 167 = BAM 574+ iii 36: *u*$_2$-⸢*ma-me*⸣ *a*-⸢*na* 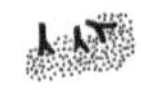

50. STO 1: 167 = BAM 574+ iii 36: [*ap-si aq-bi*]- 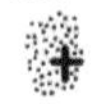

51. STO 1: 179 = BAM 574+ iii 48: *ta-mar-raq ina* 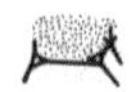

52. STO 1: 182 = BAM 574+ iii 51: KA.NA ⸢*šu* 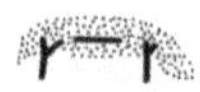

53. STO 1: 189 = BAM 574+ iii 58: *pu-luḫ-* 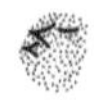

54. STO 1: 196 = BAM 574+ iii 65: *ni-ti-qam-* 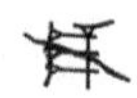

55. STO 1: 203 = BAM 574+ iv 7: *ra-ši* 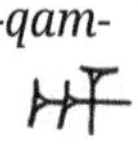

56. STO 1: 206 = BAM 574+ iv 10: *i-ne-* 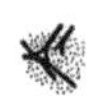

57. STO 1: 216 = BAM 574+ iv 20: KI.SIKIL 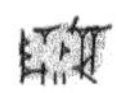 -*na*

58. STO 1: 217 = BAM 574+ iv 21: *ir-* 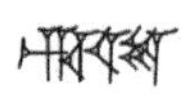 -*te-ši-ru-ma*

59. STO 1: 223 = BAM 574+ iv 27: 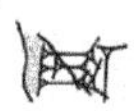 -*ru-uṣ*

60. STO 1: 225 = BAM 574+ iv 29: *di-ma-* 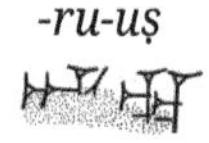 -*la*

61. STO 1: 228 = BAM 574+ iv 32: [KID$_3$ 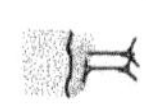

62. STO 1: 229 = BAM 574+ iv 33: *i-maḫ-ḫar* 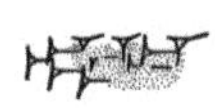

63. STO 1: 232 = BAM 574+ iv 36: x 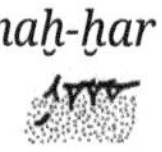 x 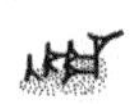 SAḪAR. 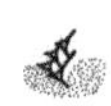 .A

64. STO 1: 235 = BAM 574+ iv 39: *ša*$_2$- 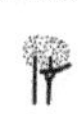 -*ru* 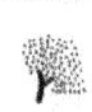

65. STO 1: 236 = BAM 574+ iv 40: [x x x] 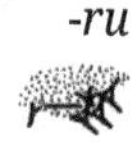 *ana* KA$_2$

66. STO 1: 238 = BAM 574+ iv 42: 3- 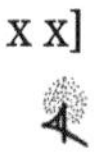

67. STO 1: 240 = BAM 574+ iv 44: SUD$_2$ *i*[*na* 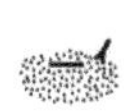 ⸢ḪI.ḪI

68. STO 1: 241 = BAM 574+ iv 45: [^{u2}IG]I.⸢NIŠ 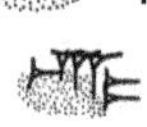 *tar-muš*

69. STO 1: 244 = BAM 574+ iv 48: *ina* GEŠTIN 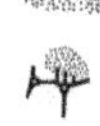 N[AG

70. STO 1: 249 = BAM 574+ iv 53: *iš-ru-* 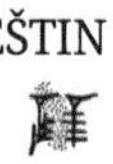 -*uš*

71. STO 2: 2 = BAM 575 i 2: *ina* KAŠ 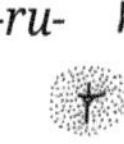

72. STO 2: 5 = BAM 575 i 5: ^{u2}*ur*$_2$- 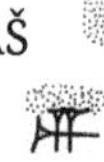 -*e*

73. STO 2: 10 = BAM 575 i 10: *ina* A GAZI 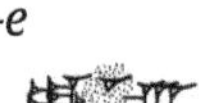 -*aš*

74. STO 2: 11 = BAM 575 i 11: [DIŠ 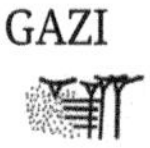

75. STO 2: 11 = BAM 575 i 11: 1/2 SILA$_3$ 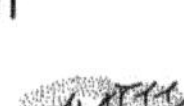

76. STO 2: 13 = BAM 575 i 13: 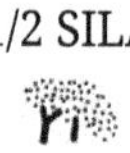 -*a*]*ṣ*

77. STO 2: 14 = BAM 575 i 14: DIŠ NA 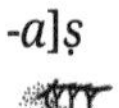 -*šu*$_2$

78. STO 2: 23 = BAM 575 i 23: *ina* U[ZU 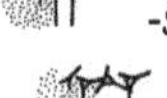 RA

79. STO 2: 24 = BAM 575 i 24: 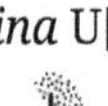 SILA$_3$ ZA$_3$.ḪI.LI

80. STO 2: 25 = BAM 575 i 25:  NA Š]A$_3$-*šu*$_2$

81. STO 2: 31 = BAM 575 i 31: *ina* I$_3$ 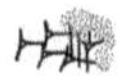

82. STO 2: 32 = BAM 575 i 32: DUB-*ak* 

83. STO 2: 34 = BAM 575 i 34: SUD$_2$ *ina* KAŠ 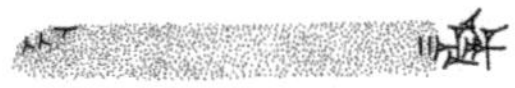

84. STO 2: 35 = BAM 575 i 35: ^{giš}DIḪ$_3$ *ina* 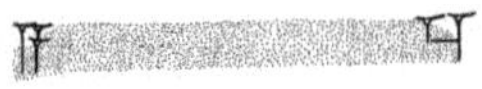

85. STO 2: 36 = BAM 575 i 36: DUB-*ak* ^{šim} 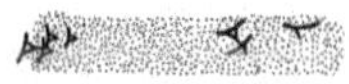

86. STO 2: 42 = BAM 575 i 42: ^{u2}SIKIL x [x x] 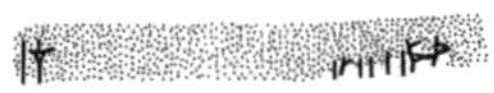

87. STO 2: 43 = BAM 575 i 43: ⸢GAZ *ina* I$_3$.UDU⸣ 

88. STO 2: 46 = BAM 575 i 46: ḪAD$_2$.DU <GAZ> 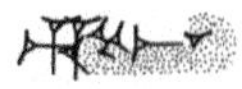

89. STO 2: 49 = BAM 575 i 49:  -*am*

90. STO 2: 51 = BAM 575 i 51: [DIŠ N]A ŠA$_3$-*šu*$_2$ GIG 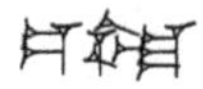 GIG

91. STO 2: 53 = BAM 575 i 53: ŠEG$_6$. 

92. STO 2: 68 = BAM 575 i 68: [. . .] 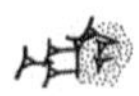 -*ma* TI

93. STO 2: 75 = BAM 575 ii 5: A.MEŠ 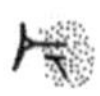 NAG A⸣. 

94. STO 2: 84 = BAM 575 ii 14: [D]UB-*ak*- 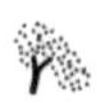

95. STO 2: 85 = BAM 575 ii 15: KUR-*i*  .ḪI⸣

96. STO 2: 86 = BAM 575 ii 16: [NAG]. 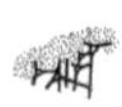

97. STO 2: 87 = BAM 575 ii 17: *ana* TI- 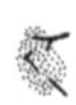

98. STO 2: 96 = BAM 575 ii 26: *u*$_2$- 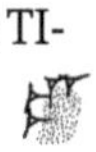 -[*lat*]

99. STO 2: 102 = BAM 575 ii 32: *ta*- 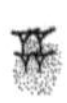 -*ru*$_3$

100. STO 2: 103 = BAM 575 ii 33: 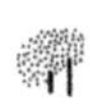 ⸢LI⸣

101. STO 2: 107 = BAM 575 ii 37: 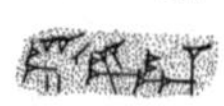 *saḫ-le*$_2$-*e*

102. STO 2: 113 = BAM 575 ii 43: *saḫ-le*$_2$- 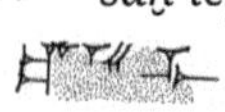

103. STO 2: 120 = BAM 575 ii 50: LAL$_3$ *u* KAŠ 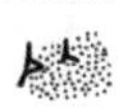

104. STO 2: 127 = BAM 575 ii 57: SUḪUŠ 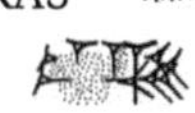 TAR

105. STO 2: 138 = BAM 575 iii 3: *es-li* 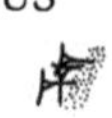 .DU$_3$. B]I 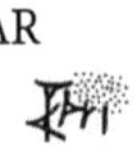

106. STO 2: 139 = BAM 575 iii 4: A ZU$_2$.⸢LUM. 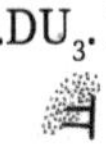

107. STO 2: 145 = BAM 575 iii 10: ŠUB-*ma* 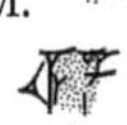 .GAL$_2$.LA (. . .) ^{u2}*a-ra-ri-ia*$_2$- 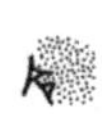

108. STO 2: 148 = BAM 575 iii 13: *tu-kaṣ*$_3$- 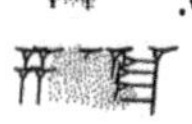 -*šu*$_2$

109. STO 2: 151 = BAM 575 iii 16: DIŠ [NA 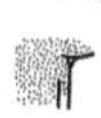 -*šu*$_2$

110. STO 2: 156 = BAM 575 iii 21: DIŠ NA *ḫa*- 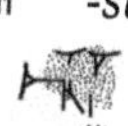

111. STO 2: 159 = BAM 575 iii 24: DIŠ KI MIN ^{u2} 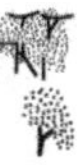

112. STO 2: 161 = BAM 575 iii 26: ḪAD$_2$.A SUD$_2$ 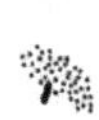

113. STO 2: 169 = BAM 575 iii 34: *ina* GE$_6$ 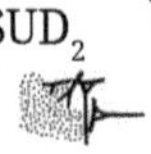 MUL$_4$

114. STO 2: 173 = BAM 575 iii 38: ⸢*i-ša*⸣- 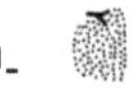

115. STO 2: 175 = BAM 575 iii 40: [. . .]  [x x x]

116. STO 2: 178 = BAM 575 iii 43: *u*$_2$-*al-lat* ḫi 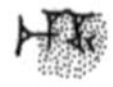

117. STO 2: 180 = BAM 575 iii 45: ^{šim}GAM. 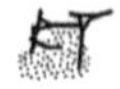

118. STO 2: 183 = BAM 575 iii 48: DUR$_2$- 

119. STO 2: 185 = BAM 575 iii 50: ŠEŠ  -*niš*

120. STO 2: 186 = BAM 575 iii 51: INIM.MEŠ- 

121. STO 2: 189 = BAM 575 iii 54:  -*am* ^{d}UTU

122. STO 2: 190 = BAM 575 iii 55: TUKU. 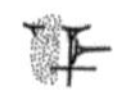 -*ši*

123. STO 2: 191 = BAM 575 iii 56: GIG  TI-*šu*$_2$

124. STO 2: 191 = BAM 575 iii 57: 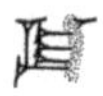 GU$_2$.TUR

125. STO 2: 196 = BAM 575 iii 61: *ina*  GAZI^{sar}

126. STO 2: 203 = BAM 575 iii 68: NUMUN ^{giš}ŠE. 

127. STO 2: 206 = BAM 575 iii 71: ŠEŠ 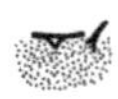 [. . .]

128. STO 2: 216 = BAM 575 iv 8: [. . .] x 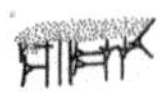 ḪAD$_2$.A

129. STO 2: 221 = BAM 575 iv 13: [GUR- 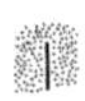 ⸢ḪAD$_2$⸣.A

130. STO 2: 223 = BAM 575 iv 15: 1/2 SILA$_3$ 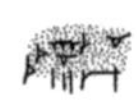 GEŠTIN

131. STO 2: 240 = BAM 575 iv 32: *tu-ša*$_2$- 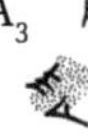 -[*ra-šu*$_2$]-⸢*ma*⸣

132. STO 2: 243 = BAM 575 iv 35: ^{šim}⸢BULUḪ 1/3 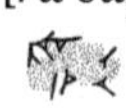 .ŠE.GIŠ.I$_3$

133. STO 2: 245 = BAM 575 iv 37: *ina* 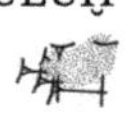 -*šu*$_2$

134. STO 2: 246 = BAM 575 iv 38: [1/2 SIL]A$_3$ [^{šim}] 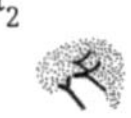 (. . .) *pa-pa-si*-⸢^{d}⸣ 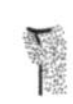

135. STO 2: 248 = BAM 575 iv 40: [1/2 SI]LA$_3$ 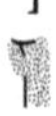 G]IB$_3$

136. STO 2: 252 = BAM 575 iv 44: $^{\text{u2}}$KUR.RA SUD$_2$ 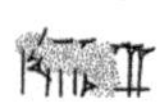

137. STO 2: 256 = BAM 575 iv 48: [DIŠ NA 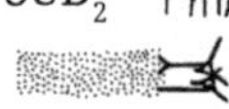 ŠA$_3$-*šu*$_2$

138. STO 2: 257 = BAM 575 iv 49: *tuš-te-mid* 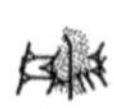

139. STO 2: 266= BAM 575 iv 58: *šip-* 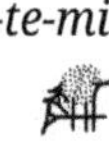

140. STO 3: 5 = BAM 578+ i 5: 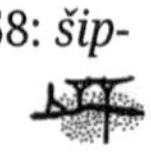 SILA$_3$ ⸢*e*⸣-*reš-ti* A.ŠA$_3$

141. STO 3: 7 = BAM 578+ i 7: 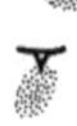 SILA$_3$ ZI$_3$.KUM

142. STO 3: 21 = BAM 578+ i 21: *ina* KAŠ 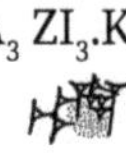

143. STO 3: 28 = BAM 578+ i 28: 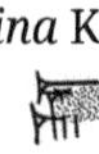 TUKU.MEŠ-*ši*

144. STO 3: 31 = BAM 578+ i 31: SIG$_7$-*su-* 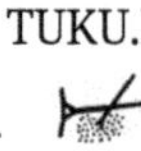 (. . .) NU *pa*-⸢*tan*⸣  -*šu*$_2$]

145. STO 3: 32 = BAM 578+ i 32: *baḫ-ra* 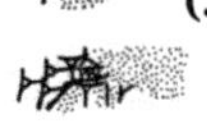 -*ra* 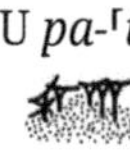 NA]G .KAM

146. STO 3: 33 = BAM 578+ i 33: *ina* KAŠ 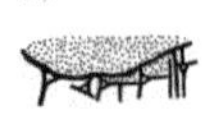 N[AG-*šu*$_2$

147. STO 3: 36 = BAM 578+ i 33: I$_3$ *ḫal-* 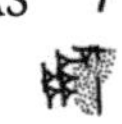

148. STO 3: 37 = BAM 578+ i 37: I_3

149. STO 3: 38 = BAM 578+ i 38: GIG (. . .) ⸢u2⸣[$UKUŠ_2$.ḪAB

150. STO 3: 39 = BAM 578+ i 39: *te-* *-er* (. . .) *ina* SAG

151. STO 3: 40 = BAM 578+ i 40: *ki* *pi-i*

152. STO 3: 41 = BAM 578+ i 41: *ta-na-k*[*ud* T]I-

153. STO 3: 43 = BAM 578+ i 43: $ŠEG_6$-*šal* ⸢*ana*⸣

154. STO 3: 45 = BAM 578+ i 45: [DIŠ] MIN⸣ (. . .) .ḪI

155. STO 3: 65 = BAM 578+ i 65: NAGA.

156. STO 3: 66 = BAM 578+ i 66: .[ḪI.A

157. STO 3: 67 = BAM 578+ i 67: AL. .NA

158. STO 3: 85 = BAM 578+ ii 15: [. . .]

159. STO 3: 86 = BAM 578+ ii 16: U_2⸣.[ḪI.A . . .]

160. STO 3: 87 = BAM 578+ ii 17: MUN

161. STO 3: 89 = BAM 578+ ii 19: NAG-

162. STO 3: 90 = BAM 578+ ii 20: *pa-*

163. STO 3: 93 = BAM 578+ ii 23: ZE_2 GIG

164. STO 3: 94 = BAM 578+ ii 24: ZE_2 *-li*

165. STO 3: 99 = BAM 578+ ii 29 .[šim.gen_7

166. STO 3: 101 = BAM 578+ ii 31: [. . .] [. . .]

167. STO 3: 103 = BAM 578+ ii 33: te.ni!(ER).

168. STO 3: 106 = BAM 578+ ii 36: [eridu] [x]

169. STO 3: 117 = BAM 578+ ii 47: *-ši*

170. STO 3: 118 = BAM 578+ ii 48: *-suk-ši*

171. STO 3: 129 = BAM 578+ ii 59: 21 *-qa*

172. STO 3: 130 = BAM 578+ ii 60: 15 ŠE *-lim*

173. STO 3: 131 = BAM 578+ ii 61: 90 u2 *-n*]*i*

174. STO 3: 132 = BAM 578+ ii 62: IGI.4.GAL_2. *ma-at-qa*

175. STO 3: 141 = BAM 578+ iii 1: *ina* A *-ma*

176. STO 3: 146 = BAM 578+ iii 6: DIŠ IGI⸣.SIG_7.SIG_7 *-ma*

177. STO 3: 147 = BAM 578+ iii 7: UZU

178. STO 3: 149 = BAM 578+ iii 9: *ina*

179. STO 3: 161 = BAM 578+ iii 21: *ina* K[AŠ

180. STO 3: 163 = BAM 578+ iii 23: UR.GI_7

181. STO 3: 166 = BAM 578+ iii 26: *ḫu-*⸢*bi-bi-*

182. STO 3: 167 = BAM 578+ iii 27: ^{giš}NU.UR$_2$.MA ^{im}SI.

183. STO 3: 170 = BAM 578+ iii 30: ⸢*saḫ*- -*e*]

184. STO 3: 214 = BAM 578+ iv 7: .MEŠ-*ma*

185. STO 3: 215 = BAM 578+ iv 8: .MEŠ-*ma*

186. STO 3: 217 = BAM 578+ iv 10: KAŠ

187. STO 3: 221 = BAM 578+ iv 14: MIN

188. STO 3: 229 = BAM 578+ iv 22: .ZU$_2$.LUM⸣.MA

189. STO 3: 242 = BAM 578+ iv 35: ^{im} .SA$_2$

190. STO 3: 244 = BAM 578+ iv 37: DIŠ (. . .) *pa-tan*

191. STO 3: 245 = BAM 578+ iv 38: DIŠ NA MIN

192. STO 3: 250 = BAM 578+ iv 43: *aḫ-ḫa-* -*šu*$_2$

193. STO 3: 257 = BAM 578+ iv 50: *e-ḫu-*⸢*uz*⸣-

194. STO 3: 260 = BAM 578+ iv 53: IGI.KAR$_2$-

195. STO 5: 4 = BAM 579+ i 4: SILA$_3$ ^{šim}ḪAB

196. STO 5: 5 = BAM 579+ i 5: *ta-* (. . .)LA[L- *ina-*⸢*eš*⸣

197. STO 5: 7 = BAM 579+ i 7: NAG-[*ma*]

198. STO 5: 18 = BAM 579+ i 18: SUD$_2$.[GEŠTIN.NA (. . .) SUR

199. STO 5: 19 = BAM 579+ i 19: ^{giš}ŠINIG ^{u2}

200. STO 5: 22 = BAM 579+ i 22: KUM$_2$ *ša*$_2$ Š]A$_3$-*šu*$_2$

201. STO 5: 23 = BAM 579+ i 23: *um-mu*

202. STO 5: 25 = BAM 579+ i 25: NINDA *u*

203. STO 5: 30 = BAM 579+ i 30: UD.DA SA$_2$.SA$_2$

204. STO 5: 40 = BAM 579+ i 40: [*mi-n*]*a-*⸢*tu-*

205. STO 5: 42 = BAM 579+ i 42: ^{u2} .NIŠ⸣

206. STO 5: 49 = BAM 579+ i 49: ^{u2} -*tam*

207. STO 5: 54 = BAM 579+ i 54: -*a*]*k-ma*

208. STO 5: 55 = BAM 579+ i 55: GAZI^{sar} *kam-mi*

209. STO 5: 57 = BAM 579+ i 57: *ina* ^{urudu}

210. STO 5: 70 = BAM 579+ ii 5: 10 GIN$_2$

211. STO 5: 117′ = BAM 579+ ii 52′: ⸢PAP 4 .[ḪI.A

212. STO 5: 118′ = BAM 579+ ii 53′: ^{u2}*ak-tam* ^{šim}

213. STO 5: 124′ = BAM 579+ ii 59′: 10 GIN$_2$ ⸢^{šim}GUR$_2$⸣.

214. STO 5: 131′ = BAM 579+ iii 2: 10 ^{u2}⸣[. . .]

215. STO 5: 137′ = BAM 579+ iii 8: 10 GIN$_2$ BAL

216. STO 5: 198′ = BAM 579+ iv 6: 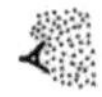 *ina* -*ri*$_3$ (. . .) *ta*-  -*ḫ*]*al*

217. STO 5: 200′ = BAM 579+ iv 8: 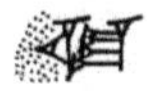

218. STO 5: 222′ = BAM 579+ iv 30: SAG-*ka* 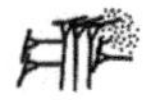 -*q*[*a-a*]

219. STO 5: 237′ = BAM 579+ iv 44 ⸢DUB. 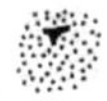 .[KAM$_2$

220. STO 5: 239′ = BAM 579+ iv 47:  -*šar-ru-t*[*i*]

221. STO 5: 241′ = BAM 579+ iv 49: 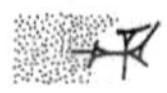 BAR.MEŠ

Chapter 3
Edition of STO 1

Manuscript A = BAM 574 + BAM 577 (+) AMT 30/6

K 191 + K 201 + K 2374 + K 2474 + K 2957 + K 3230 + K 3363 + K 5899 + K 6869 + K 10327 + K 10713 + K 11266 + K 12909 + K 13446 + K 17096 + K 21858 + K 21905 + K 22089 + K 22164 + K 22170 (+) K 2510 + K 14163 + K 20273

Manuscript B = Nougayrol 1979: 69

AO 7765

STO 1	Parallels		
	Publication number	Museum number	Parallel passage
1	AMC 29		
10	BAM 48	VAT 14157	5′–6′
24–25	STO 2: 110–112		
26–29	STO 2: 256–258		
26–30	BAM 49	VAT 7822	obverse, 9′–20′
26–27	BAM 50	VAT 14082	obverse, 11–16
27–29	BAM 51	VAT 10580	1′–8′
33–34	STO 2: 118–119 and 254–255		
35–37	BAM 558	K 2590 + K 2795	column 4, 7–9
35–37	BAM 174	VAT 13761	obverse, 11′–13′
37–38	BAM 58	VAT 13774 + VAT 14003	10–13
37–41	STO 2: 245–250		
70–71	AMT 57/3	Rm 2 260	reverse, 4–5
70–71	AMT 42/2	Sm 1895	obverse, 4–5
70–71	BAM 52	VAT 13733 + VAT 13738	reverse, 24–25
94–96	STO 2: 151–152		
98–100	BAM 564	K 5172 + K 6433 + K 8137 + K 13958 + K 16360	column 3, 2′–5′
111–116	AMT 45/5 (K 5416a)	K 5416a + BM 98584 + BM 98589	column 2, 1′–9′
111–116	BAM 489 (K 2509) + BAM 508 (K 239 + K 3261)	K 239 + K 2509 + K 3261 + K 9080	column 2, 1′–10′
111–119	BAM 509	Sm 1802	column 1′, 1′–14′
111–120	STT 252	SU 1952–69	16–25
119–122	–	K 13368	1′–4′
120–121	BAM 124	VAT 8772 + VAT 15549	column 4, 23–26
120–121	BAM 128	VAT 9955	column 4, 18′–22′
124–127	–	K 13368	6′–9′
124–130	CT 4 8	BM 92518	obverse, 1–12; reverse, 5–12 and 15–19
128–129	STVC 11	CBS 6927	obverse, 6′–8′
128–130	Gall incantation, lines 13–18 (see STO 3: 99–108)		
135–136	AMT 45/5 (K 5416a)	K 5416a + BM 98584 + BM 98589	column 2, 11′–14′
135–137	AMT 52/1	K 2537	10–14
135–137	ABRT 2 11 (K 4609a)	K 4609a + K 8211	column 3′, 27–31

https://doi.org/10.1515/9781501506574-003

135–136	Emar VI/4 737	Msk 731030	4–7
144–145	STT 252	SU 1952–69	11–13
164–169	BAM 576	Sm 1709	column 2, 2′–12′
174–175	STT 252	SU 1952–69	26
191–194	Beckman and Foster 1988: 18 no. 15	YBC 7134	2′–7′
195–199	AMT 52/1	K 2537	1–6 and 8–9
214–219	BAM 534 + BAM 535 + BAM 573	K 3484 + K 6511 + K 8792	column 1, 1′–8′
247	STO 2: 1		

1 A$_{i\,1}$ DIŠ NA *su-a-lam* GIG *ana ki-is* ŠA$_3$ GUR-<*šu*$_2$>[116] *šu-ru-*⸢*uš*⸣* ^{giš}NAM.TAR *šu-*⸢*ru-uš*⸣ ^{giš}*šu-še*

[DIŠ NA *su-a-lam* GIG *ana ki-is* ŠA$_3$ GUR-*š*]*u*$_2$ (AMC 29)

2 A$_{i\,2}$ ^{u2}*tar-muš* ^{u2}IGI-*lim* ^{u2}IGI.NIŠ ^{u2}*tu-lal* ^{u2}ŠAKIRA 7 U$_2$.⸢ḪI⸣*.A ŠEŠ TEŠ$_2$.BI SUD$_2$

3 A$_{i\,3}$ *ina* KAŠ ŠUB-*di ina* MUL *tuš-bat ina* A$_2$.GU$_2$.ZI.GA NU *pa-tan* ⸢NAG⸣.MEŠ-*ma ina-eš*

---

4 A$_{i\,4}$ DIŠ NA *ki-is* ŠA$_3$ GIG *ina* UD *ša*$_2$*-tu*[117] (eras.) ^{giš}MA$_2$.GUR$_8$ U$_5$-*šu*$_2$ ⸢E$_{11}$⸣-*šu*$_2$*-ma* TU$_6$ *ki-a-am* ŠID-*nu*

†

1 If someone suffers (*maruṣ*) from phlegm (*suālu*),[118] which has turned into (*itūršu*) gastric constriction (*kīs libbi*):[119] root from *pillû* ('mandrake'), root from *šūšu* ('liquorice'),

2 *tarmuš* ('lupin'), *imḫur-līm* ('faces a thousand' plant), *imḫur-ešrā* ('faces twenty' plant), *tullal* ('you cleanse' plant), (and) *šakirû* (a plant)—you pound (*tasâk*) these seven ingredients together,

3 you put (*tanaddi*) them in beer, you leave (the mixture) out overnight under the stars (and) in the morning, he keeps drinking (*ištanattī-ma*) it on an empty stomach; then he will get well.

---

4 If someone suffers (*maruṣ*) from gastric constriction (*kīs libbi*): on that day, you have him ride (*tušarkabšu*) on a *makūru* boat, you send him downstream (*tušerredaššū-ma*), and you recite (*tamannu*) an incantation:

---

116 Parallel catchlines and the idiom used here both suggest that—in the earlier history of our text—a haplography occurred that omitted the ŠU sign immediately following GUR, viz. GUR-*šu*, due to its repetition as the first sign of the following word, *šu-ru-uš*. Subsequent revisions would have replaced GUR-*šu* with GUR-*šu*$_2$. Other manuscripts also omit this suffix, except for the colophon of STO 5 (and possibly AMC 29), where the original spelling GUR-*šu* is preserved.

117 We take TU as a syllabic writing in the phrase *ina* UD *ša*$_2$*-tu* 'on that day', but the polyvalence of TU has inspired several more complicated proposals. Küchler (1904: 69–70) reads TU as URU$_5$ for Akk. *abūbu* 'flood', while Cadelli (2000: 68 with n. 2) suggests that TU here should be read as KU$_4$ = Akk. *erēbu* 'to enter', drawing on passages in the Diagnostic Handbook such as Sagig 17: 7, 34–35, 37–38 and 40, where *erēbu* is written either syllabically or with KU$_4$ (Heeßel 2000: 195, 198–199).

118 Although CAD S 340 translates Akk. *suālu* both as 'phlegm' and 'cough', all known examples seem to refer to a substance rather than an action and are occasionally characterized as 'white', as in AMT 50/3 rev.$^!$ 1: DIŠ NA KI MIN *su-a-lam* BABBAR ŠUB.MEŠ-*a*. For the meaning of *suālu*, see the recent discussion in Cadelli 2021: 12–13.

119 More conventionally 'colic', although most present-day English speakers tend to associate this term with infants. As Stol points out, this condition also affected horses (see Loretz 2011: 396–399).

5 A$_{i\,5}$ EN$_2$ E$_2$.NU.RU LU RA GAR[120] dam gal* kur* MIN : gi ^{d}en.lil$_2$ a$_2$.⸢e⸣ nu.ub.zum ^{d}*zar-pa-ni-tu*$_4$
6 A$_{i\,6}$ *ša* igi.gal$_2$.la gub.⸢a$^{?}$⸣ gir$_3$.a.ni gub.ba gir$_3$.a.ni dur$_2$.ra $_{:\ du\text{-}ra}$ gir$_3$ igi.gal$_2$ gub
7 A$_{i\,7}$ gir$_3$ igi.gal$_2$ TU$_6$ EN$_2$ TU$_6$ *an-ni-ta* ŠID-*nu-ma* TI

---

8 A$_{i\,8}$ DIŠ KI MIN UZU ^{d}NIN.KILIM ḪAD$_2$.A *ba-lu pa-tan* NAG-*ma* TI : DIŠ KI MIN *šu-ru-uš* ^{giš}*šu*$_2$-*še ina* A.MEŠ *ba-lu pa-tan* NAG-*ma* TI
9 A$_{i\,9}$ DIŠ KI MIN MUN SUD$_2$ *ina* A.MEŠ *ba-lu pa-tan* NAG-*ma* TI
10 A$_{i\,10}$ DIŠ KI MIN MUN *a-ma-ni*$_7$ SUD$_2$ *ba-lu pa-tan* NAG-*ma* TI

DIŠ NA MIN MUN *a-ma-n*[*i*$_7$ *t*]*a-sak*$_3$ [x x x] / *ba-lu pa-tan* EME-*šu*$_2$ D[AB-*bat* x x] (BAM 48: 5′–6′)

---

5 Enuru-incantation: '. . . the chief wife of the Mountain, DITTO (= Zarpanītu), the reed of Enlil,[121] which no one fully knows, Zarpanītu,
6 . . . establishes wisdom,[122] her feet are planted, her feet are seated, the feet stand inverted,
7 the feet are inverted'.[123] Incantation-formula. You recite (*tamannū-ma*) this incantation; then he will recover (*iballuṭ*).

---

8 If DITTO,[124] he drinks (*išattī-ma*) (an infusion of) dried mongoose meat on an empty stomach; then he will recover (*iballuṭ*). If DITTO, he drinks root from *šūšu* ('liquorice') in water on an empty stomach; then he will recover.[125]
9 If DITTO, you pound (*tasâk*) salt, (and) he drinks it in water on an empty stomach; then he will recover.
10 If DITTO, you pound *amānu* salt, (and) he drinks it on an empty stomach; then he will recover.

---

120 The reading and significance of LU RA GAR remain unclear. Cadelli (2000: 108) reads the first half of the line as LU.RA ŠA$_3$.TAM.MA NUMUN and translates 'Pour l'homme, un coeur/ventre . . .', taking LU.RA as a phonetic rendering of Sumerian lu$_2$.ra.

121 gi ^{d}en.lil$_2$ = Akk. *qan ša ellili* 'reed of Enlil' may be a playful writing of *qan šalāli*, and it might also point to the significance of nu.ub.zum: Ura IV 297 (MSL 5 p. 176) equates ^{giš}ma$_2$.gur$_8$ nu.ub.zu with *e-lep* ^{d}EN.LIL$_2$ 'the unknown barge is the boat of Enlil', so our nu.ub.zum may be a distorted form of nu.ub.zu. Attinger (2021: 1170) glosses a$_2$.bi.še$_3$ zu—perhaps analogous to our a$_2$.e . . . zum—as 'savoir à la perfection, maîtriser à la perfection'.

122 Late lexical materials, such as Malku I 149 (Hrůša 2010: 158), link IGI.GAL$_2$ with Akk. *etellu* and *mudû*, and IGI.GAL$_2$ itself loans into Akkadian as a term meaning 'wisdom'.

123 The repeated Sumerian expressions in this incantation are built up around the words IGI, IGI.GAL$_2$, GIR$_3$, GUB and DUR$_2$, which are used to express various bodily positions, such as 'seated' or 'upside-down', that reappear in the Akkadian materials that follow.

124 DIŠ KI MIN probably corresponds to Akk. *šumma ašar šanîm(-ma)* 'If DITTO' (lit. 'If — *it is the other place* —'), based on a few examples with syllabic orthography collected by Köcher (1971: xxxii); see also Böck 2003: 170–171. Kinnier Wilson (2011: 12) argues that DIŠ should be read as *ana* instead of *šumma* and translated as 'alternatively' or 'additionally' (see also BAM 10 p. 255–256). There are occurrences of *ana* followed by an infinitive in medical texts to express purpose, but even if additional symptoms follow KI MIN, the verbs are never in the infinitive. In our view, therefore, DIŠ and KI.MIN operate independently, as can also be seen when KI MIN occurs on its own as part of the therapy.

125 The two entries in this line are an expansion of a lexical equation recorded in Uruanna III 1 (1): ^{giš}*šu-šum* (the underlying plant name) = AŠ KUN ^{d}NIN.KILIM 'mongoose tail' (the cover term or *Deckname*), with KUN = Akk. *zibbatu* 'tail' confused with or transformed into UZU = Akk. *šīru* 'meat' (Böck 2011: 694; Rumor 2017: 4). This might explain the absence of a liquid carrier in the first half of the line.

11 A$_{i\,11}$ DIŠ NA *ki-is* ŠA$_3$ GIG NA BI *ina* UGU GIR$_3$.MIN-*šu$_2$ tu-še-šab-šu$_2$*

12 A$_{i\,12}$ A GAZI^{sar} *sek-ru-ti* KUM$_2$-*ti ana* UGU-*šu$_2$* DUB-*ma* TI

13 A$_{i\,13}$ DIŠ KI MIN *ina* UGU GIR$_3$.MIN-*šu$_2$ uk-tam-ma-as-ma u$_2$-šab* A SED *ana* UGU SAG-*šu$_2$ tu-qar-ra-ar$_2$*

14 A$_{i\,14}$ DIŠ KI MIN SAG.DU-*su ana šap-la-nu* GAR-*an* GIR$_3$.MIN-*šu$_2$ ana* AN.TA-*nu tu-ša$_2$-qa ina šip-ku-ti*
15 A$_{i\,15}$ TE-*su ta-ma-ḫaṣ ina šip-ku-ti tu-ma-aš-<šad>-su-ma*[126] *ana* ŠA$_3$ DU$_{10}$-*ab* DU$_{11}$.GA *ina* ŠU.SI-*ka* GAL-*ti*

11 If someone suffers (*maruṣ*) from gastric constriction (*kīs libbi*): you make that man squat over his (own) feet,[127]

12 (and) you pour (*tašappak-ma*) oven-heated (and still) warm juice from *kasû* ('tamarind')[128] over him; then he will recover (*iballuṭ*).

13 If DITTO, he kneels and sits down[129] on top of his (own) feet, (and) you drip cold water on top of his head.

14 If DITTO, you put (*tašakkan*) his head down, you lift his feet up, (and then) in (his) weakened state (*šipkūtu*)[130]
15 you strike his cheek, in (his) weakened state you rub him, and you say (*taqabbi*)[131] 'it is good (*ṭāb*) for the belly', (then) with your left thumb

126 For a similar defective spelling, with the verb *kapāru*, see the fever prescription in Bácskay 2018: 148 ln. 26. In BAM 147 obv. 26 we have the defective orthography *tu-kap-<par>*, whereas the newly identified parallel BM 35512 rev. 12′ provides the expected spelling *tu-kap-par*. See also BAM 494 ii 26 and its duplicate AMT 1/3 14′ with the instruction *ištu eliš ana šapliš tumaššad* 'you rub him from top to bottom' (Bácskay and Simkó 2017: 11).

127 The reappearance of GIR$_3$ = Akk. *šēpu* 'feet' as well as several different verbs of sitting or squatting show that this treatment is related to the preceding Sumerian incantation mentioning seated and planted feet. The patient's posture in these lines may be imitating the position of someone during a bowel movement.

128 For *kasû* as 'tamarind', see Eypper 2019. The use of two qualifications here, Akk. *sekru* and *emmu*, both of which can mean 'heated', points to *kasû sekrūtu* as a largely symbolic remedy: *kasû* and *sekrūtu* both include the two consonants (/k/ and /s/) that occur in the first word of the disease being treated here, viz. *kīs libbi*. The translation 'oven-heated' is based on the phrase *ina tinūri tesekker* 'you heat it in an oven', which occurs frequently in therapeutic texts. For further discussion, see Kinnier Wilson and Reynolds 2007: 80.

129 This example of verbal hendiadys may be an attempt to render the Sumerian of line 6, viz. gir$_3$.a.ni gub.ba gir$_3$.a.ni ⸢dur$_2$⸣.ra : $_{du\text{-}ra}$ in Akkadian. Both this expression and *tu-še-šab-šu$_2$* in line 11 above probably refer to a posture in which the patients fold their legs under themselves, often spoken of as 'sitting on one's heels' in English.

130 The word is probably *šipkūtu*, from the verb *šapāku* meaning 'to render limp, powerless' (CAD Š/1 418), and may refer to the upside-down position of the patient at the beginning of the prescription. Although we adopt this reading here, the absence of a possessive pronoun referring to the patient speaks against this interpretation. AHw 643 has instead *ina me-ku-ti* (. . .) *tamaḫḫaṣ* 'du schlägst leicht'.

131 The logographic orthography DU$_{11}$.GA allows for either the healer, in the second person (*taqabbi*), or the patient, in the third person (*iqabbi*), to be the speaker. If the patient were speaking to his own belly, however, we might expect a possessive pronoun attached to the word for 'belly', viz. *ana* ŠA$_3$-*šu$_2$*.

16 A$_{i\,16}$ *ša* GUB$_3$* 14-*šu$_2$* GU.DU-*su* TAG-*at* 14-*šu$_2$* SAG.DU-*su* TAG-*at u* ⸢*qaq*⸣-*qa-ra* TAG-*at*

---

17 A$_{i\,17}$ ⸢DIŠ⸣ KI MIN SUḪUŠ ^{giš}NAM.TAR NITA$_2$ SUḪUŠ ^{giš}*šu-šum* ^{u2}IGI-*lim* ⸢^{u2}IGI⸣.NIŠ ^{u2}*tar-muš*
18 A$_{i\,18}$ ⸢^{u2}IN.NU⸣.UŠ ^{u2}EME UR.GI$_7$ SUD$_2$ *lu ina* A *lu in*[*a* KA]Š* NAG

---

19 A$_{i\,19}$ DIŠ NA ŠA$_3$-*šu$_2$* ⸢*it-te*⸣-*net-ba-aš-šum* 10 KISAL ⸢^{u2}⸣[x x x] x
20 A$_{i\,20}$ 10 KISAL ^{u2}MA$_2$.ERIŠ$_4$.MA$_2$.⸢LA$_2$⸣-*e* SUD$_2$ ḪI.ḪI [x x x x T]I

---

21 A$_{i\,21}$ DIŠ NA *ki-is* ŠA$_3$ GIG ŠA$_3$.MEŠ-*šu$_2$* *ma-ga*[*l* M]U$_2$.MU$_2$-*ḫu mu-še-er-r*[*it*$^?$*-*ta-šu$_2$* GU$_7$-*š*]*u$_2$*[132]

†

16 you touch (*talappat*) his buttocks 14 times, you touch his head 14 times, and you touch the ground.[133]

---

17 If DITTO, you pound (*tasâk*) root from male *pillû* ('mandrake'), root from *šūšu* ('liquorice'), *imḫur-līm* ('faces a thousand' plant), *imḫur-ešrā* ('faces twenty' plant), *tarmuš* ('lupin'),
18 *maštakal* ('soapwort'), (and) *lišān kalbi* ('dog's tongue' plant),[134] (and) he drinks (*išatti*) them either in water or in beer.

---

19 If someone's belly (*libbu*)[135] keeps throbbing up against him (*ittenetbâššum*):[136] you pound (*tasâk*) ten KISAL-measures of . . .
20 (and) ten KISAL-measures of *mirišmarû* (a plant),[137] you mix (*tuballal*) them (and) . . .; (then) he will recover (*iballuṭ*).

---

21 If someone suffers (*maruṣ*) from gastric constriction (*kīs libbi*), his internal organs (*qerbū*) are extremely swollen (*napḫū*),[138] (and) his esophagus (*mušērittu*)$^?$ causes him pain (*ikkalšu*):

---

132 Our tentative reconstruction has the word for 'esophagus, gullet', Akk. *mušērittu* / *mušēridu*, which is derived from the verb *arādu* used in the sense 'that which conveys down' (von Soden 1947: 67–68). This word is only otherwise found in medical texts as an ingredient, namely the gullet of a goose in CRAN 3: 3 (AMT 102/1: 3).

133 For a similar use of the thumb to apply medicine in the Talmud, see Bavli Gittin 69a.

134 For the *lišān kalbi* plant, see the detailed discussion in Böck 2014a: 140–158.

135 The translation of Akk. *libbu* as 'belly' here is meant to emphasise its relatively non-specific character, as opposed to Akkadian *karšu* 'stomach' or *qerbū* 'internal organs'. Moreover, in line with Stol (2006), we generally distinguish the singular logogram ŠA$_3$ = Akk. *libbu* 'belly' from the plural ŠA$_3$.MEŠ = Akk. *qerbū* 'internal organs'. There are exceptions, however, as in STO 2: 96.

136 The dative pronoun is common in medical texts, presumably as the ethical dative, showing that the patient is being affected by the action of the verb, but its use here with the verb *tebû* in the Ntn-stem may, in contrast, describe a throbbing sensation in the stomach, with the ventive and third person dative pronoun pointing to the perceived direction in which the belly is moving.

137 For a recent discussion of the *mirišmarû* plant, see Stadhouders 2018.

138 The reading of MU$_2$.MU$_2$-*ḫu* as *napḫū* is based on the syllabic writing *nap-ḫu* in line 80 below, as well as in STO 2: 105, 108, 113, 115, 118, and STO 4: 56′, 62′. Elsewhere, MU$_2$.MU$_2$ is usually rendered as a finite verb in the Ntn-stem, viz. *ittananpaḫū* (Abusch and Schwemer 2011: 232 ln. 13′). However, the Ntn-stem form of the verb does not seem to be attested in a syllabic orthography in contemporary texts.

22 A$_{i 22}$ ^{u2}IGI.NIŠ SUḪUŠ ^{giš}NAM.TAR NITA$_{2}$ *a-ḫe-en-[na-a* GAZ SIM *ina* ŠA$_{3}$] ⸢*mal-ma-liš* TI-*qe*$_{2}$ *ina*⸣ K[AŠ* NAG *ina* A SED][139]

23 A$_{i 23}$ *tu-la-bak ina* MUL$_{4}$ *tuš-bat ina še-ri*$_{3}$ ⸢ŠEG$_{6}$-*šal ta-ša*$_{2}$-*ḫal ana* DUR$_{2}$⸣-*šu*$_{2}$ DUB-*ak* SI.SA$_{2}$-*m*[*a* TI]

---

24 A$_{i 24}$ ^{šim}GUR$_{2}$.GUR$_{2}$ ^{šim}LI ^{šim}GAM.MA PA ^{giš}GE$_{6}$.PAR$_{3}$ PA ^{giš}ŠE.ḪAR NUMUN ^{u2}*ur-*⸢*ba*⸣-[*ti* (x x)]*

^{šim}GUR$_{2}$.GUR$_{2}$ ^{šim}LI / ^{šim}GAM.MA PA ^{giš}ŠE.ḪAR PA ^{giš}GE$_{6}$.PAR$_{3}$ PA ^{giš}ŠE.NU$_{2}$.A NUMUN ^{u2}*ur-ba-ti* 7 U$_{2}$.ḪI.A ŠEŠ (STO 2: 110–111)

25 A$_{i 25}$ DIŠ-*niš* GAZ ⸢SIM KI$^{?}$ I$_{3}^{?}$.UDU$^{?}$* ^{šim}⸣ḪAB$^{?}$[140] ḪI.ḪI *ina* KUŠ.EDIN[141] SUR-*ri* SAG ŠA$_{3}$-*šu*$_{2}$ LAL$_{2}$-*ma* TI

TEŠ$_{2}$.BI GAZ SIM KI ⸢I$_{3}$⸣.UDU DUḪ.LAL$_{3}$ *u* ^{šim}ḪAB *tu-sa-maḫ ina* KUŠ.EDIN SUR LAL$_{2}$-*su-ma* TI (STO 2: 112)

---

22 you crush (*taḫaššal*)$^{?}$ (and) sift (*tanappi*)$^{?}$ separately *imḫur-ešrā* ('faces twenty' plant) (and) root from male *pillû* ('mandrake'), you take (*teleqqe*) equal amounts of them, (and) he drinks (*išatti*) them in beer,

23 (then) you soften (these ingredients) in cold water$^{?}$, you leave (the mixture) out overnight under the stars, in the morning you bring it to a boil (*tušabšal*), you filter it, you pour (*tašappak*) it into his anus, (and) he will have a bowel movement (*ušeššer-ma*); then he will recover (*iballuṭ*).

---

24 You crush (*taḫaššal*) (and) sift (*tanappi*) *kukru* (an aromatic), *burāšu* (a kind of juniper), *ṣumlalû* (an aromatic), leaves from *lipāru* (a fruit tree), leaves from ŠE.ḪAR (a tree),[142] (and) seed from *urbatu* ('rushes')

25 together, you mix (*tuballal*) them with fat$^{?}$ (and) *ṭūru* ('opopanax')$^{?}$, you smear (*teṭerri*) (the mixture) on a piece of leather, (and) you bandage (*taṣammid-ma*) his epigastrium (*rēš libbi*);[143] then he will recover (*iballuṭ*).

---

139 The reconstruction at the end of the line is based on the available space, as well as the fact that subsequent recipes refer to drugs to be taken in beer. For the instruction *ina* A SED *tu-la-bak*, see STO 2: 14.

140 The reconstruction is based on the available space and the remaining traces as well as the relatively close parallel STO 2: 110–112, with KI I$_{3}$.UDU DUḪ.LAL$_{3}$ *u* ^{šim}ḪAB *tu-sa-maḫ* after a similar list of drugs.

141 For the latest discussion of KUŠ.EDIN, see Maul 2019: 307. The lexical equation in Syllabary B 90 (MSL 3 p. 104) between EDIN and Akk. *e-di-nu* is a hapax and probably just an *ad hoc* loan of the Sumerian term into Akkadian, but it might also point to Akk. (*w*)*ēdēnu* 'isolated, unattached', as a qualification for a 'piece of leather' rather than an entire hide.

142 The reading and significance of ^{giš}ŠE.ḪAR is not known (Campbell Thompson 1949: 323 and Borger 2010: 375), but it is largely attested in the Stomach Treatise, viz. STO 2: 9 and 111, as well as STO 5: 6. Moreover, it occurs outside of our corpus in BAM 571 iii' 5', which is probably a manuscript of BRON. For ^{giš}ŠE.ḪAR, compare also the form [^{giš}]⸢ŠE⸣.MUR.⸢GUD⸣ in MSL SS 1 p. 15 i 52, where this form is equated with Akk. *šaššūgu* (a tree); the standard logogram for this tree is ^{giš}ŠE.MUŠ$_{5}$ as in Ura 3 52 (MSL 5 p. 97). Alternatively, the sign ḪAR can be decomposed into ḪI and AŠ$_{2}$, and ḪI, if read as DU$_{10}$, might suggest a connection to a type of juniper written as ^{giš}ŠE.DU$_{10}$ in third millennium texts (Heimpel 2011: 128–130). If so, the meaning of AŠ$_{2}$ remains unclear.

143 The term *rēš libbi* literally means 'the head of the belly', but it is often translated as 'epigastrium'. Here, the term must refer to the upper part of the abdomen as the place where the bandage was applied. This is also in line with neighbouring passages that are concerned with regurgitating food, the upper stomach and perhaps the esophagus (*mušērittu*).

26 A$_{i\,26}$ DIŠ NA *ki-i*[*s** ŠA$_3$ GIG NINDA *u* KA]Š* ŠA$_3$-*šu*$_2$ NU IGI-*ḫar-šu*$_2$ *ina* KA-*šu*$_2$ GUR.GUR-*ra* TUN$_3$-*šu*$_2$ *u*$_2$-*sa-ḫal-šu*$_2$[144]

[DIŠ NA NIND]A ⸢*u*⸣ KAŠ ŠA$_3$-*šu*$_2$ NU IGI-*šu*$_2$ (STO 2: 256)

DIŠ NA SAG ŠA$_3$-*šu*$_2$ KUM$_2$ TUKU.MEŠ-*ši* ŠA$_3$-*šu*$_2$ GIG / NINDA *u* A.MEŠ ŠA$_3$-*šu*$_2$ NU IGI-*šu*$_2$ (BAM 49 obv. 9′–10′)

DIŠ NA SAG ŠA$_3$-*šu*$_2$ KUM$_2$ [TUK]U.MEŠ-*ši* ŠA$_3$-⸢*šu*$_2$⸣ G[IG] / NINDA *u* A.MEŠ ŠA$_3$-*šu*$_2$ NU I[GI]-*šu*$_2$ (BAM 50 obv. 11–12)

27 A$_{i\,27}$ *ip-ta-na-ru* [UZU.MEŠ-*šu*$_2$ *ir*]-⸢*ta*⸣-*nam-mu-u*$_2$[145] IM *ina* DUR$_2$-*šu*$_2$ NIGIN ŠA$_3$.MEŠ-*šu*$_2$ *eb-ṭu*$_2$ *ana* TI-*šu*$_2$

UZU.MEŠ-*šu*$_2$ *ir-ta-nam-mu* IM *ina* DUR$_2$-*šu*$_2$ NIGIN-*ur*$_2$ *ana* TI-*šu*$_2$ (STO 2: 256)

DU$_8$.MEŠ-*šu*$_2$ *ir-te-nem-mu-u* / ŠA$_3$-*šu*$_2$ *ina pi-qi ana* BURU$_8$-*e* DU$_3$.DU$_3$-*uš* NU *i-par*$_5$-*ru* / IM *ina* ŠA$_3$-*šu*$_2$ *i-sa-na-ḫur i-le-eb-bu* / ŠA$_3$.MEŠ-*šu*$_2$ *eb-ṭu* NA BI ^{d}ŠU.NAM.ERIM$_2$ DAB-*su* / *ana* TI-*šu*$_2$ (BAM 49 obv. 10′–14′)

DU$_8$.MEŠ-*šu*$_2$ *ir-te-*[*nem-mu-u*] / [ŠA$_3$]-*šu*$_2$ *ina* ⸢*pi-qi*$^{?}$⸣ *ana* BURU$_8$-*e* DU$_3$.DU$_3$-*uš* NU *i-par*$_5$-[*ru*] / I[M *ina* ŠA$_3$-*šu*$_2$] ⸢*i*⸣-*sa-*[*n*]*a-ḫur i-le-eb-b*[*u*] / Š[A$_3$].MEŠ-*šu*$_2$ ⸢*eb-ṭu*$_2$⸣ NA BI NAM.ERIM$_2$ DAB-*s*[*u*] / [*ana* TI]-*šu*$_2$ (BAM 50 obv. 12–16)

[. . .] *i-*[*par*$_5$-*ru* . . .] / [. . .] *i-leb-bu* [. . .] / [NA B]I ^{d}NAM.ERI[M$_2$ DAB-*su ana* T]I-⸢*šu*$_2$⸣ (BAM 51: 1′–3′)

28 A$_{i\,28}$ 1/2 SILA$_3$ A ZU$_2$.LUM.MA 1/2 SILA$_3$ A GAZI^{sar} 10 KISAL A.GEŠTIN.NA 3 GIN$_2$ I$_3$ *ḫal-ṣa* 2 GIN$_2$ LAL$_3$ 10 GIN$_2$ ^{u2}KUR. RA[146]

1/2 SILA$_3$ A ZU$_2$.LUM.MA 1/2 SILA$_3$ A GAZI^{sar} / [2 GIN$_2$ A.GEŠTIN.N]A 2 GIN$_2$ ^{u2}KUR.RA 3 GIN$_2$ I$_3$ *ḫal-ṣa* 3 GIN$_2$ LAL$_3$ KUR-*i* (STO 2: 256–257)

1/2 SILA$_3$ A ZU$_2$.LUM.MA 1/2 SILA$_3$ A GAZI^{sar} / 1/2 SILA$_3$ *ši-qa* 1/2 SILA$_3$ A.GEŠTIN.NA 5 GIN$_2$ I$_3$ *ḫal-ṣa* / 10 GIN$_2$ LAL$_3$ 10 GIN$_2$ ^{u2}KUR.RA (BAM 49 obv. 14′–16′)

1/2 SI[LA$_3$ . . .] (BAM 50 obv. 16)

[1/2 SIL]A$_3$ A ZU$_2$.LUM.MA 1/2 SILA$_3$ A GAZI^{sar} / [1/2 SI]LA$_3$ *ši-qa* 1/2 SILA$_3$ A.GEŠTIN.NA 5 GIN$_2$ / [I$_3$ *ḫ*]*al-ṣa* 10 GIN$_2$ LAL$_3$ 10 GIN$_2$ ^{u2}KUR.R[A] (BAM 51: 4′–6′)

26 If someone suffers (*maruṣ*) from gastric constriction (*kīs libbi*), his belly (*libbu*) does not let him accept (*lā ušamḫaršu*)[147] bread and beer (and) keeps bringing them back up (*uttanarra*) into his mouth, his stomach (*tākaltu*) causes him to have a piercing pain,

27 he is constantly vomiting, his flesh continually sags, flatulence (lit. wind) circulates (*isaḫḫur*) in his anus, (and) his internal organs (*qerbū*) are cramped: in order to heal him (*ana bulluṭīšu*),

28 you pound (*tasâk*) half a litre of juice from *suluppū* ('dates'), half a litre of juice from *kasû* ('tamarind'), ten KISAL-measures of vinegar, three shekels of pressed oil,[148] two shekels of *dišpu* ('syrup'), (and) ten shekels of *nīnû* ('mint'),

---

144 For line 26, see also STO 2: 245. A version of this prescription is also known from texts dealing with *māmītu* '(broken) oath' (Maul 2019: 277–284), but with some differences.

145 Although the *māmītu* prescription provides an interesting parallel, with DU$_8$.MEŠ-*šu*$_2$ for Akk. *piṭru* 'abdominal wall$^{?}$' (Maul 2019: 280) or 'joint$^{?}$' (Cadelli 2019: 58), our reconstruction follows STO 2: 256.

146 In this line as well, STO 2 offers the closest parallel, including most of the measurements. The *lectio difficilior* 10 KISAL A.GEŠTIN.NA, however, is likely the oldest of these different versions, a formulation that is banalized to 1/2 SILA$_3$ in the parallels.

147 We take IGI-*šu*$_2$ and IGI-*ḫar-šu*$_2$ as forms of *maḫāru* in the Š-stem, viz. *ušamḫaršu*. In every example of these forms in the Stomach Treatise, ŠA$_3$-*šu*$_2$ occurs immediately before the verb, presumably to stress that the belly is the subject (i.e., causer) of the verb: 'his belly (*libbašu*) does not allow him (-*šu*) to come into contact with bread and beer'. The following verb is a Dtn-form of the verb *târu*, with the belly as the subject and the bread and beer as the objects: 'it (= his belly) makes the bread and beer return'. The idea here is probably that even if the patient forced himself to eat something, he would not be able to keep it down.

148 The ingredient *šamnu ḫalṣu* (lit. 'pressed oil') almost certainly designates the highest quality of oil, presumably extracted from sesame seeds; see CAD H 51, Stol 1985a: 121 and Waetzoldt 1985: 84.

29 A$_{i\,29}$ SUD$_2$ *ana* ŠA$_3$ ŠUB-*di ina* GE$_6$ *ana* IGI ^{mul}UZ$_3$ *tuš-bat ina* A$_2$.GU$_2$.ZI.GA NU *pa-tan* NAG-*šu*$_2$

DIŠ-*niš tuš-te-mid* ⸢GAZ⸣ *ina* GE$_6$ *ina* IGI ^{mul}UZ$_3$ *tuš-bat* / [*ina še-r*]*i*$_3$ ⸢ŠEG$_6$⸣-*šal ta-ša*$_2$*-ḫal* SED *ina* ŠA$_3$ *taḫ-ta-na-su* EGIR-*šu*$_2$ NAG (STO 2: 257–258)

SUD$_2$ DIŠ-*niš tuš-te-mid* / *ina* GE$_6$ *ana* IGI ^{mul}UZ$_3$ *tuš-bat* ZI$_3$.SUR.RA-*a* NIGIN-*mi* / NIG$_2$.NA ^{šim}LI DUB-*aq* MU ^{d}*gu-la u* DINGIR.MAḪ / *ta-zak-kar mi-iḫ-ḫa* BAL-*qi*$_2$ *ina še-ri*$_3$ ŠEG$_6$-*šal* / ⸢*ta*⸣-*ša*$_2$-⸢*ḫal*⸣ SED (BAM 49 obv. 16′–20′)

[SU]D$_2$ DIŠ-*niš tuš-te-mid ina* G[E$_6$ *ana* IGI $^{m]ul}$[UZ$_3$] / [*tuš-ba*]*t* ZI$_3$.⸢SUR⸣.R[A-*a* . . .] (BAM 51: 7′–8′)

30 A$_{i\,30}$ EGIR-*šu*$_2$ 1/2 SILA$_3$ *ši-qa* NAG-*šu*$_2$ *ina* KA-*šu*$_2$ *u* DUR$_2$-*šu*$_2$ SI.SA$_2$ *tu-ser-šu*$_2$*-ma* TI-*uṭ*

ana DUR$_2$-*šu*$_2$ DUB-*ak ina* DUR$_2$-*šu*$_2$ SI.SA$_2$-*ma* TI (BAM 49 obv. 20′)

---

31 A$_{i\,31}$ DIŠ KI MIN MUN KUR-*i* MUN *a-ma-ni*$_7$ TEŠ$_2$.BI SUD$_2$ *ina* KAŠ NU *pa-tan* NAG-*šu*$_2$ *ina* KA-*šu*$_2$ *u* DUR$_2$-*šu*$_2$ SI.SA$_2$-*ma tu-ser-šu*$_2$*-ma* TI

☨

29 you put (*tanaddi*) them all together,[149] you leave (the mixture) out for the night under the Goat Star,[150] (and) in the morning, you have him drink it (*tašaqqīšu*) on an empty stomach.

30 Afterwards, you have him drink half a litre of *šiqqu* ('garum'), he will void (*ušeššer*) from his mouth and from his anus, (and) you rub him down thoroughly (*tuseršū-ma*);[151] then he will recover (*iballuṭ*).[152]

---

31 If DITTO, you pound (*tasâk*) mountain salt (and) *amānu* salt together, you have him drink (*tašaqqīšu*) it in beer on an empty stomach, he will void (*ušeššer-ma*) from his mouth and from his anus, and you rub him down thoroughly; then he will recover (*iballuṭ*).

---

149 The only non-liquid ingredient in lines 28–29 is *nīnû* 'mint', so the use of *sâku* 'to pound' is somewhat surprising. The normal way of describing such a procedure would be to pound the solid ingredients in a liquid carrier. The verb *sâku* is omitted in the parallel in STO 2, where the drugs are first mixed together (*ištēniš tuštēmid*) and only afterward crushed (*taḫaššal*). The *māmītu* prescription in BAM 49 and 51 has a somewhat different instruction: SUD$_2$ DIŠ-*niš tuš-te-mid* 'you crush them (and) mix them together' (Maul 2019: 277–284).

150 The Goat Star, the constellation Lyra, is the celestial manifestation of the healing goddess Gula (Böck 2014a: 181).

151 CAD E 356, Š/2 336 and Cadelli 2000: 72 n. 14 interpret this verbal form as a partially logographic writing of the verb *salāḫu* 'to sprinkle' (corresponding to the Sumerogram SUD); this seems to be based on the liquid remedies that occur alongside this verb both here and in the next line. The form is also attested in AMT 16/2 obv. 2′ and 6′ as well as BAM 562: 4′: AMT 16/2 obv. 6′ reflects a similar context, with the patient drinking the remedies right before the action described by this verbal form. In line with AHw 1038 and CAD S 229, however, we read the SUD sign as a syllabic writing for /ser/ as in *tu-ser-šu*$_2$*-ma* 'you rub him down thoroughly', perhaps a euphemism for removing the expelled bodily fluids from the scene.

152 This line as well as line 32 below are cited in the Neo-Assyrian letter SAA 10 326, sent by the physician Urad-Nanaya (Heeßel 2000: 91).

32 A$_{i\,32}$ DIŠ KI MIN ^{u2}NU.LUḪ.ḪA 7 ŠE.MEŠ ^{u2}IGI-*lim* TEŠ$_2$.BI ⸢SUD$_2$* *ina** KAŠ* SAG* NU⸣* *pa-tan* NAG-*šu*$_2$ *ina* KA-*šu*$_2$ *u* DUR$_2$-*šu*$_2$ SI.SA$_2$-*ma* KI MIN

---

33 A$_{i\,33}$ [DIŠ KI MIN Z]I$_3$ ŠE.SA.A ZI$_3$ *ḫa-ru-be*[153] ⸢*di*⸣*-*ik-ta* ZU$_2$.LUM.MA TEŠ$_2$.BI SUD$_2$ *ina* KAŠ NU *pa-tan* ⸢2 UD⸣-[*me*]

[DIŠ KI MI]N ⸢ZI$_3$ ŠE.SA⸣.A ZI$_3$ ḪARUB$^!$(AMAŠ) *qi*$_2$*-lip*$_2$ ZU$_2$.LUM.MA SUD$_2$ *ina* KAŠ 2 UD-*me* / [*ba*]-*lu* ⸢*pa-tan*⸣ (STO 2: 254–255)

DIŠ NA ŠA$_3$.MEŠ-*š*[*u*$_2$ *nap*]-*ḫu* ZI$_3$ ŠE.SA.A ZI$_3$ MUNU$_6$ NUMUN ^{u2}KI.^{d}IŠKUR *di-ik-ta ša*$_2$ ZU$_2$.LUM / TEŠ$_2$.BI S[UD$_2$ NU *pa-t*]*an* GU$_7$.MEŠ (STO 2: 118–119)

34 A$_{i\,34}$ [NAG.MEŠ 2] ⸢UD*-*me*⸣*[154] *ina* A.MEŠ NU *pa-tan* NAG.MEŠ A.MEŠ SAG ŠA$_3$-*šu*$_2$ ⸢*tu*⸣-*s*[*a**-*laḫ*$_2$-*ma* TI]

NAG-*šu*$_2$ A NU NAG A SAG ŠA$_3$-*šu*$_2$ *tu-sa-laḫ*$_2$-*ma ina-eš* (STO 2: 255)

A.MEŠ NU NAG A.MEŠ SAG ŠA$_3$-*šu*$_2$ *tu-sa-laḫ*$_2$-*ma* ⸢TI⸣ (STO 2: 119)

---

32 If DITTO, you pound (*tasâk*) *nuḫurtu* ('asafoetida') (and) seven grains of *imḫur-līm* ('faces a thousand' plant) together, you have him drink (*tašaqqīšu*) them in high-quality beer[155] on an empty stomach, he will void (*uše̍šer-ma*) from his mouth and from his anus, then DITTO (= you rub him down; then he will recover).

---

33 If DITTO, you pound (*tasâk*) flour from *labtu* ('roasted barley'), flour from *ḫarūbu* ('carob'), (and) a *diktu* preparation[156] (made) from *suluppū* ('dates') together, he keeps drinking (*ištanatti*) them in beer on an empty stomach for two days,

34 for two$^?$ days$^?$ he keeps drinking them in water on an empty stomach, (and then) you sprinkle his epigastrium (*rēš libbi*) with water; then he will recover (*iballuṭ*).

---

153 Syllabic *ḫa-ru-be* seems to correspond to logographic ḪARUB$^!$(AMAŠ) in the parallel. For a discussion of this suggested reading, see STO 2: 254.

154 The tentative restoration of the passage is based on the parallel in lines 33–34, where beer is mentioned first and then water as the liquid carrier. Köcher (1980) copied UD-*me* as undamaged, but these signs are now almost entirely missing.

155 For a discussion of KAŠ SAG = Akk. *šikaru rēštû* 'high-quality beer', see Stol 1994: 161–164, who argues that in certain contexts this phrase is used interchangeably with KAŠ = Akk. *šikaru* 'beer': see, for example, KAŠ SAG in BAM 480+ i 12 and KAŠ in BAM 4 obv. 9′, both of which correspond to CRAN 1: 12.

156 Civil (1983: 238–240) explains *diktu* as 'a type of dish or food concoction whose known varieties are prepared with cereal, milk, or dates'. As a medical ingredient, it is first attested in the Old Babylonian therapeutic text UET VI/3 895 obv. 1–4, translated by Schwemer (2010) as '*dīktum*-Mehl der Dattelpalme'. Within the therapeutic corpus, the notion that *diktu* is a kind of flour (see also SAD D/T/Ṭ 30) is largely based on our passage, as well as on STO 2: 118–119, where it is listed alongside different types of flour. In the parallel STO 2: 254, *diktu* is replaced with the much more common word for 'rind, skin' (Akk. *qilpu*).

35 A$_{\text{i 35}}$ [DIŠ KI MIN ^{urudu}ŠEN.TUR]* ⸢A⸣* [*u*]* ⸢KAŠ⸣*[157] DIRI-*ma* ^{giš}*s*[*i-ḫa* ^{giš}*a*]*r*$_2$-⸢*gan*⸣-*na* ^{giš}*b*[*a-ri-ra-ta*]

DIŠ NA MUR.MIN-*šu*$_2$ KI KAK.TI-*šu*$_2$ *it-pu-qu ana* TI-*šu*$_2$ ^{urudu}ŠEN.TU[R . . .] / ^{giš}LUM.ḪA (BAM 558 iv 7–8)

[DIŠ NA MUR.MEŠ]-*šu*$_2$ KI KAK.TI-*šu*$_2$ *it-pu-qu ana* TI-*šu*$_2$ ŠEN.TUR A *u* KAŠ [DIRI-*ma*] / [^{giš}*si-ḫ*]*u* ^{giš}*ar*$_2$-*gan*-⸢*nu*⸣ ^{giš}LUM.ḪA (BAM 174 obv. 11′–12′)

36 A$_{\text{i 36}}$ [$^{\text{u2}}$ḪAR.ḪAR] ⸢$^{\text{u2}}$⸣**at**-*kam*$_2$* *ana** ⸢ŠA$_3$* ŠUB*-*di*⸣* [....................................]

$^{\text{u2}}$ḪAR.ḪAR $^{\text{u2}}$*ak-tam ana* ŠA$_3$ ŠUB-*di* ŠEG$_6$-*ša*[*l* . . .] (BAM 558 iv 8)

$^{\text{u2}}$ḪAR.ḪAR $^{\text{u2}}$*ak-tam ina* Š[A$_3$ ŠUB-*di*] / ŠEG$_6$-*šal ta-ša*$_2$-*ḫal ina* ŠA$_3$ RA-*su* E$_{11}$ (BAM 174 obv. 12′–13′)

37 A$_{\text{i 37}}$ [I$_3$ ^{giš}EREN ŠE]Š$_2$-*su* 1/2 SILA$_3$ *saḫ-le*$_2$-*e* 1/2 SILA$_3$ ^{šim}GUR$_2$.GUR$_2$ 1/2 ⸢SILA$_3$⸣ [^{šim}LI 1/2 SILA$_3$ $^{\text{u2}}$]⸢*qut-ri* 1/2 SILA$_3$⸣ GA[ZI^{sar}]

I$_3$ ^{giš}*e-re-ni* EŠ-*su* (BAM 558 iv 9)

KI I$_3$ ^{giš}*eri-īni* EŠ-*su* (BAM 174 obv. 13′)

⸢1/2⸣ SILA$_3$ *saḫ-le*$_2$-*e* / [1/2 SIL]A$_3$ ⸢^{šim}GUR$_2$.GUR$_2$ 1/2 SILA$_3$ ^{šim}LI⸣ 1/2 SILA$_3$ $^{\text{u2}}$KI.^{d}IŠKUR 1/2 SILA$_3$ *ka-si-i* (STO 2: 245–246)

⸢1/2 SILA$_3$⸣ *saḫ-le*$_2$-*e* 1/2 SILA$_3$ ^{šim}GUR$_2$.GUR$_2$ [x x x x] / [1/2 S]ILA$_3$ NUMUN $^{\text{u2}}$*qut-ri* 1/2 SILA$_3$ GAZI^{s}[^{ar}] (BAM 58: 10–11)

38 A$_{\text{i 38}}$ [1/2 SILA$_3$] ⸢ZI$_3$⸣ MUNU$_6$ 1/2 SILA$_3$ ZI$_3$ GU$_2$.GAL 1/2 SILA$_3$ ZI$_3$ GU$_2$.TUR ⸢1/2 SILA$_3$ *pa**-*pa**-*si*-^{d}ID$_2$⸣ 1/2 SILA$_3$ $^{\text{u2}}$KUR. RA 1/2 SILA$_3$ $^{\text{u2}}$AB$_2$.D[UḪ]

⸢1/2 SILA$_3$ *pa*⸣-*pa-si*-⸢^{d}⸣[ID$_2$] 1/2 SILA$_3$ $^{\text{u2}}$KUR.RA / [1/2 SILA$_3$ $^{\text{u2}}$A]B$_2$.DUḪ 1/2 SILA$_3$ ZU$_2$.LUM.MA 1/2 SILA$_3$ DIDA SIG 1/2 SILA$_3$ ZI$_3$ MUNU$_6$ ⸢1/2⸣ SILA$_3$ ZI$_3$ G[U$_2$.GA]L 1/2 SILA$_3$ ZI$_3$.KUM / ⸢1/2 SILA$_3$ ZI$_3$ GIB$_3$⸣ (STO 2: 246–248)

[x x x x x x x] / [1/2 S]ILA$_3$ $^{\text{u2}}$KUR.⸢RA 1/2 SILA$_3$⸣ NUMUN ⸢$^{\text{u2}}$⸣[AB$_2$.DUḪ x x x x] / [x x] x x x [. . .] (BAM 58: 11–13)

35 If DITTO, you fill (*tumallā-ma*) a small copper pot with water and beer, and then you put (*tanaddi*) *sīḫu* (‘wormwood’), *argannu* (a conifer), *barīrātu* (‘sagapenum’),

36 *ḫašû* (‘thyme’), (and) *aktam* (a plant) in it, you bring (the mixture) to a boil (*tušabšal*), you filter it, (and) you bathe him (*taraḫḫassu*) in it, (then) he emerges (*illi*) (from the bath),

37 (and) you anoint him (*tapaššassu*) with oil from *erēnu* (‘cedar’). Half a litre of *saḫlû* (‘cress’), half a litre of *kukru* (an aromatic), half a litre of *burāšu* (a kind of juniper), half a litre of *qutru* (a plant), half a litre of *kasû* (‘tamarind’),

38 half a litre of flour from *buqlu* (‘malt’), half a litre of flour from *ḫallūru* (‘chickpea’), half a litre of flour from *kakkû* (‘lentil’), half a litre of *pappasītu* (a mineral), half a litre of *nīnû* (‘mint’), half a litre of *kamantu* (a plant),

157 Faint traces of signs, copied both by Küchler (1904) and Köcher (1980) as A *u* KAŠ, can still be recognised at the beginning of the line. This reading can now be confirmed with the help of BAM 558 iv 7–9 and BAM 174 obv. 11′–13′, both of which provide remedies for diseases of the respiratory tract and present the same short anointment-based therapeutic procedure, preceding the long list of drugs in lines 37–40.

39 A$_{\text{i 39}}$ [1/2 SIL]A$_3$ ŠE$_{10}$ ⸢TU⸣*^{mušen} 1/2 SILA$_3$ $^{\text{u2}}$*eriš$_6$-ti* A.ŠA$_3$ 10 GIN$_2$ ^{šim}MAŠ[158] 10 GIN$_2$ KA A.AB.BA 1/2 SILA$_3$ ZI$_3$ GIB$_3$[159]

1/3 SILA$_3$ ŠE$_{10}$ TU^{mušen} 1/3 SILA$_3$ $^{\text{u2}}$*eriš$_6$-ti* GAN$_2$ 10 KISAL ^{šim}ŠEŠ 10 ⸢KISAL⸣ KA A.AB.BA (STO 2: 248)

40 A$_{\text{i 40}}$ [1/2 SIL]A$_3$ ZU$_2$.LUM.MA 1/2 SILA$_3$ DIDA SIG.GA 1/2 SILA$_3$ ZI$_3$.KUM 16 U$_2$.MEŠ *an-nu-⸢ti*⸣* TEŠ$_2$⸣*.BI GAZ SIM

[16] U$_2$.⸢ḪI.A⸣ ŠEŠ DIŠ-*niš* GAZ SIM (STO 2: 249)

41 A$_{\text{i 41}}$ [*ina* KA]Š ⸢SAG⸣ *ina* ^{urudu}ŠEN.TUR GIM *ra-bi-ki tara-bak* 3 UD-*me** SAG ŠA$_3$-*šu$_2$* LAL$_2$-*id* NINDA.⸢MEŠ* *u** KAŠ ŠA$_3$⸣-*šu$_2$** IGI*-⸢*ḫar*⸣-*šu$_2$**-*ma** TI

ina KAŠ *ina* ^{urudu}ŠEN.TUR GIM *ra-bi-ki tara-bak* / ⸢*ina* KUŠ⸣.EDIN SUR 3 UD-*me* SAG ŠA$_3$-*šu$_2$* LAL NINDA *u* KAŠ ŠA$_3$-*šu$_2$* IGI-*šu$_2$-ma ina-eš* (STO 2: 249–250)

---

39 half a litre of *zē summati* ('pigeon droppings'), half a litre of *erišti eqli* ('sown in a field' plant),[160] ten shekels of *nikiptu* ('spurge'), ten shekels of *imbū tâmti* ('algae'), half a litre of flour from *kibtu* ('wheat'),

40 half a litre of *suluppū* ('dates'), half a litre of *billat našpi* (a kind of beerwort),[161] (and) half a litre of *isqūqu* (a type of groats)—you crush (*taḫaššal*) (and) sift (*tanappi*) these 16 ingredients[162] together,

41 you stir them like a paste (*kīma rabīki tarabbak*)[163] in high-quality beer in a small copper pot, you bandage (*taṣammid*) his epigastrium (*rēš libbi*) for three days, (and) his belly (*libbu*) will let him accept (*ušamḫaršū-ma*)[164] (different) foods[165] and beer; then he will recover (*iballuṭ*).

---

158 The correct reading of ^{šim}MAŠ is not clear, but it may be an abbreviated form of $^{\text{šim.d}}$MAŠ = Akk. *nikiptu* 'spurge'. This abbreviation could, in turn, have led to uncertainty about the original plant name, perhaps with the word ^{šim}ŠEŠ in the parallel representing a banalisation.

159 For the reading of GIG as GIB$_3$ = Akk. *kibtu* 'wheat', see Powell 1984: 57 and Marchesi 2013: 285 n. 15. In line 70 below, the correct *Auslaut* is made clear by the following BA as in GIB$_3$.BA.

160 For *erišti eqli*, see especially Campbell Thompson 1944: 65–66. The word is either spelled syllabically or with the logogram KAM, which is normally only used for the homophone of *erēšu* meaning 'to desire'. So KAM is probably used here only for its phonetic value, hence *eriš$_6$*(KAM)-*ti*.

161 See the Practical Vocabulary of Assur ln. 200 (Landsberger and Gurney 1957–1958: 330): DIDA SIG.GA = MIN (= *bi-la-tu*) *na-aš$_2$-pi*, but with both SIG and SIG$_5$ being used as the logogram for *našpu*. Following Abusch and Schwemer (2011: 469), *billatu* was probably 'a dry and crumbly substance which was used as an additional (sweetening$^?$) ingredient in the beer brewing process and also as a sort of instant-beer to be mixed with water'. For the use of *billatu* as a kind of instant-beer, see Maul 1994: 54 and 121. See also Stol 1994: 165, Powell 1994: 105–106 as well as Abusch and Schwemer 2011: 53–55.

162 Nineteen ingredients are actually included in the recipe, disagreeing with the numeral '16' in our text. Even if the two ingredients marked with GIN$_2$ are not included, we still have seventeen drugs, not sixteen.

163 For the difficult verb *rabāku* and also for the idiom *kīma rabīki tarabbak*, see Heeßel 2016: 56–57. Here we follow Küchler's (1904: 103) original suggestion of translating *rabāku* as 'zu einem Brei verrühren', since the resulting substance needs to be a dense semi-liquid mixture, so that it can be smeared on leather and applied to bandages. Some attestations seem to suggest that heating was part of the operation described by *rabāku*: see, e.g., AMT 73/1+ i 44, where the verb *tukaṣṣa* 'you let it cool' follows *tarabbak*.

164 Heeßel (2016: 55) suggests that the verb is in the second person, with the physician as the subject and apparently the belly as the object: 'du lässt ihn (seinen Bauch) Speise und Trank empfangen (*tušamḫaršu*)'. However, we suspect that the verb here is identical in form to the verb in line 26 above: 'his belly will let him accept (*ušamḫaršu*) (different) foods and beer'. As part of the concluding prognosis, the passage seems to suggest that the patient will be able to eat and drink again after the treatment is completed.

165 The addition of the plural marker MEŠ after NINDA (= Akk. *akalu* 'bread') is unusual, and the parallel omits it. We retain this marker here as a possible *lectio difficilior* in reference to the patient's ability to eat a variety of foods, signalling the renewed strength of his stomach.

42 A$_{i\,42}$ [DIŠ N]A ŠA$_3$-*šu$_2$ ik-ta-na-su-šu$_2$* ^{u2}IGI-*lim* NU *pa-tan i-kal ta-sak$_3$ ina* KAŠ* ⸢NU* *pa*-*tan** NAG*.MEŠ*-*ma**⸣ TI-*uṭ*

---

43 A$_{i\,43}$ [DIŠ K]I MIN ^{u2}IGI.NIŠ SUḪUŠ ^{u2}*šur-ne$_2$-e* NU *pa-tan* GU$_7$.⸢MEŠ⸣ SUD$_2$ *ina* KAŠ NU *pa-tan* NAG.MEŠ-*ma* TI-⸢*uṭ*⸣*

---

44 A$_{i44}$ [DIŠ] KI MIN ^{u2}*ar$_2$-zal-la* ^{u2}ḪAR.ḪAR ⸢^{šim}GUR$_2$.GUR$_2$ ^{šim}⸣x x x x NU *pa-tan* KI* ⸢MIN⸣*

---

45 A$_{i\,45}$ DIŠ KI MIN I$_3$.UDU *a-a-ar* DINGIR KI I$_3$.NUN.NA *u* ⸢MUN⸣ ḪI.ḪI NU *pa*-⸢*tan* GU$_7$⸣.MEŠ*-*ma* TI

---

†

42 If someone's belly (*libbu*) constantly binds him: he eats *imḫur-līm* ('faces a thousand' plant) on an empty stomach, (and then) you pound it, (and) he keeps drinking (*ištanattī-ma*) it in beer on an empty stomach; then he will recover (*iballuṭ*).

---

43 If DITTO, he keeps eating (*ītanakkal*) *imḫur-ešrā* ('faces twenty' plant) (and) root from *šurnû* (a plant) on an empty stomach, (and then) you pound (*tasâk*) them, (and) he keeps drinking (*ištanattī-ma*) them in beer on an empty stomach; then he will recover (*iballuṭ*).

---

44 If DITTO, DITTO (= he keeps eating) *arzallu* (a plant), *ḫašû* ('thyme'), *kukru* (an aromatic) (and) . . . on an empty stomach (then he will recover).

---

45 If DITTO, you mix (*tuballal*) fat from an *ayyar ili* ('chameleon')[166] with ghee and salt (and) he keeps eating (*ītanakkal-ma*) it on an empty stomach; then he will recover (*iballuṭ*).

---

166 Uruanna III 71 (67) makes clear that fat from an *ayyar ili* 'chameleon' (though in Uruanna, the chameleon is listed under its byname *ḫurba-billu*) is a cover term for the *adamatu* plant (Rumor 2017: 15).

46 A$_{i\,46}$ DIŠ KI MIN *kak-ku-sa-*⸢*kam*$_2$⸣ *ša*$_2$ PA.MEŠ-*šu*$_2$ DAGAL.MEŠ *ina* A GAZI⸢^{sar}⸣ SUD$_2$ *ina* KAŠ *u* LAL$_3$* SIG$_3$*-⸢*aṣ** NU* *pa**-*tan** NAG⸣*.MEŠ*-*ma** TI

---

47 A$_{i\,47}$ DIŠ KI MIN *kak**-*ku-sa**-*kam*$_2$* *ša*$_2$ PA.MEŠ*-*šu*$_2$* DAGAL*.MEŠ* *u* MUN* DIŠ*-⸢*niš*⸣* S[UD$_2$* *ina* KA]Š* *u** LAL$_3$* SIG$_3$*-⸢*aṣ** NU *pa*⸣*-*tan** NAG*.MEŠ*-⸢*ma*⸣* TI

---

48 A$_{i\,48}$ ⸢DIŠ⸣ KI* MIN* ⸢KIŠI$_{16}$*.ḪAB⸣ *ša*$_2$ PA.MEŠ-*šu*$_2$ DAGAL.MEŠ GIM LU.⸢UB$_2$^{sar} *ta*⸣-*sa-laq* ⸢NAG*.MEŠ* TI⸣

---

49 A$_{i\,49}$ [DIŠ K]I ⸢MIN⸣ SUḪUŠ* ^{giš}⸢*šu**-*še*⸣* NU *pa-tan* GU$_7$ SUD$_2$ *ina* KAŠ NU *pa-tan* N[AG x x x] x x x x ⸢TI⸣

---

46 If DITTO, you pound (*tasâk*) *kakkusakku* (a plant)[167] with wide leaves in juice from *kasû* ('tamarind'), you stir (*tamaḫḫaṣ*) it into beer and *dišpu* ('syrup'), (and) he keeps drinking (*ištanattī-ma*) (the mixture) on an empty stomach; then he will recover (*iballuṭ*).

---

47 If DITTO, you pound (*tasâk*) *kakkusakku* (a plant) with wide leaves and salt together, you stir (*tamaḫḫaṣ*) them into beer and *dišpu* ('syrup'), (and) he keeps drinking (*ištanattī-ma*) (the mixture) on an empty stomach; then he will recover (*iballuṭ*).

---

48 If DITTO, you boil *dadānu* (a spiny plant) with wide leaves like *laptu* ('turnip'),[168] (and) he keeps drinking (*ištanattī*) it; (then) he will recover (*iballuṭ*).

---

49 If DITTO, he eats (*ikkal*) root from *šūšu* ('liquorice') on an empty stomach, (and then) you pound (*tasâk*) it, (and) he drinks (*išatti*) it in beer on an empty stomach . . .; (then) he will recover (*iballuṭ*).

---

167 This plant name can be etymologized as a simple phrase, perhaps *kakkû sāku* 'pounded lentil' (S. Panayotov, personal communication, December 2020), or as a playful allusion to the term *kakku sakku* in Assurbanipal's L$_4$ inscription. Parpola (1983a: 22) assumes a connection between the medicinal plant or stone *kakkusakku* and the technical term *kakku sakku*, which he sees as either the name of a medical/exorcistic compendium or that of a concrete object with a definite shape (i.e., *kakku* 'weapon'). This theory was later refuted by Lambert (1989: 220–221); see also Livingstone 2007: 101, Lenzi 2008: 89 n. 129, 188–189, and Gabbay 2016: 177–181. Like the use of the *kasû* plant to treat *kīs libbi* in line 12 above, *kakkusakku* here may be alluding to a 'sealed and stopped up' intestinal passage that the plant is meant to open. In the cover term section of Uruanna, namely Uruanna III 17b (17), a variant lists *kakkusakku* as a cover term for the 'big *ašāgu* plant' (Rumor 2017: 7), there spelled *kak-ku-ša*$_2$-*ku*.

168 The passage looks like a quote from Šammu šikinšu, with the *laptu* ('turnip') possibly used here as an object of comparison for the leaves of the *dadānu* plant: '*dadānu* plant, the leaves of which are as wide as (those of) the *laptu*', but the description may also be concerned with the nature of the boiling: 'you boil *dadānu* plant with wide leaves, like (you boil) *laptu*'. Curiously, the homophones (or near homophones) *laptu* 'turnip' (LU.UB$_2$^{sar}) and *labtu* 'roasted barley' (ŠE.SA.A) are both used in descriptions of different types of cooking processes: the verb *salāqu* ('to boil') in GIM LU.UB$_2$⸢^{sar} *ta*⸣-*sa-laq* in our line here as opposed to the verb *qalû* ('to roast') in *ki-ma* ŠE.SA.A *ta-qal-lu* in BAM 503+ iii 7.

50 A$_{i\,50}$ [DIŠ KI MIN x x x x DI]Š*-⸢*niš*⸣* SUD$_2$* UD*-*um** ŠA$_3$-*šu*$_2$ DAB-[*šu*$_2$[169] x x x x x NU *p*]*a**-⸢*tan*⸣* NAG TI

---

51 A$_{i\,51}$ [..] x [.. KA]Š ⸢MIN⸣

ten missing lines

62 A$_{i\,62'}$ [...] ⸢A$^?$⸣*

63 A$_{i\,63'}$ [...] x

64 A$_{i\,64'}$ [...] x

65 A$_{i\,65'}$ [...] ⸢UŠ⸣

---

66 A$_{ii\,1}$ [DIŠ NA ŠA$_3$-*š*]*u*$_2$ GU$_7$-*šu*$_2$ ^{u2}ḪAR.ḪAR MUN SUD$_2$ *lu in*[*a* A *l*]*u ina* KAŠ *lu ina* GEŠTIN «EN$_2$»[170] *ana* ŠA$_3$ ŠUB-*di* NAG

---

50 If DITTO, you pound (*tasâk*) . . . together, (and) when his belly (*libbu*) seizes him (*iṣabbatūšu*) . . . he drinks (*išatti*) . . . on an empty stomach; (then) he will recover (*iballuṭ*).

---

51 . . . beer$^?$, DITTO.

ten missing lines

62 . . .

63 . . .

64 . . .

65 . . .

---

66 If someone's belly (*libbu*) causes him pain (*ikkalšu*): you pound (*tasâk*) salted *ḫašû* ('thyme'),[171] you put (*tanaddi*) it in water or beer or wine, (and) he drinks (*išatti*) it.

---

169 The use of a temporal clause like this in the middle of a line is quite unusual: if the reading is correct, we assume here that it is a construct relative with *ūm* 'day, time' as the head noun.

170 The EN$_2$ sign is slightly deformed and seems to have been mistakenly added by the scribe after the line was written, presumably as a hyper-correction, in order to complement ŠUB = Akk. *nadû* 'to put'. EN$_2$ = Akk. *šiptu* 'incantation, spell' frequently occurs later in the text alongside the verb *nadû*, particularly in constructions describing the casting of a spell, viz. *šipta tanaddi*.

171 MUN = Akk. *ṭābtu* 'salt' is possibly used here in an adjectival sense, namely 'salted *ḫašû* plant', as opposed to the next prescription, where *ḫašû* occurs on its own. For the qualification *ša ṭābti* 'salted' in medical texts, see CAD Ṭ 13–14. Note as well the phrase *e-qi-di*(*-ma*) *ša*$_{(2)}$ *la* MUN 'unsalted cheese' in AMT 6/1: 3′ and 5′.

67 A$_{ii\ 2}$ DIŠ ⸢NA⸣ ŠA$_3$-*šu*$_2$ GU$_7$-*šu*$_2$ ^{u2}ḪAR.ḪAR *lu ina* A *lu ina* KAŠ NAG[172]

---

68 A$_{ii\ 3}$ DIŠ NA ŠA$_3$-*šu*$_2$ GU$_7$-*šu*$_2$ ^{u2}*ti-ia-a-ti ina* KAŠ NAG ^{u2}IGI-*lim ina* KAŠ ^{u2}IGI.NIŠ *ina* KAŠ

69 A$_{ii\ 4}$ ^{u2}*tar-muš ina* KAŠ ^{u2}DILI *ina* KAŠ ^{u2}GAMUN.GE$_6$ *ina* KAŠ ^{u2}ḪAB *ina* KAŠ ^{u2}ḪAR.ḪAR *lu ina* KAŠ *lu ina* GEŠTIN

---

70 A$_{ii\ 5}$ DIŠ ⸢NA⸣ ŠA$_3$.MEŠ-*šu*$_2$ GU$_7$.MEŠ-*šu*$_2$ ⸢1/2⸣ SILA$_3$ ZU$_2$.LUM.MA 1/2 SILA$_3$ NIG$_2$.AR$_3$.RA GIB$_3$.BA 1/2 SILA$_3$ LAGAB MUNU$_6$

[x x x x x GU$_7$.MEŠ-*š*]*u*$_2$ NA BI DUR$_2$ GIG 1/2 SILA$_3$ ZU$_2$.LUM.M[A . . .] (AMT 57/3 rev. 4)

[. . .] ⸢NA BI DUR$_2$⸣ GIG 1/2 SILA$_3$ ZU$_2$.LUM 1/2 SILA$_3$ NIG$_2$.AR$_3$.RA GIB$_3$.BA / [x x x x] (AMT 42/2 obv. 4–5)

[x x x x x] ⸢GU$_7$.MEŠ⸣-[*šu*$_2$] 1/2 SILA$_3$ ZU$_2$.LUM.MA 1/2 SILA$_3$ NIG$_2$.AR$_3$.RA GIB$_3$.BA 1/2 SILA$_3$ [x x] (BAM 52 rev. 24)

67 If someone's belly (*libbu*) causes him pain (*ikkalšu*): he drinks (*išatti*) *ḫašû* ('thyme') in water or beer.

---

68 If someone's belly (*libbu*) causes him pain (*ikkalšu*): he drinks (*išatti*) *tīyatu* (a plant)[173] in beer, *imḫur-līm* ('faces a thousand' plant) in beer, *imḫur-ešrā* ('faces twenty' plant) in beer,

69 *tarmuš* ('lupin') in beer, *ēdu* ('lone' plant) in beer, *zibû* ('black cumin') in beer, *būšānu* ('smelly' plant) in beer (and) *ḫašû* ('thyme') in beer or wine.

---

70 If someone's internal organs (*qerbū*) cause him pain (*ikkalūšu*): you bring to a boil (*tušabšal*) half a litre of *suluppū* ('dates'), half a litre of wheat *mundu* ('groats'),[174] (and) half a litre of *buqlu* ('malt') lumps

172 The gap in lines 67–73 has been filled with the help of K 21858 + K 21905, which is a direct join to MS A. The join was identified by E. Schmidtchen in 2016. K 21858 and K 21905 were pieced together by W. G. Lambert in 1991.

173 As is the case for many Akkadian plant names, Zimmern (1917^2: 58) identifies a possible cognate of Akk. *tīyatu* in Aramaic *tiyyā/tīʾā*; see also Löw 1924: 125–126.

174 The missing measurement before GIB$_3$.BA = Akk. *kibtu* 'wheat', both in the main text and the parallels, makes clear that NIG$_2$.AR$_3$.RA GIB$_3$.BA is a single expression. Even if the exact rendering of this expression in Akkadian is unclear, *kibtu* seems to be used here in an adjectival sense, specifying a type of groats.

71 A$_{ii\ 6}$ *ina* 3 SILA$_3$ KAŠ SAG ŠEG$_6$-*šal tu-kaṣ$_3$-ṣa ta-ša$_2$-ḫal* ⸢I$_3$.GIŠ *ana* IGI ŠUB-*di*⸣ *ana* DUR$_2$-*šu$_2$* DUB-*ak*

[x x x KAŠ SA]G ŠEG$_6$-*šal tu-kaṣ$_3$-ṣa ta-ša$_2$-ḫal* I$_3$.GIŠ *ana* ⸢IGI⸣ [. . .] (AMT 57/3 rev. 5)

[x x x x x ŠEG$_6$]-⸢*šal*⸣ *tu-kaṣ$_3$-ṣa ta-ša$_2$-ḫal* I$_3$.GIŠ *ana* IGI ŠUB *ana* DUR$_2$-*šu$_2$* DUB-*ak* (AMT 42/2 obv. 5)

[. . . ŠUB-*d*]*i ana* DUR$_2$-*šu$_2$* [x x] (BAM 52 rev. 25)

---

72 A$_{ii\ 7}$ UD-*ma* LU.UB$_2$ SUM^{sar} GAMUN⸢^{sar} SUD$_2$⸣ *ina* KAŠ NAG : DIŠ KI MIN ḪI.I[S^{sa}]$^{r?}$ ⸢SUM^{sar}⸣ SUD$_2$ *ana* A ŠUB *ina* MUL$_4$ *tuš-bat* ⸢NAG⸣

73 A$_{ii\ 8}$ *iš-tu* NAG-*u$_2$* NINDA.I$_3$.⸢DE$_2$.A⸣ *ina* I$_3$.NUN.NA ⸢GU$_7$: DIŠ⸣ KI MIN ^{u2}NU.LUḪ.ḪA SUD$_2$ *ina* KAŠ NAG

74 A$_{ii\ 9}$ DIŠ KI MIN ^{u2}IGI-*lim* SUD$_2$ KI MIN : DIŠ KI MIN ⸢^{u2}⸣SIKIL SIG$_7$ GU$_7$

---

75 A$_{ii\ 10}$ DIŠ NA ŠA$_3$-*šu$_2$ ka-si-šu$_2$* SUM^{sar} SIG$_7$-*su* ^{šim}G[UR$_2$.GUR$_2$ T]EŠ$_2$.BI SUD$_2$ *ina* A SIG$_3$-*aṣ* NU *pa-tan* NAG-*šu$_2$*

76 A$_{ii\ 11}$ ZU$_2$.LUM.MA *lu ina* I$_3$.ŠAḪ [*l*]*u** ⸢*ina*⸣ I$_3$.GIŠ GU$_7$

77 A$_{ii\ 12}$ DIŠ KI MIN ^{šim}ŠE.LI BABBAR SUD$_2$ *ina* KA[Š NU *pa-tan* NAG]-⸢*ma* TI⸣

71 in three litres of high-quality beer, you let (the mixture) cool, you filter it, you add (*tanaddi*) oil,[175] (and) you pour (*tašappak*) it into his anus.

---

72 When[176] you have pounded (*tassāku*) *laptu* ('turnip'), *šūmū* ('garlic') (and) *kamūnu* ('cumin'), he drinks (*išatti*) them in beer. If DITTO, you pound *ḫassū* ('lettuce')$^?$ (and) *šūmū* ('garlic'), you put (*tanaddi*) them in water, you leave (the mixture) out overnight under the stars, (and) he drinks it.

73 After he has drunk (*ištu ištatû*) it, he eats (*ikkal*) *mersu* ('honey cake') in ghee. If DITTO, you pound *nuḫurtu* ('asafoetida'), (and) he drinks it in beer.

74 If DITTO, you pound *imḫur-līm* ('faces a thousand' plant) DITTO (= he drinks it in beer). If DITTO, he eats fresh *sikillu* ('pure' plant).

---

75 If someone's belly (*libbu*) is bound up:[177] you pound (*tasâk*) *šūmū* ('garlic') while it is fresh (and) *kukru* (an aromatic)$^?$ together, you stir (*tamaḫḫaṣ*) them into water, (and) you have him drink (*tašaqqīšu*) it on an empty stomach,

76 (and then) he eats (*ikkal*) *suluppū* ('dates') in *nāḫu* ('lard') or oil.

77 If DITTO, you pound white *kikkirânu* ('juniper seeds'), (and) he drinks (*išattī-ma*) it in beer on an empty stomach; then he will recover (*iballuṭ*).

175 In line with Maul 2019: 287, the idiom *ana* IGI ŠUB-*di* = Akk. *ana pāni tanaddi* probably describes the inclusion of oil or other semi-liquid ingredients at the final stage of the manufacturing process. This additional step may have been made necessary by the way in which the drug was administered, namely as an enema (see Böck 2009: 118, citing Geller 2005: 196–197). Although both oil and oil mixed with syrup are used in this way, in our corpus *ana pāni tanaddi* almost always co-occurs with oil alone as the added ingredient. In contrast, *ana libbi tanaddi* describes the combination of ingredients with a liquid carrier as a more integral part of the manufacturing process.

176 UD-*ma* = Akk. *enūma* 'when' rarely occurs in the therapeutic literature: in BAM 3 i 15, a long list of prescriptions for bandages is followed by UD-*ma* LAL$_2$.MEŠ *an-na-ti* LAL$_2$-*uš* (= *taṣṣanduš*) 'when you have bandaged him with these bandages', whereas the parallel in CRAN 1: 10 (BAM 480+ i 10) has EGIR *na-aṣ-ma-da-ti an-na-ti* 'after these bandages' replacing the temporal clause formed with UD-*ma*.

177 For the same symptom description, see the medical text from Hattusha KUB 37 61+ rev. 8′ (Schwemer 1998: 80–81).

78 A$_{ii\,13}$ DIŠ KI MIN ^{u2}IGI-*lim* ^{u2}IGI.NIŠ ^{u2}*tar-muš* SUḪUŠ $^{giš⌜}$NAM$^{⌝}$*.T[AR NITA$_{2}$ x x x *mal-m*]*a*-⌜*liš*⌝ ḪI.⌜ḪI⌝

79 A$_{ii\,14}$ *ina* KAŠ *tara$_{3}$-sa-an ina* MUL$_{4}$ *tuš-bat ina še-ri$_{3}$ ba-lu pa*-⌜*tan*⌝ N[AG*-*šu$_{2}$* x] *šu ša$_{2}$*[178] NU NAG-*šu$_{2}$* TI

---

80 A$_{ii\,15}$ DIŠ NA ŠA$_{3}$-*šu$_{2}$ ik-ta-na-su-šu$_{2}$* ŠA$_{3}$.MEŠ-*šu$_{2}$ ma-gal nap-ḫ*[*u*] $^{⌜u2⌝}$ḪAR.ḪAR GI DU$_{10}$.GA ^{šim}MUG

81 A$_{ii\,16}$ ^{šim}LI *ana* ŠA$_{3}$-*bi* ŠUB-*di* ŠEG$_{6}$-*šal ta-ša$_{2}$-ḫal lu ba-ḫir$_{2}$ ana* DUR$_{2}$-*šu$_{2}$* DUB-*ma* TI

---

82 A$_{ii\,17}$ DIŠ NA NINDA GU$_{7}$ KAŠ NAG-*ma i-še$_{20}$-bi* ŠA$_{3}$-*šu$_{2}$ ik-ta-na-su*-⌜*šu$_{2}$*⌝ DAB.MEŠ-*su* ŠA$_{3}$.MEŠ-*šu$_{2}$* MU$_{2}$.MU$_{2}$

83 A$_{ii\,18}$ *u i-sil* ŠA$_{3}$-*šu$_{2}$ mu-še* KIN.NIM GIG *ana* TI-*šu$_{2}$* ^{giš}*e-re-na* ^{giš}ŠUR.MIN$_{3}$ GI DU$_{10}$.GA ^{šim}BAL

†

78 If DITTO, you mix (*tuballal*) *imḫur-līm* ('faces a thousand' plant), *imḫur-ešrā* ('faces twenty' plant), *tarmuš* ('lupin'), root from male *pillû* ('mandrake'), (and) . . . in equal amounts,

79 you steep (the mixture) in beer, you leave it out overnight under the stars (and) in the morning, you have him drink (*tašaqqīšu*) it on an empty stomach, (but) you should not let him drink (*lā tašaqqīšu*) . . .; (then) he will recover (*iballuṭ*).

---

80 If someone's belly (*libbu*) constantly binds him (and) his internal organs (*qerbū*) are extremely swollen (*napḫū*): you put (*tanaddi*) *ḫašû* ('thyme'), *qanû ṭābu* ('sweet reed'), *ballukku* (an aromatic),

81 (and) *burāšu* (a kind of juniper) all together, you bring (the mixture) to a boil (*tušabšal*), you filter it, (and) while it is steaming hot (*lu baḫir*),[179] you pour (*tašappak-ma*) it into his anus; then he will recover (*iballuṭ*).

---

82 If someone eats (*ikkal*) bread (and) drinks (*išattī-ma*) beer to his satisfaction (*išebbi*),[180] but then his belly (*libbu*) constantly binds (and) seizes him (*iṣṣanabbassu*), his internal organs (*qerbū*) are swollen (*napḫū*),

83 and he is constipated, he suffers (*maruṣ*) from a belly that always seeks the morning meal (*naptan šēri*):[181] in order to heal him (*ana bulluṭīšu*), *erēnu* ('cedar'), *šurmēnu* ('cypress'), *qanû ṭābu* ('sweet reed'), *ballukku* (an aromatic),

---

178 The reading of these signs is uncertain, but they may represent a unique orthography for Akk. *šūšu* 'liquorice', viz. [^{giš}]*šu-ša$_{2}$*, meaning that the patient was not allowed to consume this plant for a time. An alternative reading is offered by Küchler (1904: 6), who takes the sign sequence *šu-ša$_{2}$-nu* as a designation of Akk. *šuššān* ('one third'), whereas Cadelli (2000: 76 and 97) suggests reading ŠU GAR-*nu*, with GAR-*nu* for Akk. *šaknu* 'which is placed in . . .'.

179 For a discussion of *buḫḫuru* 'to heat', including forms like *baḫru*, see MSL 10 p. 24. In line with Landsberger, this verb may describe 'to fume', or better 'to steam' rather than simply 'to be hot'. See also CAD B 28, where *baḫru* is translated with 'as hot as can be tolerated'. For further discussion, see Labat and Tournay 1945–1946: 119.

180 The form literally means that the patient keeps eating and drinking until 'he becomes sated', but most probably over-indulging is meant here. For this verb, see also Cadelli 2019: 5 with n. 12.

181 See CAD E 329–330, with KIN.NIM as a logogram for Akk. *šēru* 'morning'. As a possible descriptive term for the belly, *mu-še* KIN.NIM could also be taken as a D-stem participle of *še'û* 'to look for' followed by KIN.NIM for Akk. *naptan šēri* as in Igituh short version 129 (CAD N/1 319). However, our translation here must remain provisional.

84 A$_{ii\ 19}$ ^{šim}GIR$_2$ ^{u2}ḪAR.ḪAR 5 U$_2$.ḪI.A ŠEŠ TEŠ$_2$.BI *ta-ka-sim ana* KAŠ ŠUB-*di* ŠEG$_6$-*šal*

85 A$_{ii\ 20}$ *ta-ša$_2$-ḫal* LAL$_3$ *u* I$_3$ *ḫal-ṣa ana* ŠA$_3$ ŠUB-*di lu ba-ḫi-ir ana* KUŠ *maš-qe$_2$-ti te-si-ip ana* DUR$_2$-*šu$_2$* DUB ⸢TI⸣

---

86 A$_{ii\ 21}$ [EN$_2$ ŠA$_3$.MEŠ *i*]*t-*⸢*ta*⸣*-nap-ša$_2$-ru zi-ir kar-*⸢*šu$_2$*⸣* ŠA$_3$ NIGIN *ku-uṣ-*⸢*ṣu-ru-u$_2$*$^?$⸣ x x [x][182]

87 A$_{ii\ 22}$ x [x x] x x *ek-le-ta ki-i me-e ḫi-ri-ti a-la-pa-a na-du-u$_2$* IGI.MEŠ-*šu$_2$*

†

84 *asu* ('myrtle'), (and) *ḫašû* ('thyme')—you chop up these five ingredients[183] all together, you put (*tanaddi*) them in beer, you bring (the mixture) to a boil (*tušabšal*),

85 you filter it, you put (*tanaddi*) *dišpu* ('syrup') and pressed oil in it, (and) while it is steaming hot, you skim it off (*tessip*)[184] into a leather (bag) for potions,[185] you pour (*tašappak*) it into his anus; (then) he will recover (*iballuṭ*).

---

86 Incantation: 'The internal organs (*qerbū*)$^?$ are constantly loosened, with the stomach (*karšu*) twisted (and) the convoluted intestines (*irrū sāḫirūtu*)[186] completely knotted up . . .

87 . . . his face is covered with darkness in the same way that water in an irrigation ditch (is covered) with algae,

---

182 Lines 86–92 are edited by Collins (1999: 166–168) as Belly 25. For a more recent discussion of the passage, see Böck 2014a: 104–106, with her emendation of the first verb as [*i*]*t-*⸢*ta*⸣*-nap-ḫa*$^!$*-ru* '(The intestines are persistently) massed together'.

183 Six drugs are actually listed in lines 83–85, although the text recognizes only five: perhaps *erēnu* and *šurmēnu* were mistakenly conflated when the editor counted up the ingredients.

184 On the basis of similar procedures in the perfume making texts (see Ebeling 1949: 405 ln. 24 and 407 ln. 22), we suggest that *esēpu* may describe a procedure in which syrup and oil are added to a mixture in order to produce a suspension of ingredients on the surface of the liquid, and this suspension was then skimmed off into a leather pouch. For an analogous procedure, see CRAN 1: 10–11 (BAM 480+ i 10–11) (. . .) 10 GIN$_2$ ZA$_3$.ḪI.LI *ša$_2$* KA ⸢*ur-ṣi*⸣ (. . .) *ina* NINDA *is-sip$_3$-ma* GU$_7$ '(. . .) he scoops up / skims off ten shekels of *saḫlû* ('cress') from the mouth of a mortar (. . .) into a loaf of bread, and then he eats it'.

185 The translation 'leather enema bag' (CAD E 331, M/1 384 and Cadelli 2000: 115) is based almost exclusively on this passage and STO 5: 202′–203′. A more parsimonious interpretation might be to separate *mašku* from *mašqītu* as in *ana maški mašqêti tessip* 'you skim it off in a leather (bag) for potions', with the orthography reflecting vowel contraction of the plural form *mašqiātu*.

186 Cadelli (2000: 97) and Collins (1999: 166) take ŠA$_3$.NIGIN as a logogram for Akk. *tīrānu* 'coils of the intestine', but this term only seems to be used in extispicy texts. In line with STO 1: 214, we read the form ŠA$_3$ NIGIN as Akk. *irrū sāḫirūtu* 'convoluted intestines'.

88 A$_{ii\,23}$ ⸢*ša*⸣-[*ar* E]DIN[187] *e-di-ip na-di*[188] *i-ta-naq-qi*$_2$ ŠU EDIN *ma-la-a* IGI.MEŠ-*šu*$_2$[189]

89 A$_{ii\,24}$ *e-t*[*a-n*]*a-ba-la* ⸢*ša-pa*⸣-*tu-šu*$_2$ *i-ta-na-pa-aṣ ki-ma* KU$_6$.MEŠ *it-ta-nak-bir ki-ma* MUŠ

90 A$_{ii\,25}$ *e-m*[*ur-m*]*a* ^{d}*gu-la na-di-na-at ba-la-ṭi* NAM.LU$_2$.U$_{18}$.LU *ina* E$_2$ ^{d}*asal-lu*$_2$-*ḫi u*$_2$-*bil eṭ-lu*

91 A$_{ii\,26}$ ⸢^{d}⸣A[MAR*.UT]U*[190] *re-me*$_2$-*nu-u ip-pa-lis-su-ma ge-ša-ma* TI-*uṭ eṭ-lu*

92 A$_{ii\,27}$ *šum*$_2$-*ma* ⸢IM⸣* *ina* DUR$_2$ *lu-ṣi šum*$_2$-*ma gi-ša-tu ina nap-ša*$_2$-*ti li-še-ṣi* TU$_6$ EN$_2$

---

88 blown up (and) thrown down by the wind of the steppe, he constantly sheds (tears), his eyes are filled with the "hand of the steppe",[191]

89 his lips are constantly parched, he keeps flopping around like fish (and) continually puffs himself up like a snake.

90 Gula, the provider of good health for mankind, saw this and brought the young man into the temple of Asalluḫi (= Marduk),

91 merciful Marduk looked upon him, and then (said): 'Belch (*gešâm-ma*) and feel better (*buluṭ*), young man!'

92 If there is flatulence (lit. wind), may it go out through the anus! If there is a belch, may he let it out through the throat!' Incantation-formula.

---

187 The reading *ša-ar* EDIN (van der Toorn 1985: 69 with n. 174) is supported by its co-occurrence with the stative form of *edēpu*, which occurs several times alongside *šāru* in the sense of 'wind blows into (somebody)' or 'to be inflated by wind' (CAD E 28). The phrase is also attested in STO 2: 175 and, as a rubric, in KAR 44 obv. 13: *e-dip* IM (Frahm 2018: 10 n. 3). In the first tablet of the zi.pa$_3$-incantations (ASKT 11+ ii 70), a similar phrase is found in connection with black magic: im nu.gi$_4$ eden.na.ke$_4$: *ša*$_2$-*ar ṣe-ri*$_3$ *la ed-pu* (Borger 1969: 6 and Steinert 2012: 321).

188 The form here is probably a stative from the verb *nadû* ('thrown down'), but it could likewise point to Akk. *nādu* 'waterskin'; if so, the genitive case is problematic. For this alternative rendering, see Collins 1999: 167, who translates 'he constantly pours out (water from) a waterskin as a libation for it', treating ŠU of ŠU EDIN as a dative suffix following the verb *i-ta-naq-qi*$_2$-.

189 Our text may be closer to the original since IGI.MEŠ is read in two different ways, first as a masculine plural *pānū* 'face' in line 87 and then as a feminine plural *īnātu* 'eyes' in line 88, in each line preceded by a stative in the appropriate gender and number (Cadelli 2000: 98 and n. 41). The metaphor is reinterpreted in line with the overall topic in the EYES treatise: GIM A.MEŠ *ša*$_2$ *a-ga-la-pe-e a-la-pa-a* ŠUB-*a* 'they (= the eyes) are spotted like the (muddy) water of a lagoon with algae' (BAM 10 pp. 81–82 and 261).

190 The reading ^{d}⸢IDIM⸣ (Cadelli 2000: 77, Collins 2000: 166 and Böck 2014a: 105) is less likely.

191 Lines 88–89 keep alluding to dryness, hence the phrase 'hand of the steppe' which is analogous to *ša-ar* EDIN at the beginning of the line and possibly works as a poetic representation of sand or rheum. The 'hand of the steppe' also occurs in the Middle Babylonian diagnostic text MDP 57 11 iii 7: ŠU EDIN *u*$_3$ *ba-ma-a-ti* 'hand of the steppe and the open country'. For the word pair 'steppe' and 'open country', but with *bēltu* 'lady' instead of ŠU = Akk. *qātu* 'hand', see Maqlû IV 22 (Abusch 2016: 117) and Šurpu VII 67–68 (Reiner 1958: 38).

93 A$_{ii\ 28}$ K[A.INI]M.MA *ana ki-is* ŠA$_3$ ŠID-*nu*

---

94 A$_{ii\ 29}$ ⌜DIŠ⌝ [NA *e-t*]*a-*⌜*na*⌝**-ša$_2$-aš$_2$*[192] NINDA *u* KAŠ *la i-maḫ-ḫar* MAŠ.SILA$_3$.MIN-*šu*$_2$ GU$_7$.MEŠ-*šu*$_2$

DIŠ [NA Š]A$_3$-*šu*$_2$ *e-ta-na-ša$_2$-aš-ma* NINDA *u* KAŠ SAG *la i-maḫ-ḫar* MAŠ.SILA$_3$.MEŠ-*šu*$_2$ GU$_7$.MEŠ-*šu*$_2$ (STO 2: 151)

95 A$_{ii\ 30}$ [SAG.DU-*su g*]*i-na-a* LAL I$_3$.NUN.NA GU$_7$ UD.7.KAM$_2$ SUM^{sar} SUM.SIKIL^{sar} GA.RAŠ^{sar} NU GU$_7$

SAG.DU-*su gi-na-a* LAL [x x x] / U[D.7.KA]M$_2$ SUM^{sar} SUM.SIKIL^{sar} GA.RAŠ^{sar} NU GU$_7$ (STO 2: 151–152)

96 A$_{ii\ 31}$ [*ina* A ^{giš}ŠE.NU] RA.MEŠ-*aṣ* NUMUN ^{u2}UKUŠ$_2$.ḪAB NUMUN ^{u2}⌜ḪAR.ḪAR⌝ SUD$_2$ *ina* KAŠ NAG-*ma* TI

ina A ^{giš}ŠE.NU RA.MEŠ NUMUN ^{u2}UKUŠ$_2$.ḪAB NUMUN ^{u2}ḪAR.ḪAR *ina* KAŠ N[AG-*ma* TI] (STO 2: 152)

---

93 An invocation for gastric constriction (*kīs libbi*). You recite (*tamannu*) it.

---

94 If someone$^{?}$ is continually distressed, does not accept bread and beer, (and) his shoulder blades cause him pain (*ikkalūšu*),

95 he keeps his head bandaged (*ginâ iṣammid*),[193] he is willing to eat (*ikkal*) ghee, (but) for seven days he would not eat *šūmū* ('garlic'), *šamaškillu* ('onion'), or *karašu* ('leek'):[194]

96 he keeps bathing (*irtanaḫḫaṣ*) in juice from *šunû* ('chaste tree'), you pound (*tasâk*) seed from *irrû* ('cucumber')[195] (and) seed from *ḫašû* ('thyme'), (and) he drinks (*išattī-ma*) them in beer; then he will recover.

---

192 There is not enough space at the beginning of the line to accommodate the full introductory phrase in the parallel STO 2: 151. According to Cadelli (2000: 77), the small space in the break precludes the possibility of a NA sign before ŠA$_3$-*šu*$_2$, but it is more likely, given these space considerations, that only NA was in the break. Moreover, the verb *ašāšu* only occasionally co-occurs with *libbu*. For the rare idiom *libbašu ītanaššaš*, see STO 2: 151.

193 The adverb *ginâ* normally means 'constantly, usually', qualifying here the state of being bandaged, viz. 'he keeps his head bandaged', rather than the act of bandaging. An on-going act of bandaging, viz. 'he keeps bandaging his head', is found in BAM 571 ii′ 21′, where LAL$_2$.MEŠ-*su* stands for a Gtn-stem of *ṣamādu*.

194 The second half of line 95 comes directly out of the hemerological tradition (Livingstone 2014: 168). These hemerological elements are situated between obvious symptom descriptions and clear therapeutic treatments, so it is difficult to know whether these elements belong to the symptomatology or the therapy. We take it as part of the symptomatology because of the psychological character of the verb *ašāšu* 'to be distressed', which may indicate that the patient was adhering, perhaps in an obsessive way, to a hemerological practice. It is also possible, however, that the actions in line 95 are part of the therapeutic procedure, similar to STO 2: 107.

195 For *irrû*, identified as wild melon, see Stol 1987: 85.

97 A$_{\text{ii 32}}$ [DIŠ KI MIN x x x NI]G$_2$*.⌜SILA$_{11}$⌝.GA$_2$ ḪAD$_2$.A SUD$_2$ *ina* KAŠ $^{\text{lu2}}$KURUN$_2$.NA NAG NUMUN $^{\text{u2}}$UKUŠ$_2$.ḪAB $_{\text{: NUMUN šimLI}}$ NUMUN ^{giš}ŠE.NU SUD$_2$ *ina* KAŠ NAG

---

98 A$_{\text{ii 33}}$ [DI]Š ⌜NA *ki-is*⌝ ŠA$_3$ GIG ⌜*ana*⌝ *ki-is* ŠA$_3$ ⌜KUD⌝-*si* $^{\text{u2}}$IGI-*lim* $^{\text{u2}}$IGI.NIŠ $_{\text{(eras.)}}$[196] $^{\text{u2}}$*tar-muš* $_{\text{: ⌜u2tar-muš}_8\text{⌝}}$[197]

[x x x x x x *ana ki-i*]*s* ŠA$_3$-*bi* KUD-*si* $^{\text{u2}}$⌜IGI-*lim*⌝ / [x x x x x x] (BAM 564 iii 2′–3′)

99 A$_{\text{ii 34}}$ ⌜$^{\text{u2}}$⌝KUR.RA SUD$_2$ *ina* I$_3$ *u* KAŠ ⌜NAG⌝

⌜$^{\text{u2}}$⌝KUR.KUR SUD$_2$ / [x x x x x] (BAM 564 iii 3′–4′)

---

100 A$_{\text{ii 35}}$ x x x ⌜*ina* KAŠ⌝ NAG PEŠ$_2$.SILA$_3$.GAZ[198] *ša$_2$-bu-la* GU$_7$

[x] x SUD$_2$ *ina* KAŠ SAG NAG / [x x x *ša$_2$-b*]*u-la* GU$_7$ (BAM 564 iii 4′–5′)

101 A$_{\text{ii 36}}$ [x x x] ⌜$^{\text{u2}}$⌝*kak-ku-sak-ku ša$_2$* PA.MEŠ-*šu$_2$* DAGAL.MEŠ $^{\text{u2}}$ḪAB $^{\text{u2}}$IGI-*lim* SUD$_2$

97 If DITTO, you dry (*tubbal*) (and) pound (*tasâk*) . . . (and) dough, (and) he drinks (*išatti*) them in brewer's beer. You pound seed from *irrû* ('cucumber') (gloss: seed from *burāšu*) (and) seed from *šunû* ('chaste tree'), (and) he drinks them in beer.

---

98 If someone suffers (*maruṣ*) from gastric constriction (*kīs libbi*): in order to stop the gastric constriction, you pound (*tasâk*) *imḫur-līm* ('faces a thousand' plant), *imḫur-ešrā* ('faces twenty' plant), *tarmuš* ('lupin'),

99 (and) *nīnû* ('mint'), (and) he drinks (*išatti*) them in oil and beer.

---

100 He drinks (*išatti*) . . . in beer, (and) he eats (*ikkal*) dried *ḫulû* ('shrew').

101 You pound (*tasâk*) . . . *kakkusakku* (a plant) with wide leaves, *būšānu* ('smelly' plant) (and) *imḫur-līm* ('faces a thousand' plant),

196 There are faint traces of a gloss with signs of intentional erasure, although a few signs are still partly legible: ⌜NUMUN $^{\text{u2}}$x⌝ (cf. Küchler 1904: pl. 2 ln. 34; Bácskay 2021a: 55–56). The gloss was presumably erased because it was deemed inconsistent to offer part of a plant as an alternative remedy, when the main text instructs us to use the whole plant. For another erased gloss on $^{\text{u2}}$IGI.NIŠ, see STO 3: 248.

197 The gap in lines 98–100 has been filled with the help of K 22170, which is a direct join to MS A. The join was identified by Zs. Földi in 2020.

198 CAD H 231 takes the SILA$_3$ and GAZ signs in this orthography as part of a single logogram for the Akkadian *ḫulû* (a type of rodent). GAZ presumably indicates that the mouse in question has already been pre-processed into an ingredient. The cover term section of Uruanna, namely Uruanna III 6 (6), equates PEŠ$_2$.SILA$_3$.GAZ *ša$_2$* GIŠ.GI with *šumuttu* 'beetroot' (Rumor 2017: 4), but there is no indication that we have this plant here.

102 A$_{ii\ 37}$ [*ina* I$_3$].⸢KUR.RA⸣ $_{:\ I_3\ SIKIL}$ NAG MUN *ina* KAŠ NAG MUN *ina* A NU *pa-tan* NAG-*ma ina-eš*

---

103 A$_{ii\ 38}$ [DIŠ N]A ⸢ŠA$_3$⸣-*bi* ŠA$_3$-*bi* GU$_3$.GU$_3$-*si*[199] ^{u2}*ur$_2$-ne$_2$-e* ^{u2}ḪAR.ḪAR ^{u2}*ti-ia-ta$_5$*
104 A$_{ii\ 39}$ ⸢^{u2}NU⸣.LUḪ.ḪA ^{u2}KUR.RA *saḫ-le$_2$-e* ^{u2}*tar-muš$_8$* ⸢^{u2}⸣IGI-*lim* ^{u2}IGI.NIŠ ^{u2}*ak-tam*
105 A$_{ii\ 40}$ ⸢^{u2}*IN*.NU⸣*.UŠ ⸢^{giš}ŠINIG 12 U$_2$.ḪI.A⸣ ŠEŠ *ba-lu pa-tan ina* KAŠ NAG.MEŠ

---

106 A$_{ii\ 41}$ DIŠ NA ŠA$_3$-*šu$_2$ ik-ta-⸢na*-ar*⸣* PA* ^{giš}ŠINIG ^{u2}IN.NU.UŠ ⸢GIŠ BUR$_2$⸣ SUD$_2$ *ina* KAŠ NU *pa-tan* NAG-*ma ina-eš*

---

102 (and) he drinks them in *napṭû* ('mountain oil')[200] (gloss: pure oil). He drinks salt in beer (and) he drinks (*išattī-ma*) salt in water on an empty stomach; then he will get well.

---

103 If someone constantly cries out (*ištanassi*), 'My belly, my belly!': *urnû* (a kind of mint), *ḫašû* ('thyme'), *tīyatu* (a plant),
104 *nuḫurtu* ('asafoetida'), *nīnû* ('mint'), *saḫlû* ('cress'), *tarmuš* ('lupin'), *imḫur-līm* ('faces a thousand' plant), *imḫur-ešrā* ('faces twenty' plant), *aktam* (a plant),
105 *maštakal* ('soapwort'), (and) *bīnu* ('tamarisk')—he keeps drinking (*ištanatti*) these twelve ingredients in beer on an empty stomach.

---

106 If someone continually rubs (*iktanâr*)[201] his belly (*libbu*): you pound (*tasâk*) leaves from *bīnu* ('tamarisk'), *maštakal* ('soapwort'), (and) *iṣ pišri* ('conjurer's tool' plant),[202] (and) he drinks (*išattī-ma*) them in beer on an empty stomach; then he will get well.

---

199 The same symptom is also recorded in the Diagnostic Handbook: see Sagig 26: 64′ and 66′ (Heeßel 2000: 284).

200 Traditionally understood as the Akkadian word for 'naphtha', which does not make much sense in this context, particularly in light of the physiological effects that the consumption of naphtha can have. The orthography might suggest it was oil from the mountains. For an analogous medical ingredient, see MUN KUR-*i* 'mountain salt' in line 31 above.

201 Based on the theme vowel, the form can only be *kâru* in the sense of 'to rub', not 'to be depressed' (Cadelli 2000: 99 n. 48), presumably used here to depict a patient with a stomach ache who continuously rubs their belly.

202 The term GIŠ BUR$_2$ = Akk. *iṣ pišri* 'wood of release' refers to a ceremonial mace or conjurer's tool that also lends its name to a plant. With BUR$_2$ = Akk. *pašāru* meaning 'to release, free', this plant must have been particularly appealing for 'loosening' constrictions within the intestines. The evidence from Uruanna II 179 suggests a connection with *terinnu* 'pinecone' (CAD T 355); see also the anti-witchcraft text RIAA 312 iii 9′, with parallels, listing the 'wood of release of the *nadītu*-priestesses' alongside the 'cone (*terinnatu*) of the *qadištu*-votaries' (Abusch and Schwemer 2011: 342 ln. 111″). For a possible difference between the lexemes *terinnu* and *terinnatu*, see Abusch and Schwemer 2009: 76.

107 A$_{\text{ii 42}}$ SUḪUŠ ^{giš}*šu-ši* SUḪUŠ ^{giš}*NAM*.TAR NITA$_{2}$ $^{\text{u2}}$*tar-muš*$_{8}$ $^{\text{u2}}$IGI-*lim* $^{\text{u2}}$IGI.NIŠ $^{\text{u2}}$IN$_{6}$.UŠ$_{2}$ NUMUN $^{\text{u2}}$IN$_{6}$.U[Š$_{2}$]

———————— [203]

108 A$_{\text{ii 43}}$ ⸢7 U$_{2}$⸣.ḪI.A *ki-is* ŠA$_{3}$*-bi ina* KAŠ N[AG]

————————

109 A$_{\text{ii 44}}$ ⸢1⸣* GIN$_{2}$* MUN* *eme*-sal*-li*$_{3}$ ⸢^{šim}⸣[GUR$_{2}$.GUR$_{2}$ ^{ši}]^{m}LI DIŠ-*niš* GAZ [SIM]

110 A$_{\text{ii 45}}$ *ina* KAŠ ŠEG$_{6}$*-šal* [x x *ana* Š]A$_{3}$ ⸢ŠUB-*di*⸣ *ana* DUR$_{2}$*-šu*$_{2}$ D[UB-*ak*]

————————

111 A$_{\text{ii 46}}$ EN$_{2}$ ⸢*mi*⸣*-na-a ma-lu-u*$_{2}$ ⸢*lib-bu*⸣-[*ka mi-na-a ma-lu*]-⸢*u*$_{2}$⸣ *lib*-⸢*bu*⸣-[*ka*][204]

[x x] ⸢mu la$^{?}$⸣ x [. . .] (AMT 45/5+ ii 1′)

[. . .] x x [. . .] (BAM 509 i′ 1′)

[. . . ŠA$_{3}$.MEŠ]-⸢*ka*⸣ / [. . . ŠA$_{3}$.ME]Š-*ka* (BAM 489+ ii 1′–2′)

EN$_{2}$ *mi-na-a* «*la*» *mal-lu-u* «aš» ŠA$_{3}$*-bu-ka* [. . .] (STT 252: 16)

112 A$_{\text{ii 47}}$ x x x ^{d}x x ⸢*lib-bu*⸣-[*ka man-nu lu-uš-pu*]*r* ⸢*ana gu-gal*[205] *lib-bi*⸣-[*ka*][206]

[*man*]-⸢*nu*⸣ *lu-uš-pur* ⸢*ana*⸣ x x x [x x x] (AMT 45/5+ ii 2′)

[. . .] *a-na* GU$_{2}$.GAL [x x x] (BAM 509 i′ 2′)

[. . .] ⸢ŠA$_{3}$⸣.MEŠ-*ka* / [. . .] ⸢*ana* GU$_{2}$.GAL *ina*⸣ ŠA$_{3}$*-bi-ka* (BAM 489+ ii 3′–4′)

x x x x / ŠA$_{3}$-⸢*bu-ka*⸣ *man-nu liš*-⸢*pur*$^{?}$⸣ «ru» *a-na* GU$_{2}$.GAL [. . .] (STT 252: 16-17)

†

107 Root from *šūšu* ('liquorice'), root from male *pillû* ('mandrake'), *tarmuš* ('lupin'), *imḫur-līm* ('faces a thousand' plant) *imḫur-ešrā* ('faces twenty' plant), *maštakal* ('soapwort'), (and) seed from *maštakal* ('soapwort').

————————

108 Seven ingredients for gastric constriction (*kīs libbi*)—he drinks (*išatti*) them in beer.

————————

109 You crush (*taḫaššal*) (and) sift (*tanappi*)$^{?}$ one shekel of *emesallu* salt, *kukru* (an aromatic),$^{?}$ (and) *burāšu* (a kind of juniper) together,

110 you bring them to a boil (*tušabšal*) in beer, you put (*tanaddi*) . . . in (the mixture), (and) you pour (*tašappak*) it into his anus.

————————

111 Incantation: 'What are your entrails (*libbū*) filled with? What are your entrails filled with?

112 . . . your entrails. Whom shall I send to the canal inspector of (var. in) your entrails?

---

203 This horizontal ruling seems to be misplaced since lines 107–108 represent a single prescription (Cadelli 2000: 99 n. 50): this type of editorial misstep may suggest that the compositional process was still underway.

204 Lines 111–113 are edited by Collins (1999: 134–137) as Belly 9. Note that the fragment BAM 577 has since been joined to MS A.

205 There seems to be some consistency in rendering the Akkadian word *gugallu* 'canal inspector' with the sign GU$_{2}$ as a frozen orthography, while the syllabic spelling in MS A is much less common (CAD G 121–122).

206 Lines 112–121 can partially be filled with the help of the fragment BAM 577, a direct joint to MS A first suggested by Köcher (1980: xxviii–xxix). The physical contact between the pertinent pieces was confirmed by M. Geller in 2007.

113 A$_{ii\ 48}$ [*liš-ša*$_2$]-⸢*a*⸣ [.. *l*]*i-pat-ta-a* ID$_2$.ME[Š]

[*l*]*i-ša*$_2$*-a* ^{giš}MAR.MEŠ *ša*$_2$ KUG.BABBAR *gi-dim-me-ti ša*$_2$ KUG.SIG$_{17}$ / ⸢*li*⸣*-pat-ta-a* ID$_2$.MEŠ (AMT 45/5+ ii 3′–4′)

[. . .] KUG.BABBAR *gi-dim-me-e-ti* [x x x] / [. . .] ID$_2$.MEŠ (BAM 509 i′ 3′–4′)

⸢*liš*⸣*-ša*$_2$*-a* ^{giš}MAR.⸢MEŠ⸣ *ša*$_2$ KUG.BABBAR *u ki-din-ne*$_2$*-e ša*$_2$ KUG.SIG$_{17}$ / *li-pat-ta-a* ID$_2$.MEŠ (BAM 489+ ii 5′–6′)

[x x x ^{gi}]^{š}⸢MAR⸣.MEŠ / *ša* KUG.BABBAR *kid*$^!$(ŠA$_3$)*-di-me-ni ša*$_2$ KUG.⸢SIG$_{17}$⸣ *lip-pa-tu-*⸢*u*$_2^?$⸣ [x x] (STT 252: 17–18)

114 A$_{ii\ 49}$ [.. *li-par-ši-d*]*u-ma li-ṣu-ni zu-u*$_2$-⸢*šu*$_2$⸣

li-pat-ta-a a-tap-pa-a-ti / [*l*]*i-par-ši-du-u*$_2$*-ni lu-ṣu-u*$_2$*-ni zu-šu*$_2$ (AMT 45/5+ ii 4′–5′)

li-pat-ta-a ⸢*a*⸣-[*tap-pa-a-ti*] / [*l*]*i*-⸢*par*⸣*-ši-du-ni lu-ṣu-u*$_2$*-ni zu*-⸢*u*$_2$⸣-[*šu*$_2$] (BAM 509 i′ 4′–5′)

li-pat-ta-a a-tap-pa-ti / *li-par-ši-du-ni lu-ṣu-u*$_2$*-ni zu-u*$_2$*-šu* (BAM 489+ ii 6′–7′)

[*lip-pa-t*]*u-u* «u$_2$» / *a-tap-pa-a-nu lu-ṣi-i* ⸢*zum*⸣*-mu-u* (STT 252: 18–19)

115 A$_{ii\ 50}$ [.. *l*]*i-mur* EN$_2$ *ul ia-tu-un*

a-šam-šu-tu$_4$ *ša*$_2$ ŠA$_3$*-bi-šu* / [*li-ṣa-a*]*m-ma* ^{d}UTU *li-mur* EN$_2$ *ul ia-tu-un* (AMT 45/5+ ii 6′–7′)

[*a-ša*]*m-šu-tu*$_4$ *ša*$_2$ ŠA$_3$*-bi-šu*$_2$ *li-ṣa-am-ma* ^{d}UTU *li*-⸢*mur*⸣ / [EN$_2$ *u*]*l ia*-⸢*ut*⸣*-tu-un* (BAM 509 i′ 6′–7′)

a-⸢*šam*⸣*-šu-tu* ⸢*ša*$_2$ ŠA$_3$⸣-[*bi-š*]*u*$_2$ *li-ṣa-am-ma* ^{d}UTU *li-mur* / ⸢EN$_2$⸣ *ul ia-tu-un* (BAM 489+ ii 8′–9′)

ša$_2^!$(A) ŠA$_3$*-bi*-[*šu*$_2$] DINGIR-*šu*$_2$ / ^{d}UTU *li*$^?$*-mur-šu* EN$_2$ ⸢*ul*⸣ *ia-tan*^{an}*-ni* (STT 252: 19–20)

116 A$_{ii\ 51}$ [..] ⸢^{d}⸣*gu-la* TI.LA[207] *qiš-ta*$_5$ TI-*e* EN$_2$

[EN$_2$ ^{d}]⸢*asal*⸣*-lu*$_2$*-ḫi* ME$^!$(AN).ME DINGIR.ME ŠUB-*ma ana-ku aš*$_2$*-ši* / [x x x TI.L]A-⸢*ma*⸣ NIG$_2$.BA-*ki* TI-*i* TU$_6$ EN$_2$ (AMT 45/5+ ii 8′–9′)

EN$_2$ ^{d}*asal-lu*$_2$*-ḫi u* ^{d}*gu-la* / [x x] x *id-di-ma a-na-ku aš*$_2$*-ši* / [^{d}*gu-l*]*a* TI.LA-*ma* NIG$_2$.BA-*ki le-qe*$_2$*-e* TU$_6$ EN$_2$ (BAM 509 i′ 7′–9′)

⸢EN$_2$⸣ [^{d}*as*]*al-lu*$_2$*-ḫi* MAŠ.MAŠ DINGIR.MEŠ ŠUB-*ma ana-ku aš*$_2$*-ši* / ⸢^{d}⸣*gu-la* TI.LA-*ma* ⸢NIG$_2$⸣.BA-*ki* TI-*i* EN$_2$ (BAM 489+ ii 9′–10′)

KI MIN (STT 252: 20)

---

113 May they bear shovels of silver (and) spades of gold! May they open up the waterways!

114 May they open up the canals so that his excrement can escape and come out,

115 so that the whirlwind in his innards can come out and see the sun (var. his god Šamaš). The incantation is not mine,

116 it is the incantation of Asalluḫi (var. and Gula), the exorcist of the gods. He cast it, and I picked it up. O Gula, cure him (and) accept the (var. your) payment!’[208] Incantation.

---

207 The conjunction *-ma* is omitted in the main text, presumably due to haplography based on the right side of LA. The conjunction may also have been dropped because it occurs between two imperatives.

208 As Böck (2014a: 114) has reiterated, based largely on Geller 2010: 93–94, the formula *Gula bulluṭī-ma qīštīki leqî* may refer to the fee the physician received, but it could also literally refer to an *ex voto* offering left at the temple of Gula.

117 A$_{ii\ 52}$ [.. G]U$_7$-*ia* ŠA$_3$-*bi* KI.SIKIL *ana* GAZ-*ia*[209]

[x x x ŠA$_3$-*b*]*u e-ki-a-am tal-lak* / [. . . GU$_7$-*i*]*a* ⸢ŠA$_3$⸣-*bi* KI.SIKIL *a-na* GAZ-*ia* (BAM 509 i′ 10′–11′)

EN$_2$ ŠA$_3$-⸢*bu*⸣ ŠA$_3$-*bu e-ka-a* ⸢*ta*⸣-^{la}*lak* ŠA$_3$-*bi* GURUŠ *ina* «*aš*» ⸢GU$_7$⸣-*ka* / ŠA$_3$-[*bi*] ⸢KI⸣.SIKIL *a-na ḫa-pi-*⸢*ka*⸣ (STT 252: 21–22)

118 A$_{ii\ 53}$ [.. Š]A$_3$-*bi* GUD *ina u$_2$-re-e li-kul*

[. . . ŠA$_3$-*b*]*i* KI.SIKIL NU ⸢GAZ⸣ / [. . .] (BAM 509 i′ 12′–13′)

ŠA$_3$-*bi* GURUŠ *la ta-*⸢*kal*⸣ / ŠA$_3$-*bi* KI.SIKIL *la* ⸢*ta-ḫa-pi*⸣ *a-kul* ŠA$_3$ GUD *a-na* ⸢*tar*⸣*-ba-ṣu* (STT 252: 22–23)

119 A$_{ii\ 54}$ [.. Š]A$_3$-*bi* ŠAḪ *ina a-sur-re-*⸢*e*⸣

[x x] x x [. . .] (K 13368: 1′)

[ŠA$_3$-*b*]*i* UDU.NITA$_2$ [x x x x] / [. . .] x x [. . .] (BAM 509 i′ 13′–14′)

ŠA$_3$-*bi* UDU.NITA$_2$ *a-na su*$^{!}$(ŠU)-*pu-ru* / ŠA$_3$-*bi* ŠAḪ *a-na a-*⸢*sur*⸣-<*re*>-⸢*e*⸣ (STT 252: 24–25)

120 A$_{ii\ 55}$ [.. ^{d}*a-sa*]*l-luḫ*[210] *u* ^{d}*gu-*[*la*]

⸢*ša*$^{?}$⸣ DU$_{11}$.GA ⸢ŠA$_3$⸣-*b*[*i* . . .] / ^{d}*a-sal-luḫ* ŠUB-*ma* x [. . .] (K 13368: 2′–3′)

ša DU$_{11}$.GA ŠA$_3$-*bi u* SAG.DU (STT 252: 25)

E[N$_2$ *ul i*]*a-ut-tu$_2$* EN$_2$ [^{d}*e$_2$-a u* ^{d}]⸢*asal*⸣-*lu$_2$-ḫi* / [EN$_2$ ^{d}]*da-mu u* [^{d}*gu-l*]*a* (BAM 124 iv 23–24)

EN$_2$ *ul ia-ut-tu-un* / EN$_2$ ^{d}*e$_2$-a u* ^{d}*asal-lu$_2$-ḫi* / EN$_2$ ^{d}*da-mu u* ^{d}*gu-la* (BAM 128 iv 18′–20′)

†

117 Incantation (as a dialogue):

117a (Head) ‘O belly, O belly! Where are you going?’

117b (Belly) ‘I’m going to inflict pain on the belly of the young man! I’m going to crush the belly of the young woman!’

118–119 (Head) ‘Do not inflict pain on the belly of the young man! Do not crush the belly of the young woman! (Instead,) may the belly of the ox in the pen be the one in pain, may the belly of the pig in the pigsty be the one in pain!’[211]

120a (Narrator) (This is) what belly and head said to each other.

120b The incantation is not mine; it is the incantation of Asalluḫi and Gula,[212]

---

209 Lines 117–120 are edited by Collins (1999: 160–162) as Belly 21. The manuscript from Sultantepe replaces the first person possessive suffixes following the infinitives with the second person. This confusion probably resulted from (i) the curious description of the belly as the agentive cause rather than the locus of pain, and (ii) the underlying ambiguity of *akālu*, between ‘to eat’ and ‘to experience pain’.

210 The unusual orthography ^{d}*a-sal-luḫ* can also be found in the parallel text K 13368: 3′. For other syllabic spellings of the name Asalluḫi in our line, including *a-sa$_3$-lu-uḫ*, *a-sa-lu-uḫ* and *a-sa-lu-uḫ$_2$*, see George 2016: 116.

211 In our text, there is a shift from first and second person to third person indicated by the use of the third person precative *līkul* ‘may it hurt’ in line 118. In the manuscript from Sultantepe, however, this change does not take place, and the corresponding verbal form is the imperative *akul* ‘hurt!’.

212 The parallels K 13368: 2′ and STT 252: 25 suggest that the narrator intervenes at the end of the incantation to explain who is participating in the dialogue (Veldhuis 1990: 39–40). Our tentative reconstruction of line 120 is based on these parallels, as well as on the occurrence of the pair of divine names Asalluḫi and Gula, presumably used here as an abbreviation for the longer list of names in BAM 124 and BAM 128. This leaves room for the comment found in K 13368 and STT 252, but the presence of this comment in our text cannot be demonstrated. For the possibility that line 120 contains a closing formula, see already BAM 9 p. 75 n. 59.

121 A$_{ii\ 56}$ [... *iq-b]u-*⸢*nim*$^{?}$*-ma a-na-ku*⸣ [x x x x]
B$_{obv.\ 1'}$ [.. *a-n]a-*⸢*ku u*$_2$⸣*-[ša*$_2$*-an-ni]*
⸢EN$_2$⸣ ^{d}NIN.GIRIM$_3$ [EN] EN$_2$ / *šu-nu iq-bu-ni-ma ana-ku u*$_2$*-ša*$_2$*-[an-ni]* (BAM 124 iv 25–26)
EN$_2$ ^{d}NIN.GIRIM$_3$ EN EN$_2$ / *šu-nu iq-bu-ma ana-ku u*$_2$*-ša*$_2$*-an-ni* (BAM 128 iv 21′–22′)

122 A$_{ii\ 57}$ [..]
B$_{obv.\ 2'}$ [...] TI-⸢*e*⸣
^{d}*gu-la* TI.L[A . . .] (K 13368: 4′)

---

123 A$_{ii\ 58}$ [.. EN$_2$ *ana* UG]U LI.DUR Š[ID-*nu*][213]
B$_{obv.\ 3'}$ [... LI.D]UR ŠID-*nu*

---

124 A$_{ii\ 59}$ [.. ^{g}]^{i}pisan$^{!}$(E$_2$).gen$_7$[214] keš$_2$.d[a]
B$_{obv.\ 4'}$ [.. ^{gi}pisa]n.gen$_7$ keš$_2$.da
[EN$_2$] ⸢ša$_3$⸣ gig.ga pisan$^{!}$(E$_2$).gen$_7$ [. . .] (K 13368: 6′)
ša$_3$ gig.ga «in» ^{gi}pisan.gen$_7$ keš$_2$.da / *li-ib-bu ma-ar-ṣu*$_2$ *ša ki-ma pi*$_2$*-ša-an-ni ka-at-m[u]* (CT 4 8 obv. 1–2)

121 it is the incantation of Ningirim, the lady of incantations. They told it to me, and I repeated it.
122 O Gula, cure him (and) accept your payment.[215]

---

123 . . . (and) you recite (*tamannu*) the incantation over his navel (*abunnatu*).

---

124 The sick$^{?}$ belly (*libbu*)$^{?}$ is bound up (Akk. covered) like a reed basket.

---

213 The gap in lines 123–144 has been filled with the help of AMT 30/6 + K 14163 + K 20273, which is an indirect join to MS A. The join was identified by K. Simkó in 2021, including K 14613 as a direct join to AMT 30/6.
214 Although most of our manuscripts have E$_2$, the GI determinative and the Akkadian translation in CT 4 8 obv. 2 (viz. *pi*$_2$*-ša-an-ni*) make clear that the sign meant here is GA$_2$, read as PISAN in ^{gi}PISAN. Certain Old Babylonian forms of E$_2$ and GA$_2$ are nearly identical, which might have led to the confusion of the two signs.
215 The line can be restored with help from the form TI-*e* as the feminine imperative of the verb *leqû*, which must belong to the standard closing formula *Gula bulluṭī-ma qīštīki leqî*, as in line 116 above.

125 A$_{ii 60}$ [...] x : ⸢a pu$_2$.gen$_7$ a⸣.ge$_6$.a nu.t[uku]
B$_{obv. 5'}$ [.. a.g]e$_6$.a nu.tuku
[a i]d$_2$.da.gen$_7$ *k[i-ma . . .]* (K 13368: 7′)
a id$_2$.da.gen$_7$ al.du.un nu.zu / *ki-ma me-e na-ri-im e-ma i-il-la-ku u$_2$-⸢ul⸣ [i-di]*
a pu$_2$.gen$_7$ a.ge$_6$.a (eras.) nu.tuku / *ki-ma me-e bu-ur-ti a-gi-a u$_2$-ul i-šu* (CT 4 8 obv. 3–6)

126 A$_{ii 61}$ [... tu]ku$^?$: u$_2$ nu.ku$_4$.ku$_4$ a nu.⸢ku$_4$.ku$_4$⸣
B$_{obv. 6'}$ [.. n]u.ku$_4$.ku$_4$
[gakk]ul$^?$.gen$_7$ dul.la x [. . .] (K 13368: 8′)
gakkul$_3$.gen$_7$ ⸢ka.bi⸣ ba.dul / *ki-ma ka-ak-ku-li [pi-šu] ka-ti-im*
a nu.mu.un.da.ku$_4$.ku$_4$ ninda nu.mu.un.da.ku$_4$.ku$_4$ / *a-ka-lu u$_3$ mu-⸢u$_2$⸣ u$_2$-ul i-ir-ru-bu-šum* (CT 4 8 obv. 7–10)

127 A$_{ii 62}$ [.................................. n]e : ^{d}asal.lu$_2$.ḫi igi : nig$_2$ ge$_{26}$.e : gen.na dumu.gu$_{10}$
B$_{obv. 7'}$ [... nig$_2$ g]e$_{26}$.e : gen.na dumu.gu$_{10}$
[x x] hun.ga$_2$ x x [. . .] (K 13368: 9′)
^{d}asal.lu$_2$.ḫi igi.ni im.ma.an.si$_3$ / ^{d}AMAR.UTU *ip-pa-li-is$_2$-su$_2$-ma*
a.a.ni ^{d}en.ki.ke$_4$ gu$_3$ mu.un.na.de$_2$.e / *a-na a-bi-šu ^{d}e$_2$-a i-⸢ša⸣-as$_2$-si* (CT 4 8 obv. 11–12)
^{d}en.«lil$_2$».ki.ke$_4$ ^{d}asal.lu$_2$.ḫi mu.un.na.ni.ib$_2$.gi.gi / ^{d}e$_2$-a ^{d}AMAR.UTU *i-ip-pa-al*
dumu.gu$_{10}$ a.na.am$_3$ nu$^{!}$(NE).zu a.na.am$_3$ ma.ra.ab.daḫ.e / *ma-ri mi-i-na la ti-di-ma mi-i-na-am lu-ṣi-ib-šu*
nig$_2$ ge$_{26}$.e zu.gu$_{10}$ u$_3$ za.e ga$_2$.zu / *ša a-na-ku i-du-u$_2$ «u$_2$» at-ta ti-di*
u$_3$ za.e ga$_2$.zu nig$_2$ ge$_{26}$.e zu.gu$_{10}$ / *ša at-ta ti-du-u$_2$ a-na-ku i-di* (CT 4 8 rev. 5–12)

125 Like water in a river, you do not know where it will go;[216] like water in a well, it does not flow.
126 Like a fermentation vat, its mouth is covered;[217] neither food nor water is able to enter.
127 . . . Asalluḫi (took) notice (and told Enki about this. Enki answered) 'What I (know, you know as well). Go, my son!'[218]

216 The first half of the line can tentatively be restored with the help of the Old Babylonian version CT 4 8 obv. 3–6.
217 Like in line 125, the first half of the line has tentatively been restored on the basis of the Old Babylonian version CT 4 8 obv. 7–10.
218 The dialogue elements of the Marduk-Ea formula, which are written in full in the Old Babylonian version CT 4 8 obv. 11–12 and rev. 5–12, are replaced with a standard abbreviation in the first millennium variant. This has resulted in a shortened version of the incantation, whereas the passage with the description of the medical condition, corresponding to CT 4 8 obv. 13–rev. 4, is not repeated. For the missing first half of the line, see K 13368: 9′ including traces of the Sumerian verb ḫun.ga$_2$.

128 A$_{ii\ 63}$ [.. n]e$^?$.ke$_4$: u$_3$ ^{u2}ḫa.šu.u$_2$ šu u.me.ti[219]
B$_{obv.\ 8'}$ [...] šu u.me.ti

lag mun u$_3$ ḫa$^!$(GIR).še.na u$_3$.un.daḫ u$_3$.bi$_2$.i[n x (x)] / *ki-ir-ba-an ṭa-ab-ti u$_3$ ḫa-ši-i uṣ-ṣa-a*[*b*$^?$ x x x] (CT 4 8 rev. 15–16)

lag mun.na šu u$_3$.me.ti (Gall: 13)

[lag mun].na šu u$_4$.me.ti (STVC 11 obv. 6')

129 A$_{ii\ 64}$ na[m.šub eridu^{ki}.ga u.m]e.ni.si$_3$: lu$_2$.u$_{18}$.lu dumu dingir.ra.na ka.bi.ta u.me.ni.gar
B$_{obv.\ 9'}$ [.. k]a.bi.ta u.me.ni.gar

nam.šub u$_3$.me.si$_3$ / [k]a.ka.na u$_3$.me.gar (Gall: 14–15)

[nam.šub er]idu^{ki}.ga u$_4$.me.si$_3$ / [k]a.ka u$_3$.me.ni.gar (STVC 11 obv. 7'–8')

130 A$_{ii\ 65}$ lu$_2$ du[mu dingir.ra.na še$_{10}$.gen$_7$ ḫe$_2$.du]r$_2$.re bu.luḫ.gen$_7$ «ri» ḫe$_2$.en.si.il.e : im.ma gu.du.a.ni.ta ḫe$_2$.em.ma.ra.⸢e$_3$⸣
B$_{obv.\ 10'-11'}$ [.. ḫ]e$_2$.en.si.il.e / [............................. ḫe$_2$.em.ma.r]a.e$_3$

še$_{10}$.<gen$_7$> ki.še$_3$ ḫe$_2$.si.il.le / *ki-ma ši-it-t*[*im li-id-di*$^?$]

bu.lu.uḫ.gen$_7$ ḫe$_2$.si.il.le / *ki-ma g*[*i-šu-tim li-ig-šu*$^?$]

im.gen$_7$ gu$^!$(ŠE).du.še$_3$ e$_3$.ib$_2$.ta / *ki-ma š*[*a-ri-im li-še-ṣi*$^?$] (CT 4 8 rev. 17–19)

še$_{10}$.gen$_7$ ḫe$_2$.dur$_2$.re / bu.lu.uḫ$_2$.gen$_7$ ḫe$_2$.si.il.le / im.gen$_7$ gu.du.ni.ta ḫe$_2$.em.ma.ra.du (Gall: 16–18)

---

131 A$_{ii\ 66}$ ⸢KID$_3$⸣.[KID$_3$.BI x x x x *ana* UG]U ⸢EN$_2$⸣ ŠUB-*di ina* KA-*šu*$_2$ *u*$_2$*-man-zaq-ma ina* KAŠ NAG-*ma ina-eš*
B$_{obv.\ 12'}$ [.. KA]Š NAG-*ma ina-eš*

☨

128 You should take a lump of salt$^?$ and *ḫašû* ('thyme'),[220]
129 you should cast the spell of Eridu over them, (and) you should place them in the mouth of the man, son of his god,
130 so that it may[221] come out like excrement, so that it may come up like a burp, so that it may pass from the anus of the man, son$^?$ of his god$^?$, like wind'.

---

131 Its ritual: . . . you cast (*tanaddi*) the incantation over it, he sucks on it in his mouth, and then he drinks (*išattī-ma*) it in beer; then he will get well.

---

219 In addition to the Old Babylonian version CT 4 8, lines 128–130 show a clear overlap with the closing section of the Gall incantation, which is known from several manuscripts, including STO 3: 99–108. Here we present a composite edition of this incantation, using BM 47859 as base text. For this incantation, see also the corresponding passage in STO 3.

220 Based on the Old Babylonian version CT 4 8 rev. 15–16, the first half of line 128 probably included salt as an ingredient alongside the *ḫašû* plant as well. In the Old Babylonian version CT 4 8 rev. 13–14, the description of medical ingredients is preceded by another reference to cattle and sheep, but this was probably not recorded in our treatise.

221 For the different uses of the subjunctive-optative ḫe$_2$- prefix in Sumerian, understood here in line with its Akkadian equivalent, see STO 3: 105.

131a B$_{\text{obv. 13'}}$ [.. Š]A$_3^?$ GIG[222]
B

---

132 A$_{\text{iii 1}}$ [.. ka.ke]š$_2$.bi ḫe$_2$.du$_8$.a
B$_{\text{rev. 1}}$ [..] ⸢ka.keš$_2$.bi⸣ ḫe$_2$.du$_8$.a
133 A$_{\text{iii 2}}$ [.................. ^{d}asal.l]u$_2$.⸢ḫi dumu⸣ eridu$^{⸢ki⸣}$.g[a.k]e$_4$ ka.keš$_2$.bi ḫe$_2$.du$_8$.a
B$_{\text{rev. 2}}$ [..] ka.keš$_2$.bi ḫe$_2$.du$_8$.a

---

134 A$_{\text{iii 3}}$ [KID$_3$.KID$_3$.BI x x x x EN$_2$] ⸢7⸣-*šu$_2$* ŠID-*nu ina* KA-*šu$_2$* ⸢*u$_2$*⸣-[*man-z*]*aq-ma ina-eš*
B$_{\text{rev. 3}}$ [KID$_3$.KID$_3$.BI .... KA-*š*]*u$_2$* *u$_2$-man-zaq-ma ina-eš*

---

135 A$_{\text{iii 4}}$ ⸢EN$_2$⸣ [^{d}ŠAKKAN$_2$ *ina* EDIN ŠA$_3$-*ba-šu$_2$*] *ka-su-šu$_2$-ma* SAḪAR SIG$_3$.SIG$_3$-*ta ma-l*[*a-a rit*]-⸢*ta-šu$_2$*⸣[223]
B$_{\text{rev. 4}}$ [.. S]IG$_3$.SIG$_3$-*ta ma-la-a rit-ta-šu$_2$*

EN$_2$ ^{d}ŠAKKAN$_2$ *ina* EDIN ŠA$_3$-*ba-šu$_2$* *ka-su-šu-m*[*a*] / [SA]ḪAR.MEŠ *mu-ti ma-la-a rit-ta-šu* (AMT 52/1: 10–11)
EN$_2$ ^{d}ŠAKKAN$_2$ *ina* ED[IN Š]A$_3$-*ba-šu$_2$* *ka-si-šu-ma* / SAḪAR.MEŠ *mu-ti* ⸢*ma*⸣-*la-a rit-ta-a-šu$_2$* (ABRT 2 11+ iii' 27–28)
[x x x x EDI]N ŠA$_3$-*ba-šu ka-si-šu-ma* / [x x x x *ma-l*]*a-a rit-ta-a-šu* (AMT 45/5+ ii 11'–12')
ša-am-ka-an i-na ṣe-r[*i-im*] / *lib$_3$-bu-šu i-ka$_4$-si$_2$-š*[*u*] (Emar VI/4 737: 4–5)

☨

131a ... sick belly$^?$.

---

132 ... may he release its blockage.
133 ... may Asalluḫi, the son of Eridu, release its blockage.

---

134 Its ritual: ... you recite (*tamannu*) the incantation seven times, (and) he sucks on it in his mouth; then he will get well.

---

135 Incantation: 'Šakkan, his belly is bound up in the steppe, his hands are filled with *murderous* dust.[224]

---

222 Line 131a probably began with a rubric like KA.INIM.MA, but it is recorded as an additional line only in MS B. Such rubrics are sometimes used inconsistently, as in EYES 1: 153', where only one of the two manuscripts, namely NA iii 29e, has a label for sick eyes (BAM 10 p. 95).
223 Lines 135–137 are edited by Collins (1999: 169–171) as Belly 27; see also Stol's discussion in Loretz 2011: 398–399.
224 The phrase SAḪAR.MEŠ *mu-ti* 'dust of death' is replaced in the main text with an obscure sign sequence that might be rendered as SAḪAR SIG$_3$.SIG$_3$-*ta*. The underlying Akkadian expression may derive from the verb *maḫāṣu*, perhaps a feminine verbal adjective in the D-stem, describing the effect that dust can have on a person caught in the steppe during a dust storm. If so, this would provide an admittedly fragile link to the 'dust of death' in the parallels. Stol (in Loretz 2011: 398–399) tentatively suggests that the form could correspond to *iš-pa-pa-ta*, a variant orthography for Akk. *išbabtu* 'grass'.

136 A$_{\text{iii 5}}$ *ul* [*um-mu pe-ta-a*]*t pa-ni-šu*$_2$ *ul a-ḫa-tu mu-š*[*e-qa-at re-ši-šu*$_2$]
B$_{\text{rev. 5}}$ [... *a*]*-ḫa-tu mu-še-qa-at re-ši-šu*$_2$
[*u*]*l um-mu pe-ta-at pa-ni-šu* / [*ul a-ḫ*]*a-tu*$_2$ *mu-še-qa-at re-ši-šu*$_2$ (AMT 52/1: 12–13)
ul um-mu ⸢*pe-ta*⸣*-at pa-ni-š*[*u*$_2$] / *ul a-ḫa-tu m*[*u-še-q*]*a-*⸢*a*⸣*-at re-ši-š*[*u*$_2$] (ABRT 2 11+ iii′ 29–30)
[. . . *pa-n*]*i*$^?$*-šu*$_2$ *ul* NIN*-su* / [. . .] (AMT 45/5+ ii 13′–14′)
iš-ši e-na-šu u$_2$*-ul um-*[*ma*] / *u*$_2$*-ul a-ḫa-ta-ma* (Emar VI/4 737: 6–7)

137 A$_{\text{iii 6}}$ ⸢*ki*⸣-[*ma* DI GI] ⸢DA⸣[225] *na-ši pat-r*[*i* TU$_6$ EN$_2$]
B$_{\text{rev. 6}}$ [....................................... *na-š*]*i pat-ri* TU$_6$ EN$_2$
[GIM] ⸢DI⸣ GI DA *na-ši* GIR$_2$ EN$_2$ (AMT 52/1: 14)
GIM DI G[I DA *na-ši pa*]*t-ri* TU$_6$ [EN$_2$] (ABRT 2 11+ iii′ 31)

---

138 A$_{\text{iii 7}}$ [KID$_3$.KID$_3$.BI] LAG MUN $^{\text{u2}}$⸢*nu-ḫur*⸣*-ta*$_5$ TI*-qe*$_2$ *ana* UGU EN$_2$ ŠUB*-d*[*i* ....]
B$_{\text{rev. 7}}$ [.. *ana* UG]U EN$_2$ ŠUB*-di ina* KA*-šu*$_2$ *u*$_2$*-man-zaq-ma ina-eš*

---

139 A$_{\text{iii 8}}$ [EN$_2$ *šam-mu ša*$_2$ Š]A$_3$*-bi ina* KUR*-i a-ṣi-*⸢*ma*⸣ *as-suḫ-šu-m*[*a* ....][226]
B$_{\text{rev. 8}}$ [... *as-su*]*ḫ-šu*$_2$*-ma iṣ-ṣa-bat* ŠA$_3$*-bi*

136 There is no mother to cheer him up. There is no sister to take care of him.
137 There is (only) him carrying a dagger like a . . .' Incantation-formula.

---

138 Its ritual: you take (*teleqqe*) lumps of salt (and) *nuḫurtu* ('asafoetida'), you cast (*tanaddi*) the incantation over them, (and) he sucks on them in his mouth; then he will get well.

---

139 Incantation: 'The Belly Plant grows in the mountains, I picked it, and it seized my belly (*libbu*).

225 The reading at the beginning of line 137 can now be confirmed with the help of M. Geller's join between ABRT 2 11 and K 8211. This reading replaces the suggested restorations of the passage by Collins (1999: 170) and Stol (in Loretz 2011: 398). The meaning of the sequence DI GI DA remains unclear. The Sumerian phrase gi.da 'with the reeds' appears in the Early Dynastic compendium CUSAS 32 1 vii 8, as part of an incantation against stomach ache (gi.da AN$_x$(UD).DUL$_3$). Analogous incantations against bile are known from both Ebla (ARET 5 11; Krebernik 1984: 64–72) and Fara (SF 46 i 1–iv 5; Krebernik 1984: 76–80).

226 Lines 139–145 are edited by Collins (1999: 151) as Belly 15. Based on the indirect join between AMT 30/6+ and MS B, it seems that the passage contained a shortened version of the 'Belly Plant' incantation. What sets this version apart from the somewhat longer version in lines 164–169 below is the absence of comparative clauses. While the short version simply asks for the belly of someone to be released (*libbi* X *lippašir*), the long version makes a comparison with another entity whose belly is also being released (*kīma libbi* X *ippaššaru libbi* Y *lippašir*). AMT 30/6+ and MS B are used by Collins (1999: 145–148), alongside BAM 576, to reconstruct the longer 'Belly Plant' incantation in lines 164–169. Pulling the two versions of the incantation apart has thus changed the distribution of the pertinent manuscripts, with lines 139–146 represented by AMT 30/6+ and MS B. BAM 576 seems to be the only parallel to lines 164–169, since it has the same comparative clauses.

140 A$_{iii\ 9}$ [*a-na* ^{d}UTU D]U$_{11}$.GA-*ma iṣ-ṣa-bat* ŠA$_3$-*b*[*i* ^{d}UT]U [...]

B$_{rev.\ 9}$ [... *a-na* AN *u* K]I DU$_{11}$.GA-*ma iṣ-ṣa-bat* ŠA$_3$-*bi* AN *u* KI

141 A$_{iii\ 10}$ ⸢*a*⸣-[*na* NENNI A NENNI D]U$_{11}$.⸢GA⸣-*ma iṣ-ṣa-bat* ŠA$_3$-*bi* N[ENNI A NENNI ....]

B$_{rev.\ 10}$ [.. *a-na u$_2$-ma*]-⸢*mi*⸣ DU$_{11}$.GA-*ma iṣ-ṣa-bat* ŠA$_3$-*bi u$_2$-ma-me*

142 A$_{iii\ 11}$ *a*-⸢*na*⸣ [^{d}*e$_2$-a*] EN-*ia aq-bi-ma* Š[A$_3$-*bi lip-pa-šir* ....]

B$_{rev.\ 11}$ [.. Š]A$_3$-*bi* ^{d}UTU *lip-pa-šir*

143 A$_{iii\ 12}$ ŠA$_3$-*b*[*i* AN *u*] ⸢KI⸣ *lip-pa-šir* Š[A$_3$-*bi* ....]

B$_{rev.\ 12}$ [................................. Š]A$_3$-⸢*bi*⸣ *u$_2$-ma-me lip-pa-šir*

144 A$_{iii\ 13}$ ŠA$_3$ NENNI [A NEN]NI *lip-pa*-⸢*šir*⸣ [..]

B$_{rev.\ 13}$ [... *šam-ma*]-*ka*

^{d}UTU *šam-me* ŠEŠ-*a šam-ma*$^{!}$(ŠU)-*ka* (STT 252: 11)

145 A$_{iii\ 14}$ NAG-⸢*šu$_2$*⸣ [..]

B$_{rev.\ 13\text{-}14}$ NAG-*šu$_2$ lib-luṭ* / [.................................] ⸢U$_2$⸣ KI KI MIN KI MIN

NAG-*šu$_2$ lib-luṭ* / NAG-*šu$_2$ li-šir* NAG-*šu$_2$* ⸢GIG⸣-*šu$_2$ lim-taš-šir* NAG-*šu$_2$ liš-lim* / ⸢NAG⸣-*šu$_2$ e-ma u$_2$-ṣa-mar* KUR-*di* (STT 252: 11–13)

---

140 I spoke to Šamaš, and it seized the belly of Šamaš, I spoke to Heaven and Earth, and it seized the belly of Heaven and Earth,

141 I spoke to so-and-so$^?$, the son of so-and-so$^?$, and it seized the belly of so-and-so$^?$, the son of so-and-so$^?$, I spoke to the beasts, and it seized the belly of the beasts.[227]

142 (Then) I spoke to Ea, my lord, (asking him) that my belly be released! May the belly of Šamaš be released!

143 May the belly of Heaven and Earth be released! May the belly of the beasts be released!

144 May the belly of so-and-so, the son of so-and-so, be released! O Šamaš$^?$, this plant$^?$ is your plant.

145 You make him drink it so that he may recover. You make him drink it so that he may become healthy. You make him drink it so that his disease may leave. You make him drink it so that he may get well. You make him drink it so that he may have success wherever he strives.'[228]

---

227 Veldhuis (1990: 37) suggests that the two entries 'Heaven and Earth' (*šamû u erṣetu*) and 'beasts' (*umāmu*) must directly follow each other, but this does not seem possible, since both *šamû u erṣetu* and *umāmu* occur in MS B, at the end of lines 9 and 10, respectively, with more than half a line missing between these two entries. We assume here that NENNI A NENNI is in the gap near the beginning of line 141, but when the chain was repeated in lines 142–144 the order of NENNI A NENNI and *umāmu* was flipped, in order to put NENNI A NENNI in final position at the end of the incantation.

228 There may not be enough room for the whole passage as it is attested in the Sultantepe parallel, which contains an extended version of the 'Belly Plant' incantation. The difficult formulation U$_2$ KI KI MIN KI MIN in MS B is probably an abbreviation for the sequence written *in extenso* in the main manuscript.

146 A$_{\text{iii 15}}$ KA.⸢INIM⸣.[MA ....]
B$_{\text{rev. 15}}$ [.......................................] ⸢ŠA$_3$⸣-*bu i-re-du-šu*

---

147 A$_{\text{iii 16}}$ KID$_3$.KID$_3$.⸢BI⸣ x x [...]
B$_{\text{rev. 16}}$ [... *ap-p*]*i*$^?$ *šil-ta-ḫi ša$_2$* 7 KA.KEŠDA.MEŠ-*šu$_2$*
148 A$_{\text{iii 17}}$ 7-*šu$_2$ u* 7-*šu$_2$* x [..]
B$_{\text{rev 16-17}}$ 7-*šu$_2$ u* 7-*šu$_2$* / [.. SAḪA]R$^?$
149 A$_{\text{iii 18}}$ TA ^{urudu}*na-a*[*ḫ-bi*$^?$ ....][229]
B$_{\text{rev. 17-18}}$ ⸢TA⸣ ^{urudu}*na-aḫ-*⸢*bi*$^?$⸣ [*ana*$^?$ ^{urud}]^{u}⸢*na-aḫ-bi*$^?$⸣ / [...]
150 A$_{\text{iii 19}}$ *ana* IGI ^{d}UTU EN$_2$ ⸢7⸣-[*šu$_2$* x x x] ⸢ŠID$^?$-*nu*⸣ [...]
151 A$_{\text{iii 20}}$ *ina* KI *ta-sa-rim* [x x x] x *ina* GIR$_3$ ⸢15 *u*$^?$ 2,30$^?$⸣ x [................................]
152 A$_{\text{iii 21}}$ *ina na-kap* GIR$_3$ [15 *u*] 2,30 *i-na-as-suk-ma* ⸢*ina*$^?$⸣-[*eš*$^?$]

---

153 A$_{\text{iii 22}}$ EN$_2$ ŠA$_3$ ^{d}UTU *ina* KUR-⸢*i*⸣ [x x G]IG-*ma* : U$_2$ ŠA$_3$ *ina ma$_2$-kan*^{ki} *a-ṣi-ma* ^{d}30 [*is-suḫ-šu*][230]

†

146 An invocation for . . . the belly pursues him.[231]

---

147 Its ritual: . . . tip$^?$ of an arrow with seven knots
148 seven times and seven times . . . dust$^?$[232]
149 from (one) brewing vessel to (another) brewing vessel$^?$ . . .
150 you recite the incantation seven times . . . while facing the sun . . .
151 you make an incision on the spot . . . on the right and left foot . . .
152 (and) he removes it with the instep (*nakkapu*)[233] of both the right and the left foot; then he will get well.

---

153 Incantation: 'The belly (*libbu*) of Šamaš grew sick in the mountains . . . but the Belly Plant had appeared in Makkan, so Sîn tore it out,

---

229 Based on the traces in the last partly legible line of MS B, the name of a copper instrument seems to be repeated. Spatial considerations suggest an instrument with a short name, such as *naḫbû* 'brewing vessel', even though this particular object does not feature elsewhere in a ritualistic context.

230 Lines 153–161 are edited by Collins (1999: 137–140) as Belly 10, with a convincing restoration of the conjugated verb form *issuḫšu* 'he tore it out' at the end of the line.

231 For the likely reconstruction of this line as KA.⸢INIM⸣.[MA *ša* DIŠ NA] ⸢ŠA$_3$⸣-*bu i-re-du-šu* 'incantation for "if Belly pursues a man"', see Collins 1999: 147.

232 This is a provisional restoration of lines 147–148 based on CAD Š/2 450. See also Steinert and Vacín 2018: 737, who suggest a more complete reconstruction of the passage as [EN$_2$ UGU$^?$ *ap*$^?$]-*pi šil-ta-ḫi ša$_2$* 7 KA.KEŠDA.MEŠ-*šu$_2$* 7-*šu$_2$ u* 7-*šu$_2$* / [ŠID-*nu*] 'you recite the incantation seven times and seven times over the tip(?) of an arrow (consisting of) seven "joints/nodes"'. However, the traces of the sign following 7-*šu$_2$ u* 7-*šu$_2$* in MS A do not support a reading like ŠID-*nu*.

233 For *nakkapu* see Cadelli 2000: 118 n. 32, who translates it as 'une partie de pied qui est en quelque sorte opposée au talon', mostly on the basis of the dream ritual tablet KAR 252 iii 35: *ki-i na-kap* GIR$_3$.MIN *a-na a-si-di la i-qar$_2$-ri-ba* 'just as the instep of the foot does not come near the heel (so the evil of the dream should not affect me)' (CAD A/2 330).

154 A$_{iii\ 23}$ *ša*$_2$ ^{d}UTU *im-me-ru p[a-n]u-šu*$_2$ ^{d}UTU *šam-ma* TA KUR-*i u*$_2$*-še-ri-dam-[ma]*
155 A$_{iii\ 24}$ *iš-kun-ma ina* ⸢*qaq*⸣*-qa-ri šur-šu-šu qaq-qa-ra* DIRI SI.MEŠ-*šu*$_2$ AN-*e nak-pa*
156 A$_{iii\ 25}$ *iṣ-bat* ŠA$_3$ ^{d}UTU *i[na l]e-qi*$_2$*-šu iṣ-bat* ŠA$_3$ ^{d}30 *ina* DUNGU.MEŠ *iṣ-bat* ŠA$_3$ GUD *ina tar-ba-ṣi*
157 A$_{iii\ 26}$ *iṣ-bat* ŠA$_3$ UDU.NIT[A$_2$ *i*]*na su-pu-ri iṣ-bat* ŠA$_3$ ANŠE *ina su-gul-li*
158 A$_{iii\ 27}$ *iṣ-bat* ŠA$_3$ UR.⸢GI$_7$⸣ *ina ši-ga-ri iṣ-bat* ŠA$_3$ ŠAḪ *ina er-re-ti*
159 A$_{iii\ 28}$ *iṣ-bat* ŠA$_3$ GURUŠ *ina me-lul-ti iṣ-bat* ŠA$_3$ KI.SIKIL *ina ur-ši-ša*$_2$
160 A$_{iii\ 29}$ *iṣ-bat* ŠA$_3$ NENNI A NENNI *tu-*⸢*mu*⸣*-re-e tu-ga-re-e*
161 A$_{iii\ 30}$ *a-na e-re-ši-šu-ma* SU-*šu*$_2$ *i-di* : *e-ma iš-ku-nu i-di* TU$_6$ EN$_2$

---

162 A$_{iii\ 31}$ KID$_3$.KID$_3$.BI ^{u2}⸢*ur*$_2$⸣*-ne*$_2$*-e* ^{u2}NU.LUḪ.ḪA ^{u2}*ti-ia-ta*$_5$ GAZI^{sar} ^{u2}KUR.RA

†

154 (and because of this) the face of Šamaš brightened. Šamaš brought the plant down from the mountains,

155 and once he had planted it in the ground, its roots filled the earth,[234] its horns gored the heavens.

156 It seized the belly of Šamaš, when he took it (*ina leqîšu*);[235] it seized the belly of Sîn in the clouds; it seized the belly of the ox in the stall.

157 It seized the belly of the ram in the fold; it seized the belly of the ass among the herd.

158 It seized the belly of the dog at the door-bolt; it seized the belly of the hog in the pigsty.

159 It seized the belly of the young man, while at play; it seized the belly of the young woman in her bedroom.

160 It seized the belly of so-and-so, the son of so-and-so — *tumurê tugarê*.[236]

161 It is according to his wish: abandon his body![237] Abandon every place where he (= Šamaš) planted (you)!' Incantation-formula.

---

162 Its ritual: you pound (*tasâk*) *urnû* (a kind of mint), *nuḫurtu* ('asafoetida'), *tīyatu* (a plant), *kasû* ('tamarind'), (and) *nīnû* ('mint')

---

234 From Šurpu V–VI 64 and 133, involving the action of roots in soil, viz. *šuršūšu qaqqara la iṣabbatū* 'its root will not take hold in the ground' (Reiner 1958: 31 and 33), it appears that the usual way of saying that 'roots take hold' was with the verb *ṣabātu* 'to seize', which appears as the leitmotif throughout the rest of the text, but here the verb used to describe the action of the roots is *malû* 'to fill'.

235 The verb *leqû* 'to take' in our version of the Belly Plant incantation possibly represents a banalisation, replacing the more appropriate *nasāḫu* 'to pull out plants or their parts' (CAD N/2 6), known from the Old Babylonian version of the same incantation, YOS 11 12 obv. 2; see Veldhuis 1990: 38–39, Collins 1999: 138–139 and Cadelli 2000: 81 with n. 45.

236 For these difficult forms, possibly representing interjections, see CAD T 450, where it is left untranslated.

237 The imperative form of the verb *nadû* is probably used here in the sense of 'to abandon' (CAD N 76–78). The command is aimed at the Belly Plant, ordering that it leave the bodies of those whom it has infected and also the place where it has been planted (cf. Collins 1999: 140). The idiom here, viz. SU-*šu*$_2$ *i-di* 'abandon his body', should be contrasted with GIG SU-*i u*$_2$*-suḫ* (from Akk. *nasāḫu*), as for example, in the recently published medical tablet in the Otago Museum E2014.6 rev. 13 (Zilberg and Horowitz 2016: 179). For the less likely reading of the verb as *i*-SILIM, viz. *išallim*, see Veldhuis 1990: 43.

163 A$_{iii\ 32}$ DIŠ-*niš* SUD$_2$ *ina* KA[Š S]IG$_3$*-*aṣ* EN$_2$ *ana* ŠA$_3$ ŠID-*nu ina* ŠU GUB$_3$-*šu*$_2$ NAG-*ma* TI

---

164 A$_{iii\ 33}$ ⸢EN$_2$ *šam-mu*⸣ [*ša*$_2$ ŠA$_3$]-*bi ina* KUR-*i a-ṣi-ma as-suḫ-šu*$_2$*-ma iṣ-ṣa-bat* ŠA$_3$-*bi*[238]

⸢EN$_2$⸣ *šam-mu ša*$_2$ ŠA$_3$-*bi ina* K[UR-*i* x x x] / *as-suḫ-šu-ma i*[*ṣ-ṣa-bat* x x] (BAM 576 ii′ 2′–3′)

[. . . *i*]*ṣ-ṣa-ba*[*t* . . .] (K 19455: 1′)

165 A$_{iii\ 34}$ [..] ⸢*aq*⸣-*bi-ma iṣ-ṣa-bat* ŠA$_3$ ^{d}UTU

ana ^{d}UTU DU$_{11}$.GA-*ma i*[*ṣ-ṣa-bat* x x x] (BAM 576 ii′ 4′)

[. . . *aq-b*]*i-ma iṣ-ṣ*[*a-bat* . . .] (K 19455: 2′)

166 A$_{iii\ 35}$ [... *aq-b*]*i*-⸢*ma*⸣ *iṣ-ṣa-bat* Š[A$_3$* A]N *u* KI

ana AN-*e u* KI-*ti*$_3$ DU$_{11}$.GA-*m*[*a* . . .] (BAM 576 ii′ 5′)

[. . . KI-*t*]*i*$_3^?$ *aq-bi-ma iṣ-ṣ*[*a-bat* . . .] (K 19455: 3′)

167 A$_{iii\ 36}$ [...................... *iṣ-ṣ*]*a-bat* ŠA$_3$ *u*$_2$-⸢*ma-me*⸣ *a*-⸢*na* ^{d}⸣*[*e*$_2$*-a* EN *ap-si aq-bi-m*]*a**

ana u$_2$*-ma-mi* DU$_{11}$.GA-[*ma* . . .] / *ana* ^{d}*e*$_2$*-a* EN *a*[*p-si* . . .] (BAM 576 ii′ 6′–7′)

[*ana u*$_2$*-ma-m*]*i*$^?$ ⸢*aq*⸣-*bi-ma iṣ-ṣa-b*[*at* . . .] / [. . .] EN-*ia* [. . .] (K 19455: 4′–5′)

168 A$_{iii\ 37}$ ŠA$_3$-*b*[*i* x x x ŠA$_3$-*b*]*i* ^{d}UTU *lip-pa-šir*$_3$ *ki-m*[*a* x x x x *ip-pa-ša*$_2$]-⸢*ru*⸣[239]

ŠA$_3$-*bi lip-pa-šir*$_3$ Š[A$_3$-*bi* . . .] / GIM ŠA$_3$-*bi* ^{d}UTU *ip-pa-ša*$_2$*-ru* (BAM 576 ii′ 8′–9′)

[. . . ŠA$_3$-*b*]*i* ^{d}UTU [. . .] / [. . .] (K 19455: 6′–7′)

†

163 together, you stir them (*tamaḫḫaṣ*) into beer, you recite (*tamannu*) the incantation over (the mixture), (and) he drinks (*išattī-ma*) it, using his left hand; then he will recover (*iballuṭ*).

---

164 Incantation: 'The Belly Plant grows in the mountains, I picked it, and it seized my belly (*libbu*).

165 I spoke to Šamaš, and it seized the belly of Šamaš.

166 I spoke to Heaven and Earth, and it seized the belly of Heaven and Earth.

167 I spoke to the beasts, and it seized the belly of the beasts. (Then) I spoke$^?$ to Ea, lord of the Apsû (asking him)

168 that my belly be released! May the belly of Šamaš be released! Just as the belly of Šamaš is released,

---

238 Lines 164–169 are edited by Collins (1999: 145–148) as Belly 13. Of the three additional manuscripts that Collins used to reconstruct this passage, only BAM 576 can still be considered a parallel. AMT 30/6+ and MS B contain a shortened version of the Belly Plant incantation recorded in lines 139–145 above. The Sultantepe manuscript STT 252 starts in much the same way as our incantation here, but it then diverges for several lines and goes on to include a number of additional lines.

239 The gap in lines 168–172 has partially been filled with the help of K 22164, which is a direct join to MS A. The join was identified by K. Simkó in 2021.

169 A$_{iii\ 38}$ ŠA$_3$-*b*[*i* AN *u* KI *lip-pa-š*]*ir*$_3$ *ki-ma* ŠA$_3$-*bi* AN *u* KI [..........................] x x x

Š[A$_3$-*bi* . . .] / GIM ŠA$_3$-*bi* AN-*e u* ⸢KI-*ti*$_3$⸣ [. . .] / ŠA$_3$ *ša*$_2$ NENNI ⸢A⸣ NE[NNI . . .] / ⸢^{d}⸣U[TU *šam-m*]*u* [. . .] (BAM 576 ii′ 9′–12′)

ŠA$_3$-*bi* AN-⸢*e*⸣ [. . .] / [. . .] x ŠA$_3$-*bi* [. . .] (K 19455: 7′–8′)

---

170 A$_{iii\ 39}$ KID$_3$.KID$_3$.B[I x x x x EN$_2$ 7-*š*]*u*$_2$ ŠID-*nu ina* KA-*šu*$_2$ *u*$_2$-[*man-zaq-ma*] *ina-eš*

---

171 A$_{iii\ 40}$ EN$_2$ ⸢ER$_2$⸣[240] IR UD LI AN x x [x x] *sa*-⸢*bi*⸣-*tu*$_4$[241]

172 A$_{iii\ 41}$ [*na*]*m-zi-tu*$_4$ *a-ši*$_{pi}$-*tu*$_4$ *ina* ⸢*a*⸣-*mat* ^{d}AMAR.⸢UTU⸣ *ina qi*$_2$-⸢*bit* ^{d}UTU⸣ LU$_2$ *lib-luṭ* TU$_6$ EN$_2$

---

173 A$_{iii\ 42}$ EN$_2$ IM *el-lu ša*$_2$ *ina* KUR-*i aš*$_2$-*bu man-nu ub-lak-ka ana* ⸢ŠA$_3$⸣ *e*[*l-l*]*i ša*$_2$ *a-me-lu-ti*[242]

✝

169 may the belly of Heaven and Earth be released! Just as the belly of Heaven and Earth is released . . . the belly of so-and-so, the son of so-and-so . . . O Šamaš, the plant . . .'[243]

---

170 Its ritual: . . . you recite (*tamannu*) the incantation seven$^?$ times (over it, and) he sucks on it in his mouth; then he will get well.

---

171 Incantation: 'Tear . . . the alewife . . .

172 the disturbed fermenting vat, by the word of Marduk (and) the utterance of Šamaš, may the man recover!' Incantation-formula.

---

173 Incantation: 'O pure wind that dwells in the mountains! Who has brought you down to the pure belly of mankind,

---

240 The traces of signs point to A.IGI, with the possible reading ER$_2$ = Akk. *dimtu* 'tear'. This reading seems to be confirmed by the fact that *ašītu* and *apītu* are derived from verbs that describe eye disease symptoms in other medical contexts, such as blurred and cloudy vision (*ešû* and *apû*, respectively): see CRAN 1: 2–3 (BAM 480+ i 2–3), which has IGI.MIN-*šu*$_2$ (. . .) *i-pi-ta*$_5$ *i-ši-ta*$_5$ *a-ša*$_2$-*a* / *u*$_3$ ER$_2$ ŠUB.ŠUB-*a* 'his eyes are made blurry by (. . .) cloudiness, confused vision (. . .), and they shed tears constantly'.

241 Lines 171–172 are edited by Collins (1999: 130–131) as Belly 7. His reading of the glossed passage in line 172, viz. *er*$_2$-*tum* '(a fermenting vat) is the chest', does not yield a clear meaning in this context. The image of the disturbed fermenting vat, on the other hand, is introduced here as a representation of an upset stomach: when closed, they both slowly fill with bubbles, foam and smelly gases.

242 The gap in lines 173–177 has partially been filled with the help of K 22089, which is a direct join to MS A. The join was identified by Zs. Földi in 2023. The incantation is also edited by Collins (1999: 126–127) as Belly 3.

243 The missing second half of the line can tentatively be restored with the help of the parallel in BAM 576. However, the size of the available space in the break at this point may not be enough to accommodate the whole passage as it stands in BAM 576.

174 A$_{iii\,43}$ *ša*$_2$ UZU-*šu*$_2$ *ša*$_2$ *la a-ka-li*$_3$ *ša*$_2$*-man-šu ša*$_2$ *la pi-it*$^!$(DA)*-šu-ši* ⸢*i-še*⸣*-er* IM *ana šu-bur-ri*
ba-lu ḫur-ru IM *a-na šu-*⸢*bur*⸣-<*ri*> (STT 252: 26)

175 A$_{iii\,44}$ *ki-ma ṣe-er ka-ra-ni*$_7$ *ta-aṣ-ṣi ana ṣi-b*[*it*$^?$ I]M$^?$ ⸢TU$_6$⸣ EN$_2$
GIM *ṣer-ri* GEŠTIN *a-na* EGIR x x x (STT 252: 26)

---

176 A$_{iii\,45}$ KID$_3$.KID$_3$.BI ^{u2}*ti-ia-ta*$_5$ GAZI^{sar} *u* MUN DIŠ-*niš* SUD$_2$ [x x x] x
177 A$_{iii\,46}$ ⸢I$_3$.GIŠ⸣ *ana pa-ni ma-aš-ti-i ta-za-ru*$_3$ 3-*šu*$_2$ EN$_2$ ŠID-*nu-ma* LU$_2$ [x x x x]

---

178 A$_{iii\,47}$ [DIŠ KI MIN ....] x [....................] x x x [...]
179 A$_{iii\,48}$ [...] ⸢*ti*⸣*-ia-ta*$_5$ GAZI⸢^{sar}⸣ *ta-mar-raq ina* ⸢KAŠ⸣* NAG

---

180 A$_{iii\,49}$ DIŠ K[I MIN ....] *ina* I$_3$.GIŠ *u* KAŠ SAG NAG

---

174 whose flesh is not to be eaten (and) whose oil not to be used to anoint oneself?[244] . . . O wind,
175 go out (*taṣṣi*)[245] through the anus just as a vineyard snake!'[246] Incantation-formula for a seizure$^?$ of wind.

---

176 Its ritual: you pound (*tasâk*) *tīyatu* (a plant), *kasû* ('tamarind'), and salt together . . .,
177 you scatter oil on the surface of the potion, you recite (*tamannu*) the incantation three times, and then the man . . .

---

178 If DITTO, . . .
179 you pulverize . . . *tīyatu* (a plant) (and) *kasû* ('tamarind'), (and) he drinks (*išatti*) them in beer.

---

180 If DITTO . . . (and) he drinks (*išatti*) it in oil and high-quality beer.

---

244 A similar formulation can be found in Lamaštu I 187–188: *iš-ta-na-at-ti da-mi naš-bu-ti ša a-me-lu-ti* / UZU *ša*$_2$ *la a-ka-li* GIR$_3$.PAD.DU *ša*$_2$ *la ka-ra-ṣi* 'she keeps drinking *blown*$^?$ blood of humans, (eats) flesh not fit for eating, (*cracks*) bone(s) not meant for *cracking*' (Farber 2014: 90 and 158–159).

245 We take this form as an anomalous Gt-stem imperative of *waṣû*, namely *taṣi*, with the unexpected doubling of /ṣ/ in our text. The only possibilities that explain the doubled /ṣ/ (a second person durative of *eṣû* 'to slit' or *neṣû* 'to tear out, to slit') are both rare and would present us with the otherwise unknown image of the wind breaking through a blocked anus.

246 The vineyard snake 'who does battle with the incantation priest' (CBS 7005: 14) is listed (without the epithet) in Ura XIV 28 (MSL 8/2 p. 8) and in Šumma ālu XXV 13–14, but it is primarily known from the incantation tradition. It already appears in Old Assyrian and Old Babylonian incantations (Finkel 1999: 223–229 and Barjamovic 2015: 58 with n. 4) and also functions as a cover term for the *daddaru* plant in Uruanna III 75 (71) (Rumor 2017: 15).

181 A$_{iii 50}$ EN$_2$ *e-sil k*[*i-ma na-d*]*i na-pi-iḫ-ma ki-ma lu-up-pi*[247]
182 A$_{iii 51}$ KA.NA ⸢*šu-u*$_2$⸣* *i*[*na*$^?$ K]A-*šu*$_2$ *šu-u*$_2$ ^{giš}PEŠ$_3$ NU E$_3$-*ma* TU$_6$ EN$_2$

---

183 A$_{iii 52}$ KID$_3$.⸢KID$_3$.BI⸣ *ina* ŠU.SI ⸢GIR$_3$-*ka*⸣ GAL-*ti ša*$_2$ GUB$_3$ EN$_2$ 7-*šu*$_2$ *ana* UGU LI.DUR-*šu*$_2$ ŠUB-*ma ina-eš*

---

184 A$_{iii 53}$ ⸢EN$_2$⸣ ŠA$_3$ *nam-zi-tu*$_4$ KAŠ *la-as-su-uḫ* TU$_6$ EN$_2$[248]

---

185 A$_{iii 54}$ KID$_3$.KID$_3$.BI *ina* ŠU.SI GIR$_3$-*ka* GAL-*ti ša*$_2$ 2,30 EN$_2$ ŠUB-*di u ina* ŠU.SI-*ka tu*$_2$-*mar-raṭ-ma*[249] *ina-eš*

---

181 Incantation: 'Inflated like a waterskin and blown up like a leather bag,
182 It is "in his mouth" (Sum.). It is "in his mouth' (Akk.)",[250] (which is like) an unopened fig.' Incantation-formula.

---

183 Its ritual: with the big toe of your left foot,[251] you cast (*tanaddī-ma*) the spell seven times over his navel (*abunnatu*); then he will get well.

---

184 Incantation: 'The belly is a fermenting vat (*namzītu*):[252] let me drain (its) beer!'

---

185 Its ritual: with the big toe of your left foot, you cast (*tanaddi*) the incantation, (and) you scratch it with your finger;[253] then he will get well.

---

247 Lines 181–182 are edited by Collins (1999: 171) as Belly 28.

248 Line 184 is edited by Collins (1999: 128) as Belly 5. We retain Cadelli's (2000: 45) reading of KAŠ *la-as-su-uḫ* as an Assyrian form of *nasāḫu* in the precative, capturing the idea that the contents of the patient's belly should be evacuated in the same way that one draws beer from the lower tap of a fermenting vat (see also CAD N/1 257). Collins (1999: 128) reads *bi-la-as-su* IM$^!$, emending UḪ to IM for Akk. *šāru* 'wind', with supporting evidence in PBS 7 87: 2 which reads *bi-il-la-as-su*$_2$ *ša-rum* (see also Farber 1984, with collations, and Stol 2006: 115).

249 AHw 610 suggests *ta*$_5$- as a possible reading of the sign UD in *tu*$_2$(UD)*-mar-raṭ-ma*, based on the variant spelling *ta-mar-raṭ* in line 199 below, but *ta*$_5$- is not otherwise used as the first syllable in verbal forms.

250 The line begins with a lexical parallel between Sumerian KA.NA 'in his mouth' and the corresponding phrase in Akkadian *ina pīšu*, with *šu-u*$_2$ following each entry, as we might expect in a lexical list. This lexical equation gives the location of the inflated waterskin or blown-up bag, as a depiction of a protruding navel or an umbilical hernia, an image that is reinforced by a comparison with an unopened fig. For the alternative reading 'string together *kanašû* plant [. . .], *šû* stone, and *ēru* wood (to make an amulet)', see Collin's 1999: 171. Except for Uruanna, the *kanašû* plant seems to have disappeared from the first millennium medical corpus (CAD K 143–144).

251 This curious use of the big toe to cast the spell may actually go back to an Old Sumerian incantation against stomach ache: CUSAS 32 1 viii 9–ix 1 reads šu.si giri$_3$.si.na ḫa.mu.ta.sar 'through his fingers and toes the spell shall flee' (George 2016: 120).

252 CUSAS 32 32 includes 'a compilation of three Old Babylonian incantations for digestive disorders, which have in common the use of the brewing jar [viz. *namzītu*] as a metaphor for the stomach and digestive tract' (George 2016: 136).

253 In AMT 73/1+ iv 26, the same verb is used in combination with fingers and toes, to describe scratching as a symptom: ⸢DIŠ NA⸣ x du šu$_2$ x x x *lu ina mim-ma lu* GIR$_3$.MIN-*šu*$_2$ *lu* ŠU.SI-*šu*$_2$ *im-ru-uṭ-ma* [. . .] 'if someone . . . has scratched it with either his feet or his fingers . . .' (Eypper 2016: 50–51).

186 A$_{iii\ 55}$ EN$_2$ *ša-ru-um-mi ša$_2$-ru ša$_2$-ru* IZI[254] DINGIR.MEŠ *at-ta$_5$ ša-ru ša bi-rit ze-e*[255]
187 A$_{iii\ 56}$ *u ši-na-a-ti at-ta$_5$ tu-ṣi-a-ma it-ti* DINGIR.MEŠ ŠEŠ.MEŠ-*ka* ⸢*na*⸣-*di-a-at* ^{giš}GU.ZA-*ka* EN$_2$

188 A$_{iii\ 57}$ KID$_3$.KID$_3$.BI ^{u2}EME UR.GI$_7$ ḪAD$_2$.A SUD$_2$ *ina* I$_3$.GIŠ ŠUB-*di* EN$_2$ ŠID-*nu* ŠEŠ$_2$-*su-ma ina-eš*

189 A$_{iii\ 58}$ EN$_2$ *lib-bu-ma* ŠA$_3$-*bu* ŠA$_3$-*bu da-an* ŠA$_3$-*bu qar-rad* GIM UR.MAḪ *ma-*⸢*li*⸣ *pu-luḫ-*⸢*ta$_5$*⸣*[256]
190 A$_{iii\ 59}$ *ki-ma* UR.BAR.RA *la-ka-da uš-šur* EN$_2$ *ul ia-at-tu$_2$* ⸢EN$_2$⸣ ^{d}*gu-la*

186 Incantation: 'Wind, they say, Wind! O Wind![257] You are the fire of the gods! O Wind, you are the one between excrement
187 and urine! You come out, and then your throne is set up with the gods, your brothers!' Incantation.

188 Its ritual: you dry (*tubbal*) (and) pound (*tasâk*) *lišān kalbi* ('dog's tongue' plant), you put (*tanaddi*) it in oil, you recite (*tamannu*) the incantation, (and) you anoint him (*tapaššassū-ma*); then he will get well.

189 Incantation: 'It is the belly! O Belly! The belly is strong! The belly is a hero! It is full of fearsomeness like a lion!
190 It is free to run (*lakāda uššur*)[258] like a wolf! The incantation is not mine; it is the incantation of Gula.'

254 There seems to be an extra horizontal wedge on the right side of IZI, which led Scurlock (in Scurlock and Andersen 2005: 124) to suggest a collation of IZI as MA. However, she ignores the left side of IZI and mistakenly transliterates the phrase as *ša$_2$-ru-ma*. The scribe who wrote our tablet may have miscopied an original NE sign as *am-ma*, yielding the ungrammatical form ***ša$_2$-ru-am-ma*.

255 Lines 186–187 are edited by Collins (1999: 125–126) as Belly 2. These two lines have been frequently translated, as for example in Ritter 1965: 312, Farber 1987 and Foster ^{3}2005: 973. Collins notes the possibility that *na-di-a-at* could be an abbreviated form of the second person stative, viz. *nadiāta*, but this is not adopted here. The line, especially the idea of placing the throne of passing gas 'with the gods, your brothers', must be a joke or perhaps an attempt to persuade the gas to leave the body and go with the other gods. These lines may also be offering a parody of a passage from the Fire Incantations, section II, lines 14–15: *na-as-pi-ḫi* GIM *im-ba-ri te-be$_2$-e* GIM *na-al-ši* / *ki-ma qut-ri e-tel-li-i a-na* AN-*e ša$_2$* ^{d}*a-nim* 'scatter like fog, rise like dew, like smoke ascend to the heaven of Anu' (Lambert 1970: 40).

256 Lines 189–190 are edited by Collins (1999: 152) as Belly 16.

257 Forms like this, with the quotative particle *-mi*, are traditionally rendered as direct speech, as in an Old Babylonian incantation containing a *historiola* for the *merḫu* kernel that starts with the phrase *erṣetum-mi erṣetum* 'The earth – they tell – was. The earth (. . .)' (Landsberger and Jacobsen 1955: 15). See generally Wasserman 2012: 179–205.

258 AHw 1486 devotes a short section to this idiom but does not cite our line. Collins (1999: 152) cites similar lines from two Old Babylonian incantations against anger (Wilcke 1985: 202–203 ln. 89; Whiting 1985: 181 ln. 6–7), which may be garbled versions of the same text. The verbal adjective *uššur* is probably the same type of *accusativus respectus* discussed by Whiting as 'he is free (with respect to running)' (Aro 1961: 108, *apud* Whiting 1985: 182).

191 A$_{iii\ 60}$ EN$_2$ *a-nam-di* EN$_2$ *ana* DUMU.MUNUS ^{d}*e*$_2$*-a a-nam-di* EN$_2$ *ana* DUMU.MUNUS ^{d}*a-nim*[259]

EN$_2$ *a-nam-di* EN$_2$ *a-*⸢*na*⸣ [. . .] / EN$_2$ *a-na* DUMU.MUNUS ^{d}*a-nim* (Beckman and Foster 1988: 18 no. 15 ln. 2′–3′)

192 A$_{iii\ 61}$ *a-nam-di ana* DUMU.MUNUS DINGIR *aš-šum mi-ni-i aš-šum mi-ni-i aš-šum ka-bat-ti aš-šum li-ib-bi*

a-⸢*nam-di a*⸣-[*na* . . .] / *aš-šum mi-ni-i aš-šum mi-*<*ni*>*-i* <*aš-šum*> *ka-bat-t*[*i* . . .] (Beckman and Foster 1988: 18 no. 15 ll. 3′–4′)

193 A$_{iii\ 62}$ *aš-šum li-ib-bi aš-šum li-ib-bi* ⸢*mar-ṣi*⸣ TU$_6$ EN$_2$

[*a*]*š-šum li-ib-bi aš-šum li-ib-bi* [. . .] (Beckman and Foster 1988: 18 no. 15 ln. 5′)

---

194 A$_{iii\ 63}$ KID$_3$.KID$_3$.BI SIG$_2$ BABBAR DUR NU.NU 7 KA.KEŠDA KE[ŠDA x x x x EGI]R-*šu*$_2$ KEŠDA-*ma ina-*⸢*eš*⸣

[DU$_3$.D]U$_3$.BI SIG$_2$ BABBAR DUR NU.NU 7 K[A.KEŠDA KEŠDA] / [EN$_2$ Š]ID-*nu ina* EGIR-*šu*$_2$ *tara-*[*kas*$_2$ x x x] (Beckman and Foster 1988: 18 no. 15 ll. 6′–7′)

---

195 A$_{iii\ 64}$ EN$_2$ *a-na li-bur-za-ni-nu qi*$_2$*-b*[*i-ma um-ma a-d*]*a-pa* ⸢ABGAL⸣-*m*[*a*][260]

EN$_2$ *a-na li-bur-za-ni-*⸢*ni*$^{?}$⸣ [. . .] / *um-ma* ⸢*a*⸣*-da-pa* ABGAL-*ma* (AMT 52/1: 1–2)

191 Incantation: 'I cast a spell; I cast a spell for the daughter of Ea; I cast a spell for the daughter of An.

192 I cast a spell for the daughter of a god. What was it about? What was it about? It was about the liver. It was about the belly

193 It was about the belly. It was about a sick belly.' Incantation-formula.

---

194 Its ritual: you spin (*ṭaṭammi*) a thread of white wool, you tie (*takaṣṣar*) seven knots, you recite (*tamannu*) the incantation, (and) you bind it (*tarakkas-ma*) on his backside; then he will get well.

---

195 Incantation: 'Speak to *Libūr-zāninu*,[261] thus says Adapa, the sage:

259 Lines 191–193 are edited by Collins (1999: 175–176) as Belly 32.

260 Lines 195–197 are edited by Collins (1999: 171–173) as Belly 29. The story of Adapa—see in particular the Sumerian version in Cavigneaux 2014—offers an alternative authorization scene, also involving Enki/Ea, that discusses how food and drink can lead to either life or death, a theme that is particular apt for the gastrointestinal diseases in our text. For a similar fictional letter sent by Adapa to Alulu, see STT 176+ 14′–22′, edited by Collins (1999: 174) as Belly 31 and discussed more recently by Annus (2016: 62 n. 97).

261 The verb *bâru* is used as a part of personal names, in the sense 'may he / she stay healthy' (CAD B 126), but both *Libūr-zāninu* here and *Libūr-nādinu* in line 200 below are probably symbolic names rather than historical individuals: the logogram for Akk. *zāninu* is U$_2$.A, namely 'food and drink' (the decisive theme in the Adapa story), while the orthography of *nādinu* here, namely NA DIN, can easily be reinterpreted in line with the logograms used in the medical texts as *amēlu iballuṭ* 'the man / patient will recover'.

196 A$_{iii\ 65}$ ⸢TA *at*⸣-*ta*$_5$ *u a-na-ku kul-lat* KUR *ni-ti-qam-ma** A ⸢PU$_2$⸣ *ḫ*[*a-li-lu-ti* x x x x]

[. . .] / *i-na kul-lat* KUR [. . .] / A PU$_2$ *ḫa-li-lu-ti* x [. . .] (AMT 52/1: 2–4)

197 A$_{iv\ 1}$ [.................. *q*]*a*$_2$*-ti mar-ṣi ṣa-bat* EN$_2$ ^{d}*e*$_2$*-a* ŠUB-*šu*$_2$*-ma* LU$_2$ *lib-luṭ* [EN$_2$][262]

<*ana*> NENNI A NENNI ŠUB-*ma* [. . .] / *qa*$_2$*-ti mar-ṣi ṣa-bat* EN$_2$ ^{d}*e*$_2$*-a* ŠUB-*š*[*u-ma* . . .] (AMT 52/1: 5–6)

---

198 A$_{iv\ 2}$ [.. ^{u2}NU.LUḪ.Ḫ]A ^{u2}*ti-ia-ta*$_5$ MUN *ta-mar-raq*

DU$_3$.DU$_3$.BI ^{u2}NU.LUḪ.ḪA ^{u2}*ti-ia*$_2$*-ta*$_5$ *ta-mar-raq* (AMT 52/1: 8)[263]

199 A$_{iv3}$ [.. GUB$_3$-*š*]*u*$_2$ *ina* ŠU-*ka ta-mar-raṭ*

ina K[AŠ ḪI.ḪI] / ŠU.SI-*šu*$_2$ GAL-*ta*$_5$ *ša* GUB$_3$-*šu*$_2$ *ina* ŠU-*ka ta-ma*[*r-raṭ*] (AMT 52/1: 8–9)

---

196 “Since you and I went through all the mountains and drew$^?$ murmuring well-water,[264]

197 Pour (*idī-ma*) it out over so-and-so, son of so-and-so . . . seize the hand of the sick man (and) cast (*idīšū-ma*) the spell of Ea on him, so that he may recover”.’ Incantation.

---

198 Its ritual: You pulverize *nuḫurtu* (‘asafoetida’) (and) salted *tīyatu* (a plant),[265]

199 you mix (*tuballal*)$^?$ them in beer$^?$, (and) you scratch his big toe of his left side with your hand.

---

262 Collins (1999: 173) offers *šipat Ea šubšûma amīlu libluṭ* ‘(this is) an incantation that Ea caused to exist so that a man would get well!’ as an alternative rendering of the end of the line, comparing it to similar formulations, such as *šiptum annītum ša Marduk ina mātim ušabšû* ‘this incantation which Marduk caused to exist in the land’ and *šipta Ea šubšīma* ‘Ea, cause an incantation to exist!’.

263 In the parallel, the rubric KA.INIM.MA ŠA$_3$-*šu*$_2$ [. . .] is added in between the incantation in lines 195–197 and the accompanying ritual in lines 198–199.

264 The verb is presumably *ḫabû* ‘to draw (water)’ as in line 209 below; for a similar reconstruction, see Collins 1999: 172. The line is reminiscent of the journey to the cedar forest and the well-digging episode in the Epic of Gilgamesh, even though the first few signs are difficult to reconstruct since they are missing from the parallel passage AMT 52/1: 2–4. Collations of the parallel in AMT 52/1: 3 have yielded a new reading *i-na kul-lat* KUR, which thus corresponds to *kul-lat* KUR of the main manuscript (Picchioni 1981: 91). Earlier editions of AMT 52/1 are based on Campbell Thompson’s hand-copy and suggest the reading *gan-na* ‘wohlan’ (Ebeling 1931: 27). For the rendering ⸢*gan-na at*⸣-*ta*$_5$ *u a-na-ku* as ‘come, you and I’, see Collins 1999: 172 and Annus 2016: 95.

265 The absence of MUN from the parallel might suggest that MUN here represents an adjective qualifying *tīyatu*. For another example of MUN used in this way, see line 66 above.

200 A$_{iv\,4}$ [EN$_2$ ....] x TIM *a-na li-bur-na-din iš-pur-an-ni*[266]
201 A$_{iv\,5}$ [..........................] *ina a-ḫi* PU$_2$ *ša$_2$* KUR-*i*
202 A$_{iv\,6}$ [..........................] *ul nu-uš-ba-am-ma*
203 A$_{iv\,7}$ [.................. NENN]I A NENNI *ra-ši* DINGIR* *ana maḫ-ri-ka*
204 A$_{iv\,8}$ [..........................] x MI AL MU TU$_6$ EN$_2$

---

205 A$_{iv\,9}$ [KID$_3$.KID$_3$.BI ....] x *ša$_2$* EN$_2$ *ana* x x ŠUB-*u$_2$*
206 A$_{iv\,10}$ [.......................... *te-d*]*e-ek-ki-šu-*⸢*ma i-ne-eš*⸣*

---

207 A$_{iv\,11}$ [EN$_2$ .... DU]MU ^{d}UTU *ina* AN-*e u* KI-*te* MIN

---

208 A$_{iv\,12}$ [KID$_3$.KID$_3$.BI ....] ⸢NI$_2$⸣-*šu$_2$* ŠID-*nu*

---

209 A$_{iv\,13}$ [EN$_2$ x x x x x] ⸢BAL$^?$ IN$^?$⸣ *e-mur-šu$_2$-ma* ^{d}*asal-lu$_2$-ḫi iḫ-ba-a* A.MEŠ ABZU[267]
210 A$_{iv\,14}$ [x x x x ^{du}]^{g}GAN$^?$ *ina qa$_2$-ti-šu is-ḫur* ŠA$_3$-*bi ana* ^{d}*e$_2$-a be-li$_2$-šu*

†

200 Incantation: '. . . he sent me to Libūr-nādin.
201 . . . by the side of a well in the mountains.
202 . . . we did not sit down and
203 . . . so-and-so, the son of so-and-so, a fortunate man (lit. possessor of a god) . . . in your presence.
204 . . .' Incantation-formula.

---

205 Its ritual: . . . of the incantation for . . . which you cast (*tanaddû*)
206 . . . you make him rise; then he will get well.

---

207 Incantation: '. . . the son of Šamaš in Heaven and Earth DITTO'.

---

208 Its ritual: . . . he recites (*tamannu*) it by himself.

---

209 Incantation: '. . . he saw it, and then Asalluḫi drew water from the *Apsû* for me,
210 I took$^?$ the *kannu* pot (with the water) from his hand, and then my belly turned to Ea, his (= Asalluḫi's) lord.[268]

266 Lines 200–204 are edited by Collins (1999: 173–174) as Belly 30.

267 Lines 209–211 are edited by Collins (1999: 168–169) as Belly 26.

268 We assume, presumably with the verb *elqe* 'I took' in the break of line 210, that the incantation records an interaction between Asalluḫi in the third person and the healer in the first person. However, no explicit first-person forms are visible in the remaining text. Alternatively, the finite verb *is-ḫur* could also be read as GIŠ.ḪUR = Akk. *uṣurtu* 'drawing', with the following ŠA$_3$-*bi* describing a representation of the belly carried in Asalluḫi's hand.

211 A$_{\text{iv 15}}$ ⌜EN$_2$ *ul*⌝ *ia-tu-un* EN$_2$ ^{d}60 *u* ^{d}*asal-lu*$_2$*-ḫi* EN$_2$ ^{d}*gu-la* GAŠAN EN$_2$ TU$_6$ EN$_2$

---

212 A$_{\text{iv 16}}$ KID$_3$.KID$_3$.BI ^{u2}NU.LUḪ.ḪA MUN TI-*qe*$_2$ EN$_2$ 3-*šu*$_2$ *ana* ŠA$_3$ ŠUB-*ma i-man-zaq-ma* TI

---

213 A$_{\text{iv 17}}$ EN$_2$ *da-an* ŠA$_3$*-bu qar-rad* ŠA$_3$*-bu ša*$_2$ ŠA$_3$*-bi ar-ra-qa* IGI.MIN-*šu*$_2$ *pur-si-it* MUD$_2$ *na-ši-ma*[269]

214 A$_{\text{iv 18}}$ *ir-ru sa-ḫi-ru-ti ul-lu-lu ina a-ḫi-šu*$_2$ *e ta-šet* ŠA$_3$*-bu e ta-tu-ra* MIN

[x x x] ⌜*sa-ḫi-ru*⌝-[*ti* . . .] (BAM 534+ i 1′)[270]

215 A$_{\text{iv 19}}$ *ana* GURUŠ *dam-qi*$_2$ *ana* KI.SIKIL *da-me-eq-tu*$_4$ *uš-šir*$_3$ GURUŠ-*ma* E$_2$ *li-pu-uš*

[x x x x x] KI.SIKIL *da-me-*⌜*eq-tu*$_4$ *uš-šir*$_3$ GURUŠ-*ma*⌝ [x x] (BAM 534+ i 2′)

†

211 The incantation is not mine; it is an incantation of Ea and Asalluḫi; it is an incantation of Gula, the lady of incantations.’[271] Incantation-formula.

---

212 Its ritual: you take (*teleqqe*) salted *nuḫurtu* (‘asafoetida’), you cast (*tanaddī-ma*) the incantation three times over it, and he sucks on it; then he will recover (*iballuṭ*).

---

213 Incantation: ‘The belly is strong! The belly is a hero! The two eyes of the belly are yellow (and) bloodshot (lit. it holds a bowl of blood)!

214 Tangled-up intestines hang from its side. You should not leave (*ē tašēt*)[272] anything, Belly! You should not return anything, DITTO (= Belly)!

215 For (the sake of) the good young man, for the good young woman: release the young man so that he can establish a household!

---

269 Lines 213–218 are edited by Collins (1999: 155–157) as Belly 19. Cadelli (2000: 87) includes a few lines in a related incantation from Emar, published by Collins (1999: 158–160) as Belly 20, at this point in the composition. However, the incantation from Emar is only parallel to line 213, where it, quite exceptionally, writes GID$_2$.DA for *ar-ra-ka*, presumably as a mistaken rendering of our *ar-ra-qa*. For further discussions of the incantation, see Farber 1990: 310 and Stol 2006: 115.

270 The corresponding passage is known from the fragment BAM 573 i 1′–7′, which is part of the same tablet as BAM 534 and 535. For these joins, see Geller 1984: 294, Collins 1999: 155, Kinnier Wilson and Reynolds 2007: 73 n. 25, as well as Abusch, Schwemer, Luukko and Van Buylaere 2020: 96.

271 As Collins (1999: 169) points out, GAŠAN EN$_2$ = Akk. *bēlet šipti* ‘lady of incantations’ is ‘usually an epithet of Ningirima, not Gula’. See, more recently, Böck 2014a: 114 for the usual wording: *šipat Damu u Gula šipat Ningirim bēlet šipti*.

272 Collins (1999: 156) transliterates the form as *e ta*-LAK but normalises it as *ē tallik*, recognising that the vetitive is based on the preterite, which for *alāku* ‘to go’ would be *tallik*; however, Borger (2004: 340) rejects the reading *lik*$_2$ for the sign LAK. In contrast, Cadelli (2000: 87) reads it as *e ta-šiṭ*, from the verb *šâṭu* ‘to be negligent’, but then the correct form would be *tašūṭ*. We tentatively suggest *ē tašēt*, from the verb *šētu* ‘to leave’, which is rare after the Old Assyrian period (CAD Š/2 343) but does occur in the Neo-Babylonian ritual text PBS 1/1 13 rev. 51: [*ḫu*]*-lu-pa-qa ta-še-et-ma šur-pu* GAR-*an* ‘you leave the brazier and perform the *šurpu* ritual’ (Reiner 1958: 3).

216 A$_{iv\ 20}$ *uš-šir$_3$* KI.SIKIL ⸢*qin*⸣**-na liq-nun ir-ru suḫ$_4$-ḫu-ru zi-ir kar-šum*

[x x KI.SIKI]L *qin-na liq-nun ir-*⸢*ru suḫ$_4$*⸣*-ḫu-ru zi-ir kar-šum* (BAM 534+ i 3′)

217 A$_{iv\ 21}$ *u$_3$ ši-i ri-qi$_2$-tu$_2$ bu-up-pa-ni-ša$_2$ saḫ-pat liš-lim kar-šum ir-ri liš*-te-ši-ru-ma*

⸢*u$_3$*?⸣ [x x *r*]*i-qi$_2$-tu$_2$ bu-*⸢*up-pa*⸣*-ni-ša$_2$ saḫ-pat* / *liš*!-[*lim kar-š*]*um ir-ru* [*li*]*š-te-še-ru-ma* (BAM 534+ i 4′–5′)

218 A$_{iv\ 22}$ *ri-qi$_2$-tu$_4$ lit-ru-uṣ* GIM IM *ina šu-bur-*⸢*ri* GIM⸣ *ge-šu-ti ina na-piš-ti li-ṣa-a* EN$_2$

ri-qi$_2$-tu$_2$ [*lit-r*]*u-uṣ* GIM [I]M *ina šu-bur-ri* / GIM *ge-š*[*u-ti*] *ina* ZI-*ti* ⸢*li*⸣*-ṣa-a* EN$_2$ (BAM 534+ i 6′–7′)

---

219 A$_{iv\ 23}$ KID$_3$.KID$_3$.BI 7 LAG MUN *ina* ŠA$_3$-*bi* ŠUB EN$_2$ 7-*šu$_2$* ŠID-*nu* NAG-*šu$_2$-ma ina-eš*

DU$_3$.DU$_3$.BI 7 L[AG MUN] *ina* ŠA$_3$-*bi* ŠUB-*di* EN$_2$ 7-*šu$_2$* ŠID-*nu* NAG-*šu$_2$-ma ina-eš* (BAM 534+ i 8′)

---

220 A$_{iv\ 24}$ ⸢EN$_2$⸣ ŠA$_3$-*bu* ŠA$_3$-*bu e-ki-il* ŠA$_3$-*bu* GIM *mu-ši-ti$_3$ ma-li nam-ri-ri*[273]

216 Release the young woman so that she can make a nest! The intestines are tangled up, the stomach is twisted,

217 and even the large intestine (*riqītu*)[274] lies flat face down! May the stomach be healed! May the intestines straighten themselves out!

218 May the large intestine stretch out! May it (= the gas) come out like wind from the anus, like a belch from the throat!' Incantation.

---

219 Its ritual: you put (*tanaddi*) seven lumps of salt into it, you (*tamannu*) recite the incantation seven times, (and) you have him drink (*tašaqqīšu*) it; then he will get well.

---

220 Incantation: 'Belly, O Belly! The belly is as dark as night, full of terror!

273 Lines 220–227 are edited by Collins (1999: 153–154) as Belly 17. The phraseology in line 220 exhibits a number of similarities to VS 17 9 obv. 2–4: ⸢*e-ki*⸣*-il li-ib-bu-um i*[*m*-mi*?*-ir*?] *nam-ri-ri ma-li ki-i-ma w*[*a-ar-ḫi-im*] / *a-na a-ap-ti-šu ma-am-ma u$_2$-ul* [*iṭeḫḫi*] '(The belly) is dark, the belly is bloated (and) full of luminosity like the moon. Nobody can approach its opening' (these reconstructions follow, with minor differences, SEAL no. 7204). Given the surrounding context, however, the usual meaning of *namrīrrū* as 'luminosity' makes little sense in our passage, whereas in the late lexical text LTBA 2 2: 58–59 the term is equated with *pulḫu* 'terror, fearsomeness' (CAD N/1 237).

274 Strictly speaking, *riqītu* corresponds to the third compartment of the stomach, viz. omasum, in ruminants (Stol 2006: 106), but it is used here to describe the folds of the large intestine in a human being, perhaps because it is below and larger than the stomach. The idiom involving *buppanīšu saḫpat* probably refers to the large intestine folding back against itself, imagined as two curves of the intestine facing (and in contact with) one another.

221 A$_{iv 25}$ [*i-n*]*a qab-li-ti ul i-šu a-pa-tu*$_2$*-ma ul u*$_2$*-šer*$_3$*-šu ma-am-ma*

222 A$_{iv 26}$ [*ir*]*-ru su-ḫu-ru zi-ir kar-šum u*$_3$ *ši-i ri-qi*$_2$*-tu bu-up-pa-ni-ša*$_2$ *saḫ-pat*

223 A$_{iv 27}$ [*li*]*-*it-ru-uṣ kar-šu*$_2$ *ri-qi*$_2$*-tu*$_2$ *lit-ru-uṣ*

224 A$_{iv 28}$ [*ki-m*]*a ša*$_2$*-a-ri a-na šu-bur-ri ki-ma ge-šu-te a-na* ZI.MEŠ

225 A$_{iv 29}$ [*ki-m*]*a zu-ʾ-ti u*$_2$*-pa-ṭi u di-ma-*⸢*ti ka*⸣*-*la* SU-*šu*$_2$ *na-šal-li-la-ni*

226 A$_{iv 30}$ [E]N$_2$ *ul ia-ut-tu* EN$_2$ ^{d}*e*$_2$*-a u* ^{d}*asal-*⸢*lu*$_2$⸣*-ḫi* EN$_2$ ^{d}*da-mu u* ^{d}*gu-la*

227 A$_{iv 31}$ [EN$_2$] ⸢^{d}NIN.GIRIM$_3$⸣ EN EN$_2$ TU$_6$ EN$_2$

---

228 A$_{iv 32}$ [KID$_3$.KID$_3$]*.⸢BI⸣* *ana* ŠA$_3$-*bi* 10 LAG MUN 7.TA.AM$_3$ EN$_2$ ŠID-*nu-ma*

229 A$_{iv 33}$ [*ina* GU]B$_3$-*ka* KAŠ$_3$-*šu* IGI *ina* GUB$_3$-*šu i-maḫ-ḫar* ⸢*ka**-*la*$^{?}$* NAG⸣-*ma ina-eš*

---

230 A$_{iv 34}$ [EN$_2$ Š]A$_3$-⸢*bu*⸣-*ma* ŠA$_3$-*bu qar-rad* ŠA$_3$ KAS$_4$ *ša* ŠA$_3$ *zi-ra* IGI.MIN-*šu*$_2$ *pur-sit*$_2$ *da-a-me*[275]

231 A$_{iv 35}$ [ŠA$_3$-*b*]*u* ⸢ŠA$_3$⸣-*bu a-ia-ša*$_2$ *ta-lak* ŠA$_3$-*bu a-ia-ša*$_2$ *ta-ṣa-bur* ŠA$_3$-*bu*

†

221 It has no windows in its interior; no one leans out of it![276]

222 The intestines are tangled up, the stomach is twisted, and even the large intestine lies flat face down.

223 May the stomach stretch out! May the large intestine stretch out!

224 Like wind through the anus, like belch through the throat!

225 Like sweat, snot and tears that slither out from his entire body![277]

226 The incantation is not mine, it is the incantation of Ea and Asalluḫi, it is the incantation of Damu and Gula,

227 it is the incantation of Ningirim, the lady of incantations.' Incantation-formula.

---

228 Its ritual: you recite (*tamannū-ma*) the incantation over ten lumps of salt, seven times over each,

229 and then you inspect (*tammar*) his urine on your left, he collects it up on his left, and he drinks (*išattī-ma*) it all$^{?}$ (with the salt); then he will get well.[278]

---

230 Incantation: 'It is the belly! The belly is a hero! The belly is a runner! The belly's two eyes are twisted and bloodshot!

231 O Belly! O Belly! Where are you going?[279] O Belly! Where are you rushing? O Belly!

---

275 Lines 230–236 are edited by Collins (1999: 163–164) as Belly 22.

276 This is probably an allusion to Kilili, the demoness who stereotypically leans out the window (Schwemer 2004: 73–75).

277 For lines 224–225, compare Muššu'u V 57–62 (Böck 2007: 195–196, 210 and 219). Incidentally, a very similar passage in Muššu'u goes on to mention urine, which is missing from our incantation but shows up in the following ritual in lines 228–229.

278 This difficult passage was emended by Cadelli (2000: 88 with n. 66), presumably in order to avoid the obscure reference to urine. However, a similar instruction to collect animal urine can be found in BAM 323 obv. 40: KAŠ$_3$ ANŠE.KUR.RA *tu-šam-ḫar-šu*$_2$ 'you have him collect the urine of a horse' (Scurlock 2006: 507–508). The verb IGI = Akk. *amāru* is probably used here in the sense 'to inspect': the physician somehow inspects the urine before allowing the patient to combine it with the lumps of salt. The repetition of *ina* GUB$_3$-*ka* and *ina* GUB$_3$-*šu*$_2$, with the change from the second to third person, makes it unlikely that IGI (for Akk. *īnu* or *pānu*) and the verb *maḫāru* represent a single idiom meaning 'to be acceptable' (CAD M/1 64–65).

279 The phraseology recalls *a-i-iš li-ib-b*[*a-k*]*a* [(x x)] *i-il-la-ak* 'Wohin geht dein Herz!' in Wilcke 1985: 202 rev. 63, but of course in a love incantation, the context (and consequently the meaning) is quite different.

232 A$_{iv\ 36}$ [……………………………………] x ⸢ŠA$_3$⸣* x ⸢tu* SAḪAR⸣.ḪI*.⸢A⸣[280] x x x x [x]
233 A$_{iv\ 37}$ [………………………………………………………………] x x [x]
234 A$_{iv\ 38}$ [……………………………………………………………] x pad su x
235 A$_{iv\ 39}$ [x x x] *ša*$_2$-⸢*a**-*ru*⸣ x* [x x x x x x x] *i-pa-šar pi-šir*$_3$-⸢*šu*⸣
236 A$_{iv\ 40}$ [x x x] *lip-šur ki*-⸢*ši*⸣-[*ia*[281] x x x] ⸢mu⸣* *ana* KA$_2$ *li-še-ṣi* TU$_6$ EN$_2$

---

237 A$_{iv\ 41}$ [KA.INIM.M]A ⸢IM⸣[282] *ša*$_2$ ŠA$_3$ DAB-*šu*$_2$

---

238 A$_{iv\ 42}$ [KID$_3$.KID$_3$.BI I$_3$].GIŠ ŠA$_3$-*šu*$_2$ EŠ.MEŠ EN$_2$ *an-ni-ta*$_5$ 3-⸢*šu*$_2$⸣* ŠID-*nu*

---

239 A$_{iv\ 43}$ [DIŠ NA LI.D]UR-*su* DU$_8$-*at* ^{na4}PEŠ$_4$ ⸢ANŠE⸣ ^{u2}SIKIL ^{u2}ŠAKIRA ^{šim}LI
240 A$_{iv\ 44}$ [x x x] ⸢5⸣ U$_2$.ḪI.A ŠEŠ TEŠ$_2$.BI SUD$_2$ *i*[*na* KA]Š* ⸢ḪI.ḪI *ina* LI⸣.DUR-*šu*$_2$ *tu-na-tak*

232 … O Belly! … dust …
233 …
234 …
235 … wind … he brings about its release,[283]
236 … may he release my pain … may he make it leave through the door'. Incantation-formula

---

237 An invocation for flatus (lit. wind) that the belly (*libbu*) holds (*ṣabtūšu*).[284]

---

238 Its ritual: You keep anointing (*taptanaššaš*) his belly (*libbu*) with oil, (and) you recite (*tamannu*) this incantation three times.

---

239 If someone's navel (*abunnatu*) is loose (*paṭrat*):[285] *biṣṣūr atāni* ('donkey vulva' shell), *sikillu* ('pure' plant), *šakirû* (a plant), *burāšu* (a kind of juniper),
240 (and) …—you pound (*tasâk*) these five ingredients together, you mix (*tuballal*) them in beer$^?$, (and) you drip (the mixture) into his navel.

---

280 Collins (1999: 164) notes that the logogram SAḪAR.ḪI.A recalls the *Šakkan ina ṣēri* element in lines 135–137 above and similar passages in a related incantation from Emar published as Belly 20 (pp. 158–160). Collins also suggests that there are traces of a line division after line 230, but no such traces are visible on the tablet.

281 For this reading, see AHw 1569.

282 This fragmentary passage is restored after Collins 1999: 163. The passage was read by Cadelli (2000: 88 and 122) as [KA.INIM].MA ⸢EN$_2$⸣ *ša*$_2$ ŠA$_3$ DAB-*šu*$_2$ '[Incantati]on: incantation pour celui dont le ventre est atteint'.

283 This is a tentative translation of Akk. *ipaššar piširšu*, which is left untranslated in CAD P 430.

284 For the belly containing wind, see also Diagnostic Handbook Sagig 36: 19, with the syllabic rendering of the verb as ŠA$_3$-*ša*$_2$ IM *ṣa-bit* (Labat 1951: 214–215).

285 For the symptom description in line 239, compare BAM 240 obv. 30′: DIŠ MUNUS MIN-*ma* LI.DUR-*sa* DU$_8$-*at* IR *a-la-ka la i-kal-la* 'If a woman DITTO (= gives birth), subsequently her navel becomes loose (and) cannot stop sweating'.

241 A$_{iv\ 45}$ [U$_2$.ḪI.A Š]EŠ-*ma ina* KAŠ SILA$_{11}$-*aš tara-bak* [x x x x ^{u2}IG]I.⸢NIŠ ^{u2}⸣**tar-muš*
242 A$_{iv\ 46}$ [x x x x SU]D$_2$ SUR *tuš-ta-na-as-*[*sa$_3$-qam$_2$* ....] TI

---

243 A$_{iv\ 47}$ [DIŠ KI MIN ^{u2}*ṣ*]*i-bu-ra* ^{u2}DILI ⸢TEŠ$_2$.BI SUD$_2$⸣ x [....................................]

---

244 A$_{iv\ 48}$ [DIŠ KI MIN ^{u2}]IGI-*lim* SUD$_2$ *ina* GEŠTIN ⸢SUR⸣* N[AG-*ma* TI]

---

245 A$_{iv\ 49}$ [DIŠ NA LI.DU]R-*su* ŠUB.MEŠ-*su ana* TI-*šu$_2$* ^{u2}*im-ḫur-aš-na*[286] ⸢SUḪUŠ⸣ x x x
246 A$_{iv\ 50}$ [x x] x TI *ina* KAŠ *ina* GEŠTIN DU$_{10}$.GA NAG.MEŠ-*ma* TI

---

241 It is these (same) ingredients: you knead (*talâš*) them in beer, you stir them into a paste . . . (afterwards) you pound (*tasâk*) . . . *imḫur-ešrā* ('faces twenty' plant), *tarmuš* ('lupin')
242 (and) . . . you squeeze (their) liquid out (*taṣaḫḫat*), you prepare it (*tuštanassaqam*)[287] . . .; (then) he will recover (*iballuṭ*).

---

243 If DITTO, you pound (*tasâk*) *ṣibaru* ('aloe')[288] (and) *ēdu* ('lone' plant) together . . .

---

244 If DITTO, you pound (*tasâk*) *imḫur-līm* ('faces a thousand' plant), (and) he drinks (*išattī-ma*) it in pressed wine; then he will recover (*iballuṭ*).

---

245 If someone's navel (*abunnatu*) is continually collapsed (*muqqutassu*): in order to heal him (*ana bulluṭīšu*), you take (*teleqqe*) *imḫur-ešrā* ('faces twenty' plant), root from . . .
246 . . . (and) he keeps drinking (*ištanattī-ma*) them in beer (and) in good wine; then he will recover (*iballuṭ*).

---

286 The phonetic writing *im-ḫur-aš-na* is a variant reading of the logogram ^{u2}IGI.NIŠ, replacing the expected *ešrā*, the usual word for the number 20 in Akkadian (viz. the dual form of the number 10), with a dual form of the number 2, viz. **ešnā*, built on the syllabic pattern of *ešrā*. This orthography is also attested in a lone variant of Uruanna III 24 (24) (Rumor 2017: 8). For other variant readings of the plant, such as ^{u2}*im-ḫur-aš$_2$-na*, see Abusch and Schwemer 2011: 37.

287 The only attested verbal form that fits here is *tu-uš-ta-na-as-sa$_3$*-KAM/QAM$_2$, which is attested in AbB 10 148: 26, with the translation 'vorbereiten' (see also CAD N/2 22); see also AbB 12 30: 10 with the spelling *tu-uš-ta-na-sa-aq*. The preceding logogram, SUR, should probably be read as *taṣaḫḫat*, as in AMT 28/6: 2′.

288 For the *ṣibaru* plant, see Fronzaroli 1998: 238.

247 A$_{iv\ 51}$ ⸢DIŠ NA⸣ ŠA$_3$-*šu$_2$* GIG GA AB$_2$ KUG.GA I$_3$.NUN.NA UD.2.KAM$_2$ NAG
DIŠ NA ŠA$_3$-*šu$_2$* GIG GA ^{gud}AB$_2$ KUG.GA I$_3$.NUN UD.2.KAM$_2$ N[AG] (STO 2: 1)

248 A$_{iv\ 52}$ DUB.1.KAM$_2$ DIŠ NA *su-a-lam* GIG *ana ki-is* ŠA$_3$ GUR-<*šu$_2$*>

249 A$_{iv\ 53}$ E$_2$.GAL ^{m}AN.ŠAR$_2$-DU$_3$-A LUGAL ŠU$_2$ MAN KUR AN.ŠAR$_2^{ki}$ *ša* ^{d}AG ^{d}*taš-me-tu$_4$* GEŠTU.MIN DAGAL-*tu$_4$ iš-ru-*⸢*ku*⸣*-*uš*

250 A$_{iv\ 54}$ *e-ḫu-uz-zu* IGI.MIN *na-mir-tu$_4$ ni-siq ṭup-sar-ru-*⸢*ti*⸣

251 A$_{iv\ 55}$ *ša ina* LUGAL.MEŠ-*ni a-lik maḫ-ri-ia mam$_2$-ma šip-ru šu-a-tu la e-ḫu-uz-*⸢*zu*⸣

252 A$_{iv\ 56}$ *bul-ṭi* TA *muḫ-ḫi* EN UMBIN *liq-ti* BAR.MEŠ *ta-ḫi-zu nak-la*

253 A$_{iv\ 57}$ *a-zu-gal-lu-ut* ^{d}*nin-urta u* ^{d}*gu-la ma-la ba-aš-mu*

254 A$_{iv\ 58}$ *ina ṭup-pa-a-ni aš$_2$-ṭur as-niq* IGI.KAR$_2$-*ma*

255 A$_{iv\ 59}$ *a-na ta-mar-ti ši-ta-si-ia qe$_2$-reb* E$_2$.GAL-*ia u$_2$-kin*

247 (Catchline:) If someone's belly (*libbu*) is sick (*maruṣ*): he drinks (*išatti*) pure cow milk (and) ghee for two days.

248 (Tablet designation:) First tablet of 'If someone suffers (*maruṣ*) from phlegm (*suālu*), which has turned into (*itūršu*) gastric constriction (*kīs libbi*)'.

249 (Colophon:) Palace of Assurbanipal, ruler of everything, king of the land of Assur, on whom Nabû and Tašmētu have bestowed wisdom (lit. wide ears),

250 He acquired for himself shining eyes, the pinnacle of scholarship,

251 Of the kings who came before me, none were able to comprehend this task.

252 Prescriptions (organized) from head to foot, gleanings from extraneous materials, technical lore

253 (And) whatever pertains to the great medical expertise of Ninurta and Gula,

254 I have written on tablets, checked and double-checked, and

255 I deposited them in the middle of my palace for my reading and recitation.

Chapter 4
Edition of STO 2

Manuscript A = BAM 575

K 71B + K 238 + K 6253 + K 11622 + Sm 1491

STO 2	Parallels		
	Publication number	**Museum number**	**Parallel passage**
1	AMC 29		
1	STO 1: 247		
3–4	BAM 403	VAT 14532	obverse, 1–3
21–22	BAM 52	VAT 13733 + VAT 13738	reverse, 9–11
57	Stadhouders and Johnson 2018	BM 78963	34–35
77	AMT 38/3 (K 9066)	K 9066 + K 17154	obverse, 4′
101–102	STO 5: 4–5		
110–112	STO 1: 24–25		
118–119	STO 2: 254–255		
118–119	STO 1: 33–34		
125	BAM 240	VAT 8881	obverse, 26′ and 28′
139–140	STO 5: 9–10		
141	STO 5: 8		
145	STO 3: 132, 134 and 136		
145	BAM 72	Ass 13956/ct	8′–9′
146	STO 3: 131		
146	BAM 72	Ass 13956/ct	3′–4′
151–152	STO 1: 94–96		
160–161	BAM 158	VAT 13789	column 4, 14–17
163–164	BAM 54	VAT 8027	obverse, 1–3
165–168	BAM 56	A 251	reverse, 8′–12′
165–171	BAM 55	VAT 13890 + VAT 13895	1–17
166–171	BAM 57	A 270	obverse, 1′–reverse, 6
177	AMC 32		
184	AMC 33–34		
186–188	BAM 59	A 212	reverse, 6–14
200–210	STO 3: 1–13		
245	AMC 34		
245–250	STO 1: 37–41		
245–247	BAM 58	VAT 13774 + VAT 14003	8–13
251	AMC 34		
252	STO 1: 30		
254–255	STO 1: 33–34		
254–255	STO 2: 118–119		
256–258	STO 1: 26–29		
256–258	BAM 49	VAT 7822	obverse, 9′–20′
256	BAM 50	VAT 14082	obverse, 11–15
256–257	BAM 51	VAT 10580	1′–8′
262	STO 3: 1		

https://doi.org/10.1515/9781501506574-004

1 A$_{i1}$ DIŠ NA ŠA$_3$-*šu*$_2$ GIG GA ^{gud}AB$_2$ KUG.GA I$_3$.NUN UD.2.KAM$_2$ N[AG ....]

DIŠ NA ŠA$_3$-*šu*$_2$ ⸢GIG⸣ (AMC 29)

⸢DIŠ NA⸣ ŠA$_3$-*šu*$_2$ GIG GA AB$_2$ KUG.GA I$_3$.NUN.NA UD.2.KAM$_2$ NAG (STO 1: 247)

---

2 A$_{i2}$ DIŠ NA ŠA$_3$-*šu*$_2$ GIG ^{u2}GEŠTIN KA$_5$.A ⸢SUD$_2$⸣ *ina* KAŠ NAG ^{u2}*im*-[*ḫur*-NIŠ$^?$ SUD$_2$ *ina* KAŠ NA]G*[289]

3 A$_{i3}$ ^{u2}*šiz-ba-na*$_7$ SUD$_2$ *ina* ⸢KAŠ⸣ NAG 1/2 SILA$_3$ *s*[*aḫ-le*$_2$-*e* 1/2 SILA$_3$ NAGA] SI

[. . .] 1/2 SILA$_3$ *saḫ-le*$_2$-*e* 1/2 SILA$_3$ ⸢NAGA⸣ SI (BAM 403 obv. 1)

4 A$_{i4}$ 1/2 SILA$_3$ IM.GU$_2$ EN.NA 1/2 SILA$_3$ [^{giš}Š]E.NU 1/2 SILA$_3$ ZI$_3$.KUM 1/2 SILA$_3$ ^{š}[^{im}LI 1/2 SILA$_3$ ^{šim}]GUR$_2$.GUR$_2$

[. . .] ⸢SILA$_3$ ^{giš}ŠE⸣.NU$_2^{!}$.A 1/2 SILA$_3$ ZI$_3$.KUM 1/2 SILA$_3$ ^{šim}LI / [. . .] (BAM 403 obv. 2–3)

5 A$_{i5}$ 1/2 SILA$_3$ ZI$_3$ GU$_2$.GAL 1/2 SILA$_3$ ZI$_3$ G[U$_2$.TUR] 1/2 SILA$_3$ ^{u2}SIKIL 1/2 SILA$_3$ ^{u2}NIG$_2$ ⸢GIDRU 1/2 SILA$_3$ ^{u2}*ur*$_2$-*ne*$_2$⸣*-*e*

6 A$_{i6}$ GAZ *ina* KAŠ SAG *ina* ^{urudu}Š[EN.T]UR *tara-bak ina* TUG$_2$ *te-ṭer*$_5$-*ri* IGI *u* MAŠ.SILA$_3$ LAL-*id*

---

†

1 If someone's belly (*libbu*) is sick (*maruṣ*): he drinks (*išatti*) pure cow milk (and) ghee for two days . . .

---

2 If someone's belly (*libbu*) is sick (*maruṣ*): you pound (*tasâk*) *karān šēlebi* ('fox-vine'), (and) he drinks (*išatti*) it in beer. You pound *imḫur-ešrā* ('faces twenty' plant)$^?$, (and) he drinks it in beer.

3 You pound *šizbānu* ('milkweed'), (and) he drinks it in beer. You crush (*taḫaššal*) half a litre of *saḫlû* ('cress'), half a litre of *uḫūlu qarnānû* ('horned alkali'),

4 half a litre of *qadūt šikāni* ('river mud'), half a litre of *šunû* ('chaste tree'), half a litre of *isqūqu* (a type of groats), half a litre of *burāšu* (a kind of juniper), half a litre of *kukru* (an aromatic),

5 half a litre of flour from *ḫallūru* ('chickpea'), half a litre of flour from *kakkû* ('lentil'), half a litre of *sikillu* ('pure' plant), half a litre of *ḫaṭṭi rēʾî* ('shepherd's staff' plant), (and) half a litre of *urnû* (a kind of mint),

6 you stir them into a paste in high-quality beer in a small copper pot, you smear (the mixture) on a piece of fabric (*lubāru*),[290] (and) you bandage (*taṣammid*) him front and back (lit. shoulder blades).[291]

---

289 The tentative restoration at the end of line 2 is based on the parallel instructions in lines 2–3: in both lines single ingredients are processed and consumed in the same way. For the syllabic spelling ^{u2}*im-ḫur*-NIŠ, see line 52 below.

290 TUG$_2$ and TUG$_2$.ḪI.A seem to alternate freely in our corpus, but both orthographies probably represent Akkadian *lubāru* (CAD L 230 and Ṭ 103).

291 For the same instruction, see STO 5: 5, BAM 564 ii 17′ and BAM 571 ii′ 3′, as well as BAM 555 iii 6′, 9′ and 12′, where KI MIN probably corresponds to the verb LAL-*su* included in line 2 of the same column. This is an unusual way of applying a bandage in the context of gastrointestinal diseases but probably refers to the bandaging of the front and the back of the upper body in line with Cadelli's (2000: 169) 'devant et derrière' (see also CAD N/1 119 and P 85). For a similar procedure, where the upper part of the abdomen, viz. *rēš libbi* 'epigastrium', is bandaged, see STO 1: 25.

7 A$_{i\,7}$ DIŠ KI MIN 1/3 SILA$_3$ *saḫ-le$_2$-e* 1/3 SILA$_3$ ŠE$_{10}$ ⸢TU⸣^{mušen} 1/3 SILA$_3$ ŠE.SA.A 1/3 SILA$_3$ ^{šim}LI 1/3 SILA$_3$ ^{šim}GUR$_2$.GUR$_2$
8 A$_{i\,8}$ ḪI.ḪI *ma-la na-aṣ-ma-ti tu-šam-ṣa ina* KAŠ SAG SILA$_{11}$-*aš* LAL-*id*

9 A$_{i\,9}$ ⸢DIŠ⸣ KI MIN 1 MA.NA PA ^{giš}ŠE.ḪAR SUD$_2$ *ina* A GAZI^{sar} ŠEG$_6$-*šal tu-kaṣ$_3$-ṣa* LAL-*id*

10 A$_{i\,10}$ [DIŠ K]I MIN 1/2 SILA$_3$ ZA$_3$.ḪI.LI 1/2 SILA$_3$ ŠE.SA.A SUD$_2$ *ina* A GAZI⸢^{sar}* SILA$_{11}$⸣*-*aš* ^{šim}GUR$_2$.GUR$_2$ ^{šim}LI *ana* IGI *ta-za-ru$_3$* IGI *u* MAŠ.SILA$_3$ (eras.) LAL

11 A$_{i\,11}$ [DIŠ K]I* MIN 1/2 SILA$_3$ ZI$_3$ MUNU$_6$ 1/2 SILA$_3$ ZI$_3$ DUḪ.ŠE.GIŠ.I$_3$ 1/2 SILA$_3$ ZI$_3$ GIB$_3$ 1/2 SILA$_3$ ⸢^{šim}*GUR$_2$*.GUR$_2$⸣* 1/2 SILA$_3$ ^{šim}LI SUD$_2$ ḪI.ḪI *ina* A GAZI^{sar} *ta-la-aš* LAL-*id*

12 A$_{i\,12}$ [DIŠ N]A ŠA$_3$-*šu$_2$* GIG PA ^{u2}*er-re-e* ḪAD$_2$.A GAZ SIM *ina* LAL$_3$ KAŠ SAG *u* I$_3$ *ḫal-ṣi*

7 If DITTO, you mix (*tuballal*) a third of a litre of *saḫlû* ('cress'), a third of a litre of *zē summati* ('pigeon droppings'), a third of a litre of *labtu* ('roasted barley'), a third of a litre of *burāšu* (a kind of juniper) (and) a third of a litre of *kukru* (an aromatic),
8 you take enough (of the mixture) for an entire bandage, you kneed (*talâš*) it in high-quality beer, (and) you bandage (*taṣammid*) him.

9 If DITTO, you pound (*tasâk*) one mina of leaves from the ŠE.ḪAR (a tree), you bring it to a boil (*tušabšal*) in juice from *kasû* ('tamarind'), you let (the mixture) cool, (and) you bandage (*taṣammid*) him.

10 If DITTO, you pound (*tasâk*) half a litre of *saḫlû* ('cress') (and) half a litre of *labtu* ('roasted barley'), you knead (*talâš*) them in juice from *kasû* ('tamarind'), you strew *kukru* (an aromatic) (and) *burāšu* (a kind of juniper) over it, (and) you bandage (*taṣammid*) him front and back (lit. shoulder blades).

11 If DITTO, you pound (*tasâk*) (and) mix (*tuballal*) half a litre of flour from *buqlu* ('malt'), half a litre of flour from *kupsu* ('sesame pomace'),[292] half a litre of flour from *kibtu* ('wheat'), half a litre of *kukru* (an aromatic), (and) half a litre of *burāšu* (a kind of juniper), you kneed (the mixture) in juice from *kasû* ('tamarind'), (and) you bandage (*taṣammid*) him.

12 If someone's belly (*libbu*) is sick (*maruṣ*): you dry (*tubbal*), crush (*taḫaššal*) (and) sift (*tanappi*) leaves from *irrû* ('cucumber'), you stir (*tamaḫḫaṣ*) it into *dišpu* ('syrup'), high-quality beer and pressed oil,

292 DUḪ.ŠE.GIŠ.I$_3$ = Akk. *kupsu* probably describes the sesame cake that is left over after the extraction of oil (see Stol 1985a: 122 and 2009a: 404, as well as Abusch and Schwemer 2016: 512).

13 A$_{i 13}$ S[IG$_3$*-*a*]*ṣ ba-lu pa-tan* NAG-*šu*$_2$ *ina* DUR$_2$-*šu*$_2$ SI.SA$_2$-*ma* TI

---

14 A$_{i 14}$ DIŠ NA ⸢ŠA$_3$⸣*-*šu*$_2$ GIG ^{šim}*su-a-di tu-ḫa-sa ina* A SED *tu-la-bak* NU *pa-tan* NAG

---

15 A$_{i 15}$ DIŠ NA ⸢ŠA$_3$⸣-*šu*$_2$ GIG-*ma* DUB$_2$ NUMUN GIŠ.GI.ZU$_2$.LUM.MA ⸢SUD$_2$⸣ *ina* KAŠ SAG NAG 1/2 SILA$_3$ *saḫ-le*$_2$*-e* 1/2 SILA$_3$ NAGA SI

16 A$_{i 16}$ 1/2 ⸢SILA$_3$ ZI$_3$⸣ GIB$_3$ 1/2 SILA$_3$ ZI$_3$.KUM GAZ *ina* KAŠ SAG [SIL]A$_{11}$-*aš ina* TUG$_2$ SUR IGI *u* MAŠ.SILA$_3$ LAL

---

†

13 you have him drink (*tašaqqīšu*) it on an empty stomach, (and) he will void (*uše̮šser-ma*) from his anus; then he will recover (*iballuṭ*).

---

14 If someone's belly (*libbu*) is sick (*maruṣ*): you mince (*tuḫassa*) *suādu* (a kind of sedge),[293] you soften (*tulabbak*) it in cold water, (and) he drinks (*išatti*) it on an empty stomach.

---

15 If someone's belly (*libbu*) is sick (*maruṣ-ma*), and more specifically,[294] it throbs (*itarrak*):[295] you pound (*tasâk*) seed from *kūru*[296] (a plant), (and) he drinks (*išatti*) it in high-quality beer. You crush (*taḫaššal*) half a litre of *saḫlû* ('cress'), half a litre of *uḫūlu qarnānû* ('horned alkali'),

16 half a litre of flour from *kibtu* ('wheat'), (and) half a litre of *isqūqu* (a type of groats), you kneed (*talâš*) them in high-quality beer, you smear (*teṭerri*) (the mixture) on a piece of fabric, (and) you bandage (*taṣammid*) him front and back (lit. shoulder blades).

---

293 For the identification of the plant *suādu* as 'chufa (yellow nutsedge)', see Abusch and Schwemer 2011: 472.

294 The idiom DIŠ NA ŠA$_3$-*šu*$_2$ GIG-*ma*, followed by a more specific symptom in the trunk of the body, occurs here as well as in lines 21, 25, 37 and 50. As Eran Cohen (2015) has argued, the stative followed by *-*ma* (here *maruṣ-ma*) often represents a circumstantial clause that is specified by what follows. Lines 15, 21, 25, 37 and 50 all seem to exhibit this pattern (although line 37 is broken). The orthography DIŠ-*ma* in the second column probably represents a further abbreviation of DIŠ (NA ŠA$_3$-*šu*$_2$ GIG)-*ma*, for which see the commentary on line 84 below.

295 The Sumerogram DUB$_2$ probably corresponds to the Akkadian verb *tarāku* which can describe a throbbing sensation in various parts of the body (CAD T 204–205, Küchler 1904: 16, and Cadelli 2000: 149 n. 7). The verb *tarāku* can also occur alongside *libbu* in order to express someone's fearfulness, although not in medical texts (see Leichty 2011: 21 ln. 85).

296 Although GIŠ.GI.ZU$_2$.LUM.MA and GI.ZU$_2$.LUM.MA may represent orthographic variants of a single logogram, presumably corresponding to Akk. *kūru*, other Akkadian equivalents like *buṣinnu* and *kurṣiptu* are also possible. The two orthographies are carefully separated in STO: GIŠ.GI.ZU$_2$.LUM.MA is only found in STO 2, while GI.ZU$_2$.LUM.MA is only found in STO 3 and 4. In Uruanna II 381 (351), the plant also has the descriptive name *kurṣipti eqli* 'field butterfly' (CAD K 568). BAM 10 pp. 273 and 282 translates it as 'date reed', while Abusch and Schwemer (2011: 469) suggest 'mullein'.

17 A$_{i\,17}$ DIŠ NA ŠA$_3$-*šu*$_2$ GIG ^{u2}IGI-*lim* SUD$_2$ *ina* KAŠ SAG ⸢*tara-muk*⸣ *ina* MUL$_4$ *tuš-bat* NU *pa-tan* NAG
18 A$_{i\,18}$ PA ^{giš}ŠE.NU GAZ *ina* ZI$_3$.KUM ḪI.ḪI *ina* A GAZI$^{⸢sar⸣}$ *tara-bak ina* TUG$_2$.ḪI.A SUR IGI *u* MAŠ.SILA$_3$ LAL

---

19 A$_{i\,19}$ DIŠ KI MIN GA.RAŠ^{sar} *bu-ut-ta-ti ta-sak*$_3$ *ina* GA NAG

---

20 A$_{i\,20}$ 1/2 SILA$_3$ ZA$_3$.ḪI.LI 1/2 SILA$_3$ ŠE.SA.A *ina* GA SILA$_{11}$-*aš ina* TUG$_2$ SUR LAL

☨

17 If someone's belly (*libbu*) is sick (*maruṣ*): you pound (*tasâk*) *imḫur-līm* ('faces a thousand' plant), you soak it in high-quality beer, you leave (the mixture) out overnight under the stars, (and) he drinks (*išatti*) it on an empty stomach.

18 You crush (*taḫaššal*) leaves from *šunû* ('chaste tree'), you mix (*tuballal*) it with *isqūqu* (a type of groats), you stir them into a paste in juice from *kasû* ('tamarind'), you smear (*teṭerri*) (the mixture) on a piece of fabric, (and) you bandage (*taṣammid*) him front and back (lit. shoulder blades).

---

19 If DITTO, you pound (*tasâk*) *karašu* ('leek') that has been left out overnight (*buttāti*),[297] (and) he drinks (*išatti*) it in milk.

---

20 You knead (*talâš*) half a litre of *saḫlû* ('cress') (and) half a litre of *labtu* ('roasted barley') in milk, you smear (*teṭerri*) (the mixture) on a piece of fabric, (and) you bandage (*taṣammid*) him.

---

297 Stol (2020a: 106) has recently suggested that forms like A.MEŠ *bu-ut-tu-ti* in BAM 152 iv 8 and KAŠ *bu-ut-ti* in BAM 122 rev. 7′ are D-stem adjectives derived from *biātu* 'to spend the night', hence our translation of GA.RAŠ^{sar} *bu-ut-ta-ti* as '*karašu* that has been left out overnight', replacing GA.RAŠ^{sar} *pu-ut-ta-ti* 'a sectioned(?) leek' in CAD K 213. While *karašu* seems to be a masculine noun, the word for 'leek' in Neo-Assyrian administrative documents is either KUR-(*i*-)*sa-a-te* or KUR.MI$_2$.MEŠ (SAA 7 161 and 162). These are clearly feminine plural forms, indicated by the phonetic rendering *-issāte* and its logographic equivalent MI$_2$.MEŠ, meaning 'women' in Neo-Assyrian (Postgate 1987: 98 and Parpola 1988: 74). According to Postgate, the corresponding Akkadian form might have been *kurissāte*, which has nearly the same consonantal elements as *karašu*. Although it would be surprising for a Nineveh scribe, well-versed in Standard Babylonian, to mix his native language into a Standard Babylonian text, perhaps he misinterpreted GA.RAŠ^{sar} as a feminine plural and modified it with the correspondingly feminine plural adjective, viz. *bu-ut-ta-ti*.

21 A$_{i\,21}$ DIŠ NA ŠA$_3$-*šu*$_2$ GIG-*ma* ŠA$_3$ GIR$_3$.PAD.DU-*šu*$_2$ SIG$_7$ Š[A$_3$-*šu*$_2$[298] GI]G.MEŠ DIRI UD.DA SA$_2$.SA$_2$
DIŠ NA ŠA$_3$-*šu*$_2$ GIG-*ma* ŠA$_3$ GIR$_3$.PAD.DA-*šu*$_2$ SIG$_7$ ŠUB-*a* ŠA$_3$-*šu*$_2$ [x x x] / NA BI UD.DA SA$_2$.SA$_2$ (BAM 52 rev. 9–10)

22 A$_{i\,22}$ I$_3$.UD[U UK]UŠ$_2$.ḪAB *ina* ZI$_3$ ŠE.SA.A ḪI.ḪI 14 *ku-pa-tin-n*[*i* LA]L$_3$ ⸢SUD⸣ *u*$_2$*-al-lat*
I$_3$.UDU UKUŠ$_2$.ḪAB *ina* ZI$_3$ ŠE.SA.A [x x] / 14 *ku-pa-tin-nu* LAL$_3$ SUD ⸢*u*$_2$⸣-[*al-lat*] (BAM 52 rev. 10–11)

---

23 A$_{i\,23}$ ⸢1/2⸣ S[ILA$_3$ Z]A$_3$.ḪI.LI ^{giš}*si-ḫa* SUD$_2$ *ina* U[ZU GU]D* ⸢GUR$_4$⸣.RA[299] GU$_7$.MEŠ

24 A$_{i\,24}$ ⸢1/2⸣* [SIL]A$_3$ ZA$_3$.ḪI.LI *ṭe*$_4$*-ne-ti*$_3$ *ina* [x x x] ⸢SILA$_{11}$⸣-*aš* LAL

---

†

21 If someone's belly (*libbu*) is sick (*maruṣ-ma*), and more specifically, it has yellow 'subcutaneous bruises',[300] his belly is full (*mali*) of lesions, (and) he is . . . by fever (*ṣēta* SA$_2$.SA$_2$):[301]

22 you mix (*tuballal*) pulp from *irrû* ('cucumber') with flour from *labtu* ('roasted barley'), you sprinkle (*tusallaḫ*)[302] the fourteen pills with *dišpu* ('syrup'), (and) he swallows them.

---

23 You pound (*tasâk*) half a litre of *saḫlû* ('cress') (and) *sīḫu* ('wormwood'), (and) he keeps eating (*ītanakkal*) them with fatty beef$^?$.

24 You knead (*talâš*) half$^?$ a litre of ground *saḫlû* ('cress') in . . . (and) you bandage (*taṣammid*) him.

---

298 Although the parallel might suggest reading ŠUB-*a* instead of ŠA$_3$-*šu*$_2$, there are enough traces of ŠA$_3$ before the break to exclude this possibility.

299 See STO 3: 208, with the syllabic orthography UZU GUD *kab-ra*.

300 The literal translation of ŠA$_3$ GIR$_3$.PAD.DU-*šu*$_2$ SIG$_7$ as 'the inside (*libbu*) of his bone is yellow' makes little sense, and even if we were to assume a pun (*libbu* for *lipû*, written I$_3$.UDU, the usual term for 'marrow'), it is unlikely that a physician could assess this condition. The phrase ŠA$_3$ GIR$_3$.PAD.DU/DA reappears in BAM 580 iii 20′–25′, which also deals with *simmu* 'wound', and there a distinction is made between signs of the disease on the surface of the skin (*pān šīri*) and signs under the skin's surface (*libbi eṣemti*). This suggests that the idiom refers to subcutaneous bruising of some kind. For the expression *ina libbi eṣemti* in a similar context and also in connection with fever, see SAA 10 242 as well as Cadelli 2019: 59.

301 The correct Akkadian rendering of *ṣēta* SA$_2$.SA$_2$ is unclear, although it should be distinguished from *ṣēta kašid*, usually written UD.DA KUR-*id*. See Johnson 2014b: 23–26 and further discussion in STO 4, where the two orthographies occur in different sections.

302 According to CAD S 86, there is a distinct use of *salāḫu* for softening pills and other carriers with oil or other substances like syrup, hence the restoration [LA]L$_3$ SUD above, which is also confirmed by the parallel BAM 52 rev. 11 (Cadelli 2000: 125–126). Other passages give somewhat different formulations, such as 7 *u* 7 *ku-pa-ti-ni* DU$_3$-*uš* LAL$_3$ KUR-*i u-ṣap-pa u*$_2$*-al-lat* in BAM 159 ii 14–15.

25 A$_{\text{i }25}$ D[IŠ* NA Š]A$_3$-*šu*$_2$ GIG-*ma di-ik-ša*$_2$ TUKU-*ši* NINDA GU$_7$ K[AŠ NAG *ana* DUR$_2$-*šu*$_2$ DUB]-⸢*ak*[303] *ru*⸣-*pu-uš-ta ina* A.GAR$_3$ NAG$^?$.NAG$^?$[304]

26 A$_{\text{i }26}$ [^{u2}N]U.LUḪ.ḪA SUD$_2$ *ina* A NAG ⸢U$_2$ BABBAR⸣ [*ina* I$_3$.GIŠ *tara-bak ana*][305] DUR$_2$-*šu*$_2$ DUB-*ak*

27 A$_{\text{i }27}$ ⸢GEŠTIN⸣ SUR NAG ^{šim}LI ⸢ŠIM⸣.Š[AL x x x *ina* ^{urudu}ŠE]N.TUR *tara-bak ina* TUG$_2$ SUR LAL

---

28 A$_{\text{i }28}$ [DIŠ KI MIN U$_2$] BABBAR *ina* I$_3$.GIŠ NAG *i-ar*$_2$*-ru*$_3$ x [x x x x x x ^{u2}I]N$_6$.UŠ$_2$ ^{u2}EME UR.GI$_7$

29 A$_{\text{i }29}$ [*ina* A ŠE]G$_6$.GA$_2$ *tara-ḫas*$_2$*-su* A GAZI^{sar} [x x x x x x GIŠIM]MAR[306] PA ^{giš}*šu-še*

†

25 If someone's belly (*libbu*) is sick (*maruṣ-ma*), and more specifically, he has (*iraššī*) a pressing pain (*dikšu*),[307] he eats (*ikkal*) bread (and) drinks (*išatti*) beer, (but then) he voids (*utabbak*) it through his anus, (and) he keeps swallowing (*ištanatti*) (lit. drinking) (his own) phlegm (*rupuštu*) . . . :

26 you pound (*tasâk*) *nuḫurtu* ('asafoetida'), (and) he drinks it in water. You stir into a paste *šammu peṣû* ('white plant') in oil, (and) you pour (*tašappak*) (the mixture) into his anus.

27 He drinks pressed wine. You stir into a paste *burāšu* (a kind of juniper) (and) *šimiššallû* ('box tree') . . . in a small copper pot, you smear (*teṭerri*) (the mixture) on a piece of fabric, (and) you bandage (*taṣammid*) him.

---

28 If DITTO, he drinks (*išatti*) *šammu peṣû* ('white plant') in oil, (and) he will vomit. You bring to a boil (*tušabšal*) . . . *maštakal* ('soapwort') (and) *lišān kalbi* ('dog's tongue' plant)

29 in water, (and) you bathe him in it. . . . juice from *kasû* ('tamarind') . . . *gišimmaru* ('date palm')$^?$, leaves from *šūšu* ('liquorice'),

---

303 The fragmentary passage was restored by using BAM 88 obv. 13′–14′ as a distant parallel: [DIŠ NA DUR$_2$ GI]G-*ma di-ik-ša*$_2$ TUKU-*ši* / [NINDA *u* A ŠA$_3$-*šu*$_2$ *la i*]-*ma-ḫar* UḪ$_2$ *ina*$^!$ DUR$_2$-*šu*$_2$ *u*$_2$-[*tab-bak*].

304 The damaged passage at the end of the line only allows for a provisional restoration, based on the occurrence of 'piercing pain' (Akk. *dikšu*) in conjunction with phlegm (Akk. *rupuštu*) in STO 4: 54′–55′. The end of the line could also be read, however, as BURU$_8$ GIGURU$_3$ 'he vomits (and) swallows phlegm . . .'. GIGURU$_3$ (KA×LAG) = Akk. *alātu* or *la'ātu* 'to swallow' is only otherwise attested, outside of the lexical tradition, in BM 78963 rev. 26 (Stadhouders and Johnson 2018: 581–582 ln. 72, and 605).

305 The tentative restoration of the passage is based on line 34 below.

306 Only the end of the sign is visible after the break, perhaps either TIR or GIŠIMMAR. If it were GAMUN (= DIN.TIR), as Cadelli (2000: 126) suggests, we would expect SAR as a following determinative.

307 For the meaning 'bulge' of *dikšu*, see already AHw 169. We take *dikšu* 'bulge' as a description of 'pressure' felt within the body of the patient rather than 'piercing pain' as in CAD D 137–138. In line 163 below, *dikšu* appears in connection with the build-up of gases within the abdominal cavity, which is often described in terms of abdominal pressure.

30 A$_{i\,30}$ [^{šim}ŠE.L]I PA ^{giš}ŠE.NU ^{šim}LI ^{šim}G[UR$_2$.GUR$_2$ x x x x x *ina* KU]Š *te-ṭer*$_5$*-ri* LAL

---

31 A$_{i\,31}$ [DIŠ KI MIN] ⸢^{u2}⸣GEŠTIN KA$_5$.A *ina* KAŠ NAG U$_2$ BABBAR *ina* I$_3$ ⸢NAG⸣* x [x x x *ina*] LAL$_3$ GU$_7$

32 A$_{i\,32}$ [A ^{giš}ŠE].NU A GAZI^{sar} *ana* DUR$_2$*-šu*$_2$ DUB-*ak* ⸢PA⸣* [x x x x] ⸢^{u2}⸣SIKIL

33 A$_{i\,33}$ [P]A ^{u2}ŠAKIRA PA ^{u2}IN$_6$.UŠ$_2$ GAZ x [x x x x SU]R LAL

---

34 A$_{i\,34}$ [DIŠ] ⸢KI⸣ MIN ^{u2}NU.LUḪ.ḪA ^{u2}*ti-ia*$_2$*-ta*$_5$ SUD$_2$ *ina* KAŠ ⸢NAG⸣* [U$_2$ BABBAR *ina* I$_3$.GIŠ *tara-bak ana* DUR$_2$*-šu*$_2$ DU]B-*ak*[308]

35 A$_{i\,35}$ [PA ^{u2}]GUR$_2$.UŠ PA ^{giš}KIŠI$_{16}$ PA ^{giš}DIḪ$_3$ *ina* ⸢A⸣* [ŠEG$_6$.GA$_2$ *tara-ḫas*$_2$*-su* A ^{giš}ŠE.NU A GAZI^{sa}]⸢[309]

✝

30 *kikkirânu* ('juniper seeds')$^?$, leaves from *šunû* ('chaste tree'), *burāšu* (a kind of juniper), (and) *kukru* (an aromatic) . . . you smear (the mixture) on a piece of leather, (and) you bandage (*taṣammid*) him.[310]

---

31 If DITTO, he drinks (*išatti*) *karān šēlebi* ('fox-vine') in beer, he drinks *šammu peṣû* ('white plant') in oil, (and) he eats (*ikkal*) . . . in *dišpu* ('syrup').

32 You pour (*tašappak*) juice from *šunû* ('chaste tree') (and) juice from *kasû* ('tamarind') into his anus. You crush (*taḫaššal*) leaves from . . . *sikillu* ('pure' plant),

33 leaves from *šakirû* (a plant) (and) leaves from *maštakal* ('soapwort') . . . you smear (*teṭerri*) (the mixture) on a . . . (and) you bandage (*tasammid*) him.

---

34 If DITTO, you pound (*tasâk*) *nuḫurtu* ('asafoetida') (and) *tīyatu* (a plant) (and) he drinks (*išatti*) them in beer. You stir into a paste *šammu peṣû* ('white plant') in oil, (and) you pour (*tašappak*) (the mixture) into his anus.

35 You bring to a boil (*tušabšal*) leaves from *šarmadu* (a plant),[311] leaves from *ašāgu* ('acacia'), (and) leaves from *baltu* (a thornbush) in water, (and) you bathe him in it. You pour juice from *šunû* ('chaste tree') (and) juice from *kasû* ('tamarind')

---

308 The middle of line 34, namely NAG U$_2$ BABBAR *ina* I$_3$.GIŠ, which is still present in Küchler's (1904) and Köcher's (1980) copies, is now missing from the tablet.

309 As with the preceding line, the middle of line 35, namely A ŠEG$_6$.GA$_2$ *tara-ḫas*$_2$-⸢*su*⸣, which Küchler (1904) and Köcher (1980) included in their copies, is now missing. The restoration of the rest of the line is based on line 32 above.

310 Several key expressions are missing from this passage, which has the same overall structure as the prescription in lines 34–36 below. Based on this parallel, the missing part of our passage may have included a *kasû* juice enema and a paste-based bandage made of several ingredients in a small copper pot.

311 In line with Böck 2003: 181, ^{u2}GUR$_2$.UŠ is probably a variant orthography for ^{u2}GUR$_5$.UŠ = Akk. *šarmadu*; see also Attia 2015: 110. The logogram is rendered the same way in EYES 2: 112′ (BAM 10 pp. 133–134).

36 A$_{i\,36}$ [*ana* DU]R$_2$-*šu*$_2$ DUB-*ak* ^{šim}L[I* ^{šim}GUR$_2$].GUR$_2$* x [x x *ina* ^{urudu}ŠEN.TUR *tara-bak ina* TUG$_2$ *te-ṭer*$_5$*-ri* LAL][312]

---

37 A$_{i\,37}$ [DIŠ N]A ŠA$_3$-*šu*$_2$ GIG-*ma* Š[A$_3$-*šu*$_2$ ....]

38 A$_{i\,38}$ [x x] x x x [x] x [...]

two missing lines

41 A$_{i\,41}$ ⸢DIŠ KI MIN U$_2$ BABBAR⸣ x [..] x

42 A$_{i\,42}$ $^{\text{u2}}$SIKIL x [x x] ⸢A$^?$⸣* [............] x* x* x* x* [.............. *ana* DUR$_2$-*šu*$_2$ DU]B-*ak*

43 A$_{i\,43}$ ^{šim}LI ⸢^{šim}ŠE.LI⸣ ^{šim}GAM.MA ILLU ⸢^{šim}⸣BULUḪ ŠIM.ḪI.A ⸢GAZ *ina* I$_3$.UDU⸣ Ḫ[I*.ḪI *ina* KUŠ SUR] LAL

---

44 A$_{i\,44}$ DIŠ KI MIN ^{šim}ŠE.LI BABBAR *ina* KAŠ NAG-*ma i-ar*$_2$*-ru*$_3$ SUḪUŠ ^{giš}NAM.TAR NITA$_2$ *ina* KAŠ NAG-*ma i-ar*$_2$*-ru*$_3$ ⸢LAL$_3$⸣ [KUR.RA ḪAD$_2$].DA

†

36 into his anus. You stir into a paste *burāšu* (a kind of juniper) (and) *kukru* (an aromatic) . . . in a small copper pot, you smear (the mixture) on a piece of fabric, (and) you bandage (*taṣammid*) him.

---

37 If someone's belly (*libbu*) is sick (*maruṣ-ma*), and more specifically, his belly . . .

38 . . .

two missing lines

41 If DITTO, . . . *šammu peṣû* ('white plant') . . .

42 *sikillu* ('pure' plant) . . . (and) you pour (*tašappak*) them into his anus$^?$.

43 *burāšu* (a kind of juniper), *kikkirânu* ('juniper seeds'), *ṣumlalû* (an aromatic), (and) resin from *baluḫḫu* ('galbanum')[313]—you crush (*taḫaššal*) (these) aromatics, you mix (*tuballal*) them in fat, you smear (*teṭerri*) (the mixture) on a piece of leather, (and) you bandage (*taṣammid*) him.

---

44 If DITTO, he drinks (*išattī-ma*) white *kikkirânu* ('juniper seeds') in beer, and then he will vomit. He drinks root from male *pillû* ('mandrake') in beer, and then he will vomit. You dry (*tubbal*) *dišpu* ('syrup') from the mountains,

---

312 Three signs, namely LI, ŠIM and GUR$_2$, as well as traces of URUDU are still present in Küchler's (1904) and Köcher's (1980) copies, but they are now largely missing from the tablet. The restoration of the rest of the line is based on line 27 above.

313 Our translation of *baluḫḫu* and *ḫīl baluḫḫi* as 'ferula gummosa' and 'galbanum', respectively, follows Abusch and Schwemer 2011: 469.

45 A$_{i\,45}$ *ina* A ^{giš}ŠE.NU *tara-ḫas$_2$-su* A.GEŠTIN.NA I$_3$.GIŠ KUM$_2$*-am ana* DUR$_2$*-šu$_2$* DUB*-ak* PA ^{giš}*šu-še* PA ⸢GIŠ⸣.[GI.ZU$_2$.L]UM.MA

46 A$_{i\,46}$ PA ^{u2}ŠAKIRA PA ^{u2}EME UR.GI$_7$ ^{šim}LI ZU$_2$.LUM.MA[314] SUD$_2$ *ina* KAŠ ḪI.ḪI GUR*-ma* ḪAD$_2$.DU <GAZ> ⸢SIM*⸣ *ina** x* [x x *ina* KU]Š SUR LAL

---

47 A$_{i\,47}$ ⸢DIŠ KI MIN⸣ ^{u2}KUR.KUR *ina* KAŠ NAG*-ma i-ar$_2$-ru$_3$* U$_2$ BABBAR *ina* I$_3$.GIŠ NAG*-ma i-ar$_2$-ru$_3$* ^{u2}PEŠ.TUR.Z[I GIŠIM]MAR[315]

48 A$_{i\,48}$ [^{u2}N]AM.TAL ^{šim}LI GAZI^{sar} *ina* A ŠEG$_6$.GA$_2$ *tara-ḫas$_2$-su* ^{šim}GUR$_2$.GUR$_2$ *ta-sak$_3$ i*[*na* LAL$_3$].ḪAD$_2$[316]

45 (and) you bathe him in it with juice from *šunû* ('chaste tree'). You heat (*tummam*) vinegar (and) oil, (and) you pour (*tašappak*) them into his anus. You pound (*tasâk*) leaves from *šūšu* ('liquorice'), leaves from *kūru* (a plant),

46 leaves from *šakirû* (a plant), leaves from *lišān kalbi* ('dog's tongue' plant), *burāšu* (a kind of juniper), (and) *suluppū* ('dates'), you mix (*tuballal*) them in beer, (then) you dry, crush (*taḫaššal*) (and) sift (*tanappi*) (the mixture) over and over again (*tatâr-ma*),[317] . . . in . . ., you smear (*teṭerri*) (the mixture) on a piece of leather, (and) you bandage (*taṣammid*) him.

---

47 If DITTO, he drinks (*išattī-ma*) *atā'išu* (a plant) in beer, and then he will vomit. He drinks *šammu peṣû* ('white plant') in oil, and then he will vomit. You bring to a boil (*tušabšal*) *liblibbi gišimmari* ('offshoot of date palm'),

48 *pillû* ('mandrake'), *burāšu* (a kind of juniper), (and) *kasû* ('tamarind') in water, (and) you bathe him in it. You pound *kukru* (an aromatic),

314 Although the MA following ZU$_2$.LUM is, historically speaking, a Sumerian genitive case, it is not used consistently in the medical corpus to mark the second term of a genitive construction. Curiously, however, PA for Akk. *aru* 'leaf' occurs as part of the four ingredients that precede ^{šim}LI and ZU$_2$.LUM.MA. Similarly, two other lists of ingredients end with the same phrase, but with ZI$_3$ for Akk. *qēmu* 'flour' as the repeating element: AMT 96/1 obv. 9 has ZI$_3$ ^{šim}MAN.DU ZI$_3$ ^{šim}GUR$_2$.GUR$_2$ ZI$_3$ ^{šim}LI ZU$_2$.LUM.MA, while BAM 217 rev. 2–3 has ZI$_3$ ŠE ⸢ŠEŠ⸣ ZI$_3$ MUNU$_6$ ZI$_3$ ^{šim}⸢MAN.DU⸣ [. . .] / ŠEŠ ^{šim}LI ZU$_2$.LUM.MA.

315 See Cadelli 2000: 127, with the reading ^{u2}GIR.TUR ⸢x⸣ [. . . ^{giš}GIŠ]IMMAR. A more probable rendering of this fragmentary passage may be ^{u2}PEŠ.TUR.ZI = Akk. *liblibbu*, which is used in connection with date palms in the sense of 'heart' (CAD L p. 175) or 'young and productive offshoot' (Landsberger 1967: 28–29).

316 The medical substance LAL$_3$.ḪAD$_2$, typically rendered as LAL$_3$.BABBAR, for Akk. *lallāru*, also features in EYES 2: 195′ and EYES 3: 1 (BAM 10 pp. 147 and 158). See also BAM 494 iii 4, for the somewhat different LAL$_3$ KUR*-i* BABBAR 'white mountain honey' (Bácskay and Simkó 2017: 44–45). As Stol (2021: 443) points out, MSL 14 p. 334 ln. 87 suggests that the correct reading of UD in this word, according to the first-millennium lexical tradition, is actually ḪAD$_2$ rather than BABBAR: ḫa-ad = UD = *ša$_2$* LAL$_3$.UD *lal-la-ru*.

317 Used as a hendiadys, the form *tatâr-ma* seems to describe the repetition of a series of actions as a sequence, viz. ACTION A$_1$ and ACTION B$_1$ followed by ACTION A$_2$ and ACTION B$_2$, rather than the separate repetition of the individual actions, which would normally have been expressed with a Gtn verbal form. In STO 2, the sequence of actions following *tatâr-ma* usually consists of ḪAD$_2$.DU = Akk. *tubbal* ('you dry') and GAZ = Akk. *taḫaššal* ('you crush'), twice with the addition of SIM = Akk. *tanappi* ('you sift') here and in line 231 below. The logic of the procedure in this line, viz. drying and sifting the ingredients without crushing, makes an emendation necessary, namely the addition of GAZ = Akk. *taḫaššal*.

49 A$_{i\,49}$ [KU]M$_2$*-*am* I$_3$.GIŠ *ana* ŠA$_3$ *tu-na-tak ana* DUR$_2$-*šu*$_2$ DUB-*ak* PA ^{giš}ŠENNUR PA ^{giš}MA.NU PA ^{giš}ŠE.NU PA ^{g}[^{iš}GE$_6$.PA]R$_7$

50 A$_{i\,50}$ [P]A$^{?}$ $^{giš.šim}$LI[318] ^{šim}GUR$_2$.GUR$_2$ GAZ *ina* KAŠ ḪI.ḪI GUR-*ma* ḪAD$_2$.A GAZ *ina* I$_3$.UDU ḪI.ḪI *ina* KUŠ *te-ṭer*$_5$-⸢*ri* LAL⸣[319]

---

51 A$_{i\,51}$ [DIŠ N]A ŠA$_3$-*šu*$_2$ GIG-*ma*$^{!}$(GIŠ)* *mim**-*ma**[320] GIG ^{u2}KUR.RA ^{u2}ḪAR.ḪAR ^{u2}KUR.KUR ^{u2}GAM[UN.G]E$_6$

52 A$_{i\,52}$ [^{u2}]⸢*ur*$_2$⸣-*ne*$_2$-*e* ^{u2}*tar-muš*$_8$ ^{u2}IGI-*lim* ^{u2}*eli-kul-la* ^{u2}SIKIL ^{u2}*im-ḫur*-NIŠ GURUN ^{gi}[^{š}DI]Ḫ$_3$

53 A$_{i\,53}$ [x] ⸢^{u2}⸣x x[321] PA ^{u2}UKUŠ$_2$.ḪAB SUD$_2$ *ina* KAŠ NAG *ina* DUR$_2$-*šu*$_2$ SI.SA$_2$ *ina* GE$_6$ *ina* A GAZI^{sar} ŠEG$_6$.G[A$_2$]*

☨

49 you heat it (*tummam*) in *lallāru* ('white honey')$^{?}$, you drip oil in (the mixture), (and) you pour (*tašappak*) it into his anus. You crush (*taḫaššal*) leaves from *šallūru* ('plum tree'), leaves from *ēru* (a tree), leaves from *šunû* ('chaste tree'), leaves from *lipāru* ('a fruit tree'),

50 leaves$^{?}$ from *burāšu* (a kind of juniper), (and) *kukru* (an aromatic), you mix (*tuballal*) them in beer, (then) you dry (*tubbal*) (and) crush (the mixture) over and over again (*tatâr-ma*), you mix it in fat, you smear it on a piece of leather, (and) you bandage (*taṣammid*) him.

---

51 If someone's belly (*libbu*) is sick (*maruṣ-ma*), and in addition, he has any (other) illness (*mimma murṣu*):[322] you pound (*tasâk*) *nīnû* ('mint'), *ḫašû* ('thyme'), *atā'išu* (a plant), *zibû* ('black cumin'),

52 *urnû* (a kind of mint), *tarmuš* ('lupin'), *imḫur-līm* ('faces a thousand' plant), *elikulla* (a plant), *sikillu* ('pure' plant), *imḫur-ešrā* ('faces twenty' plant), fruit from *baltu* (a thornbush)$^{?}$,

53 . . . (and) leaves from *irrû* ('cucumber'), he drinks (*išatti*) them in beer, (and) he will void (*ušeššer*) from his anus. At night, in hot juice from *kasû* ('tamarind'),

---

318 For this tentative reading, see already Küchler 1904: 18. The logogram LI for Akk. *burāšu* (a kind of juniper) only occurs a few times accompanied by both the determinatives GIŠ and ŠIM, although this is the only occurrence in the medical corpus (CAD B 327). This odd form may be related to the omission of PA from the list of ingredients in line 46 above.

319 Compare the very similar passage in BAM 99 rev. 16–17: GAZ *ina* KAŠ *ta-la-aš* GUR-*ma* ḪAD$_2$.DU ⸢GAZ⸣ / *ina* I$_3$.UDU ḪI.ḪI *ina* KUŠ *te-ṭer*$_5$-*ri* [LAL].

320 Cadelli (2000: 127 and 172) reads the passage as [DIŠ N]A ŠA$_3$-*šu*$_2$ GIG *ma-dam* GIG 'si un homme présente une maladie grave du ventre', but collations suggest that the text has a somewhat malformed GIŠ rather than MA and perhaps NIN rather than DAM. In line with the other occurrences of the same phrase earlier in the column, we emend GIŠ to MA and read it as [DIŠ N]A ŠA$_3$-*šu*$_2$ GIG-*ma*$^{!}$(GIŠ) *mim-ma* GIG.

321 Cadelli's (2000: 127) reconstruction [PA] ⸢^{u2}GIR.TUR⸣ does not seem plausible: the plant ^{u2}GIR.TUR is not otherwise attested in the medical corpus. The only phrase that would seem to correspond partly to the remaining traces of signs is PA ^{giš}GIŠIMMAR.TUR, as in BAM 124 i 43, but this is also unlikely due to the limited space available.

322 The expression *mimma murṣu* is probably a catch-all phrase that takes the place of the more specific symptoms found in earlier lines of the text, namely 15, 21, 25 and 37. The expression *mimma murṣu* also appears as a concluding remark in KAR 73 obv. 20: *mim-ma mur-ṣu ša*$_2$ *mar-ṣa-ku-ma* '(and) any illness that I am suffering from'; see also ln. 5 of the same text (BAM 7 pp. 104–105).

54 A$_{i\,54}$ [x] x x [...] x x x UZU *kab-ra ša* ŠAḪ GU$_7$ [TI]

---

55 A$_{i\,55}$ [.......................................] ⸢SUD$_2$⸣ *ina* I$_3$.GIŠ NU *pa-tan* EME-*šu*$_2$ DAB-[*bat*]
56 A$_{i\,56}$ [..] x *šu*$_2$ *u*$_2$*-sak*$_6$*-k*[*a*]

---

57 A$_{i\,57}$ [...............................] x x *ina* I$_3$.GIŠ ḪI.ḪI *ta-kan-nak-ma* UD.3.KAM$_2$ GAR

ŠIM *šu-a-ti* / *ana* ŠA$_3$ ḪI.ḪI *pa-ṣu-u*$_2$ *ana* UGU ŠUB-*ma* 3 UD *ka-nik*$_2$ *ina* UD.3.KAM BAD-*ma* (eras.) *ana* ^{d}GAŠAN BAL (Stadhouders and Johnson 2018: 574 lines 34–35)

58 A$_{i\,58}$ [...] ⸢*i-ar*$_2$⸣*-ru*$_3$ UD.7.KAM$_2$ NAG.MEŠ

---

59 A$_{i\,59}$ [..] *ina* KAŠ SAG NAG

---

60 A$_{i\,60}$ [..] PA ^{giš}NU.UR$_2$.MA

†

54 . . . (and) he eats (*ikkal*) fatty pork; (then) he will recover (*iballuṭ*)$^?$.

---

55 . . . you pound (*tasâk*) it, (and) you put (*tušaṣbat*) it with oil on his tongue (lit. have his tongue seize it) on an empty stomach,
56 . . . (and) he retches it up (*usakka*).[323]

---

57 . . . you mix (*tuballal*) it in oil, you seal up (the mixture), and then you let it stand (*tašakkan*) for three days,
58 . . . he will vomit. He keeps drinking (*ištanatti*) it for seven days.

---

59 . . . he drinks (*išatti*) it in high-quality beer.

---

60 . . . leaves from *nurmû* ('pomegranate'),

---

323 Most occurrences of this and similar orthographies, including *tu*-ZAK and *tu-zak-ka* in STO 3: 151, 153, 156, 245 and 246, represent a D-stem of *zakû* used to describe the purification of liquids by removing particulate matter. In our passage, however, this interpretation seems unlikely since the verb occurs at the end of the recipe. The gastric focus in our passage might allow for a different analysis, with the form *u*$_2$*-sak*$_6$(ZAG)*-ka* derived from Akk. *sâku*, which is sometimes used with the ventive in D-stem, in the sense 'to bring something up, to retch (but not necessarily to vomit)': CRAN 1: 12 (BAM 480+ i 12 and parallels) has *ina šikari rēštî* (var. *šikari*) *tamaḫḫaṣ-ma tašaqqīšu usakkā-ma tuša'râššu* (var. *iparra*) 'you stir (the ingredients) into high-quality beer, you have him drink it, he retches, and then you make him vomit'. For a discussion of this verb, see also CAD S 84 and Worthington 2006: 34.

61 $A_{i\,61}$ [………………………… *i*]*na* KAŠ SAG NAG

62 $A_{i\,62}$ […………………………] x *ina* I_3.GIŠ *u* KAŠ SAG GAZ
63 $A_{i\,63}$ […………………………] x x ad

64 $A_{i\,64}$ […………………………] x
65 $A_{i\,65}$ […………………………] x
66 $A_{i\,66}$ [………………………… $SILA_{11}$]-*aš*
67 $A_{i\,67}$ [………………………… T]U_5.⸢MEŠ⸣-*šu*$_2$-*ma* TI

68 $A_{i\,68}$ […………………………] ⸢NAG⸣*-*ma* TI

69 $A_{i\,69}$ […………………………] ⸢TI?-*uṭ*⸣

three missing lines

73 $A_{ii\,3}$ x […………………………]

†

61 … he drinks (*išatti*) it in high-quality beer.

62 … you crush (*taḫaššal*) it in oil and high-quality beer,
63 …

64 …
65 …
66 … you knead (*talâš*)? it
67 … you bathe him repeatedly (*tartanammukšū-ma*); then he will recover (*iballuṭ*).

68 … he drinks (*išattī-ma*) it; then he will recover (*iballuṭ*).

69 … he will recover (*iballuṭ*)?

three missing lines

73 …

74 A$_{ii\,4}$ NA$_4$ Z[U$_2$.LUM.MA][324] x x [..]
75 A$_{ii\,5}$ A.MEŠ ⸢NU* NAG A⸣.M[EŠ* ....]

---

76 A$_{ii\,6}$ ^{u2}KUR.RA SUD$_2$ *ina* A [...]

---

77 A$_{ii\,7}$ BAR ^{giš}NU.UR$_2$.MA-*a ša* ^{im}SI.SA$_2$ *ina* [...]
[. . . ^{giš}NU.UR$_2$].⸢MA⸣ *ša$_2$* ^{im}SI.SA$_2$ *ina* KAŠ ^{lu2}K[URUN$_2$.NA . . .] (AMT 38/3+ obv. 4′)

---

78 A$_{ii\,8}$ SUM^{sar} SIG$_7$-*su ḫi-bi-iš ḫi-bi-iš*[325] *u$_2$-al-lat* [...]

---

79 A$_{ii\,9}$ NUMUN ^{u2}*a-zu-ki-ra-ni*[326] SUD$_2$ [...]

---

74 *aban suluppi* (‘date stone’)$^?$ . . .
75 He should not drink (*lā išatti*) water, . . . water . . .

---

76 You pound (*tasâk*) *nīnû* (‘mint’) . . . in water . . .

---

77 . . . rind from *nurmû* (‘pomegranate’) from the north side in brewer’s$^?$ beer$^?$ . . .

---

78 He swallows very finely chopped fresh *šūmū* (‘garlic’) . . .

---

79 You pound (*tasâk*) seed from *azupirānu* (‘saffron-like’ plant) . . .

---

324 See already Cadelli 2000: 129 for this reconstruction; less likely alternatives are ^{na4}K[A.GI.NA] for Akk. *šadânu* ‘haematite’ or ^{na4}Z[U$_2$] for Akk. *ṣurru* ‘obsidian’.

325 We follow CAD Š/3 300, viz. ‘finely chopped fresh garlic’, likely from the verb *ḫabāšu*, from which *ḫibištu* for ‘crushed pieces (of aromatic wood)’ also derives. The form here is problematic because the ŠIM sign consists of BI followed by IŠ as a single sign, so the sequence *ḫi-bi-iš* could also be read *ḫi-riq*(ŠIM): this form is not attested in Akkadian, but Mandaic uses √HRQ for ‘to grind’ (Drower and Macuch 1963: 153), corresponding to √ḤRQ in Jewish Aramaic and Hebrew.

326 Cadelli (2000: 129 n. 14) suggests a link to the fairly common noun *azupirānu*, with the suggested cognates *zaʿfarān* (AHw 93) or *ʿuṣfur* in Arabic (Landsberger 1966: 260 n. 56). Our form may have arisen via folk etymology, replacing /pi/ with either /ka/ (see already the Old Babylonian letter AbB 9 276 obv. 5) or /ki/ in our text, in order to arrive at *asû* ‘physician’ + *karānu* ‘vineyard’. The fact that *kirānu* is a by-form of *karānu* would further strengthen this folk etymology.

80 A$_{ii\ 10}$ 1/3 SILA$_3$ A.GEŠTIN.NA 1/3 SILA$_3$ GAZI^{sar} 10 KISAL MUN 1/2 SILA$_3$ I$_3$.GIŠ BA[RA$_2$.GA ....]

81 A$_{ii\ 11}$ A UZU GUR$_4$ 5 GIN$_2$ MUN *ana* ŠA$_3$ ŠUB-*ma* NU *pa-tan* NAG : SUḪ[UŠ ....]

82 A$_{ii\ 12}$ I$_3$.UDU ^{u2}UKUŠ$_2$.ḪAB GAZ 1 SILA$_3$ A.⸢GEŠTIN.NA⸣ ŠEG$_6$.GA$_2$ *ana* ŠA$_3$ ⸢ŠUB⸣ [...]

83 A$_{ii\ 13}$ ^{šim}LI SUD$_2$ *ina* ⸢I$_3$.GIŠ⸣ [...]

84 A$_{ii\ 14}$ DIŠ-*ma*[327] UḪ$_2$ TUKU.TUKU ^{u2}LAG GAN$_2$ SUD$_2$ *ina* A ^{giš}NU.UR$_2$.MA ⸢SED⸣ [*ina* DUR$_2$-*šu$_2$* D]UB-*ak-m*[*a** TI]

80 A third of a litre of vinegar, a third of a litre of *kasû* (‘tamarind’), 10 KISAL-measures of salt, half a litre of pressed oil . . .

81 You put (*tanaddī-ma*) five shekels of salt in broth from fatty meat, and he drinks (*išatti*) it on an empty stomach. Root from . . .

82 You crush (*taḫaššal*) pulp from *irrû* (‘cucumber’), you put (*tanaddi*) one litre of boiled vinegar in it . . .

83 You pound (*tasâk*) *burāšu* (a kind of juniper) . . . in oil . . .

84 If (someone’s belly is sick), and more specifically, he continually has (*irtanašši*) phlegm (*rupuštu*):[328] you pound (*tasâk*) *kirbān eqli* (‘field clod’ plant), you let it cool (*tukaṣṣa*) in juice from *nurmû* (‘pomegranate’), (and) you pour (*tašappak-ma*) it into his anus; then he will recover (*iballuṭ*).

327 DIŠ-*ma* is probably an abbreviation for DIŠ (NA ŠA$_3$-*šu$_2$* GIG)-*ma*, since the symptoms that follow here and in the analogous lines in column 2 are similar to the symptoms found following DIŠ NA ŠA$_3$-*šu$_2$* GIG-*ma* in column 1. Other possibilities, such as that DIŠ-*ma* is a pleonastic orthography for Akk. *šumma* ‘if’ or a previously unattested orthography for *enūma* ‘when’ do not explain the alternation between DIŠ-*ma* and DIŠ NA ŠA$_3$.MEŠ-*šu$_2$* MU$_2$.MU$_2$ here in lines 84 and 87, and again (but in reverse order) in lines 98 and 101.

328 The logogram UḪ$_2$ corresponds to four different Akkadian words: *ru’tu* ‘spittle’, *illātu* ‘saliva’, *rupuštu* ‘phlegm’ and *ḫaḫḫu* ‘mucus’, but syllabic spellings in the witchcraft literature suggest that UḪ$_2$ here corresponds to *rupuštu*. See, for example, the incipit DIŠ NA SAG ŠA$_3$-*šu$_2$* *ru-pul$_2$-ta* TUKU.MEŠ-*ši*, with variants, in Abusch and Schwemer 2011: 227 ln. 22, and 231 ln. 1′. For an overview of the different Akkadian words corresponding to UḪ$_2$, see also Stol 1993: 8–9 and Cadelli 2021: 9–12.

85 A$_{\text{ii 15}}$ *ša-ru-ra*[329] *ša* $^{\text{u2}}$UKUŠ$_2$.ḪAB ḪAD$_2$.DU GAZ *ana* ŠA$_3$ NIG$_2$.SILA$_{11}$.GA$_2$ *u* LAL$_3$ KUR-*i* ⸢ḪI*.ḪI⸣ [ŠE$_{10}$ T]U$^{\text{muš[en}}$.MEŠ]

86 A$_{\text{ii 16}}$ *u*$_2$*-al-lat* KAŠ SAG ZU$_2$.LUM NAG $^{\text{u2}}$ḪAB SUD$_2$ *ina* I$_3$.GIŠ ⸢BARA$_2$.GA⸣ [NAG].⸢NAG⸣*

---

87 A$_{\text{ii 17}}$ DIŠ NA ŠA$_3$.MEŠ-*šu*$_2$ MU$_2$.MU$_2$ *it-ta-ne*$_2$*-bi-ṭu* ŠA$_3$-*šu ana pa-re-e e-ta-ne*$_2$*-pa-aš*$_2$ *ana* TI-⸢*šu*$_2$⸣*

88 A$_{\text{ii 18}}$ SUM^{sar} $^{\text{u2}}$GAMUN.GE$_6$ TEŠ$_2$.BI SUD$_2$ *ina* KAŠ SAG NU *pa-tan* NAG.MEŠ ⸢TI⸣

---

89 A$_{\text{ii 19}}$ DIŠ KI MIN $^{\text{u2}}$SIKIL SIG$_7$-*su* SUD$_2$ KI I$_3$.ŠAḪ ḪI.ḪI NU *pa-tan u*$_2$*-na-ṣab* KAŠ BIL$_2$.LA$_2$ NAG T[I]

---

90 A$_{\text{ii 20}}$ DIŠ NA ŠA$_3$.MEŠ-*šu*$_2$ MU$_2$.MU$_2$ *it-te-ne*$_2$*-bi-ṭu* IM *ina* ŠA$_3$-*šu*$_2$ NIGIN-*ur i-le-bu* I$_3$.UDU $^{\text{u2}}$UKUŠ$_2$.ḪAB *ana* DUR$_2$-*šu*$_2$ ⸢GAR⸣-[*an*]

†

85 You dry (*tubbal*) (and) crush (*taḫaššal*) tendrils from *irrû* ('cucumber'), you mix (*tuballal*) it into dough and *dišpu* ('syrup') from the mountains, he swallows (the mixture) (with) *zē summati* ('pigeon droppings'),

86 (and then) he drinks (*išatti*) beer from *suluppū* ('dates').[330] You pound (*tasâk*) *būšānu* ('smelly' plant), (and) he keeps drinking (*ištanatti*) it in pressed oil.

---

87 If someone's internal organs (*qerbū*) are swollen (*napḫū*) (and) continually have cramps, his belly (*libbu*) continually acts like it is going to vomit: in order to heal him (*ana bulluṭīšu*),

88 you pound (*tasâk*) *šūmū* ('garlic') (and) *zibû* ('black cumin') together, (and) he keeps drinking (*ištanatti*) them in high-quality beer on an empty stomach; (then) he will recover (*iballuṭ*).

---

89 If DITTO, you pound (*tasâk*) fresh *sikillu* ('pure' plant), you mix (*tuballal*) it with lard, he sucks on it on an empty stomach, (and) he drinks (*išatti*) sour beer; (then) he will recover (*iballuṭ*).

---

90 If someone's internal organs (*qerbū*) are swollen (*napḫū*) (and) continually have cramps, flatulence (lit. wind) circulates (*isaḫḫur*) (and) rumbles in his belly (*libbu*): you put (*tašakkan*) pulp from *irrû* ('cucumber') into his anus.

---

329 This seems to be the only syllabic spelling of the word *šarūru* 'sprout, tendril', which otherwise occurs only rarely in the therapeutic literature. For a discussion of the different orthographies, see Heeßel 2018a: 332. In all likelihood, *šarūru* is an Aramaic loanword, presumably a precursor to the later Syriac term *šrūrā* (see Küchler 1904: 111 and Sokoloff 2009: 1603).

330 This rare ingredient probably is beer made from dates (CAD S 376), but then the logogram KAŠ.SAG must be a single logogram for *šikaru* rather than Akk. *šikaru rēštû*.

91 A$_{ii\,21}$ ^{u2}SUM^{sar} ^{u2}*zi-ba-a* SUD$_2$ *ina* KAŠ NAG.MEŠ 2 UD.MEŠ 1/2 SILA$_3$.TA.AM$_3$ I$_3$.GIŠ *ana* ⸢DUR$_2$⸣-*šu$_2$* DUB-⸢*ak* TI⸣

---

92 A$_{ii\,22}$ DIŠ NA ŠA$_3$.MEŠ-*šu$_2$* MU$_2$.MU$_2$-*ḫu it-te-ne$_2$-bi-ṭu* NU *pa-tan* KAŠ LAL$_3$ *baḫ-*⸢*ra* NAG⸣-*šu$_2$ i-ar$_2$-ru* A.GEŠTIN.[NA]

93 A$_{ii\,23}$ ŠEG$_6$-*šal* ^{u2}KUR.RA MUN TEŠ$_2$.BI SUD$_2$ *ana* ŠA$_3$ GAZ LAL$_3$ *u* I$_3$ *ḫal-*⸢*ṣa*⸣ ŠUB *ana* DUR$_2$-*šu$_2$* DUB-*ak* T[I]

---

94 A$_{ii\,24}$ DIŠ NA ŠA$_3$.MEŠ-*šu$_2$ it-te-nen-bi-ṭu$_3$* NU *pa-tan* KAŠ *ina* ^{dug}LA.⸢ḪA.AN⸣ NAG A.GEŠTIN.NA ŠEG$_6$.GA$_2$ ^{u2}KUR.RA MUN *e*[*me-sal*]

95 A$_{ii\,25}$ *ana* ŠA$_3$ ŠUB I$_3$.GIŠ *ana* ŠA$_3$ *tu-na-tak ana* ŠA$_3$ *na-aš-pak-ti* DUB-⸢*ak*⸣ I$_3$.GIŠ *ina* ŠU.SI GUB$_3$-*ka* <*ka*>[331]-*lu-šu$_2$* ŠEŠ$_2$-*s*[*u*]

---

91 You pound (*tasâk*) *šūmū* ('garlic') (and) *zibû* ('black cumin'), (and) he keeps drinking (*ištanatti*) them in beer. For two days you pour (*tašappak*) half a litre of oil each (day) into his anus; (then) he will recover (*iballuṭ*).

---

92 If someone's internal organs (*qerbū*) are swollen (*napḫū*)[332] (and) continually have cramps: you have him drink (*tašaqqīšu*) hot beer (and) *dišpu* ('syrup') on an empty stomach, (and then) he will vomit. You bring vinegar to a boil (*tušabšal*),

93 you pound (*tasâk*) *nīnû* ('mint') (and) salt together, you crush (*taḫaššal*) them into[333] (the vinegar), you put (*tanaddi*) *dišpu* ('syrup') and pressed oil into it, (and) you pour (*tašappak*) it into his anus; (then) he will recover (*iballuṭ*).

---

94 If someone's internal organs (*qerbū*) continually have cramps: he drinks (*išatti*) beer from a flask on an empty stomach. You bring vinegar to a boil (*tušabšal*) , you put (*tanaddi*) *nīnû* ('mint') (and) *emesallu* salt

95 in it, you drip oil into it, (and) you pour (*tašappak*) it into the middle of the 'vessel' (*našpaktu*) (viz. the anus).[334] You anoint (*tapaššassu*) him in his entirety with oil, using your left finger.

---

331 We assume a haplography of KA here and have, consequently, reconstructed the missing occurrence of the sign.

332 For the use of reduplicated logograms to code a G-stem plural, in contrast to the traditional rendering of MU$_2$.MU$_2$ as the Ntn-stem *ittananpaḫū*, see STO 1: 21.

333 The relatively rare phrase *ana* ŠA$_3$ GAZ = Akk. *ana libbi taḫaššal* 'you crush them into' is used here in much the same way as the more frequent expression *ana* ŠA$_3$ ŠUB = Akk. *ana libbi tanaddi* 'you put them into'. The same construction occurs in a few other places in the medical corpus, such as BAM 49 rev. 7, BAM 57 rev. 4 and BAM 159 ii 48, as well as in line 170 below.

334 As a figura etymologica, the phrase *ana libbi našpakti tašappak* includes a feminine **mapras*-form of the verb *šapāku*, namely *našpaktu*, hence the location or instrument of pouring (CAD N/2 66). Given the well-developed vocabulary for vessels in Akkadian, this type of cognate noun is probably a euphemism, presumably for the anus. For a similar euphemism, see lines 122 and 183.

96 A$_{ii\ 26}$ DIŠ NA ŠA$_3$-*šu*$_2$ *it-te-ne*$_2$*-bi-ṭu* I$_3$.UDU UKUŠ$_2$.⸢ḪAB⸣ *ana* DUR$_2$-*šu*$_2$ GAR-*an* SUM^{sar} 7 *u* 7 *u*$_2$-⸢*al*⸣*-[*lat*]

---

97 A$_{ii\ 27}$ SUM^{sar} ^{u2}GAMUN.GE$_6$ SUD$_2$ *ina* KAŠ NAG L[AL$_3$ KUR]-⸢*i*⸣ I$_3$.GIŠ *ana* DUR$_2$-*šu*$_2$ DUB NUMUN ^{u2}*a-zu-ki-ra-a-ni* SUD$_2$ G[U$_7$][335]

---

98 A$_{ii\ 28}$ DIŠ-*ma* UḪ$_2$ TUKU.TUKU *gan-ḫa* ḪAD$_2$.⸢DA⸣ KUR A ^{giš}NU.UR$_2$.MA SUR [NAG]

---

96 If someone's internal organs (*qerbū*)[336] continually have cramps: you place (*tašakkan*) pulp from *irrû* ('cucumber') into his anus,[337] (and then) he swallows *šūmū* ('garlic') seven and seven times.

---

97 You pound (*tasâk*) *šūmū* ('garlic') (and) *zibû* ('black cumin'), (and) he drinks (*išatti*) them in beer. You pour (*tašappak*) *dišpu* ('syrup') from the mountains (and) oil into his anus. You pound seed from *azupirānu* ('saffron-like' plant), (and) he eats (*ikkal*)$^?$ it.

---

98 If (someone's belly is sick), and more specifically, he continually has (*irtanašši*) phlegm (*rupuštu*) (and) is overwhelmed (*kašid*) by a hacking cough (*gaḫḫa šābula*):[338] you press out (*taṣaḫḫat*) juice from *nurmû* ('pomegranate'),[339] (and) he drinks (*išatti*) it.

---

335 Cadelli (2000: 131 and 155) restores T[I] = Akk. *i[balluṭ]* at the end of the line, but then the last procedure has no indication of how the medicine is delivered to the body of the patient. One would rather expect a verb like GU$_7$ = Akk. *ikkal* 'he eats it', since no liquid carrier is mentioned here.

336 Although ŠA$_3$ alone, without MEŠ, normally codes *libbu* 'belly' (see Stol 2006), the masculine plural agreement on the verb, both here and frequently below (including lines 101, 126, 147 and 172), suggests that ŠA$_3$ in these lines can also represent the masculine plural noun *qerbū* 'internal organs' (as is the norm in UGU.MU, see Couto-Ferreira 2009: 270–271). Exceptions like this are acknowledged in Stol 2007: 27.

337 The statement *ana šuburrīšu tašakkan* 'you place it into his anus' might be an abbreviation of the instructions for making suppositories, usually rendered with the form *allāna teppuš . . . ana šuburrīšu tašakkan* 'you make an acorn-shaped suppository . . . (and) you place it into his anus'. For this and other methods of suppository making, see Böck 2009: 124–125.

338 Since fever is one of the main medical conditions discussed in STO 4, the reading of UD.DA KUR for Akk. *ṣēta kašid* (Cadelli 2000: 156) in this passage seems to be out of place. The nominal form *gan-ḫa* derives from Akk. *ganāḫu* 'to have fits of coughing', for which compare the assimilated form in line 147 below with *ga-aḫ-ḫa* TUKU. In line with Cadelli's (2000: 131 n. 20, and 2021: 21) alternative, we take *gan-ḫa* ḪAD$_2$.DA with the stative form of the verb KUR = Akk. *kašādu*, viz. *kašid*, as a single symptom, namely of a patient with a hacking (lit. dry) cough.

339 For pomegranate juice, used as an aphrodisiac in the Babylonian Talmud, see Geller 1991: 110–111.

99 A$_{\text{ii 29}}$ GA I$_3$.GIŠ EME-*šu*$_2$ DAB-*bat* ⸢NAG⸣ 1 SILA$_3$ KAŠ NAG ^{šim}LI SUD$_2$ *ina* KAŠ [NAG]

100 A$_{\text{ii 30}}$ $^{\text{u2}}$GAMUN.GE$_6$^{sar} SUD$_2$ [*ina*] KAŠ NAG $^{\text{u2}}$GAMUN.GE$_6$^{sar} SUD$_2$ *ina* GEŠTIN NAG I$_3$.GIŠ *u*$_2$-*a*[*l-lat*]

101 A$_{\text{ii 31}}$ DIŠ NA SAG ŠA$_3$-*šu*$_2$ KUM$_2$ ⸢ŠA$_3$⸣-*š*[*u*$_2$ M]U$_2$.MU$_2$-*ḫu* 1/2 SILA$_3$ ^{šim}ḪAB *ina šur-šum-me* KAŠ *ta-r*[*ab-bak*]

DIŠ NA SAG ŠA$_3$-*šu*$_2$ KUM$_2$ ŠA$_3$-*šu*$_2$ MU$_2$.MU$_2$ *ana* TI-*šu*$_2$ 1/2 SILA$_3$ ⸢^{šim}⸣ḪAB *ina š*[*ur-šu*]*m-me* KAŠ / *tara-bak* (STO 5: 4–5)

102 A$_{\text{ii 32}}$ *ina* TUG$_2$ *te*-<(*ṭer-ri*)> LAL-*id ana* ⸢*na*⸣-[*aṣ*]-*ma-ti* GAZI^{sar} ŠIM.ŠAL *ta*-⸢*za**-*ru*$_3$ IGI *u* MAŠ.SILA$_3$⸣ [LAL]

ina TUG$_2$ SUR-*ri* GAZI^{sar} ^{šim}BULUḪ SUD$_2$ *ana* IGI SUR *ta*-⸢*za*⸣-*ru*$_3$ ⸢IGI⸣ *u* MAŠ.SILA$_3$ LA[L-*m*]*a ina*-⸢*eš*⸣ (STO 5: 5)

103 A$_{\text{ii 33}}$ [x x] x [x x x] x [x x x] x [x x x ^{ši}]^{m}*⸢LI⸣ ^{šim}ŠE.LI $^{\text{u2}}$⸢ḪAR.ḪAR⸣ *ana* KAŠ ŠUB

104 A$_{\text{ii 34}}$ [x x x] x x x x ⸢GAZ *lu ba*⸣-*ḫir*$_2$ ⸢NAG⸣-*šu*$_2$ *ina* A$_2$ MUŠEN *tu-šap-ra-šu-ma* TI

99 You put (*tušaṣbat*) milk (and) oil on his tongue (lit. have his tongue seize it),[340] he drinks (*išatti*) them, (and then) he drinks one litre of beer. You pound (*tasâk*) *burāšu* (a kind of juniper), (and) he drinks it in beer.

100 You pound (*tasâk*) *zibû* ('black cumin'), (and) he drinks (*išatti*) it in beer. You pound *zibû* ('black cumin'), he drinks it in wine, (and then) he swallows oil.

101 If someone's epigastrium (*rēš libbi*) is hot (*ēm*) (and) his internal organs (*qerbū*) are swollen (*napḫū*): you stir into a paste half a litre of *ṭūru* ('opopanax') in beer dregs,

102 you smear (*teṭerri*) (the mixture) on a piece of fabric, (and) you bandage (*taṣammid*) him. You scatter *kasû* ('tamarind') (and) *šimiššalû* ('box tree') over the bandage, (and) you bandage him front and back (lit. shoulder blades)

103 You put (*tanaddi*) . . . *burāšu* (a kind of juniper), *kikkirânu*, ('juniper seeds'), (and) *ḫašû* ('thyme') in beer,

104 you crush (*taḫaššal*) . . . you have him drink (*tašaqqīšu*) it while it is steaming hot, (and) you make him vomit with the feather of a bird; then he will recover (*iballuṭ*).

340 The idiom EME-*šu*$_2$ DAB-*bat* can only be translated here in the causative Š-stem due to the presence of two objects: the milk and the oil (direct object) as opposed to the patient's tongue (causee). Consequently, this line demonstrates that the tongue was not grasped by the physician (*ṣabātu* in the G-stem), but rather was made to grasp the ingredients (*ṣabātu* in the Š-stem), hence our translation 'you put them on his tongue'. For a discussion of this idiom, with a possible Greek parallel, see Stol 2004: 73–74.

105 A$_{ii\,35}$ ⸢DIŠ NA⸣ ŠA$_3$.MEŠ-*šu*$_2$ *ma-gal nap-ḫu* ⸢NINDA⸣.MEŠ KAŠ.MEŠ *ina* KA-*šu*$_2$ GUR.GUR-*ra* SAG.DU-*su* GABA-*su* LAL$_2$-*id*

106 A$_{ii\,36}$ *ra-bi-ik* ZI$_3$.KUM ⸢ŠEG$_6$⸣-*šal ina* LAL$_3$.MEŠ I$_3$.UDU *u* I$_3$.NUN.NA GU$_7$.MEŠ SUM^{sar} SUM.SIKIL^{sar}

107 A$_{ii\,37}$ ⸢GA*.RAŠ*^{sar}⸣* *saḫ-le*$_2$*-e* ^{u2}*u*[*r*$_2$*-n*]*e*$_2$*-e* 3 UD-*me* NU GU$_7$ A NU TU$_5$-*ma* TI

---

108 A$_{ii\,38}$ DIŠ NA ŠA$_3$.MEŠ-*šu*$_2$ *nap-ḫu* x [x KU]M$_2$ ŠUB.MEŠ-*su*[341] NINDA *u* KAŠ LAL UḪ$_2$ TUKU.TUKU-*ši ana* TI-*šu*$_2$ ^{u2}IGI-*lim*

109 A$_{ii\,39}$ ^{u2}IGI.NIŠ SUḪUŠ ^{giš}NAM.[TAR] *a-ḫe-nu-u*$_2$ SUD$_2$ *ina* KAŠ NAG-*šu*$_2$ *i-par-ru-ma* EGIR *an-ne*$_2$*-e*

110 A$_{ii\,40}$ I$_3$ *ḫal-ṣa u* KAŠ NAG-*šu*$_2$ A GA[ZI^{sa}]^{r} *u* A.GEŠTIN.NA ŠEG$_6$-*šal ana* DUR$_2$-*šu*$_2$ DUB-*ak-ma* ^{šim}GUR$_2$.GUR$_2$ ^{šim}LI ^{šim}GUR$_2$.GUR$_2$ ^{šim}LI (STO 1: 24)

105 If someone's internal organs (*qerbū*) are extremely swollen, he constantly regurgitates (*uttanarra*) (different) foods (and) beer into his mouth, (and) he constantly bandages (*iṣṣanammid*) his head (and) chest:[342]

106 you bring a porridge (made) from *isqūqu* (a type of groats) to a boil (*tušabšal*), (and) he keeps eating (*ītanakkal*) it in *dišpu* ('syrup'), fat, and ghee.

107 He should not eat (*lā ikkal*) *šūmū* ('garlic'), *šamaškillu* ('onion'), *karašu* ('leek'), *saḫlû* ('cress'), (and) *urnû* (a kind of mint) for three days, (and) he should not bathe (*lā irammuk-ma*);[343] then he will recover (*iballuṭ*).

---

108 If someone's internal organs (*qerbū*) are swollen . . . heat$^{?}$ keeps afflicting him (*imtanaqqussu*), he has a diminished appetite (*muṭṭu*) for bread and beer, (and) he keeps having (*irtanašši*) phlegm (*rupuštu*): in order to treat him,

109 you pound (*tasâk*) separately *imḫur-līm* ('faces a thousand' plant), *imḫur-ešrā* ('faces twenty' plant), (and) root from *pillû* ('mandrake'), you have him drink (*tašaqqīšu*) them in beer so he will vomit, and, after this,

110 you have him drink pressed oil and beer. You bring to a boil (*tušabšal*) juice from *kasû* ('tamarind') and vinegar, (and) you pour (*tašappak-ma*) them into his anus. *Kukru* (an aromatic), *burāšu* (a kind of juniper),

341 For the symptom KUM$_2$ ŠUB.MEŠ-*su* = Akk. *ummu imtanaqqussu* 'heat keeps afflicting him', see line 130 below as well as CTN 4 72 vi 9′-10′, where phlegm is also mentioned: DIŠ GIG-*ma* KUM$_2$ ŠUB.[ŠUB-*su*]-*ma u*$_2$*-ta-ṣal u* UḪ$_2$ NU [T]UK[U] 'if he is sick, and more specifically heat constantly affects him, he becomes numb and has no saliva' (Stadhouders 2011: 45). The restoration *š*[*e-er-šu*$_2$] ŠUB.MEŠ-*su* for Akkadian *šēršu imtanaqqussu* 'his flesh is constantly flabby'—proposed by Cadelli (2000: 132 with n. 23) as an alternative to the reading *abunnassu imtanaqqussu* 'his navel is constantly collapsed' in CAD M 245—is unlikely because *šēru* usually occurs as a plural noun as in STO 2: 256. The reading *q*[*u*$_{(2)}$*-l*]*u* ŠUB.MEŠ-*su* for Akkadian *qūlu imtanaqqussu* 'silence constantly befalls him' (CAD Q 304) is incompatible with the available space and the traces before the break.

342 Compare STO 1: 94–95 and STO 2: 151–152, where the patient's bandaging of himself seems to be part of a longer symptom description. Another possible symptom in the same sequence is his unwillingness to eat *šūmū* ('garlic'), *šamaškillu* ('onion') and *karašu* ('leek') for seven days; a similar reference occurs in this passage, but here the admonition to the patient, not to eat garlic, onion and leek for three days, is part of the therapy. The verb form describing the act of bandaging is *gi-na-a* LAL 'he keeps his head bandaged' as in STO 1: 95 and STO 2: 151. This form is replaced here with LAL$_2$, which probably captures the same continuous action on the orthographic level: LAL$_2$ consists of two LAL signs, and as such it may represent the Gtn form of LAL, viz. LAL.LAL = Akk. *ṣitammudu*.

343 Restrictions that include not eating garlic, onion and leek, along with not bathing, are of a hemerological nature (Geller 2004: 222). See the partial parallel in lines 151–152 below and its duplicate in STO 1: 94–95.

111 A$_{\text{ii 41}}$ ^{šim}GAM.MA PA ^{giš}ŠE.ḪAR PA ^{giš}GE$_6$.PAR$_3$ PA ^{giš}ŠE.NU$_2$.A NUMUN $^{\text{u2}}$*ur-ba-ti* 7 U$_2$.ḪI.A ŠEŠ
^{šim}GAM.MA PA ^{giš}GE$_6$.PAR$_3$ PA ^{giš}ŠE.ḪAR NUMUN $^{\text{u2}}$*ur-⸢ba⸣-[ti* (x x)] (STO 1: 24)

112 A$_{\text{ii 42}}$ TEŠ$_2$.BI GAZ SIM KI ⸢I$_3$⸣.UDU DUḪ.LAL$_3$ *u* ^{šim}ḪAB *tu-sa-maḫ ina* KUŠ.EDIN SUR LAL$_2$-*su-ma* TI
DIŠ-*niš* GAZ ⸢SIM KI$^?$ I$_3^?$.UDU$^?$ ^{šim}⸣ḪAB$^?$ ḪI.ḪI *ina* KUŠ.EDIN SUR-*ri* SAG ŠA$_3$-*šu*$_2$ LAL$_2$-*ma* TI (STO 1: 25)

---

113 A$_{\text{ii 43}}$ DIŠ NA ŠA$_3$.MEŠ-*šu*$_2$ *nap-⸢ḫu⸣ gu-ḫa u* UḪ$_2$ TUKU.MEŠ-*ši* NINDA *u* KAŠ LAL *ana* TI-*šu*$_2$ $^{\text{u2}}$KUR.RA *saḫ-le*$_2$-⸢*e** DIŠ*-*niš** SUD$_2$⸣*

114 A$_{\text{ii 44}}$ *ina* KAŠ NAG-*šu*$_2$ $^{\text{u2}}$⸢*ur*$_2$⸣-*ne*$_2$-*e ina* A GAZI^{sar} ŠEG$_6$-*šal ta-ša*$_2$-*ḫal* SED *lu ba-ḫir*$_2$ *ana* DUR$_2$-*šu*$_2$ DUB TI

---

115 A$_{\text{ii 45}}$ DIŠ NA ŠA$_3$.MEŠ-*šu*$_2$ *nap-⸢ḫu⸣* SAG ŠA$_3$-*šu*$_2$ *ru-pu-ul-ta*[344] TUKU.MEŠ-*ši ana* TI-*šu*$_2$ U$_5$ ARGAB^{mušen} $^{\text{u2}}$*tu-lal* GI.ŠUL.ḪI

111 *ṣumlalû* (an aromatic), leaves from ŠE.ḪAR (a tree),[345] leaves from *lipāru* (a fruit tree), leaves from *šunû* ('chaste tree'), (and) seed from *urbatu* ('rushes')—you crush (*taḫaššal*) (and) sift (*tanappi*) these seven ingredients

112 together, you mix them with fat, wax, and *ṭūru* ('opopanax'), you smear (*teṭerri*) (the mixture) on a piece of leather, (and) you bandage him (*taṣammissū-ma*); then he will recover (*iballuṭ*).

---

113 If someone's internal organs (*qerbū*) are swollen, he continually has (*irtanašši*) fits of coughing (*guḫḫa*)[346] and phlegm (*rupuštu*), (and) he has a diminished appetite (*muṭṭu*) for bread and beer: in order to heal him (*ana bulluṭīšu*), you pound (*tasâk*) *nīnû* ('mint'), (and) *saḫlû* ('cress') together, (and)

114 you have him drink (*tašaqqīšu*) them in beer. You bring to a boil (*tušabšal*) *urnû* (a kind of mint) in juice from *kasû* ('tamarind'), you filter it, (and) you pour (*tašappak*) it into his anus (either) cold or steaming hot; (then) he will recover (*iballuṭ*).

---

115 If someone's internal organs (*qerbū*) are swollen (and) his epigastrium (*rēš libbi*) keeps having (*irtanašši*) phlegm (*rupuštu*):[347] in order to heal him (*ana bulluṭīšu*), you fix (*tukān*)[348] *rikibti arkabi* ('bat guano'), *tullal* ('you cleanse' plant), *qān šalāli* (a type of reed)

---

344 For the mistaken reading *šup-pu-ul-ta* in our passage, see CAD Š/3 326; the corrected reading is already in Stol 2013: 127. The word *šuppultu*, with the straightforward syllabic spelling *šu-pul-ti*, seems to be limited to the physiognomic corpus, where it co-occurs with ŠA$_3$ = Akk. *libbu* (Cadelli 2021: 24–25).

345 For the tree ^{giš}ŠE.ḪAR, see STO 1: 24.

346 For a discussion of *guḫḫu* and the related term *gaḫḫu* in line 147 below, see Cadelli 2021: 13.

347 The parallel in BAM 90 obv. 10′ has the logographic form UḪ$_2$, which led Schwemer (2007: 177) to read it as *ru'tu* 'saliva'. Other instances of this idiom suggest, however, that the Akkadian word meant here is *rupuštu* 'phlegm': see AMT 48/2: 1, STT 102 obv. 7 and BAM 190 obv. 22. For a discussion of the idiom *rēš libbīšu rupušta irtanašši*, see Stol 2006: 104–105, with the translation of *rupuštu* as 'foam', as well as Stol 2013: 127.

348 The D-stem of *kânu*, used to describe mixing ingredients, is rare in the therapeutic corpus but occurs in the culinary texts (Bottéro 1995: 205; Lassen, Frahm and Wagensonner 2019: 123–124). Its use here may be due to the fact that both cedar sap and *kasû* ('tamarind') juice are low viscosity semi-liquids, requiring a process where solid substances are being worked into a gooey dough-like substance.

116 A$_{ii\ 46}$ PA ^{giš}*šu-še i*[*na* MU]D$_2$ EREN *u* A GAZI^{sar} *tu-ka-an* LAL$_3$ I$_3$ *ḫal-ṣa* I$_3$.NUN *u* KAŠ SAG

117 A$_{ii\ 47}$ *ana* ŠA$_3$ ŠUB-*d*[*i*] *ina* MUL$_4$ *tuš-bat ina še-ri*$_3$ *ta-ša*$_2$*-ḫal* NU *pa-tan* NAG-*ma* TI

---

118 A$_{ii\ 48}$ DIŠ NA ŠA$_3$.MEŠ-*š*[*u*$_2$ *nap*]-*ḫu* ZI$_3$ ŠE.SA.A ZI$_3$ MUNU$_6$ NUMUN ^{u2}KI.^{d}IŠKUR *di-ik-ta ša*$_2$ ZU$_2$.LUM

[DIŠ KI MI]N ⸢ZI$_3$ ŠE.SA⸣.A ZI$_3$ ḪARUB!(AMAŠ) *qi*$_2$*-lip*$_2$ ZU$_2$.LUM.MA (STO 2: 254)

[DIŠ KI MIN Z]I$_3$ ŠE.SA.A ZI$_3$ *ḫa-ru-be* ⸢*di*⸣-*ik-ta* ZU$_2$.LUM.MA (STO 1: 33)

119 A$_{ii\ 49}$ TEŠ$_2$.BI S[UD$_2$ NU *pa-t*]*an*[349] GU$_7$.MEŠ A.MEŠ NU NAG A.MEŠ SAG ŠA$_3$-*šu*$_2$ *tu-sa-laḫ*$_2$*-ma* ⸢TI⸣

SUD$_2$ *ina* KAŠ 2 UD-*me* / [*ba*]-*lu* ⸢*pa-tan*⸣ NAG-*šu*$_2$ A NU NAG A SAG ŠA$_3$-*šu*$_2$ *tu-sa-laḫ*$_2$*-ma ina-eš* (STO 2: 254–255)

TEŠ$_2$.BI SUD$_2$ *ina* KAŠ NU *pa-tan* ⸢2 UD⸣-[*me*] / [NAG.MEŠ 2] ⸢UD-*me*⸣ *ina* A.MEŠ NU *pa-tan* NAG.MEŠ A.MEŠ SAG ŠA$_3$-*šu*$_2$ ⸢*tu*⸣-*s*[*a-laḫ*$_2$*-ma* TI] (STO 1: 33–34)

---

120 A$_{ii\ 50}$ [DIŠ] NA ŠA$_3$-⸢*šu*$_2$⸣ [*e-m*]*e-er* 10 KISAL A ^{giš}ŠE.NU 10 KISAL A MUN *ina* LAL$_3$ *u* KAŠ N[AG]*

---

116 (and) leaves from *šūšu* ('liquorice') in *erēnu* ('cedar') sap and juice from *kasû* ('tamarind'), you put (*tanaddi*) *dišpu* ('syrup'), pressed oil, ghee, and high-quality beer

117 in it, you leave (the mixture) out overnight under the stars, you filter it in the morning, (and) he drinks (*išattī-ma*) it on an empty stomach; then he will recover (*iballuṭ*).

---

118 If someone's internal organs (*qerbū*) are swollen: you pound (*tasâk*)$^{?}$ flour from *labtu* ('roasted barley'), flour from *buqlu* ('malt'), seed from *qutru* (a plant) (and) a *diktu* preparation[350] (made) from *suluppū* ('dates')

119 together, (and) he keeps eating (*ītanakkal*) them on an empty stomach, (but) he should not drink (*lā išatti*) any water (with them). You sprinkle his epigastrium (*rēš libbi*) with water; then he will recover (*iballuṭ*).

---

120 If someone's belly (*libbu*) is bloated: he drinks (*išatti*) ten KISAL-measures of juice from *šunû* ('chaste tree') (and) ten KISAL-measures of salt water in *dišpu* ('syrup') and beer.

---

349 Cadelli (2000: 133) reconstructs TEŠ$_2$.BI N[U *pa*]-*tan* GU$_7$.MEŠ at the beginning of the line, but the full form normally includes SUD$_2$ = Akk. *sâku* 'to pound' following TEŠ$_2$.BI = Akk. *ištēniš* 'together'. There may not be enough room in the break to accommodate the whole sign sequence.

350 For a discussion of *diktu*, see STO 1: 33.

121 A$_{ii\ 51}$ [DIŠ K]I MIN ^{gi}[^{š}NU.U]R$_2$.MA GU$_7$ A ^{giš}NU.UR$_2$.MA N[AG]

---

122 A$_{ii\ 52}$ [DIŠ K]I MIN ^{ši}[^{m}L]I SUD$_2$ *ina* KAŠ NAG : DIŠ KI MIN SIG$_2$ GAL$_4$.LA ^{munus}ŠU.GI *ina* MURUB$_4$ KA-*šu*$_2$ G[AR-*an*]

---

123 A$_{ii\ 53}$ [DIŠ KI MIN PA ^{giš}NU.U]R$_2$.MA PA ^{giš}MA$_2$.RI$_2$.IŠ.MA$_2$.RA SUD$_2$ *ina* A NA[G]

---

124 A$_{ii\ 54}$ [DIŠ NA ŠA$_3$-*šu*$_2$ I]M *ṣe-en* $^{urudu!}$ŠUM$^{!}$(DIM$_3$).GAM.ME[351] ZABAR *lu* GIR$_2$ ZABAR *i-lek-ma* TI

121 If DITTO, he eats (*ikkal*) *nurmû* ('pomegranate') (and) drinks juice from *nurmû* ('pomegranate').

---

122 If DITTO, you pound (*tasâk*) *burāšu* (a kind of juniper)$^{?}$, (and) he drinks (*išatti*) it in beer. If DITTO, you put (*tašakkan*) pubic hair from an old woman in the middle of his 'mouth' (viz. the anus).[352]

---

123 If DITTO, you pound (*tasâk*) leaves from *nurmû* ('pomegranate') (and) leaves from *mirišmarû* (a plant), (and) he drinks (*išatti*) them in water.

---

124 If someone's belly (*libbu*) is loaded (*ṣēn*)[353] with flatulence (lit. wind): he licks a bronze saw or a bronze knife; then he will recover (*iballuṭ*).

351 Based on a Geers collation, CAD Š/2 174 claims that the sign is ŠUM, but new collation of the passage shows that it is actually DIM$_3$. The incoherent use of the DIM$_3$ sign as part of the orthography for Akk. *šaššāru* may have resulted from miscopying the traditional sign sequence URUDU+ŠUM at the beginning of the logogram ^{urudu}ŠUM.GAM.ME, particularly since the saw in question is explicitly described as made of bronze (Sum. ZABAR) rather than copper (Sum. URUDU).

352 In agreement with Böck 2009: 123, we see this as a euphemism here, as well as in line 183 below, for the anus. For a similar euphemism, see line 95 above.

353 For the verb *ṣênu*, see the discussion in STO 5: 27.

125 A$_{ii\ 55}$ [SAḪAR ^{urudu}NIG$_2$.KAL]AG.GA[354] *tu-uš-ṣe-en-šu*$_2$ *i-še*$_{20}$*-ḫi-iq-ma* TI

DIŠ MUNUS U$_3$.TU-*ma ṣe-em-rat u* IM *ud-du-pat* SAHAR ^{urudu}NIG$_2$.KALAG.GA *tu-še-ṣe-en-ši-ma ina-eš* (BAM 240 obv. 26′)

DIŠ MUNUS *e'-re-et-ma u* IM *ud-du-pat* DIM$_{10}$.ME DAB SAHAR ^{urudu}NIG$_2$.KALAG.GA-*e tu-še-ṣe-en-ši* (BAM 240 obv. 28′)

---

126 A$_{ii\ 56}$ DIŠ NA ŠA$_3$-⸢*šu*$_2$⸣ [*em-r*]*u* 10 KISAL PA ^{giš}*šu-nim* 10 KISAL LAL$_3$ *ana* ŠA$_3$ KAŠ ⸢ŠUB⸣[355] *ina* MUL$_4$ *tuš-bat ina še-ri*$_3$ NU *pa-tan* NAG.MEŠ-*ma* TI

---

127 A$_{ii\ 57}$ DIŠ NA ŠA$_3$-*šu*$_2$ *e*[*m-ru* M]U$_2$.⸢MU$_2$-*ḫu*⸣ Š[A$_3$-*š*]*u*$_2$ *iš-ta-na-si* NINDA *u* A GUR SUḪUŠ ⸢^{giš}*NAM⸣*.TAR NITA$_2$ ^{šim}ḪAB *ina* KA-*šu*$_2$ *i-na-'-is*

†

125 You have him smell (*tušeṣṣeššu*)[356] dust from a bronze bell, (and) he will sneeze (*išeḫḫiq-ma*);[357] then he will recover.

---

126 If someone's internal organs (*qerbū*) are bloated$^?$: you put (*tanaddi*) ten KISAL-measures of leaves from *šunû* ('chaste tree') (and) ten KISAL-measures of *dišpu* ('syrup') in beer, you leave (the mixture) out overnight under the stars, (and) he keeps drinking (*ištanattī-ma*) it in the morning on an empty stomach; then he will recover (*iballuṭ*).

---

127 If someone's internal organs (*qerbū*) are bloated (and) swollen (*napḫū*), his belly (*libbu*) constantly makes noises (and) brings food and drink back up (*utār*): he chews root from male *pillû* ('mandrake') (and) *ṭūru* ('opopanax') in his mouth,

---

354 Reiner (1963: 171) suggests that ^{urudu}NIG$_2$.KALAG.GA is a cryptogram for the Akkadian word *tigû*, because the Sumerogram is followed by -*u*$_2$ or occasionally by -*gu-u*$_2$ as a complement, whereas a straightforward calque of ^{uruda}NIG$_2$.KALAG.GA should regularly end in -*ku*. For ^{urudu}NIG$_2$.KALAG.GA denoting a type of copper bell that was used in exorcistic rituals, see now Panayotov 2013.

355 Cadelli (2000: 133) reads here *ana lib*$_3$*-bi* ŠUB-*di*, but there is no DI sign on the tablet.

356 Cadelli (2000: 157 with n. 30), following AHw 252, acknowledges the odd spelling of the Š-stem of *eṣēnu* and convincingly suggests that the spelling has been influenced by *ṣe-en*, the stative form of the verb *ṣênu* 'to load', in the preceding line. In BAM 240 obv. 26′ and 28′, the formulation is much simpler, with the grammatically correct form *tu-še-ṣe-en-ši-ma*. In BM 78963 rev. 7, the verb is also misspelled, namely *tu-še-en-ṣe-šu-ma* in place of the expected *tu-še-ṣe-en-šu-ma* (Stadhouders and Johnson 2018: 578–579 ln. 53). For an analysis of the verb, see Stadhouders and Johnson 2018: 600–601.

357 That *i-še*$_{20}$*-ḫi-iq* is a hapax for *šeḫēqu* 'to sneeze' was first proposed in AHw 1209, in part based on West Semitic *ś/ṣḥq* 'to laugh'. See also Stol 1991–1992: 60, CAD Š/2 263 and Cadelli 2000: 133.

128 A$_{\text{ii 58}}$ LAL$_3$ KUR-*i ina* K[AŠ SAG NA]G ^{šim}ḪAB *ina* KAŠ SAG ŠEG$_6$.GA$_2$ *ana* DUR$_2$-*šu*$_2$ DUB-*ak* PA ^{giš}GE$_6$.PAR$_3$ ^{šim}LI ^{šim}KU$_7$.KU$_7$

129 A$_{\text{ii 59}}$ ILLU *a-bu-k*[*a-ti* ^{giš}Š]E.NU GAZ *ina* I$_3$.UDU ḪI.ḪI *ina* KUŠ *te-*<(*ṭer-ri*)> LAL *ina* A ^{giš}ŠE.NU *ir-ta-na-ḫaṣ*

---

130 A$_{\text{ii 60}}$ DIŠ NA ŠA$_3$-*šu*$_2$ [x x x x K]UM$_2$ ŠUB.ŠUB-*su* IM TUKU.TUKU NINDA A GUR $^{\text{u2}}$IGI.NIŠ SUḪUŠ ^{giš}NAM.TAR NITA$_2$

131 A$_{\text{ii 61}}$ *ina* KAŠ SAG S[UD$_2$ NAG-*šu*$_2$ EG]IR-*šu*$_2$ I$_3$ *ḫal-ṣa ina* KAŠ NAG SI.SA$_2$ GAZI^{sar} A.GEŠTIN.NA ŠEG$_6$-*šal ana* DUR$_2$-*šu*$_2$ DUB

132 A$_{\text{ii 62}}$ ^{šim}L[I x x x ^{ši}]^{m}ḪAB PA ^{giš}GE$_6$.PAR$_3$ PA ^{giš}ŠE.NU GAZ *ina* I$_3$.UDU ḪI.ḪI *ina* KUŠ *te-*<(*ṭer-ri*)> LAL KI MIN

---

133 A$_{\text{ii 63}}$ DIŠ NA ŠA$_3$-*šu*$_2$ [x x x NIND]A *u* A *ina* KA-*šu*$_2$ GUR.GUR-*ra* SAG.KI.MEŠ-*šu*$_2$ *up-ta-ṭa-*<<TA>>-*ra* x x x x

†

128 (and then) he drinks (*išatti*)$^?$ *dišpu* ('syrup') from the mountains in high-quality beer$^?$. You bring to a boil (*tušabšal*) *ṭūru* ('opopanax') in high-quality beer, (and) you pour (*tašappak*) it into his anus. You crush (*taḫaššal*) leaves from *lipāru* ('a fruit tree'), *burāšu* (a kind of juniper), *kukru* (an aromatic),

129 resin from *abukkatu* (a tree), (and) resin from *šunû* ('chaste tree'), you mix (*tuballal*) them in fat, you smear (*teṭerri*) (the mixture) on a piece of leather, (and) you bandage (*taṣammid*) him. He keeps bathing in juice from *šunû* ('chaste tree').

---

130 If someone's belly (*libbu*) . . . (and) heat keeps afflicting him (*imtanaqqussu*), he continually has (*irtanašši*) flatulence (lit. wind), (and) he regurgitates (*utār*) food (and) drink: you pound (*tasâk*) *imḫur-ešrā* ('faces twenty' plant) (and) root from male *pillû* ('mandrake')

131 in high-quality beer, (and) you have him drink (*tašaqqīšu*)$^?$ it. Afterwards, he drinks (*išatti*) pressed oil in beer, (and) he will have a bowel movement (*ušeššer*). You bring to a boil (*tušabšal*) juice from *kasû* ('tamarind') (and) vinegar, (and) you pour (*tašappak*) them into his anus.

132 You crush (*taḫaššal*) *burāšu* (a kind of juniper) . . . *ṭūru* ('opopanax'), leaves from *lipāru* (a fruit tree), (and) leaves from *šunû* ('chaste tree'), you mix (*tuballal*) them in fat, you smear (*teṭerri*) (the mixture) on a piece of leather, (and) you bandage (*taṣammid*) him. DITTO (= he keeps bathing in juice from *šunû* ('chaste tree')).

---

133 If someone's belly (*libbu*) . . . (and) keeps bringing food and drink back up (*uttanarra*) into his mouth, his temples are splitting apart (*uptaṭṭarā*)[358] . . .

358 For this uncertain verbal form, probably *paṭāru* in the Dt-stem, compare BAM 248 ii 66: *up-te-eṭ-ṭi-ra meš-re-*[*ti-ša*$_2$]. However, the symptom in our line is not concerned with relaxed limbs (cf. CAD M/2 41), but rather with a medical condition of the temples, seemingly unique in the gastrointestinal materials; a similar symptom is found only in line 136 below. Idioms with SAG.KI = Akk. *nakkaptu* 'temple' and the verb *paṭāru* are otherwise attested in the physiognomic corpus (Böck 2000: 92). See also Diagnostic Handbook Sagig 11: 21–25 (Labat 1951: 90–91; BAM 13 pp. 459, 465 and 471–472), which connects a patient pressing his hands in pain against his head with various medical problems, including a gastrointestinal condition.

134 A$_{\text{ii 64}}$ x x x [................] x x *ina* ⸢I$_3$.ŠAḪ⸣ GU$_7$.MEŠ SUM^{sar} SUM.SI[KIL^{sar} x x x x]
135 A$_{\text{ii 65}}$ [...] x [............] x [.................................]

---

136 A$_{\text{iii 1}}$ DIŠ NA ŠA$_3$-*šu*$_2$ *e-sil* SAG.DU G[U$_7$-*šu*$_2$ ....]
137 A$_{\text{iii 2}}$ a.ba ḫi.ši.in a.ba [...]

---

138 A$_{\text{iii 3}}$ KA.INIM.MA LU$_2$ *es-li* D[U$_3$*.DU$_3$.B]I ⸢EN$_2$* 3-*šu*$_2$ *ana*⸣ Š[A$_3$ ŠID-*nu* ....]

---

139 A$_{\text{iii 4}}$ DIŠ NA ŠA$_3$-*šu*$_2$ NINDA *u* KAŠ *la i-*⸢*maḫ*⸣-*ḫar* 1/3 SILA$_3$ A ZU$_2$.⸢LUM.MA* 1/3 SILA$_3$⸣ [A] ⸢GAZI^{sar}⸣ [x x x x x x][359]

DIŠ KI MIN 1/3 SILA$_3$ A ZU$_2$.LUM.MA 1/3 SILA$_3$ A ⸢GAZI⸣^{sar} 1/3 SILA$_3$ [. . .] / NU *pa-tan* 1-*šu*$_2$ 2-*šu*$_2$ 3-*šu*$_2$ NAG (STO 5: 9–10)

134 . . . he keeps eating (*ītanakkal*) . . . in lard . . . *šūmū* ('garlic'), *šamaškillu* ('onion') . . .
135 . . .

---

136 If someone's belly (*libbu*) is constipated, the head causes him pain (*ikkalšu*) . . .
137 a.ba ḫi.ši.in a.ba[360] . . .

---

138 An invocation for a constipated man. Its ritual: you recite (*tamannu*) the incantation three times over the belly (*libbu*) . . .

---

139 If someone's belly (*libbu*) does not accept bread and beer: he drinks on an empty stomach a third of a litre of juice from *suluppū* ('dates'), a third of a litre of juice from *kasû* ('tamarind'), (and) a third of a litre of . . .

---

359 The distant parallel from STO 5 is included here to offer a possibility for the verbs missing at the end of this line, but there is not enough room in the break to accommodate all of the instructions in the STO 5 parallel (see also Bácskay 2018: 63 n. 224, and 83 for these parallels).

360 This short spell is unintelligible at the moment, but if rendered in Akkadian, the underlying word could be *abahšinnu* 'green barley stalk'. In the context of an incantation like this, one might also consider a Sumerian reading that starts with a.ba for Akk. *mannu* 'who' (cf. Küchler 1904: 116), perhaps as a humorous Sumerian version of the *mannam lušpur* formula.

140 A$_{iii 5}$ EGIR-*šu*$_2$ AL.US$_2$.SA A.GEŠTIN.NA NAG-*ma* KUM$_2$ *ša*$_2$ ŠA$_3$-*šu*$_2$ *i-ša*$_2$*-ḫaṭ*^{at}[361] *im-me-*⸢*si*⸣ [x x x x]

AL.US$_2$.SA ⸢A⸣.GEŠTIN.NA NAG *ana* DUR$_2$-[*šu*$_2$ DUB-*ak-ma* TI] (STO 5: 10)

---

141 A$_{iii 6}$ DIŠ NA ŠA$_3$-*šu*$_2$ NINDA *la i-maḫ-*⸢*ḫar*⸣ NUMUN ^{giš}ŠINIG SUD$_2$ *ina* LAL$_3$ *u* I$_3$.NUN ḪI.ḪI *ba-lu pa-tan* N[AG-*šu*$_2$-*ma* TI]

DIŠ NA ŠA$_3$-*šu*$_2$ KUM$_2$ *u*$_2$*-kal* NINDA *u* A *la i-maḫ-ḫar* NUMUN ^{giš}ŠINIG SUD$_2$ *ina* LAL$_3$ *u* [. . .] (STO 5: 8)

---

142 A$_{iii 7}$ DIŠ NA NINDA *u* KAŠ LAL-*ṭu* ^{u2}ḪAR.ḪAR ^{u2}NU.LUḪ.ḪA ^{u2}*ur*$_2$*-nu-u* GAZI^{sar} ^{u2}*ti-ia*$_2$*-ta*$_5$ ^{u2}SUMUN.DAR ^{u2}x x [x]

140 Afterwards, he drinks (*išattī-ma*) *šiqqu* ('garum')[362] (and) vinegar, and then the heat in his belly will be drained (*iššaḫḫaṭ*)[363] (and) washed off (*immessi*) . . .

---

141 If someone's belly (*libbu*) does not accept food: you pound (*tasâk*) seed from *bīnu* ('tamarisk'), you mix (*tuballal*) it in *dišpu* ('syrup') and ghee, (and) you have him drink (*tašaqqīšū-ma*)$^?$ it on an empty stomach; then he will recover (*iballuṭ*).

---

142 If someone has a diminished appetite (*muṭṭu*) for bread and beer: you soak *ḫašû* ('thyme'), *nuḫurtu* ('asafoetida'), *urnû* (a type of mint), *kasû* ('tamarind'), *tīyatu* (a plant), *šumuttu* ('beetroot') . . .

---

361 For the same expression, with the straightforward spelling of the verb in the N-stem *iš-ša*$_2$*-ḫa-aṭ*, see STO 5: 24 and 29, as well as the second-person form in *um-mi ša*$_2$ ŠA$_3$-*šu*$_2$ *ta-ša*$_2$*-ḫaṭ-ma* 'you drain the heat from his belly' in line 218 below. The sign AD, viz. *aṭ*, is rendered here as a pronunciation gloss, even though the sign is not actually written as a gloss. The scribe probably did not recognize the form *i-ša*$_2$*-ḫaṭ*^{at} and re-interpreted the PA sign as *pa* rather than *ḫaṭ*, which has resulted in the incorrect spelling *i-ša*$_2$*-pa-aṭ*. For a similar misstep involving the sign AD, see the parallel in line 133 above.

362 The sequence AL.US$_2$.SA : *ši-iq* : *ṭa-ba-a-tu*$_2$ occurs in the commentary SpTU 1 47 obv. 17, which largely comments on SpTU 1 46; see Frahm 2010 and 2015. Without any *Glossenkeil* in our line, it is unlikely that garum is being equated with vinegar, as Frahm suggests. For garum, see the discussion in Curtis 1984.

363 Although CAD Š/1 94 derives this from *šaḫāṭu* B 'to remove, to take away', its juxtaposition with *immessi*, from Akk. *mesû* 'to wash', suggests instead that it is a by-form of *šaḫātu* A (CAD Š/1 84–86) meaning 'to drain, to rinse'; see Böck 2009: 118–119 n. 63, as well as Maul 1994: 72, who suggests that *šaḫāṭu* B, corresponding to his 'Abstreifen des Gewandes', and *šaḫātu* A, meaning 'Abspülen des Bösen mit dem Wasser', are actually a single verb.

143 A$_{\text{iii 8}}$ ^{šim}GUR$_2$.GUR$_2$ ^{šim}GAM.MA (eras.)[364] ^{šim}MAN.DU ^{giš}EREN ^{giš}EREN.SUMUN ^{šim}MUG ZU$_2$.LUM.MA LAGAB MUNU$_6$ MUN ^{giš}ŠE.[NU]

144 A$_{\text{iii 9}}$ A.GEŠTIN.NA KALAG.GA *ina* KAŠ *tara-muk ina* MUL$_4$ *tuš-bat ina še-ri$_3$ ina* ^{urudu}ŠEN.TUR ŠEG$_6$-*šal* 5 GIN$_2$ I$_3$ *ḫal-ṣa ana* IGI ŠUB *ana* DUR$_2$-*šu$_2$* DU[B-*ak*]

---

145 A$_{\text{iii 10}}$ *ana* ŠA$_3$ UTUL$_2$ ŠUB-*ma*[365] ⸢IGI*.4⸣*.GAL$_2$.LA U$_2$ *mat-qa* IGI.4.GAL$_2$.LA U$_2$ TUR *mat-*⸢*qu*⸣ IGI.4.GAL$_2$.LA $^{\text{u2}}$*a-ra-ri-ia$_2$-*⸢*nu*⸣* : $^{\text{u2}}$*mer-gi-ra-a-nu*

IGI.4.GAL$_2$.[LA] ⸢U$_2$⸣ *ma-at-qa ina* 10 GIN$_2$ A NAG-*šu$_2$* (STO 3: 132)

1/2 GIN$_2$ $^{\text{u2}}$*a-ra-ri-a-nu ina* 10 GIN$_2$ A NAG-*šu$_2$* (STO 3: 134)

IGI.4.GAL$_2$.LA $^{\text{u2}}$*me-er-gi-ra-nu ina* 10 GIN$_2$ KAŠ [NAG-*šu$_2$*] (STO 3: 136)

[1/2 GI]N$_2$ $^{\text{u2}}$*a-*⸢*ra*⸣*-ri-a-nu* / [. . .] (BAM 72: 8′–9′)

146 A$_{\text{iii 11}}$ 90 $^{\text{u2}}$*si-sin-ni* ŠA$_3$ *mal-ma-liš* SUD$_2$ *ina* KAŠ $^{\text{lu2}}$KURUN$_2$.NA NU *pa-tan* NAG-*ma ina* ⸢DUR$_2$⸣-*šu$_2$* SI.SA$_2$-*ma* TI

90 $^{\text{u2}}$[*sis-sin-n*]*i* ŠA$_3$-*bi ina* 10 GIN$_2$ A NAG-*šu$_2$* (STO 3: 131)

⸢4$^?$⸣-*ut* $^{\text{u2}}$*sis-sin-nu* ŠA$_3$-[*bi*] / [. . .] (BAM 72: 3′–4′)

---

†

143 *kukru* (an aromatic), *ṣumlalû* (an aromatic), *suādu* (a kind of sedge), *erēnu* ('cedar'), *šupuḫru* ('old cedar'), *ballukku* (an aromatic), *suluppū* ('dates'), *buqlu* ('malt') lumps, salt, *šunû* ('chaste tree'),

144 (and) strong vinegar in beer, you leave them out overnight under the stars, you bring them to a boil (*tušabšal*) in the morning in a small copper pot, you add (*tanaddi*) five shekels of pressed oil, (and) you pour (*tašappak*) it into his anus.

---

145 You put (*tanaddī-ma*) (the following) into a pot: a fourth of a shekel of *šammu matqu* ('sweet plant'), a fourth of a shekel of *šammu ṣeḫru matqu* ('small sweet plant'),[366] a fourth of a shekel of *arariānu* (a plant) (gloss: *mergirānu*),

146 (and) ninety (grains of)[367] *sissinni libbi* ('date spadix for the innards' plant), you pound (*tasâk*) them in equal amounts, and he drinks (*išattī-ma*) them in brewer's beer on an empty stomach, and he will void (*ušeššer-ma*) from his anus; then he will recover (*iballuṭ*).

---

364 It appears that the scribe wrote ^{šim}GAM.MA a second time and then tried to erase his mistake.

365 The fronting of *ana* ŠA$_3$ UTUL$_2$ ŠUB-*ma*, before the list of ingredients and with the addition of the connective -*ma*, is unique to this passage and probably results from confusing the *ana* ŠA$_3$ ŠUB idiom (normally an instruction that follows the ingredients) with the purpose clauses that occasionally appear at the beginning of recipes.

366 That U$_2$ is not a determinative, but a logogram here, is made clear by the passage in Uruanna I 681–682, where the syllabic spelling *ša$_2$-mu mat-qu* for Akk. *šammu matqu* 'sweet plant' co-occurs with *arariānu* (CAD M/1 413).

367 The phrase literally means 'ninety (grains of) *sissinni libbi*', with the ninety grains corresponding to half of a shekel. This measurement seems to be out of place here, since all other drugs in the prescription are given in the amount of a fourth of a shekel.

147 A$_{iii\ 12}$ DIŠ NA ŠA$_3$-*šu*$_2$ *qa*$_2$*-an-nu ga-aḫ-ḫa* TUKU NINDA *u* A *muṭ-ṭu*$_2$ UḪ$_2$ TUKU.MEŠ-*ši* ^{u2}KUR.RA SUD$_2$ ⸢*ina* I$_3$⸣.GIŠ NAG-*ma i-ar*$_2$*-ru*$_3$

148 A$_{iii\ 13}$ ^{u2}KUR.RA *saḫ-le*$_2$*-e* SUD$_2$ *ina* KAŠ NAG ^{u2}*ur*$_2$*-ne*$_2$*-e ina* A ŠEG$_6$-*šal tu-kaṣ*$_3$*-ṣa** ⸢*ana** DUR$_2$⸣*-*šu*$_2$ DUB-*a*[*k*]

149 A$_{iii\ 14}$ PA ^{giš}GE$_6$.⸢PAR$_3$⸣ PA ^{u2}KI.^{d}IŠKUR PA ^{giš}*bi-ni* ^{šim}LI ^{šim}GUR$_2$.GUR$_2$ ^{šim}GAM.MA ⸢^{šim}⸣ḪAB ^{š}[^{im}x x]

150 A$_{iii\ 15}$ *ina* ⸢A⸣ [ZU$_2$].LUM.MA *tara-bak* GUR-*ma* ḪAD$_2$.A GAZ *ina* I$_3$.UDU ḪI.ḪI *ina* KUŠ *te-*<(*ṭer-ri*)> LAL *ina* A ^{giš}ŠE.NU *ir-ta-na-*[*ḫaṣ-ma* TI][368]

---

151 A$_{iii\ 16}$ DIŠ [NA Š]A$_3$*-*šu*$_2$ *e-ta-na-ša*$_2$*-aš-ma* NINDA *u* KAŠ SAG *la i-maḫ-ḫar* MAŠ.SILA$_3$.MEŠ-*šu*$_2$ GU$_7$.MEŠ-*šu*$_2$ SAG.DU-*su gi-na-a* LAL [x x x]

⸢DIŠ⸣ [NA *e-t*]*a-*⸢*na*⸣*-ša*$_2$*-aš*$_2$ NINDA *u* KAŠ *la i-maḫ-ḫar* MAŠ.SILA$_3$.MIN-*šu*$_2$ GU$_7$.MEŠ-*šu*$_2$ / [SAG.DU-*su g*]*i-na-a* LAL I$_3$.NUN.NA GU$_7$ (STO 1: 94–95)

147 If someone's internal organs (*qerbū*) are twisted (*qannū*),[369] he has (*iraššī*) fits of coughing (*gaḫḫu*) (and) a diminished appetite for food and drink, he continually has (*irtanaššī*) phlegm (*rupuštu*):[370] you pound (*tasâk*) *nīnû* ('mint'), he drinks (*išattī-ma*) it in oil, and he will vomit.

148 You pound *nīnû* ('mint') (and) *saḫlû* ('cress'), (and) he drinks them in beer. You bring to a boil (*tušabšal*) *urnû* (a kind of mint) in water, you let (the mixture) cool, (and) you pour (*tašappak*) it into his anus.

149 You stir into a paste leaves from *lipāru* (a fruit tree), leaves from *qutru* (a plant), leaves from *bīnu* ('tamarisk'), *burāšu* (a kind of juniper), *kukru* (an aromatic), *ṣumlalû* (an aromatic), *ṭūru* ('opopanax'), (and) . . .

150 in juice from *suluppū* ('dates'), (then) you dry (*tubbal*) (and) crush (*taḫaššal*) (the mixture) over and over again (*tatâr-ma*), you mix (*tuballal*) it in fat, you smear (*teṭerri*) it on a piece of leather, (and) you bandage (*taṣammid*) him. He keeps bathing in juice from *šunû* ('chaste tree'); then he will recover (*iballuṭ*).

---

151 If someone's belly (*libbu*) is continually upset[371] and does not accept bread and high-quality beer, his shoulder blades constantly cause him pain (*ītanakkalšu*), he keeps his head bandaged (*ginâ iṣammid*), he is willing to eat (*ikkal*) ghee,

368 The restoration is based on the phrase *ina mê šunî irtanaḫḫaṣ(-ma iballuṭ)*, which occurs several times in STO 2. As a less likely alternative, one might also read *ir-ta-na-*[*muk-ma* TI].

369 The spelling may also suggest the reading *ganānu* 'to confine' for this verb, as suggested in CAD G 40. In line with Cadelli 2000: 136 and Cadelli 2019: 60, the verb is probably a by-form of *kanānu* 'to twist, to roll up'.

370 There are a number of similarities between these lines in our text and the illnesses classified as A.GA ZI in the medical texts from Assur, such as BAM 49, BAM 55, BAM 72, BAM 73, BAM 74, BAM 75, BAM 76 and BAM 176. However, A.GA ZI does not seem to occur in the Nineveh Medical Encyclopaedia.

371 In this line, we seem to have a reinterpretation of the idiom found in STO 1: 94, viz. [NA *e-t*]*a-*⸢*na*⸣*-ša*$_2$*-aš*$_2$ 'if someone is continually distressed', with the belly replacing the patient as the subject of the verb. Consequently, the focus here is probably placed on a physical problem in the patient's belly rather than an emotional condition, as was the case in STO 1: 94.

152 A$_{iii\ 17}$ U[D.7.KA]M$_2$ SUM^{sar} SUM.SIKIL^{sar} GA.RAŠ^{sar} NU GU$_7$ *ina* A ^{giš}ŠE.NU RA.MEŠ NUMUN ^{u2}UKUŠ$_2$.ḪAB NUMUN ^{u2}ḪAR.ḪAR *ina* KAŠ N[AG-*ma* TI]

UD.7.KAM$_2$ SUM^{sar} SUM.SIKIL^{sar} GA.RAŠ^{sar} NU GU$_7$ / [*ina* A ^{giš}ŠE.NU] RA.MEŠ-*aṣ* NUMUN ^{u2}UKUŠ$_2$.ḪAB NUMUN ^{u2}⸢ḪAR.ḪAR⸣ SUD$_2$ *ina* KAŠ NAG-*ma* TI (STO 1: 95–96)

---

153 A$_{iii\ 18}$ DIŠ ⸢NA⸣ ŠA$_3$-*šu*$_2$ *ḫa-aḫ-ḫa* DIRI *ana* TI-*šu*$_2$ GI DU$_{10}$ ^{šim}BAL ^{šim}LI ^{u2}ḪAR.ḪAR ^{šim}ŠE.L[I BABBAR][372]

154 A$_{iii\ 19}$ *i*[*na* K]AŠ SAG ŠUB ŠEG$_6$-*šal ta-ša*$_2$-*ḫal lu ba-ḫir*$_2$ 10 KISAL LAL$_3$ *ana* ŠA$_3$ GAZ NU *pa-tan* NAG-*šu*$_2$ *i-ar*$_2$-[*ru*$_3$-*ma*]

155 A$_{iii\ 20}$ [*ina*] A$_2$.GU$_2$.ZI.GA LAL$_3$ I$_3$ *ḫal-ṣa u* KAŠ TEŠ$_2$.BI ḪI.ḪI NU *pa-tan* EME-*šu*$_2$ DAB-*bat* NAG-*šu*$_2$ [TI]

---

156 A$_{iii\ 21}$ DIŠ NA *ḫa*-⸢*ḫu*⸣* DAB-*su* NUMUN ^{u2}SIKIL NUMUN ^{giš}GEŠTIN KA$_5$.A ^{u2}AB$_2$.DUḪ ^{u2}NIGIN^{sar} ^{u2}TAL$_2$.TAL$_2$ 5 U$_2$.MEŠ ŠEŠ TEŠ$_2$.B[I SUD$_2$]

†

152 but for seven days he would not eat (*lā ikkal*) *šūmū* ('garlic'), *šamaškillu* ('onion'), or *karašu* ('leek'):[373] he keeps bathing (*irtanaḫḫaṣ*) in juice from *šunû* ('chaste tree'), (and) he drinks (*išattī-ma*) seed from *irrû* ('cucumber') (and) seed from *ḫašû* ('thyme') in beer; then he will recover (*iballuṭ*).

---

153 If someone's belly (*libbu*) is full (*malī*) of mucus (*ḫaḫḫu*): in order to heal him (*ana bulluṭīšu*), you put (*tanaddi*) *qanû ṭābu* ('sweet reed'), *ballukku* (an aromatic), *burāšu* (a kind of juniper), *ḫašû* ('thyme'), (and) white *kikkirânu* ('juniper seed')$^?$,

154 in high-quality beer, you bring (the mixture) to a boil (*tušabšal*), you filter it, you crush (*taḫaššal*) ten KISAL-measures of *dišpu* ('syrup') into it while it is steaming hot, you have him drink (*tašaqqīšu*) it on an empty stomach, he will vomit,

155 and then in the morning, you mix (*tuballal*) *dišpu* ('syrup'), pressed oil and beer together, you put (*tušaṣbat*) (the mixture) on his tongue (lit. have his tongue seize it) on an empty stomach, (and) you have him drink (*tašaqqīšu*) it; (then) he will recover (*iballuṭ*).

---

156 If someone has been seized (*iṣbassu*)[374] by mucus (*ḫaḫḫu*): seed from *sikillu* ('pure' plant), seed from *karān šēlebi* ('fox-vine'), *kamantu* (a plant), *supālu* (a kind of juniper),[375] (and) *urânu* ('anise')[376]—you pound (*tasâk*)$^?$ these five ingredients together,

---

372 Köcher (1980) copied a trace of one wedge from the sign LI, which is now missing from the tablet. The passage is tentatively restored in line with Köcher's copy, but we cannot exclude other possibilities.

373 For a discussion of this unusual symptom description, see STO 1: 94–95.

374 See line 182 below for the syllabic orthography *iṣ-bat-su-ma*. Elsewhere in the therapeutic corpus, as in CRAN 2: 88 and 94 (BAM 482+ ii 24 and 30), the verb is also found in the stative: DIŠ NA SAG.KI.MIN-*šu*$_2$ *ṣab-ta-šu*$_2$-*ma* 'if someone's temples are seized'.

375 The plant name ^{u2}NIGIN^{sar} is unusual, but its equation with *supālu* seems to be confirmed by a parallel between CRAN 1: 57 (BAM 480+ i 57) and BAM 12 rev. 41′, with the standard orthography ^{u2}ZA.BA.LAM in the CRAN passage, but ^{u2}NIGIN^{sar} in the BAM 12 parallel. This orthography is also found in CT 41 45: 8, a commentary on Uruanna I 426 (CAD S 390).

376 ^{u2}TAL$_2$.TAL$_2$ = Akk. *urânu* is a rare ingredient but also appears in BAM 15 iv 10 and 13, which immediately precede the parallel passage in lines 160–161 below.

157 A$_{iii\ 22}$ *ina* A GAZI^{sar} ⸢*tara*⸣-*bak ina* TUG$_2$.ḪI.A SUR SAG ŠA$_3$-*šu*$_2$ LAL$_2$-*id* U$_2$ BABBAR SUD$_2$ *ina* A.MEŠ NU *pa-tan* NAG T[I]

---

158 A$_{iii\ 23}$ DIŠ KI MIN ILLU ^{š}[^{im}BUL]UḪ SUD$_2$ *ina* GEŠTIN SUR.RA NU *pa-tan* NAG [TI]

159 A$_{iii\ 24}$ DIŠ KI MIN ^{u2}x* [x] x SUD$_2$ *ina* KAŠ SAG NU *pa-tan* NAG [TI]

---

160 A$_{iii\ 25}$ DIŠ NA IM *ina* ŠA$_3$-*š*[*u*$_2$ NIGIN-*ḫ*]*ar ana* TI-*šu*$_2$ SUḪUŠ ^{u2}EME UR.GI$_7$ *ša ina* ZI-*ka* ^{d}UTU NU IGI-[*ru*][377]

[DIŠ N]A IM *ina* ŠA$_3$-*šu*$_2$ *u*$_2$-*sa-na-ḫar* / ^{u2}EME UR.GI$_7$ *ša*$_2$ *ina* ZI-*ka* / ^{d}UTU NU IGI.DU$_8^{!}$(BI) (BAM 158 iv 14–16)

161 A$_{iii\ 26}$ ḪAD$_2$.A SUD$_2$ *i*[*na** KAŠ SA]G NU *pa-tan* NAG T[I]

ḪAD$_2$.A SUD$_2$ / *ina* KAŠ SAG NAG-*šu*$_2$ (BAM 158 iv 16–17)

---

162 A$_{iii\ 27}$ DIŠ NA IM *ina* ŠA$_3$-*šu*$_2$ *i*-⸢*le*⸣-[*eb-bu* ^{u2}EME U]R.GI$_7$ NUMUN ^{u2}EME UR.GI$_7$ DIŠ-*niš* SUD$_2$ *ina* KAŠ NU *pa-tan* NAG TI

157 you stir them into a paste in juice from *kasû* ('tamarind'), you smear (*teṭerri*) (the mixture) on a piece of fabric, (and) you bandage (*taṣammid*) his epigastrium (*rēš libbi*). You pound *šammu peṣû* ('white plant'), (and) he drinks (*išatti*) it in water on an empty stomach; (then) he will recover (*iballuṭ*).

---

158 If DITTO, you pound (*tasâk*) resin from *ballukku* (an aromatic), (and) he drinks (*išatti*) it in pressed wine on an empty stomach; (then) he will recover (*iballuṭ*).

159 If DITTO, you pound . . . (and) he drinks it in high-quality beer on an empty stomach; (then) he will recover.

---

160 If flatulence (lit. wind) keeps circulating (*ussanaḫḫar*) in someone's belly (*libbu*): in order to heal him (*ana bulluṭīšu*), you dry (*tubbal*) (and) pound (*tasâk*) root from *lišān kalbi* ('dog's tongue' plant), which has not yet seen the sun when you picked it,[378]

161 (and) he drinks (*išatti*) it in high-quality beer on an empty stomach; (then) he will recover (*iballuṭ*).

---

162 If flatulence (lit. wind) rumbles in someone's belly (*libbu*): you pound (*tasâk*) *lišān kalbi* ('dog's tongue' plant) (and) seed from *lišān kalbi* ('dog's tongue' plant) together, (and) he drinks (*išatti*) them in beer on an empty stomach; (then) he will recover (*iballuṭ*).

377 The restoration here follows Cadelli 2000: 137.

378 For a discussion of collecting ingredients before sunrise, see Reiner 1995: 36–37 and Böck 2014a: 158.

163 A$_{iii\ 28}$ DIŠ NA IM GIM *di-ik-ši ina* ⸢ŠA$_3$⸣-[*šu*$_2$ x x x 1/2 GIN$_2$ ^{giš}E]REN 1/2 GIN$_2$ ^{giš}ŠUR.MIN$_3$ 1/3 GIN$_2$ ^{šim}GIR$_2$ 10 GIN$_2$ ^{giš}EREN.SUMUN

[DIŠ N]A ⸢IM⸣ [GI]M *di-ik-ši* ⸢*ina* ŠA$_3$-*šu*$_2$⸣ TAG.MEŠ-*su* 1/3 GIN$_2$ ^{giš}*eri-nu* 1/3 GIN$_2$ ^{giš}ŠUR.MIN$_3$ / 1/3 GIN$_2$ ^{šim}GIR$_2$ 1/3 GIN$_2$ ^{giš}EREN.SUMUN (BAM 54 obv. 1–2)

164 A$_{iii\ 29}$ 10 GIN$_2$ MUN *eme-sal-li*$_3$ ^{šim}L[I x x x x x x x] *ina* KAŠ SAG ŠEG$_6$-*šal* I$_3$.GIŠ *ana* IGI ŠUB *ana* DUR$_2$-*šu*$_2$ DUB-*ak*

10 GIN$_2$ MUN *eme-sal-li*$_3$ ^{giš}LI ^{giš}GUR$_2$.GUR$_2$ DIŠ-*niš* ⸢GAZ⸣ / SIM *ina* KAŠ ŠEG$_6$-*šal ta-ša*$_2$-*ḫal* I$_3$.GIŠ *ana* IGI ŠUB-*di ana* DUR$_2$-*šu*$_2$ DUB-*ak-ma* TI (BAM 54 obv. 2–3)

---

165 A$_{iii\ 30}$ DIŠ NA IM *ina* ŠA$_3$-*šu*$_2$ *uš-tar-'-ab* [x x x x x] x SU *šu*$_2$[379] *še-pi-*BI[380] GABA-*su u* MAŠ.SILA$_3$.MEŠ-*šu*$_2$

[DIŠ] NA IM *ina* ŠA$_3$-*šu*$_2$ *uš-tar-'-ab i-le-ḫi-ib ni-i*[*p-še* . . .] (BAM 56 rev. 8′)

[DIŠ N]A IM *ina* ŠA$_3$-*b*[*i-šu*$_2$ . . .] / *u*$_3$ *i-le*$_3$-*ḫi-ib* [. . .] / GABA-*su* MAŠ.SILA$_3$.MEŠ-[*šu*$_2$] (BAM 55: 1–3)

†

163 If flatulence (lit. wind) continually afflicts him (*iltanappassu*) like a pressing pain (*dikšu*): half$^?$ a shekel$^?$ of *erēnu* ('cedar'), half a shekel of *šurmēnu* ('cypress'), a third of a shekel of *asu* ('myrtle'), ten shekels of *šupuḫru* ('old cedar'),

164 ten shekels of *emesallu* salt, *burāšu* (a kind of juniper) . . . you bring them to a boil (*tušabšal*) in high-quality beer, you add (*tanaddi*) oil, (and) you pour (*tašappak*) (the mixture) in his anus.

---

165 If flatulence (lit. wind) churns (and) growls in someone's belly (*libbu*), . . . of his feet, his chest and his shoulder blades

379 One might consider reconstructing [*ki-ib*]-*su-šu*$_2$, for Akk. *kibsu*, but this word normally occurs in construct before *šēpu* to denote the soles of the feet. If so, the body parts in this line are listed in a reversed order, starting with the feet and moving upwards until it reaches the shoulder blades.

380 The correct reading of *še-pi-*BI remains unclear. Cadelli (2000: 138 and 160 with n. 36) reads it as *še-pi-iš*$_2$/BI and argues, following Küchler (1904: 117), that both readings point to the same possible meaning, viz. *šēpāšu* 'his legs'. Neither the value *iš*$_2$ nor *šu*$_{13}$ of the sign BI is normally used in first-millennium medical texts. See, however, the Middle Assyrian manuscript BAM 66 rev. 21′ with *tu-šap-ra-*BI*-ma*. For further discussion, see STO 4: 4.

166 A$_{iii\ 31}$ GU$_7$.MEŠ-*šu$_2$* UZU.MEŠ-*šu$_2$*[381] *u$_2$-šam-ma-[mu-šu$_2$ u* GIR$_2$.GI]R$_2$-*šu$_2$* UZU.MIN-*šu$_2$ ma-ṭu-u ni-ip-še* DIRI SAG.MEŠ-*šu$_2$ i-ta-na-nu-u$_2$*

UZU.[MEŠ-*šu$_2$* . . .] / UZU.MEŠ-*šu$_2$* [x x x] *ni-ip-še* [x] / SAG.MEŠ-*šu$_2$* [*i*]-⸢*ta*$^?$⸣-[*na-nu-u$_2$*] (BAM 57 obv. 1′–3′)

[. . .] / UZU.MEŠ-*šu$_2$ u$_2$-šam-ma-mu-šu$_2$ u* GIR$_2$.GIR$_2$-*šu$_2$ ši-ri-*[*šu$_2$* . . .] (BAM 56 rev. 8′–9′)

[. . .] / UZU.MEŠ-*šu$_2$* GIR$_2$.GIR$_2$-[*šu$_2$* . . .] / UZU.MEŠ-*šu$_2$ aš$_2$-ṭu* [. . .] / SAG.MEŠ-*šu$_2$ i-te-ne$_2$-*[*en-nu-u$_2$*] (BAM 55: 3–6)

167 A$_{iii\ 32}$ KUM$_2$.MEŠ *ina kal* UD-*me u$_2$-kil$_2$-š*[*u* x x x x x x ^{ši}]^{m}LI ^{u2}KUR.KUR ^{u2}ḪAR.ḪAR *saḫ-le$_2$-e* GAZI^{sar}

KUM$_2$ *ina kal* UD-*me* ⸢*u$_2$*⸣-[*kal-šu$_2$*] / *ana* TI-*šu$_2$* ^{šim}GUR$_2$.GUR$_2$ ^{šim}⸢LI⸣ [x x x] / ^{u2}ḪAR.ḪAR (BAM 57 obv. 4′–6′)

[. . .] / [x x] x x [x] su *ana* TI-*šu$_2$* ^{giš}GUR$_2$.GUR$_2$ ^{giš}LI ^{u2}[KUR.KUR x x x] / [*saḫ-le$_2$*]-*e* GAZI^{sar} (BAM 56 rev. 9′–11′)

[. . .] / *u$_2$-kal-šu$_2$ ana* TI-[*šu$_2$* . . .] / ^{u2}KUR.KUR ^{u2}ḪA[R.ḪAR . . .] (BAM 55: 6–8)

168 A$_{iii\ 33}$ MUN *a-ma-ni$_7$* ^{u2}*ur$_2$-ne$_2$-e* PA ^{giš}*b*[*i-ni* 9 U$_2$.ḪI].⸢A⸣ ŠEŠ TEŠ$_2$.BI SUD$_2$ *ina* GEŠTIN DU$_{10}$.GA *u* KAŠ SAG *ta-ra-sa-an*

^{u2}⸢*ur$_2$-ni*⸣-*i* PA [^{giš}*bi-ni*] / [*saḫ*]-*li$_2$-i* GAZI^{sar} / MUN *a-ma-ni$_7$* 9 U$_2$.MEŠ Š[EŠ] / DIŠ-*niš* SUD$_2$ *ina* GEŠTIN DU$_{10}$.GA *u* KAŠ SAG *tara-*⸢*sa*⸣-[*an*] (BAM 57 obv. 6′–rev. 1)

MUN *a-ma-ni$_7$* x x [. . .] / [. . .] x [. . .] *u* ⸢KAŠ⸣ [. . .] (BAM 56 rev. 11′–12′)

[. . .] / PA ^{giš}*bi-ni saḫ-le$_2$-*[*e* . . .] / 9 U$_2$.ḪI.A ŠEŠ [. . .] / *u* KAŠ SAG *tara-bak* (BAM 55: 8–11)

⸸

166 constantly cause him pain (*ītanakkalšu*), his flesh is paralyzed and causes him a stinging pain (*uzaqqatūšu*), his flesh is wasting away (and) full (*malû*) of stench (*nipšu*), his appearance (*zīmū*)[382] constantly changes,

167 he is continually hot (*ītenemmim*) (and) it (= the heat) has affected him (*ukīlšu*)[383] for an entire day: in order to heal him (*ana bulluṭīšu*), *kukru* (an aromatic), *burāšu* (a kind of juniper), *atā'išu* (a plant), *ḫašû* ('thyme'), *saḫlû* ('cress'), *kasû* ('tamarind'),

168 *amānu* salt, *urnû* (a kind of mint), (and) leaves from *bīnu* ('tamarisk')—you pound (*tasâk*) these nine drugs together, you steep them in good wine and high-quality beer,

---

381 In comparison with CRAN 2: 185 (BAM 482+ iii 61), it seems clear that UZU.MEŠ in our line and UZU.MIN in CRAN are in free variation with each other: both of them occur as the subject of the verb *ušammamūšu*. In our line UZU.MIN reappears later in the same line as the subject of *ma-ṭu-u*; the parallel in BAM 55: 5 with the variant *aš$_2$-ṭu* '(his flesh) is hard' is probably a misreading of *ma-ṭu-u* (see Cadelli 2019: 58). The repetition of *šīrū*, in spite of variations between UZU.MEŠ and UZU.MIN, also seems to be confirmed by the parallel texts: BAM 56 rev. 9′ has UZU.MEŠ-*šu$_2$* followed by the syllabic orthography *ši-ri-*[*šu$_2$*], and BAM 55 4–5 repeats UZU.MEŠ-*šu$_2$* in both places.

382 As Cadelli (2000: 161 n. 38) notes, the expression here is parallel with STO 3: 29, viz. MUŠ$_2$.MEŠ-*šu$_2$ i-te-nen-nu-u*, suggesting that SAG.MEŠ stands here for *zīmū* 'appearance'. See also the lexical passage in Idu I 122, equating *zīmu* with the singular SAG (CAD Z 119).

383 Taking KUM$_2$.MEŠ as a finite verb meaning 'he is constantly hot' resolves the grammatical problem identified by Cadelli (2000: 138 n. 43): if KUM$_2$.MEŠ were understood as a plural noun (viz. *ummātu*), the following verb *ukīlšu* should be in the plural, not the singular.

169 A$_{iii 34}$ *ina* GE$_6$ ⸢*ana** IGI⸣* MUL$_4$ *tuš-bat ina* ⸢A$_2$.GU$_2$⸣.Z[I.GA ŠEG$_6$-*šal t*]*a-ša$_2$-ḫal* SED 7 ŠE.MEŠ ḪENBUR$_2$ ^{u2}UKUŠ$_2$.ḪAB
ina GE$_6$ *ana* IGI MUL *tuš-bat ina še-ri$_3$* ŠEG$_6$-*šal* / *ta-ša$_2$-ḫal* SED 5 ŠE ḪENBUR$_2$ ^{u2}UKUŠ$_2$.ḪAB (BAM 57 rev. 2–3)
[. . .] / ^{d}UTU NU IGI.LAL *ina* [. . .] / *ta-ša$_2$-ḫal* SE[D . . .] (BAM 55: 11–13)

170 A$_{iii 35}$ 7 ŠE.MEŠ ^{na4}AN.ZAḪ TEŠ$_2$.BI SUD$_2$ *a*[*na* ŠA$_3$ GA]Z *la-am* ^{d}UTU *na-pa-ḫi* NAG-*šu$_2$*
7 ŠE ^{na4}AN.ZAḪ DIŠ-*niš* SUD$_2$ *ana* ŠA$_3$ GAZ / *la-am* ^{d}UTU KUR-*ḫi* NAG-*šu$_2$* (BAM 57 rev. 4–5)
7 ŠE AN.ZAḪ DIŠ-*niš* [. . .] / *ina še-ri$_3$ la-am* ⸢^{d}⸣[UTU . . .] (BAM 55: 14–15)

171 A$_{iii 36}$ *ina* A$_2$ *tu-šap-ra-šu$_2$ šum$_4$-ma* DU$_{10}$.G[A N]U IGI-*mur ana* DUR$_2$-*šu$_2$* DUB-*ak* TI
ina A$_2$ *tu-ša*[*p-ra-šu$_2$*] / *šum$_4$*-[*ma* x x x x] x *ana* DUR$_2$-*šu$_2$* DUB-*ma* [TI] (BAM 57 rev. 5–6)
ina A$_2$ [. . .] / *šum$_4$-ma* DU$_{10}$.GA NU [. . .] (BAM 55: 16–17)

---

172 A$_{iii 37}$ DIŠ NA NINDA GU$_7$ KAŠ NAG-*ma la i-še-eb-bi* ŠA$_3$-*šu$_2$* MU$_2$.MU$_2$-*ḫ*[*u* ŠA$_3$-*šu$_2$* N]U ⸢IGI-*ḫar*⸣[384] GIM *it-ta-šu bi-bik-ta$_5$* GIG

†

169 in the evening you leave (the mixture) out overnight under the stars, in the morning you bring it to a boil (*tušabšal*), you filter it, you let it cool (*tukaṣṣa*), (and then) you pound seven grains of shoots from *irrû* ('cucumber')

170 (and) seven grains of *anzaḫḫu* ('frit') together, you crush (*taḫaššal*) them into (the mixture), you have him drink (*tašaqqīšu*) it before sunrise,

171 you make him vomit with a feather, (and) if you have not seen (*tāmur*) any improvement,[385] you pour (*tašappak*) it into his anus; (then) he will recover (*iballuṭ*).

---

172 If someone eats (*ikkal*) bread (and) drinks (*išattī-ma*) beer, but he is not satisfied, his internal organs (*qerbū*) are swollen (*napḫū*) (and) his belly (*libbu*) cannot accept (*lā imaḫḫar*) anything, according to its sign(s), he suffers from *bibiktu* disease:[386]

---

384 The reading of the signs after the break is unclear: based on the partially similar passages [*ki-a*]*m it-ta-šu$_2$-nu* in AMT 30/2 i 15′ and *ki-a it-ta-ši-na* in BAM 582 i 3′, both in fragmentary contexts, the reading UR$_5$.GIM has been suggested (Ritter 1965: 301 n. 11). Our rendering of the passage as [N]U ⸢IGI-*ḫar*⸣ lines up with the traces and seems to fit the context: the patient first eats a large amount of food, without ever feeling full, which then leads to swollen intestines and a stomach that cannot tolerate any more food.

385 Cadelli (2000: 161 n. 43), following AHw 1393, equates DU$_{10}$.GA with Akk. *ṭūbu* and sees this word as an expression for 'improvement' or perhaps 'signs of improvement'. The same idiom can be found in the Middle Assyrian medical text published in Lambert 1969: 29 ln. 13 and 19, as well as in BAM 548 iv 6′ and BAM 558 iv 15.

386 Küchler's (1904: 30–31 and 118) reading of the disease name as *bišiktu*, with a cognate in Aramaic meaning 'boil', does not seem to be supported by the context. Rendered as *bibiktu*, the word might be compared to *bibītu* / *bibiḫtu* which, according to CAD B 219, can be the name of both a disease and a demon.

173 A$_{iii\ 38}$ ŠURUN GUD *ina* A *ta-maḫ-ḫa-aḫ* ŠEŠ$_{2}$ ^{giš}ZU$_{2}$.LUM.MA GA.RAŠ^{sar} U[KUŠ$_{2}$.ḪAB x x] x ⸢NINDA *u*⸣ KAŠ *la i-lem* UD.7.KAM$_{2}$ A *ša*$_{2}^{!}$(7) PU$_{2}$ ⸢*i-ša*⸣-*t*[*i*]*

---

174 A$_{iii\ 39}$ DIŠ NA *ḫu-šaḫ-ḫu* DAB-*su* 1 SILA$_{3}$ KAŠ SAG *ina* MUL$_{4}$ *tuš-bat ina š*[*e-ri*$_{3}$ x x x x] x x [x x x]

---

175 A$_{iii\ 40}$ DIŠ NA *ma-ʾ-di-iš e-na-aḫ-ma* IM *e-dip-ma* ⸢NU⸣ [..................] ⸢ud$^{?}$⸣* [x x x]

176 A$_{iii\ 41}$ *ina* A GAZI^{sar} *ir-ta-na-ḫaṣ* MUN DUR$_{2}$.⸢NU⸣.[LUḪ.ḪA ....] x [x x x]

---

177 A$_{iii\ 42}$ DIŠ NA U$_{2}$ NAG-*ma la i-ar*$_{2}$-*ru*$_{3}$ *ṣe-me-er a-za-pi* Š[AḪ ....]
[. . .] x U$_{2}$ NAG-*ma* ⸢*la*⸣ *i-ar*$_{2}$-⸢*ru*⸣ (AMC 32)

178 A$_{iii\ 43}$ A *u* I$_{3}$.GIŠ ŠEG$_{6}$-*šal* EN *še*$_{20}$-*bi-šu*$_{2}$[387] *u*$_{2}$-*al-lat ḫi*-⸢*iq*$^{?}$⸣* [KAŠ$^{?}$ ....]

---

173 you soften (*tamaḫḫaḫ*) ox dung in water, you anoint (*tapaššaš*) him (and then) . . . *suluppū* ('dates'), *karašu* ('leek'), (and) *irrû* ('cucumber')$^{?}$. (If) he cannot eat (*lā ilêm*) bread or beer, he drinks (*išatti*) well-water for seven days.

---

174 If ravenous hunger (*ḫušaḫḫu*)[388] has seized (*iṣbassu*) him: you leave one litre of high-quality beer out overnight (*tušbāt*) under the stars, in the morning . . .

---

175 If someone is extremely tired, and more specifically, he is inflated (*edip-ma*)[389] with flatulence (lit. wind), and he does not . . .

176 he keeps bathing (*irtanaḫḫaṣ*) in juice from *kasû* ('tamarind'), . . . salt, *tīyatu* (a plant) . . .

---

177 If someone took (lit. drank) (*ištī-ma*) a drug, and subsequently, he does not throw up, (and) he is distended: hog bristles . . .

178 you bring to a boil (*tušabšal*) water and oil, he swallows them until he can swallow no more (lit. until he is satisfied), (then) . . . diluted beer$^{?}$ . . .

---

387 CAD A/1 337 renders the passage as 'he swallows (water and oil) seven times', but then the expected form would be *se-bi-šu*$_{2}$, not *še*$_{20}$-*bi-šu*$_{2}$ which derives from the verb *šebû* 'to become sated'; see also Cadelli 2019: 5.

388 The translation of *ḫušaḫḫu* as 'ravenous hunger' follows CAD H 261, a suggestion that seems to be supported by its placement here after a symptom that describes someone who is initially unsatiated, and later on cannot tolerate any food or drink. For this term, see also Cadelli 2019: 6.

389 The term *edip* can also be found in one of the medical incantations in STO 1: 88, used in a metaphorical sense for someone who has been blown up by the wind of the steppe.

179 A$_{iii\ 44}$ DIŠ NA U$_2$ NAG-*ma la ip-ru la iṣ-nu-uḫ* NA BI *ze-e-ze-na* GIG *ana* TI-*šu*$_2$ ⸢^{giš}*si*⸣-[*ḫu* ^{giš}*ar*$_2$*-ga-nu*]

180 A$_{iii\ 45}$ ^{giš}*ba-ri-ra-ta*$_5$ ^{šim}GUR$_2$.GUR$_2$ ^{šim}LI ^{šim}GAM.⸢MA⸣* ^{šim}GIG ^{giš}EN.DI *ina* A PU$_2$ [x x x x]

181 A$_{iii\ 46}$ NE-*su ana* DUR$_2$-*šu*$_2$ DUB-*ak* 10 KISAL ^{šim}GUR$_2$.GUR$_2$ ŠEŠ$_2$-*su-ma* ŠA$_3$.MEŠ-*šu*$_2$ [SI.SA$_2$-*ma* TI]

---

182 A$_{iii\ 47}$ DIŠ NA *an-šu*$_2$*-tu*$_4$ *iṣ-bat-su-ma la u*$_2$*-šar-da* KAŠ SAG *ina* ŠEN.TUR ŠEG$_6$-*šal* MUN *ana* ŠA$_3$ ŠUB *ana* DU[R$_2$-*šu*$_2$ DUB]

183 A$_{iii\ 48}$ ŠU.SI-*ka* ^{tug2}GADA NIGIN MUN *ta-ṣap-pu* DUR$_2$-⸢*šu*$_2$⸣* *ta-kar* SIG$_2$ GAL$_4$.LA ^{munus}ŠU.GI *ina* MURUB$_4$ KA-*šu*$_2$ GAR [*ina-eš*]

---

179 If someone took (lit. drank) (*ištī-ma*) a drug, and subsequently, he did not throw up (*lā ipru*), (and) he did not excrete liquid (*lā iṣnuḫ*), that man suffers from *zēzēnu* disease:[390] in order to heal him (*ana bulluṭīšu*), . . . *sīḫu* ('wormwood'), *argannu* (a conifer),

180 *barīrātu* ('sagapenum'), *kukru* (an aromatic), *burāšu* (a kind of juniper), *ṣumlalû* (an aromatic), *kanaktu* (an aromatic), (and) *suādu* (a kind of sedge) in well water,

181 you pour (*tašappak*) it into his anus while it is steaming hot, you anoint (*tapaššassū-ma*) him with ten KISAL-measures of *kukru* (an aromatic), and he will void (*ušeššer-ma*) his internal organs (*qerbū*); then he will recover (*iballuṭ*).

---

182 If paralysis (*anšūtu*)[391] seizes someone, so that he cannot void (*ušarda*):[392] you bring high-quality beer to a boil (*tušabšal*) in a small copper pot, you put (*tanaddi*) salt in it, (and) you pour (*tašappak*) it into his anus.

183 You wrap (*talammi*) your finger in linen, you coat it with salt, you rub his anus, (and) you put (*tašakkan*) pubic hair from an old woman in the middle of his 'mouth' (viz. the anus);[393] (then) he will get well.

---

390 The disease name *zēzēnu* is otherwise attested only in the rectal disease text BAM 7 30 rev. 1-2: [DIŠ NA] *šit-ta-šu*$_2$ *ina* ŠA$_3$*-bi-šu*$_2$ *i-ta-nab-bal* / [NA B]I *ze-ze-na* GIG 'if someone's stool keeps drying up inside him, that man suffers from *zēzēnu* disease'.

391 The meaning and derivation of *anšūtu* is unclear: it may derive from *amāšu* 'to be paralyzed' (CAD A/2 80) or *enēšu* 'to be weak' (AHw 220). For a discussion of *anšūtu*, see Cadelli 2000: 323–324 with n. 84 and 2019: 14.

392 The verbal form here *u*$_2$*-šar-da* is a Š-stem of *redû*, which CAD R 243 translates as 'to make (a fluid) flow'. For this meaning, compare line 179 above, where the verb *ṣanāḫu* is used in much the same way to describe the excretion of liquid. The two verbs, viz. *redû* in the Š-stem and *ṣanāḫu*, are equated in KADP 32 iii 12 (CAD R 244).

393 For this euphemism, see line 122 above.

184 A$_{\text{iii 49}}$ DIŠ NA KAŠ SAG NAG-*ma* SUḪUŠ.MEŠ-*šu*$_2$ *pa-al-qa di-ig-la ma-a-ṭi ana* TI-*šu*$_2$ NUMUN ^{u2}SIKIL NUMUN ^{u2}DILI NUMUN ^{giš}⸢*bi*⸣-[*ni*]

[. . . DIŠ NA KA]Š NAG-*ma* SUḪUŠ.MEŠ-*šu*$_2$ *pa-al-qa* / [. . .] (AMC 33–34)

185 A$_{\text{iii 50}}$ NUMUN ^{u2}*am-ḫa-ra* NUMUN ^{u2}IN$_6$.UŠ$_2$ 5 U$_2$.ḪI.A ŠEŠ ⸢DIŠ⸣*-*niš* SUD$_2$ *ina* GEŠTIN SIG$_3$-*aṣ* NU *pa-tan* NAG-*ma ina*-⸢*eš*⸣

---

186 A$_{\text{iii 51}}$ DIŠ NA KAŠ NAG-*ma* SAG.DU-*su* DAB.DAB-*su* INIM.MEŠ-⸢*šu*$_2$⸣* *im-ta-na-aš*$_2$-*ši ina* DU$_{11}$.DU$_{11}$-*šu*$_2$ *u*$_2$-*pa-aš*$_2$-*šaṭ*

DIŠ NA KAŠ SAG NAG-*ma* SAG.[DU-*su* x x x] / INIM.MEŠ-*šu*$_2$ *im-ta-na-aš*-⸢*ši*⸣ *ina* D[U$_{11}$.DU$_{11}$-*šu*$_2$ x x x x] (BAM 59 rev. 6–7)

187 A$_{\text{iii 52}}$ *ṭe*$_4$-*en-šu*$_2$ *la ṣa-bit* LU$_2$ BI IGI.MIN-*šu*$_2$ GUB-*za ana* TI-*šu*$_2$ ^{u2}IGI-*lim* ^{u2}IGI.NIŠ ^{u2}*tar-muš* ^{u2}ḪAR.ḪAR

ṭe$_4$-*en-šu*$_2$ *la ṣa-bit* ⸢NA⸣ BI I[GI.MIN-*šu*$_2$ x x] / [x x x] ^{u2}IGI-*lim* ^{u2}IGI.N[IŠ x x x] / [. . .] x [. . .] (BAM 59 rev. 8–10)

188 A$_{\text{iii 53}}$ ^{u2}SIKIL ^{u2}DILI KA A.AB.BA ^{u2}NU.LUḪ.ḪA NUMUN ^{u2}NIG$_2$.GAN$_2$.GAN$_2$ ^{u2}*kam-ka-du* ^{u2}*eli-kul-la* 11 U$_2$.ḪI.A ŠEŠ

[^{u2}]SIKIL ^{u2}[DILI . . .] / [. . . ^{u2}N]U$^?$.⸢LUḪ$^?$⸣.Ḫ[A . . .] / [. . . ^{u2}*eli-kul-l*]*a* 11 ⸢U$_2$.MEŠ$^?$ ŠEŠ⸣ (BAM 59 rev. 10–12)[394]

184 If someone drinks (*išattī-ma*) high-quality beer, and then his lower extremities are impaired (lit. shattered),[395] (and his) vision is diminished:[396] in order to heal him (*ana bulluṭīšu*), seed from *sikillu* ('pure' plant), seed from *ēdu* ('lone' plant), seed from *bīnu* ('tamarisk'),

185 seed from *amḫaru* (a plant), (and) seed from *maštakal* ('soapwort')—you pound (*tasâk*) these five ingredients together, you stir (*tamaḫḫaṣ*) them into wine, (and) he drinks (the mixture) on an empty stomach; then he will get well.

---

186 If someone drinks (*išattī-ma*) beer, and then his head seizes him continually (*iṣṣanabbassu*), he keeps forgetting his words, in the midst of speaking he constantly corrects himself,

187 (and) he cannot form a thought,[397] that man has 'constantly starring eyes' (*īnāšu ittanazzazzā*):[398] in order to heal him (*ana bulluṭīšu*), *imḫur-līm* ('faces a thousand' plant), *imḫur-ešrā* ('faces twenty' plant), *tarmuš* ('lupin'), *ḫašû* ('thyme'),

188 *sikillu* ('pure' plant), *ēdu* ('lone' plant), *imbū tâmti* ('algae'), *nuḫurtu* ('asafoetida'), seed from *egingīru* ('rocket'),[399] *kamkadu* (a plant), (and) *elikulla* (a plant)—you pound (*tasâk*) these eleven ingredients

---

394 For a collation of BAM 59 rev. 10–14, with additional lines not included in Köcher's (1963) copy, see Abusch and Schwemer 2011: 226 and plate 131 no. 40.

395 The verb *palāqu* is usually rendered in this context as 'unsteady' (CAD I/J 240; Steinert 2018: 231; Cadelli 2000: 181; 2021: 24 with n. 614), but see also AHw 314 with the meaning 'zerschlagen' in connection with drunkenness.

396 As Küchler (1904: 120–121) first pointed out, the patient here probably shows symptoms of drunkenness, including the inability to stand on his feet and see clearly; see also Heeßel 2002 and Cadelli 2021: 23–24 for more recent discussions of the passage.

397 For *ṭēma ṣabātu*, see Stol 2009: 3–4.

398 Based on the discourse pattern LU$_2$ BI, the form is understood here as a disease name, but the expression literally means: 'that man's eyes continually stand firm'. The same expression can be found in CRAN 3: 65 (AMT 13/5 obv. 12), as part of a longer symptom description which also includes *amâtīšu imtanaššî*.

399 For the suggestion that *egingīru* goes back to ^{u2}NIG$_2$.NAGAR, see Civil 1982: 15–16.

189 A$_{iii\ 54}$ DIŠ-*niš* SUD$_2$ *ina* I$_3$.GIŠ *u* KAŠ *ana* IGI ^{d}*gu-la tuš-bat ina še-ri*$_3$ ⸢*la*⸣*-*am* ^{d}UTU MU$_2$-*ḫi la-am ma-am-ma iš-ši-qu-šu*$_2$ NAG-*ma ina-eš*

[. . .] / [. . . *tu*]*š-bat* [. . .] / [. . .] *iš-*[*ši-qu-šu*$_2$ . . .] (BAM 59 rev. 12–14)

---

190 A$_{iii\ 55}$ DIŠ NA GABA-*su* GIG-*ma* GIM *ši-ne*$_2$*-e-ti* SAḪAR TUKU.⸢TUKU⸣*-*ši ina da-ba-bi-šu*$_2$ *ik-ka-šu*$_2$ *ik-ta-ner-ru*
191 A$_{iii\ 56}$ ⸢*u*$_3$⸣ ZE$_2$ *ip-te-nar-ru* (eras.)[400] NA BI *bi-šit* ŠA$_3$ GIG ⸢*ana*⸣* TI-*šu*$_2$ ^{u2}EME UR.GI$_7$ *ina* KAŠ NU *pa-tan* NAG-*šu*$_2$
192 A$_{iii\ 57}$ *ina* A GAZI^{sar} RA.MEŠ A ^{giš}ŠE.NU *ana* DUR$_2$-*šu*$_2$ DUB ⸢ZI$_3$⸣* GU$_2$.TUR ^{giš}*ur*$_2$*-ne*$_2$*-e ina* ^{gi}SAG.KUD *ina* KA-*šu*$_2$ GID$_2$-*ad*
193 A$_{iii\ 58}$ ^{šim}ḪAB I$_3$.UDU ZU$_2$.LUM ^{šim}LI ^{šim}⸢KU$_7$⸣.KU$_7$ DIŠ-*niš* ḪI.ḪI *ina* KUŠ SUR LAL

☤

189 together, you leave them out overnight in oil and beer before Gula, (and) he drinks them in the morning, before sunrise, before anyone has kissed him; then he will get well.

---

190 If someone's chest is diseased (*marṣat-ma*) and he continually has (*irtanašši*) particles (*eperu*)[401] (in his throat) as if there were an obstruction (*šini'tu*),[402] he is short tempered[403] whenever he speaks

191 (and) he continually vomits up bile, that man suffers from 'stuff in the belly' (*bišīt libbi*):[404] in order to heal him (*ana bulluṭīšu*), you have him drink (*tašaqqīšu*) *lišān kalbi* ('dog's tongue' plant) in beer on an empty stomach,

192 he keeps bathing (*irtanaḫḫaṣ*) in juice from *kasû* ('tamarind'), you pour (*tašappak*) juice from *šunû* ('chaste tree') into his anus, he sucks up (*išaddad*) flour from *kakku* ('lentil') (and) *urnû* (a kind of mint) through a reed straw into his mouth,

193 you mix (*tuballal*) *ṭūru* ('opopanax'), fat, *suluppū* ('dates'), *burāšu* (a kind of juniper), (and) *kukru* (an aromatic) together, you smear (*teṭerri*) (the mixture) on a piece of leather, (and) you bandage (*taṣammid*) him.

---

400 Traces of a single horizontal wedge, presumably part of an erasure, are still legible between RU and NA.

401 For SAḪAR = Akk. *eperu* 'dust', which in our context describes the feeling that there are particles caught in the windpipe, see Kienast 1961: 60 n. 13. A possibly analogous use of the word *eperu* can be found in PBS 2/2: 7 (see Rutz 2011: 297 n. 15 with further literature).

402 The form *šini'tu* derives from the verb *šanā'u*, which reappears in line 200 below and means 'to block up (the throat)'. For a discussion of the verb, see Heeßel 2000: 263–264 and Cadelli 2021: 16.

403 The idiom *ikku karû* occurs in the Neo-Assyrian letters SAA 10 43 obv. 10 and SAA 10 226 rev. 4 in the sense 'to be short tempered'. For this idiom, see Cadelli 2021: 16.

404 The term *bišīt libbi* is also known from a bilingual cultic text, SBH 47 rev. 20, with the straightforward orthography *bi-ši-it* ŠA$_3$*-bi-*⸢*ia*⸣ (CAD B 270). The term *bišīt libbi* 'stuff in the belly', as a disease name, however, probably refers to the source of the particles obstructing the throat.

194 A$_{iii\ 59}$ U$_2$ BABBAR *ina* I$_3$.GIŠ KI MIN <A> GAZI^{sar} KI MIN[405] A ^{u2}*ur*$_2$*-ne*$_2$*-*⸢*e*⸣ *u* GAZI^{sar} ^{šim}GUR$_2$.GUR$_2$ KI MIN ^{šim}LI ^{šim}GUR$_2$.GUR$_2$ MIN

195 A$_{iii\ 60}$ PA ^{giš}GE$_6$.PAR$_3$ PA ^{giš}ŠE.NU PA ^{giš}MA.NU E$_2$ NIM *lab-bi-ni* DIŠ-*niš* ḪI.ḪI ŠU.BI.AŠ.AM$_3$

---

196 A$_{iii\ 61}$ U$_2$ BABBAR *ina* I$_3$.GIŠ NAG-*šu*$_2$ *ina* ⸢A⸣* GAZI^{sar} RA-*su-ma* A ^{giš}NU.UR$_2$.MA *ana* DUR$_2$-*šu*$_2$ DUB-*ak-ma* GU$_2$.GAL ^{šim}GUR$_2$.GUR$_2$

197 A$_{iii\ 62}$ GID$_2$-*ad-ma* ^{šim}LI ^{šim}ḪAB ILLU ^{šim}BULUḪ ^{giš}*bi-nu* ^{u2}SIKIL DIŠ-*niš* SUD$_2$ *ina* I$_3$.UDU ḪI.ḪI GABA-*su* LAL-*ma ina-eš*

---

198 A$_{iii\ 63}$ ^{u2}EME UR.GI$_7$ *ina* KAŠ NAG *ina* A GAZI^{sar} KI MIN GAZI^{sar} ^{šim}LI ^{šim}GUR$_2$.GUR$_2$ ^{šim}GAM.MA

†

194 DITTO (= you have him drink) *šammu peṣû* ('white plant') in oil, DITTO (= he keeps bathing) in juice from *kasû* ('tamarind'), DITTO (= you pour into his anus) *urnû* (a kind of mint) and juice from *kasû* ('tamarind') (as well as) *kukru* (an aromatic), DITTO (= he sucks up through a reed straw into his mouth) *burāšu* (a kind of juniper) (and) *kukru* (an aromatic),

195 you mix (*tuballal*) leaves from *lipāru* (a fruit tree), leaves from *šunû* ('chaste tree'), leaves from *ēru* (a tree), (and) *bīt zumbi labbini* ('wasp's nest')[406] together, (and) DITTO (= you smear them on a piece of leather, and you bandage him).

---

196 You have him drink (*tašaqqīšu*) *šammu peṣû* ('white plant') in oil, you bathe him (*taraḫḫassū-ma*) in juice from *kasû* ('tamarind'), and then you pour (*tašappak-ma*) juice from *nurmû* ('pomegranate') into his anus, and then he sucks up (*išaddad-ma*) *ḫallūru* ('chickpea') (and) *kukru* (an aromatic),

197 and then you pound (*tasâk*) *burāšu* (a kind of juniper), *ṭūru* ('opopanax'), resin from *baluḫḫu* ('galbanum'), *bīnu* ('tamarisk') (and) *sikillu* ('pure' plant) together, you mix (*tuballal*) them in fat, (and) you bandage (*taṣammid-ma*) his chest; then he will get well.

---

198 He drinks (*išatti*) *lišān kalbi* ('dog's tongue' plant) in beer, DITTO (= you bathe him) in juice from *kasû* ('tamarind'), DITTO (= you bandage him with) *burāšu* (a kind of juniper), *kukru* (an aromatic), *ṣumlalû* (an aromatic),

---

405 Based on the preceding prescription, the second DITTO should refer to the bathing of the patient, here probably with the juice of the *kasû* plant ('tamarind'). The sign A might have been dropped due to its subsequent occurrence as part of the nominal phrase *mê urnê u kasê*, which denotes the juice of two different plants, including the previously mentioned *kasû*.

406 This rare ingredient is only attested a couple of times in the medical literature: see Buisson 2009: 150–151 and Bácskay 2015: 21–22.

199 A$_{iii\ 64}$ ŠIM.ḪI.A DU$_3$.A.BI PA ^{giš}GE$_6$.PAR$_3$ PA ^{giš}*šu-še* K[I MIN]

---

200 A$_{iii\ 65}$ DIŠ NA *di-ik-šu ina* GABA-*šu*$_2$ TAG.TAG-*su-ma* GIM *ši-ne*$_2$*-'-ti* SAḪAR *i-ša*$_2$*-an-na-'-šu ina g*[*e-ši-šu*][407]

DIŠ NA SAG ŠA$_3$-*šu*$_2$ GU$_7$-*šu*$_2$ *ina ge-ši-šu* (STO 3: 1)

201 A$_{iii\ 66}$ ZE$_2$ *i-par-ru ina da-ba-bi-šu*$_2$ *ik-ka-šu ik-t*[*e-ne*]*r-ru* NA BI <*bi*>[408]*-šit* ŠA$_3$-*bi* GIG KU$_6$ SUM^{sar} UZU GU[D UZU ŠAḪ]

ZE$_2$ *im-ta-na-'a* NA BI *qer-be*$_2$-⸢*na*⸣ GIG / SUM^{sar} GA.RAŠ^{sar} UZU GUD UZU ŠAḪ (STO 3: 1–2)

202 A$_{iii\ 67}$ *u* KAŠ ^{lu2}KURUN$_2$.NA *la uš-ta-maḫ-ḫar ut-ta-šar* [1/2 SILA$_3$ Z]A$_3$.ḪI.LI 1/2 SILA$_3$ ^{šim}GUR$_2$.GUR$_2$ 1/2 SILA$_3$ ^{giš}L[I x x x x]

KAŠ ^{lu2}KURUN$_2$.NA NU *uš-ta-maḫ-*⸢*ḫar*⸣ *ana* TI-*šu*$_2$ / 1/2 SILA$_3$ ZA$_3$.ḪI.LI 1/2 SILA$_3$ ^{šim}LI 1/2 SILA$_3$ ^{šim}GUR$_2$.GUR$_2$ 1/2 SILA$_3$ NUMUN GADA (STO 3: 2–3)

203 A$_{iii\ 68}$ 1/2 SILA$_3$ ^{giš}GIG 1/2 SILA$_3$ ^{giš}EN.DI 1/2 SILA$_3$ NUMUN ^{u2}[*qut-ra-ti* 1/2] SILA$_3$ GAZI^{sar} 1/2 SILA$_3$ NUMUN ^{giš}ŠE.N[U* x x x x x x]

1/2 SILA$_3$ *pa-pa-si* ⸢MUNU$_6$⸣ 1/2 SILA$_3$ ^{šim}IM.DI / 1/2 SILA$_3$ NUMUN ^{u2}*qut-ra-ti* 1/2 SILA$_3$ GAZI^{sar} 1/2 SILA$_3$ ^{giš}ŠE.NU 1/2 SILA$_3$ GU$_2$.NIG$_2$.AR$_3$.RA (STO 3: 3–4)

†

199 all (these) aromatics (as well as) leaves from *lipāru* (a fruit tree) (and) leaves from *šūšu* ('liquorice').

---

200 If pressing pain (*dikšu*) continually afflicts him (*iltanappassū-ma*) in the chest and particles (lit. dust) continually block up (his throat) like an obstruction,[409] he vomits up bile whenever he belches,

201 (and) he is short tempered whenever he speaks, that man suffers from 'stuff in the belly' (*bišīt libbi*), (and consequently) he cannot stand (*lā uštamaḫḫar*)[410] fish, *šūmū* ('garlic'), beef, pork,

202 or brewer's beer, (and) he ends up weakening himself (*uttaššar*):[411] half a litre of *saḫlû* ('cress'), half a litre of *kukru* (an aromatic), half a litre of *burāšu* (a kind of juniper), half a litre seed from *kitû* ('flax')$^?$,

203 half a litre of *kanaktu* (an aromatic), half a litre of *suādu* (a kind of sedge), half a litre of seed from *qutrātu* ('smoke' plant), half a litre of *kasû* ('tamarind'), half a litre of seed from *šunû* ('chaste tree'), half a litre of *kiššanu* ('bitter vetch')$^?$,[412]

---

407 For a discussion of lines 200–210, in comparison with STO 3: 1–13, see Heeßel 2016: 45–49 with n. 53.

408 A haplography may have occurred here that omitted the second BI sign following directly after the discourse pattern NA BI. For the complete phrase, compare line 191 above.

409 For this symptom, see also line 190 above.

410 In our corpus, the Š-stem of *maḫāru* seems to be reserved for cases where the belly acts as the subject (viz. causer), with the patient as the causee indicated by the object pronoun *-šu*, as in *libbašu ušamḫaršu*. Here, however, the Št-stem—without any reference to the belly or the use of an object pronoun—is probably used to form a reflexive construction with the patient as both the causer and the causee: 'he (the patient) does not allow himself to come into contact with fish, *šūmū* ('garlic'), beef, pork or brewer's beer'. In our passage, the weakness clearly results from the patient not consuming strong food and drink. This may also explain why the description is not part of the symptomology, but rather appears in an unusual position otherwise reserved for the prognosis or results of treatment. For a discussion of this passage, see also Heeßel 2016: 55.

411 For a discussion of the form *uttaššar*, from the verb *našāru* in the Dt-stem meaning 'to be weakened', see Cadelli 2019: 58.

412 For a discussion of *kiššanu*, see Stol 1985b: 130–132.

204 A$_{iii\ 69}$ 1/2 SILA$_3$ BA.BA.ZA.^{d}ID$_2$ 1/2 SILA$_3$ NUMUN ^{u2}*ka-man-[ta* ....]

1/2 SILA$_3$ *pa-*⸢*pa*⸣*-si-*^{d}ID$_2$ / 1/2 SILA$_3$ U$_2$ *a-ši-i* 1/2 SILA$_3$ ^{u2}KUR.RA 1/2 SILA$_3$ ŠE$_{10}$ TU^{mušen} 1/3 SILA$_3$ NUMUN ^{u2}AB$_2$.DUḪ ⸢1/3⸣ SILA$_3$ ⸢*e*⸣*-reš-ti* A.ŠA$_3$ (STO 3: 4–5)

205 A$_{iii\ 70}$ 10 KISAL ILLU ^{šim}BULUḪ 10 KISAL KA A.A[B.BA ....]

10 KISAL ILLU ^{šim}BULUḪ 10 KISAL KA A.AB.BA 1 SILA$_3$ ZI$_3$ GIB$_3$ 1 SILA$_3$ ZU$_2$.LUM.MA 1 SILA$_3$ ⸢DIDA⸣ SIG / ⸢1⸣ SILA$_3$ ZI$_3$.KUM (STO 3: 6–7)

206 A$_{iii\ 71}$ 21 ⸢U$_2$.ḪI.A ŠEŠ DIŠ⸣*-*n[iš** ....]

TEŠ$_2$.BI GAZ SIM *ina* KAŠ GIM *ra-bi-ki ta-rab-bak ina* TUG$_2$.ḪI.A SUR-*ri šu-lu-uš-ti* 9 ⸢UD-*me*⸣ LAL / *ina* 4 UD-*me* DU$_8$*-ma ta-mar* (STO 3: 7–8)

207 A$_{iii\ 72}$ ⸢*šum*⸣*-m[a* ....]

šum$_2$-ma U$_3$.BU$_2$.BU$_2$.UL BABBAR ŠA$_3$*-šu$_2$ i-pa-*⸢*šaḫ*⸣ / *šum$_2$-ma* U$_3$.BU$_2$.BU$_2$.UL SA$_5$ ŠA$_3$*-šu$_2$* KUM$_2$ *u$_2$-kal* (STO 3: 8–9)

208 A$_{iii\ 73}$ [..]

šum$_2$-ma U$_3$.BU$_2$.BU$_2$.UL SIG$_7$ UD.DA KUR-*id* / GUR.GUR-*šu šum$_2$-ma* U$_3$.BU$_2$.BU$_2$.UL GE$_6$ *u$_2$-šam-ra-su-ma* NU TI (STO 3: 9–10)

209 A$_{iv\ 1}$ [.. U]D.DA SA$_2$.SA$_2$ GAZ SIM

ana U$_3$.BU$_2$.BU$_2$.UL *bu-le-e* ^{u2}LAG A.ŠA$_3$ IM.GU$_2$ *ša$_2$* UD.DA SA$_2$*-kat$_3$* / GAZ SIM (STO 3: 11–12)

204 half a litre of *pappasītu* (a mineral), half a litre of seed from *kamantu* (a plant) . . .

205 ten KISAL-measures of resin from *baluḫḫu* ('galbanum'), ten KISAL-measures of *imbū tâmti* ('algae'), one litre of flour from *kibtu* ('wheat'), one litre of *suluppū* ('dates'), one litre *billat našpi* (a kind of beerwort), (and) one litre of *isqūqu* (a type of groats)—

206 you crush (*taḫaššal*) and sift (*tanappi*) these twenty-one[413] ingredients together, you stir them as a paste in beer, you smear (*teṭerri*) (the mixture) on a piece of fabric, you bandage (*taṣammid*) him for one-third of nine days, on the fourth day you remove (*tapaṭṭar-ma*) it, and you examine him.[414]

207 If the boil is white (*peṣiat*), his belly will calm down. If the boil is red (*sāmat*), his belly will retain heat.

208 If the boil is green-yellow (*arqat*), he will be overwhelmed by fever (*ṣēta kašid*), (and) it will keep coming back to him (*uttanarrāšu*). If the boil is black (*ṣalmat*), it will make him sick, and he will not recover (*lā iballuṭ*).

209 In order to soothe the boil, you crush (and) sift *kirbān eqli* ('field clod' plant) (and) mud that . . . fever (*ṣēta* SA$_2$.SA$_2$),[415]

413 The number of drugs in line 204 is unclear because of the differences between our line and the parallel in STO 3: 4–5: if it contains five drugs (as opposed to the six drugs in the parallel), the total would add up to 21 drugs as indicated in line 206, but it is unclear which drugs follow *kamantu* in the break.

414 Lines 206–208, which run parallel with STO 3: 8–10, seem to record a skin test to predict the outcome of the disease. For this skin test, see also Cadelli 2019: 4 n. 1.

415 For the different interpretations of IM.GU$_2$ (*ša$_2$*) UD.DA SA$_2$.SA$_2$ / SA$_2$*-kat$_3$*, see Heeßel 2016: 59.

210 A$_{iv 2}$ [... $^{gi]š}$*bi-nu* ^{u2}IN$_6$.UŠ$_2$ RA-*ma* TI
ina A GAZI^{sar} *ta-la-aš$_2$* LAL-*id* EGIR-*šu$_2$* *saḫ-le$_2$-e* *ina* KAŠ NAG / UD-*ma* NAG-*u$_2$* *ina* A ^{giš}*šu-nu* ^{giš}ŠINIG ^{u2}*ak-tam* ^{u2}IN$_6$.UŠ$_2$ *ir-ta-na-ḫaṣ* (STO 3: 12–13)

---

211 A$_{iv 3}$ [DIŠ KI MIN .... *ina* K]AŠ NU *pa-tan* NAG-*ma* TI

---

212 A$_{iv 4}$ [DIŠ KI MIN .... ^{u2}NAG]A SI TEŠ$_2$.BI SUD$_2$ *ina* KAŠ SAG SILA$_{11}$-*aš* *ina* KUŠ SUR-*ri* LAL-*id*[416]

213 A$_{iv 5}$ [DIŠ KI MIN .... SILA$_{11}$-*a*]*š* *ina* KUŠ MIN

214 A$_{iv 6}$ [DIŠ KI MIN .... SILA$_{11}$-*a*]*š* *ina* SAG ŠA$_3$-*šu$_2$* LAL-*ma* TI

215 A$_{iv 7}$ [DIŠ KI MIN ....] x *ina* A.GEŠTIN.NA KALAG.GA SILA$_{11}$-*aš* SAG ŠA$_3$-*šu$_2$* LAL-*ma* TI

216 A$_{iv 8}$ [DIŠ KI MIN ....] x ⌜^{u2}*ḪA*⌝[417] ḪAD$_2$.A GAZ SIM *ina* KAŠ SILA$_{11}$-*aš* KI MIN

---

†

210 you knead them in juice from *kasû* ('tamarind'), (and) you bandage (*taṣammid*) him. Afterwards, he drinks (*išatti*) *saḫlû* ('cress') in beer, (and) while he drinks (*enūma išattû*) it, he bathes (*iraḫḫaṣ-ma*) in juice from *ēru* (a tree), *bīnu* ('tamarisk'), (and) *maštakal* ('soapwort'); then he will recover (*iballuṭ*).[418]

---

211 If DITTO$^?$, . . . (and) he drinks (*išattī-ma*) it in beer on an empty stomach; then he will recover.

---

212 If DITTO$^?$, you pound (*tasâk*) . . . (and) *uḫūlu qarnānû* ('horned alkali') together, you kneed (*talâš*) them in high-quality beer, you smear (*teṭerri*) (the mixture) on a piece of leather, (and) you bandage (*taṣammid*) him.

213 If DITTO$^?$ . . . you knead it . . . DITTO (= you smear it) on a piece of leather (and you bandage him).

214 If DITTO$^?$ . . . you knead it . . . (and) you bandage (*taṣammid-ma*) him on the epigastrium (*rēš libbi*); then he will recover (*iballuṭ*).

215 If DITTO$^?$ . . . you knead it in strong vinegar, (and) you bandage his epigastrium (*rēš libbi*); then he will recover.

216 If DITTO$^?$ . . . you dry (*tubbal*), crush (*taḫaššal*) (and) sift (*tanappi*) . . . (and) *urânu* ('anise'), you knead them in beer, DITTO (= you bandage his epigastrium; then he will recover).

---

416 Lines 212–216 each contain an individual prescription, without any horizontal ruling separating them from each other.

417 The correct reading of this logogram for *urânu* ('anise') is still unknown; see Maul 2019: 309.

418 Lines 205–210 are tentatively restored with the help of the parallel in STO 3: 6–13, which diverges from our main text at several points.

217 A$_{iv 9}$ [DIŠ KI MIN x x x x x] ^{u2}ḪAR.ḪAR ^{u2}KUR.KUR ^{u2}GAMUN.GE$_6$ ^{u2}*tar-muš*$_8$

218 A$_{iv 10}$ [x x x x x] x ⸢DIŠ⸣-*niš* SUD$_2$ *ina* KAŠ NAG *um-mi ša*$_2$ ŠA$_3$-*šu*$_2$ *ta-ša*$_2$-*ḫaṭ-ma* TI

---

219 A$_{iv 11}$ [DIŠ NA x x x x x K]I ⸢UḪ$_2$⸣-*šu*$_2$ MUD$_2$ ŠUB.ŠUB-*a ki-ṣir-te* ŠA$_3$ GIG UD.DA SA$_2$.SA$_2$ ŠA$_3$-*šu*$_2$ *qer-be*$_2$-*na*$_7$ GIG

220 A$_{iv 12}$ [^{u2}*u*]*r*$_2$-⸢*ne*$_2$⸣-*e* A.GAR.GAR MAŠ.DA$_3$ NUMUN ^{u2}KI.^{d}IŠKUR NUMUN ^{u2}IN$_6$.UŠ$_2$ ^{šim}GUR$_2$.GUR$_2$ 2 KISAL KA A.AB.BA GAZ *ina* A PU$_2$ *tara-bak*

221 A$_{iv 13}$ [GUR-*m*]*a** ⸢ḪAD$_2$⸣.A GAZ *ina* A ZU$_2$.LUM.MA *ina* ^{dug}GAN *tara-bak ina* TUG$_2$ SUR-*ri* SAG ŠA$_3$-*šu*$_2$ *ur-ra u* GE$_6$ LAL-*id* DU$_8$-*šu*$_2$-*ma*

222 A$_{iv 14}$ [x] x x[419] *ta-ḫab-bu* U$_2$ BABBAR SUD$_2$ *ina* I$_3$ *ḫal-ṣa* EME-*šu*$_2$ DAB-*bat* NAG *i-ar*$_2$-*ru* LAL$_2$-*su* NAG.NAG-*šu*$_2$ *iš-tu* NAG-*u*$_2$

217 If DITTO$^{?}$, you pound (*tasâk*) . . . *ḫašû* ('thyme'), *atā'išu* (a plant), *zibû* ('black cumin'), *tarmuš* ('lupin'),

218 . . . together, he drinks (*išatti*) them in beer, (and thereby) you drain the heat from his belly (*libbu*);[420] then he will recover (*iballuṭ*).

---

219 If someone . . . he regularly spits up (*ittanaddâ*) blood along with his phlegm (*rupuštu*), he suffers from clots in the belly (*kiṣirti libbi*),[421] he is . . . by fever (*ṣēta* SA$_2$.SA$_2$), (and) his belly suffers internally:

220 you crush (*taḫaššal*) *urnû* (a kind of mint), gazelle dung, seed from *qutru* (a plant), seed from *maštakal* ('soapwort'), *kukru* (an aromatic), (and) two KISAL-measures of *imbū tâmti* ('algae'), you stir them into a paste in well water,

221 (then) you dry (*tubbal*) (and) crush (the mixture) over and over again (*tatâr-ma*), you stir it into a paste in juice from *suluppū* ('dates') in a jar, you smear (*teṭerri*) it on a piece of fabric, (and) you bandage (*taṣammid*) his epigastrium (*rēš libbi*) for a day and a night, you remove it (*tapaṭṭaršū-ma*),

222 and then you draw . . . you pound (*tasâk*) *šammu peṣû* ('white plant'), you put (*tušaṣbat*) it on his tongue (lit. have his tongue seize it) with pressed oil, he drinks (*išatti*) it, (and) he will vomit. You bandage him (*taṣammissu*) (again, and) you have him continually drink (*taštanaqqīšu*) (the well water). After he has finished drinking (*ištatû*) it,

---

419 A liquid carrier may have been mentioned at the beginning of the line, preceding the verb *taḫabbu* 'you draw'. This verb usually occurs with well- or river-water as the object, as in STO 1: 196 and AMT 73/1+ i 18 (see also CAD H 19), but the fragmentary traces in our line do not support reading A PU$_2$ or A ID$_2$. For the reading of these fragmentary signs as ḪU and UŠ, see also Küchler 1904: 36–37 with plate XII.

420 For the same idiom, expressed with the verb *šaḫāṭu* in the third person, see line 140.

421 For the possible meanings of *kiṣirtu*, see BAM 13 p. 92 and Cadelli 2021: 14–15. See also Aramaic *q/kîrṣâ*, 'sting, bite', once written *kîṣrâ* (Sokoloff 2002: 578b).

223 A$_{iv\ 15}$ [1/2] SILA$_3$ ⸢NUMUN ^{giš}*bi*⸣-*ni* 1/2 SILA$_3$ (eras.)* ⸢^{giš}⸣*GEŠTIN[422] KA$_5$.A 1/2 SILA$_3$ ^{šim}LI 1/2 SILA$_3$ ZU$_2$.LUM.MA 1/2 SILA$_3$ ZI$_3$ GIB$_3$ GAZ *ina* A GAZI^{sar} *tara-bak*

224 A$_{iv\ 16}$ [GUR-*ma* ḪA]D$_2$.A GAZ *ina* A ZU$_2$.LUM *ina* ^{dug}GAN *tara-bak ina* TUG$_2$.ḪI.A SUR-*ri ur-ri u* GE$_6$ LAL

---

225 A$_{iv\ 17}$ [DIŠ KI MIN] ⸢PA⸣ ^{giš}NU.UR$_2$.MA PA ^{giš}GE$_6$.PAR$_3$ PA ^{giš}NAM.TAR NITA$_2$ ŠIKA NIG$_2$.BUN$_2$.NA^{ku6} ILLU ^{šim}BULUḪ GAZ

226 A$_{iv\ 18}$ [*ina* A Z]U$_2$.LUM.MA *ina* ^{dug}GAN *tara-bak* GUR-*ma* ḪAD$_2$.A GAZ *ina* KAŠ *u* I$_3$.GIŠ *ina* ^{dug}GAN *tara-bak ina* TUG$_2$ SUR

227 A$_{iv\ 19}$ ⸢*ur-ri*⸣ *u* GE$_6$ LAL-*id* EḪ$_3$[423] ^{u2}*ti-ia$_2$-ta$_5$ ina* KAŠ NU *pa-tan* NAG 1/3 SILA$_3$ ŠE$_{10}$ TU^{mušen}.MEŠ

⸸

223 you crush half a litre of seed from *bīnu* ('tamarisk'), half a litre of *karān šēlebi* ('fox-vine'), half a litre of *burāšu* (a kind of juniper), half a litre of *suluppū* ('dates'), (and) half a litre of flour from *kibtu* ('wheat'), you stir them into a paste in juice from *kasû* ('tamarind'),

224 (then) you dry (and) crush (the mixture) over and over again, you stir it into a paste in juice from *suluppū* ('dates') in a jar, you smear it on a piece of fabric, (and) you bandage him for a day and a night.

---

225 If DITTO, you crush (*taḫaššal*) leaves from *nurmû* ('pomegranate'), leaves from *lipāru* (a fruit tree), leaves from male *pillû* ('mandrake'), turtle shell, (and) resin from *baluḫḫu* ('galbanum'),

226 you stir them into a paste in juice from *suluppū* ('dates') in a jar, (then) you dry (*tubbal*) (and) crush (the mixture) over and over again (*tatâr-ma*), you stir it into a paste in beer and oil in a jar, you smear (*teṭerri*) it on a piece of fabric,

227 (and) you bandage (*taṣammid*) him for a day and a night. (Next) he drinks (*išatti*) powder from *tīyatu* (a plant) in beer on an empty stomach. You crush a third of a litre of *zē summati* ('pigeon droppings'),

---

422 There are traces of a sign before the GIŠ of ^{giš}GEŠTIN KA$_5$.A: Küchler (1904: 36 with plate 12) and Cadelli (2000: 144) read U$_2$ here, which they take as the determinative for GEŠTIN KA$_5$.A, instead of GIŠ. However, GIŠ is the expected determinative for GEŠTIN KA$_5$.A, and the traces immediately before GEŠTIN cannot be read as U$_2$, nor as NUMUN ('seed'), PA ('leaf') or A ('juice'). We take the traces that immediately precede GEŠTIN as the expected determinative GIŠ, perhaps written over an erased U$_2$ sign.

423 Schwemer (2021) has recently suggested the Sumerian reading /ḫeḫe/ for KU.KU (Akk. *supāndu*), based on the commentary BRM 4 32 obv. 20 (Frazer 2017), with the glossed form KU$^{ḫe\text{-}ḫe}$KU : *su-pan-du*. We suggest, however, that the Sumerian reading of the sign sequence KU.KU is EḪ$_3$, which is found in Diri Ugarit I 85–86 along with the Akk. equivalent *pi$_2$-ṣu$_2$-u$_2$*; this probably derives from Akkadian *pa'āṣu* 'to grind (into powder)' (MSL 15 p. 70). The editor of the commentary may have pronounced EḪ$_3$ as /eḫe/ and this might have led them to gloss of KU.KU with ḫe-ḫe, influenced by the common logogram ḪE.ḪE for Akk. *balālu* 'to mix'.

228 A$_{\text{iv 20}}$ 1/3 SILA$_3$ NUMUN ^{u2}AB$_2$.DUḪ 1/3 SILA$_3$ GURUN ^{u2}MAŠ.ḪUŠ *ta-ḫaš-šal ina* A GAZI^{sar} *tara-bak* GUR-*ma* ḪAD$_2$.A GAZ
229 A$_{\text{iv 21}}$ *ina* A ZU$_2$.LUM.MA *ina* ^{dug}GAN *tara-bak ina* TUG$_2$ SUR-*ri ur-ri u* GE$_6$ LAL-*id*

---

230 A$_{\text{iv 22}}$ DIŠ KI MIN 1/2 SILA$_3$ NUMUN ^{u2}DILI 1/2 SILA$_3$ ^{u2}LAG GAN$_2$ SIG$_7$ 1/2 SILA$_3$ U$_5$ ARGAB^{mušen} 1/2 SILA$_3$ ZI$_3$ ZIZ$_2$.A.AN
231 A$_{\text{iv 23}}$ GAZ *ina* A ID$_2$ *tara-bak* GUR-*ma* ḪAD$_2$.A GAZ SIM *ina* A ZU$_2$.LUM.MA *ina* ^{dug}GAN *tara-bak ina* TUG$_2$ SUR-*ri*
232 A$_{\text{iv 24}}$ *ur-ra u* GE$_6$ LAL-*id* NUMUN ^{giš}GEŠTIN KA$_5$.A *ina* KAŠ NU *pa-tan* NAG *ina* A ŠEG$_6$-*šal tara-*⌜*ḫas-su*⌝

---

233 A$_{\text{iv 25}}$ DIŠ KI MIN ZA$_3$.ḪI.LI *ina* KAŠ NAG NUMUN ^{u2}KI.^{d}IŠKUR-*ri*[424] NUMUN ^{giš}MA.NU NUMUN ^{giš}ŠINIG ^{šim}GUR$_2$.GUR$_2$ G[AZ]
234 A$_{\text{iv 26}}$ *ina* A GAZI^{sar} *tara-bak* GUR-*ma* ḪAD$_2$.A GAZ *ina* A ZU$_2$.LUM.MA *ina* ^{dug}GAN *tara-bak ina* TUG$_2$.ḪI.A SUR-*ri ur-ri u* GE$_6$ [LA]L

---

†

228 a third of a litre of seed from *kamantu* (a plant), (and) a third of a litre of fruit from *kalbānu* (a plant), you stir them into a paste in juice from *kasû* ('tamarind'), (then) you dry (and) crush (the mixture) over and over again (*tatâr-ma*),
229 you stir it into a paste in juice from *suluppū* ('dates') in a jar, you smear it on a piece of fabric, (and) you bandage him for a day and a night.

---

230 If DITTO, you crush (*taḫaššal*) half a litre of seed from *ēdu* ('lone' plant), half a litre of fresh *kirbān eqli* ('field clod' plant), half a litre of *rikibti arkabi* ('bat guano'), (and) half a litre of flour from *kunāšu* ('emmer'),
231 you stir them into a paste in river water, (then) you dry (*tubbal*), crush (and) sift (*tanappi*) (the mixture) over and over again (*tatâr-ma*), you stir it into a paste in juice from *suluppū* ('dates') in a jar, you smear (*teṭerri*) it on a piece of fabric,
232 (and) you bandage (*taṣammid*) him for a day and a night. He drinks (*išatti*) seed from *karān šēlebi* ('fox-vine') in beer on an empty stomach, (then) you bring it to a boil (*tušabšal*) in water, (and) you bathe him in it.

---

233 If DITTO, he drinks (*išatti*) *saḫlû* ('cress') in beer, (and then) you crush (*taḫaššal*) seed from *qutru* (a plant), seed from *ēru* (a tree), seed from *bīnu* ('tamarisk'), (and) *kukru* (an aromatic),
234 you stir them into a paste in juice from *kasû* ('tamarind'), (then) you dry (*tubbal*) (and) crush (the mixture) over and over again (*tatâr-ma*), you stir it into a paste in juice from *suluppū* ('dates') in a jar, you smear (*teṭerri*) it on a piece of fabric, (and) you bandage him for a day and a night.

---

424 The phonetic complement *-ri* following the logogram KI.^{d}IŠKUR in this line clearly shows that the reading is *qutru* rather than *qutrātu*; the logogram for *qutrātu* in Ura XVII 125 (MSL 10 p. 87) adds NIM, yielding KI.^{d}IŠKUR.NIM. Uruanna II 183–185 and the Practical Vocabulary of Assur, ll. 101–102 (Landsberger and Gurney 1957–1958: 329), use KI.^{d}IŠKUR for *qutrātu* and equate it with U$_2$ I.BI$_2$ 'smoke plant' (CAD Q 323).

235 A$_{\text{iv }27}$ DIŠ KI MIN ^{šim}LI ^{šim}GUR$_2$.GUR$_2$ ^{šim}ḪAB ^{šim}GAM.MA $^{\text{u2}}$*ba-ri-ra-ta*$_5$ ^{šim}BULUḪ ^{giš}EREN ^{giš}ŠUR.[MIN$_3$]

236 A$_{\text{iv }28}$ ^{šim}BAL GAZ *ina* A GAZI^{sar} *tara-bak* GUR-*ma* ḪAD$_2$.A GAZ *ina* A ZU$_2$.LUM.MA *u* KAŠ *ina* ^{dug}GAN *tara-*⸢*bak*⸣

237 A$_{\text{iv }29}$ *ina* TUG$_2$.ḪI.A *te-ṭer*$_5$*-ri ur-ra u* GE$_6$ LAL-*id* IM.SAḪAR.NA$_4$.KUR.RA *ina* KAŠ ⸢NAG⸣

---

238 A$_{\text{iv }30}$ DIŠ KI MIN PA GIŠ.GI.ZU$_2$.LUM.MA PA $^{\text{u2}}$SIKIL PA $^{\text{u2}}$IN$_6$.UŠ$_2$ GURUN GA.RAŠ^{sar} GURUN ^{giš}NU.UR$_2$.MA NUMUN ^{giš}ḪA.LU.UB$_2$

239 A$_{\text{iv }31}$ PA ^{giš}ASAL$_2$ GAZ *ina* A GAZI^{sar} ⸢*ina* ^{dug}GAN *tara-bak*⸣ *ina* TUG$_2$ SUR *ur-ra u* GE$_6$ LAL *ina* A ŠEG$_6$*-šal tara-ḫas*$_2$*-su* [U$_2^{?}$] ŠEŠ

240 A$_{\text{iv }32}$ ⸢*ina* I$_3$ *u*⸣ [x x] x x ⸢NAG⸣ *tu-ša*$_2$-⸢⸣*-[*ra-šu*$_2$]-⸢*ma*⸣[425] DU$_{10}$.GA GU$_7$ DU$_{10}$.GA NAG *ka-la* UD *u* GE$_6$ *ina* K[A$_2$ GU]B.GUB

☨

235 If DITTO, you crush (*taḫaššal*) *burāšu* (a kind of juniper), *kukru* (an aromatic), *ṭūru* ('opopanax'), *ṣumlalû* (an aromatic), *barīrātu* ('sagapenum'), *baluḫḫu* ('ferula gummosa'), *erēnu* ('cedar'), *šurmēnu* ('cypress'),

236 (and) *ballukku* (an aromatic), you stir them into a paste in juice from *kasû* ('tamarind'), (then) you dry (*tubbal*) (and) crush (the mixture) over and over again (*tatâr-ma*), you stir it into a paste in juice from *suluppū* ('dates') and beer in a jar,

237 you smear it on a piece of fabric, (and) you bandage (*taṣammid*) him for a day and a night, (then) he drinks (*išatti*) *aban gabî* ('alum') in beer.

---

238 If DITTO, you crush (*taḫaššal*) leaves from *kūru* (a plant), leaves from *sikillu* ('pure' plant), leaves from *maštakal* ('soapwort'), stalk from *karašu* ('leek'),[426] fruit from *nurmû* ('pomegranate'), seed from *ḫaluppu* (a tree),[427]

239 (and) leaves from *ṣarbatu* ('poplar'), you stir them into a paste in juice from *kasû* ('tamarind') in a jar, you smear (*teṭerri*) (the mixture) on a piece of fabric, (and) you bandage (*taṣammid*) him for a day and a night, (then) you bring (the mixture) to a boil (*tušabšal*) in water, (and) you bathe him in it. He drinks (*išatti*) these drugs$^?$

240 in oil and . . . you make him vomit, and then he eats (*ikkal*) (and) drinks good things,[428] while standing constantly (*ittanazzaz*)$^?$ in the doorway$^?$ for a whole day and night,

---

425 We reconstruct the verb *arû* in the Š-stem, viz. 'to make (someone) vomit', following Cadelli 2000: 145 with n. 56, who cites STO 3: 16 and 92 as parallels for the same procedure. The identity of the sign at the end of the verb is somewhat uncertain, but we expect the connective *-ma* here.

426 The phrase literally means 'the fruit from *karašu* (= 'leek')', which in the case of leeks probably denotes the edible stalk. Murgud B IV 114 as well as Murgud E III 19 (MSL 10 p. 33) equate *inib karaši* with the stone *ašgikû*, usually identified as turquoise (Schuster-Brandis 2008: 400–401) because of its bluish green colour, and this presumably corresponds to the green colour of the stalk rather than the white bulb.

427 For the long history of the *haluppu* tree, see Gadotti 2014: 27–48.

428 For a similar idiom involving the consumption of 'good things', see the DINGIR.ŠA$_3$.DIB.BA incantation in Lambert 1974: 276 ln. 49: *šaptāka ṭūba limḫurā* 'may your lips receive good things', presumably referring to the fat and oil that are mentioned in the preceding line.

241 A$_{\text{iv 33}}$ *ina* ^{giš}NA$_2$-⸢*šu*$_2$⸣ *l*[*a*$^?$ NU$_2$ *ina š*]*e-ri*$_3$ A KUM$_2$-*ti*$_3$ TU$_5$-*šu*$_2$ I$_3$.GIŠ KUM$_2$ ŠEŠ$_2$ UD.3.KAM$_2$ G[UR.GUR-*š*]*um*[429]

---

242 A$_{\text{iv 34}}$ DIŠ NA KI ⸢UḪ$_2$-*šu*$_2$⸣ MUD$_2$ ŠUB.MEŠ-*a* NA BI *ta-aš*$_2$*-ni-qa* GIG *ana* TI-*šu*$_2$ 1/3 SILA$_3$ I$_3$.UDU 1/3 SILA$_3$ ZU$_2$.LUM.⸢MA 1/3⸣ SILA$_3$ ^{šim}ḪAB

243 A$_{\text{iv 35}}$ 1/3 SILA$_3$ ^{šim}⸢GUR$_2$⸣.GUR$_2$ 1/3 SILA$_3$ ^{šim}LI 1/3 SILA$_3$ ^{šim}⸢BULUḪ 1/3 SILA$_3$* DUḪ⸣*.ŠE.GIŠ.I$_3$ 1/3 SILA$_3$ NUMUN ^{giš}*bi-ni* 8 ⸢U$_2$⸣.[ḪI.A] ŠEŠ DIŠ-*niš* GAZ

244 A$_{\text{iv 36}}$ *ina* I$_3$.NUN *tal-*[*ta*]*p-pat ina* KUŠ SUR IGI *u* MAŠ.SILA$_3$ EN DU$_{10}$.GA-*šu*$_2$ 3 ITI.MEŠ LAL$_2$-*su-ma* LAL-*ta ina* K[A-*šu*$_2$][430] ⸢*u*$_2$⸣-*še-ṣa-am-ma ina-eš*

---

†

241 without lying down (*lā inâl*) in his bed. In the morning you bathe him (*tarammukšu*) in warm water, (and) you anoint (*tapaššaš*) him with warm oil. You repeat (*tutāršu*) (this procedure) on him for three days.

---

242 If someone regularly spits up (*ittanaddâ*) blood along with his phlegm (*rupuštu*), that man suffers from *tašnīqu* disease:[431] in order to heal him (*ana bulluṭīšu*), a third of a litre of fat, a third of a litre of *suluppū* ('dates'), a third of a litre of *ṭūru* ('opopanax'),

243 a third of a litre of *kukru* (an aromatic), a third of a litre of *burāšu* (a kind of juniper), a third of a litre of *baluḫḫu* ('ferula gummosa'), a third of a litre of *kupsu* ('sesame pomace'), (and) a third of a litre of seed from *bīnu* ('tamarisk'), you crush (*taḫaššal*) these eight ingredients together,

244 you moisten (the mixture) with ghee, you smear (*teṭerri*) it on a piece of leather, you bandage him (*taṣammissū-ma*) front and back (lit. shoulder blades) over the next three months, until he gets better and expels the . . . from his mouth;[432] then he will get well.

---

429 This may be an abbreviated writing of GUR.GUR-*šum-ma* TI(-*uṭ*), which is attested in BAM 503+ iii 63, 67 and 73, alongside the variant spelling GUR.GUR-*šu*$_2$-*ma* TI in line 60 of the same column.

430 Cadelli (2000: 167) reconstructs *ina p*[*îka*] here, but there does not seem to be enough room in the break for a second KA sign. For the reading *p*[*îšu*], see already CAD A/2 375.

431 For the disease name *tašnīqu*, see von Soden 1968: 268, who initially derived this form from Aramaic *šanneq* 'to suffocate', but later turned to Izi V 148 (von Soden 1977: 196), arguing that it derives from *šunnuqu*, presumably a Š-stem of *enēqu* 'to suck' (cf. CAD Š/3 304). The *taprīs*-form is normally based on the D-stem, however, not the Š-stem. In line with CAD T 295, *tašnīqu* probably derives from the verb *sanāqu* in the D-stem, viz. *sunnuqu* 'to harass, to plague'. As a disease name, *tašnīqu* also features in Diagnostic Handbook Sagig 29: 8, 29 and 41 (Heeßel 2000: 319–321), sometimes accompanied by the qualification KUR.RA 'from the mountains'.

432 In line with CAD A/2 375, the passage may be part of a prognosis, describing that some kind of obstruction should leave the patient's body through his mouth. The meaning of LAL-*ta* is unknown, but it might correspond to the hitherto unattested Akkadian form *nenbettu*, presumably a *mapras* from Akk. *ebēṭu* 'to have cramps', which is equated with LAL in MSL 9 p. 127 ln. 122.

245 A$_{iv 37}$ ⸢DIŠ NA⸣ *ki*-⸢*ṣir*⸣ ŠA$_3$ GIG NINDA *u* KAŠ ⸢ŠA$_3$-*šu*$_2$⸣ *la* IGI-*šu*$_2$ *ina* ⸢KA⸣*-*šu*$_2$ GUR.GUR ⸢TUN$_3$-*šu*$_2$ *i*⸣-*sa*-⸢*ḫal*⸣-*šu*$_2$[433] *ana* TI-[*šu*$_2$] ⸢1/2⸣ SILA$_3$ *saḫ-le*$_2$*-e*

ki-ṣir ŠA$_3$ GIG (AMC 34)

1/2 SILA$_3$ *saḫ-le*$_2$*-e* (STO 1: 37)

DIŠ ⸢NA⸣ [*ki*]-*ṣir* ŠA$_3$ GIG NINDA *u* KA[Š x x x] / ⸢*ina* KA⸣-*šu*$_2$ GUR.GUR TUN$_3$-*šu*$_2$ *u*$_2$-*s*[*a-ḫal-šu*$_2$] / ⸢1/2 SILA$_3$⸣ *saḫ-le*$_2$*-e* (BAM 58: 8–10)

246 A$_{iv 38}$ [1/2 SIL]A$_3$ [^{šim}]⸢GUR$_2$*.GUR$_2$⸣* [1/2 SI]LA$_3$ ^{šim}LI 1/2 SILA$_3$ ^{u2}KI.^{d}IŠKUR 1/2 SILA$_3$ *ka-si-i* 1/2 SILA$_3$ *pa-pa-si*-⸢^{d}⸣I[D$_2$]* 1/2 SILA$_3$ ^{u2}KUR.RA

1/2 SILA$_3$ ^{šim}GUR$_2$.GUR$_2$ 1/2 ⸢SILA$_3$⸣ [^{šim}LI 1/2 SILA$_3$] ⸢^{u2}*qut-ri* 1/2 SILA$_3$⸣ GA[ZI^{sar}] / [1/2 SILA$_3$] ⸢ZI$_3$⸣ MUNU$_6$ 1/2 SILA$_3$ ZI$_3$ GU$_2$.GAL 1/2 SILA$_3$ ZI$_3$ GU$_2$.TUR ⸢1/2 SILA$_3$ *pa-pa-si*-^{d}ID$_2$⸣ 1/2 SILA$_3$ ^{u2}KUR.RA (STO 1: 37–38)

1/2 SILA$_3$ ^{šim}GUR$_2$.GUR$_2$ [x x x x] / [1/2 S]ILA$_3$ NUMUN ^{u2}*qut-ri* 1/2 SILA$_3$ GAZI^{s}[^{ar} x x x x x x x x] / [1/2 S]ILA$_3$ ^{u2}KUR.⸢RA⸣ (BAM 58: 10–12)

247 A$_{iv 39}$ [1/2 SILA$_3$ ^{u2}A]B$_2$.DUḪ 1/2 SILA$_3$ ZU$_2$.LUM.MA 1/2 SILA$_3$ DIDA SIG 1/2 SILA$_3$ ZI$_3$ MUNU$_6$ 1/2 SILA$_3$ ZI$_3$ G[U$_2$.GA]L 1/2 SILA$_3$ ZI$_3$.KUM

1/2 SILA$_3$ ^{u2}AB$_2$.D[UḪ] / [1/2 SIL]A$_3$ ŠE$_{10}$ ⸢TU⸣^{mušen} 1/2 SILA$_3$ ^{u2}*eriš*$_6$*-ti* A.ŠA$_3$ 10 GIN$_2$ ^{šim}MAŠ 10 GIN$_2$ KA A.⸢AB.BA⸣ (STO 1: 38–39)

⸢1/2 SILA$_3$⸣ NUMUN ⸢^{u2}⸣[AB$_2$.DUḪ x x x x] / [x x] x x x [. . .] (BAM 58: 12–13)

248 A$_{iv 40}$ [1/2 SI]LA$_3$ Z[I$_3$* G]IB$_3$ 1/3 SILA$_3$ ŠE$_{10}$ TU^{mušen} 1/3 SILA$_3$ ^{u2}*eriš*$_6$*-ti* GAN$_2$ 10 KISAL ^{šim}ŠEŠ 10 ⸢KISAL⸣ KA A.AB.BA

1/2 SILA$_3$ ZI$_3$ GIB$_3$ / [1/2 SIL]A$_3$ ⸢ZU$_2$.LUM⸣.MA 1/2 SILA$_3$ DIDA SIG.GA 1/2 SILA$_3$ ZI$_3$.KUM (STO 1: 39–40)

245 If someone suffers (*maruṣ*) from a knotted-up belly (*kiṣir libbi*),[434] his belly (*libbu*) does not let him accept (*lā ušamḫaršu*) bread and beer (and) keeps bringing them back up (*uttanarra*) into his mouth, (and) his stomach (*tākaltu*) pierces him: in order to heal him (*ana bulluṭīšu*), half a litre of *saḫlû* ('cress'),

246 half a litre of *kukru* (an aromatic), half a litre of *burāšu* (a kind of juniper), half a litre of *qutru* (a plant), half a litre of *kasû* ('tamarind'), half a litre of *pappasītu* (a mineral), half a litre of *nīnû* ('mint'),

247 half a litre of *kamantu* (a plant), half a litre of *suluppū* ('dates'), half a litre of *billat našpi* (a kind of beerwort), half a litre of flour from *buqlu* ('malt'), half a litre of flour from *ḫallūru* ('chickpea'), half a litre of *isqūqu* (a type of groats),

248 half a litre of flour from *kibtu* ('wheat'), a third of a litre of *zē summati* ('pigeon droppings'), a third of a litre of *erišti eqli* ('sown in a field' plant), ten KISAL-measures of *murru* ('myrrh'),[435] (and) ten KISAL-measures of *imbū tâmti* ('algae')—

433 For this line compare STO 1: 26, with the same symptom description, except that the disease in question is *kīs libbi* rather than *kiṣir libbi* and the final verb is in the D-stem rather than the G-stem (Cadelli 2021: 15).

434 For a recent discussion of *kiṣir libbi*, see Steinert and Vacín 2018: 722–723 with n. 47.

435 We maintain the conventional translation of *murru* as 'myrrh', although this has been challenged by Jursa (2003–2005: 336) in line with an argument put forward by Farber (1993).

249 A$_{iv\ 41}$ [16] U$_2$.⸢ḪI.A⸣ ŠEŠ DIŠ-*niš* GAZ SIM *ina* KAŠ *ina* ^{urudu}ŠEN.TUR GIM *ra-bi-ki tara-bak*

16 U$_2$.MEŠ *an-nu-⸢ti⸣* TEŠ$_2$.BI GAZ SIM / [*ina* KAŠ] ⸢SAG⸣ *ina* ^{urudu}ŠEN.TUR GIM *ra-bi-ki tara-bak* (STO 1: 40–41)

250 A$_{iv\ 42}$ [*ina*] ⸢KUŠ⸣.EDIN SUR 3 UD-*me* SAG ŠA$_3$-*šu*$_2$ LAL NINDA *u* KAŠ ŠA$_3$-*šu*$_2$ IGI-*šu*$_2$-*ma ina-eš*

3 UD-*me* SAG ŠA$_3$-*šu*$_2$ LAL$_2$-*id* NINDA.⸢MEŠ *u* KAŠ ŠA$_3$⸣-*šu*$_2$ IGI-⸢*ḫar*⸣-*šu*$_2$-*ma* TI (STO 1: 41)

---

251 A$_{iv\ 43}$ [DIŠ N]A *ki-ṣir* ŠA$_3$-*bi* GIG ⸢NINDA *u* KAŠ⸣ ŠA$_3$-*šu*$_2$ NU IGI-*šu*$_2$ *ina* KA-*šu*$_2$ GUR.GUR *ip-te-ne*$_2$-*ru ana* TI-*šu*$_2$ 1/2 SILA$_3$ A ZU$_2$.LUM.MA

ki-ṣir ŠA$_3$ GIG (AMC 34)

252 A$_{iv\ 44}$ [1/2 SIL]A$_3$ A ⸢GAZI⸣^{sar} 10 KISAL ^{u2}KUR.RA SUD$_2$ ⸢*ana** ŠA$_3$* ŠUB⸣* *ba-lu pa-tan* NAG-*šu*$_2$ EGIR-*šu*$_2$ 1/3 SILA$_3$ AL.US$_2$.SA ⸢NAG⸣ *ina* DUR$_2$-*šu*$_2$ GIŠ-*ma*[436] NINDA *u* KAŠ ŠA$_3$-*šu*$_2$ KI MIN

EGIR-*šu*$_2$ 1/2 SILA$_3$ *ši-qa* NAG-⸢*šu*$_2$⸣ *ina* KA-*šu*$_2$ *u* DUR$_2$-*šu*$_2$ SI.SA$_2$ *tu-ser-šu*$_2$-*ma* TI-*uṭ* (STO 1: 30)

---

249 you crush (*taḫaššal*) and sift (*tanappi*) these sixteen[437] ingredients together, you stir them as a paste in beer in a small copper pot,

250 you smear (*teṭerri*) (the mixture) on a piece of leather, you bandage (*taṣammid*) his epigastrium (*rēš libbi*) for three days, (and) his belly will let him accept (*ušamḫaršu*) bread and beer; then he will get well.

---

251 If someone suffers (*maruṣ*) from a knotted-up belly (*kiṣir libbi*), his belly (*libbu*) does not let him accept bread and beer, it keeps bringing them back up (*uttanarra*) into his mouth, (and) he constantly vomits: in order to heal him (*ana bulluṭīšu*), you pound (*tasâk*) half a litre of juice from *suluppū* ('dates'),

252 half a litre of juice from *kasû* ('tamarind'), (and) ten KISAL-measures of *nīnû* ('mint'), you put (*tanaddi*) them all together, (and) you have him drink (*tašaqqīšu*) it on an empty stomach. Afterwards, he drinks (*išatti*) a third of a litre of *šiqqu* ('garum'), he will void (*ušeššer-ma*) from his anus, then his belly DITTO (= will let him accept) bread and beer; (then he will get well).

---

436 For the reading of GIŠ-*ma* as a Š-stem of *ešēru*, 'to void', see CAD E 253. This rendering seems to be confirmed by the parallel with SI.SA$_2$ in STO 1: 30.

437 If we do not count the ingredients listed with 10 KISAL-measures, we arrive at 16 ingredients, which is the number indicated in the parallel in STO 1: 40, even though in STO 1: 40 that number is clearly mistaken.

253 A$_{\text{iv 45}}$ [DIŠ KI MIN M]UN KUR-*i* MUN *a-ma-ni*$_7$ DIŠ[438]*-niš* SUD$_2$ *ina* KAŠ NU *pa-*⸢*tan*⸣ NAG-*ma ina-eš*

---

254 A$_{\text{iv 46}}$ [DIŠ KI MI]N ⸢ZI$_3$ ŠE.SA⸣.A ZI$_3$ ḪARUB$^!$(AMAŠ)[439] *qi*$_2$*-lip*$_2$ ZU$_2$.LUM.MA SUD$_2$ *ina* KAŠ 2 UD-*me*

[DIŠ KI MIN Z]I$_3$ ŠE.SA.A ZI$_3$ *ḫa-ru-be* ⸢*di*⸣*-ik-ta* ZU$_2$.LUM.MA TEŠ$_2$.BI SUD$_2$ *ina* KAŠ NU *pa-tan* ⸢2 UD⸣-[*me*] (STO 1: 33)

DIŠ NA ŠA$_3$.⸢MEŠ⸣-*š*[*u*$_2$ *nap*]*-ḫu* ZI$_3$ ŠE.SA.A ZI$_3$ MUNU$_6$ NUMUN ^{u2}KI.^{d}IŠKUR *di-ik-ta ša*$_2$ ZU$_2$.⸢LUM⸣ / TEŠ$_2$.BI SU[D$_2$ NU *pa-t*]*an* GU$_7$.MEŠ (STO 2: 118–119)

255 A$_{\text{iv 47}}$ [*ba*]*-lu* ⸢*pa-tan*⸣ NAG-*šu*$_2$ A NU NAG A SAG ŠA$_3$*-šu*$_2$ *tu-sa-laḫ*$_2$*-ma ina-eš*

[NAG.MEŠ 2] ⸢UD-*me*⸣ *ina* A.MEŠ NU *pa-tan* NAG.MEŠ A.MEŠ SAG ŠA$_3$*-šu*$_2$ ⸢*tu*⸣*-s*[*a-laḫ*$_2$*-ma* TI] (STO 1: 34)

A.MEŠ NU NAG A.MEŠ SAG ŠA$_3$*-šu*$_2$ *tu-sa-laḫ*$_2$*-ma* ⸢TI⸣ (STO 2: 119)

---

†

253 If DITTO, you pound (*tasâk*) salt from the mountains (and) *amānu* salt together, (and) he drinks (*išattī-ma*) them in beer on an empty stomach; then he will get well.

---

254 If DITTO, you pound (*tasâk*) flour from *labtu* ('roasted barley'), flour from *ḫarūbu* ('carob'), (and) skin from *suluppū* ('dates'),

255 you have him drink (*tašaqqīšu*) them in beer on an empty stomach for two days. He should not drink (*lā išatti*) water, (but) you sprinkle his epigastrium (*rēš libbi*) with water; then he will get well.

---

438 The DIŠ sign is written over a partially erased horizontal wedge.

439 Cadelli (2000: 146 with n. 63) emends the passage as [ZI$_3$ ŠE.SA].A <I$_3$>.UDU UDU AMAŠ. It seems more probable, however, based on the parallel with the syllabically written *ḫarūbu* 'carob' (CAD Ḫ 120), that the scribe confused the sign ḪARUB (DAG.KISIM$_5$×U$_2$.GIR$_2$) with AMAŠ (DAG. KISIM$_5$×LU.MAŠ$_2$), which then led him to include UDU as the standard determinative that usually accompanies AMAŠ when used to render the Akkadian word *puḫālu* 'stud, breed animal, ram'. The logogram ḪARUB is extremely rare and *ḫarūbu* 'carob' is normally written syllabically in the medical texts, so this probably led to the confusion of ḪARUB and AMAŠ.

256 A$_{iv\ 48}$ [DIŠ NA NINDA *u* K]AŠ* ŠA$_3$-*šu*$_2$ NU IGI-*šu*$_2$ UZU.MEŠ-*šu*$_2$ *ir-ta-nam-mu* IM *ina* DUR$_2$-*šu*$_2$ NIGIN-*ur*$_2$ *ana* TI-*šu*$_2$ 1/2 SILA$_3$ A ZU$_2$.LUM.MA 1/2 SILA$_3$ A GAZI^{sar}

DIŠ NA *ki-i*[*s* ŠA$_3$ GIG NINDA *u* KA]Š ⸢ŠA$_3$⸣-*šu*$_2$ NU IGI-*ḫar-šu*$_2$ *ina* KA-*šu*$_2$ GUR.GUR-*ra* TUN$_3$-*šu*$_2$ *u*$_2$-*sa-ḫal-šu*$_2$ / *ip-ta-na-*⸢*ru*⸣ [UZU.MEŠ-*šu*$_2$ *ir*]-⸢*ta*⸣-*nam-mu-u*$_2$ IM *ina* DUR$_2$-*šu*$_2$ NIGIN ŠA$_3$.MEŠ-*šu*$_2$ *eb-ṭu*$_2$ *ana* TI-*šu*$_2$ / 1/2 SILA$_3$ A ZU$_2$.LUM.MA 1/2 SILA$_3$ A GAZI^{sar} (STO 1: 26–28)

DIŠ NA SAG ŠA$_3$-*šu*$_2$ KUM$_2$ TUKU.MEŠ-*ši* ŠA$_3$-*šu*$_2$ GIG / NINDA *u* A.MEŠ ŠA$_3$-*šu*$_2$ NU IGI-*šu*$_2$ DU$_8$.MEŠ-*šu*$_2$ *ir-te-*⸢*nem*⸣-*mu-u* / ŠA$_3$-*šu*$_2$ *ina pi-qi ana* BURU$_8$-*e* DU$_3$.DU$_3$-*uš* NU *i-par*$_5$-*ru* / IM *ina* ŠA$_3$-*šu*$_2$ *i-sa-na-ḫur i-le-eb-bu* / ŠA$_3$.MEŠ-*šu*$_2$ *eb-*⸢*ṭu*$_2$⸣ NA BI ^{d}ŠU.NAM.ERIM$_2$ DAB-*su* / *ana* TI-*šu*$_2$ 1/2 SILA$_3$ A ZU$_2$.LUM.MA 1/2 SILA$_3$ A GAZI^{sar} (BAM 49 obv. 9′–14′)

DIŠ NA SAG ŠA$_3$-*šu*$_2$ KUM$_2$ [TUK]U.MEŠ-*ši* ŠA$_3$-⸢*šu*$_2$⸣ G[IG] / NINDA *u* A.MEŠ ŠA$_3$-*šu*$_2$ NU I[GI]-*šu*$_2$ DU$_8$.MEŠ-*šu*$_2$ *ir-te-*[*nem-mu-u*] / [ŠA$_3$]-*šu*$_2$ *in*[*a pi-qi*] *ana* BURU$_8$-*e* DU$_3$.DU$_3$-*uš* ⸢NU *i*⸣-*par*$_5$-[*ru*] / I[M *ina* ŠA$_3$-*šu*$_2$] ⸢*i*⸣-*sa-*⸢*na*⸣-*ḫur i-le-eb-*[*bu*] / [ŠA$_3$].MEŠ-*šu*$_2$ ⸢*eb-ṭu*$_2$⸣ NA BI NAM.ERIM$_2$ DAB-*s*[*u*] (BAM 50 obv. 11–15)

[x x x] *i-*[*par*$_5$-*ru* x x x] / [x x] *i-lib-bu* [x x x x] / [NA B]I ^{d}NAM.ERI[M$_2$ DAB-*su ana* T]I-*šu*$_2$ / [1/2 SIL]A$_3$ A ZU$_2$.LUM.MA 1/2 SILA$_3$ A GAZI^{sar} (BAM 51: 1′–4′)

257 A$_{iv\ 49}$ [2 GIN$_2$ A.GEŠTIN.N]A 2 GIN$_2$ ^{u2}KUR.RA 3 GIN$_2$ I$_3$ *ḫal-ṣa* 3 GIN$_2$ LAL$_3$ KUR-*i* DIŠ-*niš tuš-te-mid* ⸢GAZ⸣* *ina* GE$_6$ *ina* IGI ^{mul}UZ$_3$ *tuš-bat*

10 KISAL A.GEŠTIN.NA 3 GIN$_2$ I$_3$ *ḫal-ṣa* 2 GIN$_2$ LAL$_3$ 10 GIN$_2$ ^{u2}KUR.RA / SUD$_2$ *ana* ŠA$_3$ ŠUB-*di ina* GE$_6$ *ana* IGI ^{mul}UZ$_3$ *tuš-bat* (STO 1: 28–29)

1/2 SILA$_3$ *ši-qa* 1/2 SILA$_3$ A.GEŠTIN.NA 5 GIN$_2$ I$_3$ *ḫal-ṣa* / 10 GIN$_2$ LAL$_3$ 10 GIN$_2$ ^{u2}KUR.RA SUD$_2$ DIŠ-*niš tuš-te-mid* / *ina* GE$_6$ *ana* IGI ^{mul}UZ$_3$ *tuš-bat zi*$_2$-*sur-ra-a* NIGIN-*mi* / NIG$_2$.NA ^{šim}LI DUB-*aq* MU ^{d}*gu-la u* DINGIR.MAḪ / *ta-zak-kar mi-iḫ-ḫa* BAL-*qi*$_2$ (BAM 49 obv. 15′–19′)

[1/2 SI]LA$_3$ *ši-qa* 1/2 SILA$_3$ A.GEŠTIN.NA 5 GIN$_2$ / [I$_3$ *ḫ*]*al-ṣa* 10 GIN$_2$ LAL$_3$ 10 GIN$_2$ ^{u2}KUR.R[A] / [SU]D$_2$ DIŠ-*niš tuš-te-mid ina* G[E$_6$ *ana* IGI ^{m}]^{ul}[UZ$_3$] / [*tuš-b*]*at zi*$_3$-⸢*sur*⸣-*r*[*a-a* x x x x x x] (BAM 51: 5′–8′)

†

256 If someone's belly (*libbu*) does not let him accept bread and beer (*lā ušamḫaršu*), his flesh continually sags, (and) flatulence (lit. wind) circulates (*isaḫḫur*) in his anus: in order to heal him (*ana bulluṭīšu*), you mix (and) crush (*taḫaššal*) half a litre of juice from *suluppū* ('dates'), half a litre of juice from *kasû* ('tamarind'),

257 two$^?$ shekels$^?$ of vinegar, two shekels of *nīnû* ('mint'), three shekels of pressed oil, (and) three shekels of *dišpu* ('syrup') from the mountains together, you leave (the mixture) out in the evening overnight under the Goat Star,

258 A$_{iv 50}$ [*ina še-r*]*i*$_3$ ⌜ŠEG$_6$⌝-*šal ta-ša*$_2$-*ḫal* SED *ina* ŠA$_3$ *taḫ-ta-na-su*[440] EGIR-*šu*$_2$ NAG A *u* KAŠ DIRI ^{giš}*si-ḫa* ^{giš}*ar-ga-nu* *ina* A$_2$.GU$_2$.ZI.GA NU *pa-tan* NAG-*šu*$_2$ (STO 1: 29)
ina še-ri$_3$ ŠEG$_6$-*šal* / *ta-ša*$_2$-*ḫal* SED *ana* DUR$_2$-*šu*$_2$ DUB-*ak ina* DUR$_2$-*šu*$_2$ SI.SA$_2$-*ma* TI-*uṭ* (BAM 49 obv. 19′–20′)

259 A$_{iv 51}$ ⌜^{giš}⌝LUM.ḪA GAZI^{sar} PA GAZI^{sar} NUMUN ^{giš}ŠE.NU$_2$.A *ana* ŠA$_3$ ŠUB ŠEG$_6$-*šal ta-ša*$_2$-*ḫal mar-ḫa-ṣi tu-ša*$_2$-*at-tam-ma*
260 A$_{iv 52}$ *ina* ŠA$_3$ RA-*su* I$_3$ SU-*šu*$_2$ EŠ-*aš* ^{giš}GEŠTIN KA$_5$.A ^{u2}EME UR.GI$_7$ SUD$_2$ *ina* KAŠ NAG-*šu*$_2$
261 A$_{iv 53}$ PA ^{giš}GE$_6$.PAR$_3$ PA ^{giš}*šu-še* ḪAD$_2$.A DIŠ-*niš* GAZ SIM *ina* I$_3$.UDU ḪI.ḪI *ina* KUŠ.EDIN SUR LAL$_2$-*su-ma ina-eš*

---

†

258 in the morning, you bring it to a boil (*tušabšal*), you filter it, you let it cool (*tukaṣṣa*), you keep it . . . (and) afterwards, he drinks (*išatti*) it. You fill (*tumalli*) (a small copper pot)[441] with water and beer, you put (*tanaddi*) *sīḫu* ('wormwood'), *argannu* (a conifer),

259 *barīrātu* ('sagapenum'), *kasû* ('tamarind'), leaves from *kasû* ('tamarind'), (and) seed from *šunû* ('chaste tree') in it, you bring it to a boil (*tušabšal*), you filter it, you bring it together (*tušattam-ma*)[442] into a lotion,

260 and then you bathe him (*taraḫḫassu*) in it, (and) you anoint (*tapaššaš*) his body with oil. You pound (*tasâk*) *karān šēlebi* ('fox-vine') (and) *lišān kalbi* ('dog's tongue' plant), (and) you have him drink (*tašaqqīšu*) them in beer.

261 You dry (*tubbal*) leaves from *lipāru* (a fruit tree) (and) leaves from *šūšu* ('liquorice'), you crush (*taḫaššal*) (and) sift (*tanappi*) them together, you mix (*tuballal*) them in fat, you smear (*teṭerri*) (the mixture) on a piece of leather, (and) you bandage him (*taṣammissū-ma*); then he will get well.

---

440 Cadelli (2000:168 n. 58) notes the two formal possibilities: either reading *taḫ-ta-na-su* as a Gtn of *ḫiātu* 'to supervise, to watch over' (base form **iḫtana''aṭ*, with the addition of an object pronoun *-šu*, hence, in the second person, *taḫtanâssu*), or reading *tuh*$_2$*-ta-na-su* as a Dtn of *ḫesû* 'to cover,' hence *tuḫtanassa*, but in this latter case, the final vowel seems to be incorrect. Unfortunately, neither verb makes much sense here.

441 This passage seems to be roughly analogous to STO 1: 35–37 and parallels, where the text specifies that a small copper pot needs to be filled with water and beer first. This is followed by a similar set of instructions.

442 The unusual form *tu-ša*$_2$*-at-tam-ma* should be compared with *tu-uš-te-te-ma*, which occurs four separate times in the Old Babylonian medical compendium BAM 393 and is analysed differently in the major dictionaries: AHw 1494 treats *tu-uš-te-te-ma* as a Št form of *(w)atû* 'to meet one another, to combine ingredients', while CAD E 383 books it as a Št of *etēmu* 'to mix'. Proto Izi I 82–86 (MSL 13 p. 19) lists five Akkadian glosses for ḪI.ḪI: *ba-la-lum*, *e-te-mu*, *šu-te-tu-mu*, *šu-ta-ab-lu-lu* (this term often confused or conflated with *šutābulu*, Št-stem of *wabālu*) and *du-šu-u*$_2$, suggesting that both the G-stem (transitive) and Št-stem (middle) of the verbs *balālu* and *etēmu* are relatively standard (and that the CAD interpretation is likely correct). Our form, however, is a Š-stem of *etēmu*, with the expected doubling of the middle radical in the durative, apparently based on a by-form *atāmu*.

262 A$_{iv\ 54}$ DIŠ NA SAG ŠA$_3$-*šu*$_2$ GU$_7$-*šu*$_2$ *ina ge-ši-šu*$_2$ ZE$_2$ *im-ta-na-'a* NA BI *qer-be*$_2$*-na* GIG
DIŠ NA SAG ŠA$_3$-*šu*$_2$ GU$_7$-*šu*$_2$ *ina ge-ši-šu* ZE$_2$ *im-ta-na-'a* NA BI *qer-be*$_2$-⸢*na*⸣ GIG (STO 3: 1)

263 A$_{iv\ 55}$ DUB.2.KAM$_2$ DIŠ NA *su-a-lam* GIG *ana ki-is* ŠA$_3$ GUR

264 A$_{iv\ 56}$ E$_2$.GAL ^{m}AN.ŠAR$_2$-DU$_3$-A MAN ŠU$_2$ MAN KUR AN.ŠAR$_2$^{ki} *ša* ^{d}AG *u* ^{d}*taš-m*[*e-t*]*u*$_4$ GEŠTU.MIN *ra-pa-aš*$_2$*-tu*$_4$ *iš-ru-ku-uš*

265 A$_{iv\ 57}$ *e-ḫu-uz-zu* IGI.MIN *na-mir-tu*$_4$ *ni-siq ṭup-šar-ru-ti*

266 A$_{iv\ 58}$ *ša ina* LUGAL.MEŠ-*ni a-lik maḫ-ri-ia mam*$_2$*-ma šip-*⸢*ru*⸣* *šu-a-tu la e-ḫu-uz-zu*

267 A$_{iv\ 59}$ *bul-ṭi* TA *muḫ-ḫi* EN UMBIN *liq-ti* BAR.MEŠ *ta-ḫi-zu nak-la*

268 A$_{iv\ 60}$ *a-zu-gal-lu-ut* ^{d}*nin-urta u* ^{d}*gu-la ma-la ba-aš*$_2$*-mu*

269 A$_{iv\ 61}$ *ina ṭup-pa-a-ni aš*$_2$*-ṭur as-niq* IGI.KAR$_2$*-ma*

270 A$_{iv\ 62}$ *a-na ta-mar-ti ši-ta-as-*⸢*si*⸣-[*ia qe*$_2$*-reb*] ⸢E$_2$⸣.GAL-*ia u*$_2$*-kin*

†

262 (Catchline:) If someone's epigastrium (*rēš libbi*) causes him pain (*ikkalšu*), (and) he vomits up (*imtana''a*) bile (*martu*) whenever he belches, that man suffers (*maruṣ*) internally.

263 (Tablet designation:) Second tablet of 'If someone suffers (*maruṣ*) from phlegm (*suālu*), which has turned into (*itūršu*) gastric constriction (*kīs libbi*)'.

264 (Colophon:) Palace of Assurbanipal, ruler of everything, king of the land of Assur, on whom Nabû and Tašmētu have bestowed wisdom (lit. wide ears),

265 He acquired for himself shining eyes, the pinnacle of scholarship,

266 Of the kings who came before me, none were able to comprehend this task.

267 Prescriptions (organized) from head to foot, gleanings from extraneous materials, technical lore

268 (And) whatever pertains to the great medical expertise of Ninurta and Gula,

269 I have written on tablets, checked and double-checked, and

270 I deposited them in the middle of my palace for my reading and recitation.

Chapter 5
Edition of STO 3

Manuscript A = BAM 578 + AMT 5/4 + AMT 9/5 + AMT 17/7 + AMT 58/8

K 61 + K 161 + K 390 + K 2476 + K 3273 + K 5032 + K 5683 + K 5762 + K 13344 + K 13384 + K 16429 + K 16444 + K 16454 + K 16459 + K 17699 + K 22008

STO 3	Parallels		
	Publication number	Museum number	Parallel passage
1	AMC 30		
1	STO 2: 262		
1–13	STO 2: 200–210		
14	STO 3: 140		
14–15	BAM 60	VAT 10612	1′–2′
14–18	BAM 64	A 207	column 1[!], 9′–13′
18–19	BAM 60	VAT 10612	3′–6′
19	STO 3: 128–129	VAT 10612	5′–6′
19	BAM 246	VAT 13896	11–13
26	BAM 1	VAT 8256	column 1, 30
33	BAM 558	K 2590 + K 2795	column 1, 21′
34	STO 3: 76		
36	STO 3: 76		
37	BAM 92	VAT 10085 + VAT 10850 + VAT 11056 + VAT 11080 + VAT 11606 + VAT 12199 + VAT 12265 (+) VAT 10793	column 2′, 33′
38–41	BAM 159	A 198	column 1, 29–37
38–41	BAM 60	VAT 10612	7′–12′
50–52	BAM 159	A 198	column 1, 38–42
59	STO 5: 113′		
65–66	STO 5: 34–37		
65–66	BAM 174	VAT 13761	reverse, 1–3
70–71	BAM 52	VAT 13733 + VAT 13738	reverse, 43–46
70–71	BAM 62	VAT 11148	obverse, 1–4
76	STO 3: 34		
76	STO 3: 36		
76	AMT 69/1	K 9156	16′
83	Labat and Tournay 1945–1946: 116	–	obverse, 1–3
86	STO 5: 114′–115′		
99–101	RA 53 p. 123 (K 9141)	K 2841 + K 9141 + K 16783	obverse, 1–10
99–108	Alster and van Dijk 1972: 357 Fig. 1	BM 47859	
99–108	Alster and van Dijk 1972: 358 Fig. 2	N 1266	
99–108	Alster and van Dijk 1972: 358 Fig. 3	IM 44468	
99–107	CUSAS 32 7	MS 3097	column 4, 20′–column 5, 8
99–108	Michalowski 1981: 14	CBS 10474	
106–108	STO 1: 128–130		
106–108	CT 4 8	BM 92518	reverse, 15–19

https://doi.org/10.1515/9781501506574-005

106–107	STVC 11	CBS 6927	obverse, 6′–8′
127	BAM 72	Ass 13956/ct	2′–3′
128–129	STO 3: 19		
128–129	BAM 60	VAT 10612	5′–6′
129	BAM 246	VAT 13896	11–13
131	STO 2: 146		
131	BAM 72	Ass 13956/ct	3′–4′
132	STO 2: 145		
134	STO 2: 145		
134	BAM 72	Ass 13956/ct	8′–9′
136	STO 2: 145		
140	STO 3: 14		
140	BAM 60	VAT 10612	1′
144–145	STO 3: 250–251		
146	STO 3: 252–253		
147	Sagig 33: 92–93		
147	Sagig 18: 24		
147	STO 3: 233		
153–156	STO 3: 246–249		
156–164	BAM 64	A 207	column 2!, 2′–13′
157–160	STO 3: 238–241		
159	STO 3: 254		
159	STO 4: 2		
159	BAM 66	VAT 9475 + VAT 10753 (+) VAT 9499	reverse, 4′–5′
161	Schmidtchen 2018	BM 38583	obverse, 12′ and 14′–15′
162	Schmidtchen 2018	BM 38583	reverse, 1 and 3
163	Schmidtchen 2018	BM 38583	reverse, 2 and 4
165	Schmidtchen 2018	BM 38583	reverse, 5–6
212	IGI 2: 115		
233	Sagig 33: 92		
233	Sagig 9: 13 and Sagig 33: 93		
233	STO 3: 147		
238–239	STO 3: 157–158		
238–239	BAM 64	A 207	column 3, 4′–5′
239	AMT 30/2	Sm 1524	7′
240	STO 4: 2		
240–241	STO 3: 159–160		
240–241	BAM 64	A 207	column 3, 6′–7′
246	STO 3: 153		
247–248	STO 3: 153–155		
249	STO 3: 156		
249	BAM 64	A 207	column 3, 2′–3′
250–251	STO 3: 144–145		
252–253	STO 3: 146		
254	STO 4: 1		

1 A$_{i\,1}$ DIŠ NA SAG ŠA$_3$-*šu*$_2$ GU$_7$-*šu*$_2$ *ina ge-ši-šu* ZE$_2$ *im-ta-na-'a* NA BI *qer-be*$_2$-⸢*na*⸣ GIG

[DIŠ NA SAG ŠA$_3$-*šu*$_2$ GU$_7$-*šu*$_2$] (AMC 30)

DIŠ NA SAG ŠA$_3$-*šu*$_2$ GU$_7$-*šu*$_2$ *ina ge-ši-šu*$_2$ ZE$_2$ *im-ta-na-'a* NA BI *qer-be*$_2$*-na* GIG (STO 2: 262)

2 A$_{i\,2}$ SUM^{sar} GA.RAŠ^{sar} UZU GUD UZU ŠAḪ KAŠ ^{lu2}KURUN$_2$.NA NU *uš-ta-maḫ-*⸢*ḫar*⸣ *ana* TI-*šu*$_2$

KU$_6$ SUM^{sar} UZU G[UD UZU ŠAḪ] / *u* KAŠ ^{lu2}KURUN$_2$.NA *la uš-ta-maḫ-ḫar ut-ta-šar* (STO 2: 201–202)

3 A$_{i\,3}$ 1/2 SILA$_3$ ZA$_3$.ḪI.LI 1/2 SILA$_3$ ^{šim}LI 1/2 SILA$_3$ ^{šim}GUR$_2$.GUR$_2$ 1/2 SILA$_3$ NUMUN GADA 1/2 SILA$_3$ *pa-pa-si* ⸢MUNU$_6$⸣ 1/2 SILA$_3$ ^{šim}IM.DI

[1/2 SILA$_3$ Z]A$_3$.⸢ḪI⸣.LI 1/2 SILA$_3$ ^{šim}GUR$_2$.GUR$_2$ 1/2 SILA$_3$ ^{giš}L[I x x x x] / 1/2 SILA$_3$ ^{giš}GIG 1/2 SILA$_3$ ^{giš}EN.DI (STO 2: 202–203)

4 A$_{i\,4}$ 1/2 SILA$_3$ NUMUN ^{u2}*qut-ra-ti* 1/2 SILA$_3$ GAZI^{sar} 1/2 SILA$_3$ ^{giš}ŠE.NU 1/2 SILA$_3$ GU$_2$.NIG$_2$.AR$_3$.RA 1/2 SILA$_3$ *pa-*⸢*pa*⸣*-si-*^{d}ID$_2$

1/2 SILA$_3$ NUMUN ^{u2}[*qut-ra-ti* 1/2] SILA$_3$ GAZI^{sar} 1/2 SILA$_3$ NUMUN ^{giš}ŠE.N[U x x x x x x] / 1/2 SILA$_3$ BA.BA.ZA.^{d}ID$_2$ (STO 2: 203–204)

5 A$_{i\,5}$ 1/2 SILA$_3$ U$_2$ *a-ši-i* 1/2 SILA$_3$ ^{u2}KUR.RA 1/2 SILA$_3$ ŠE$_{10}$ TU^{mušen} 1/3 SILA$_3$ NUMUN ^{u2}AB$_2$.DUḪ ⸢1/3⸣* SILA$_3$ ⸢*e*⸣*-reš-ti* A.ŠA$_3$

1/2 SILA$_3$ NUMUN ^{u2}*ka-man-*[*ta* . . .] (STO 2: 204)

1 If someone's epigastrium (*rēš libbi*) causes him pain (*ikkalšu*), (and) he vomits up (*imtana''a*) bile (*martu*) whenever he belches, that man suffers (*maruṣ*) internally,[443]

2 (and consequently) he cannot stand *šūmū* ('garlic'), *karašu* ('leek'), beef, pork, (or) brewer's beer: in order to heal him,

3 you crush (*taḫaššal*) (and) sift (*tanappi*) half a litre of *saḫlû* ('cress'), half a litre of *burāšu* (a kind of juniper), half a litre of *kukru* (an aromatic), half a litre of seed from *kitû* ('flax'), half a litre of *pappāsi buqli* ('malt porridge'), half a litre of *suādu* (a kind of sedge),

4 half a litre of seed from *qutrātu* ('smoke' plant), half a litre of *kasû* ('tamarind'), half a litre of *šunû* ('chaste tree'), half a litre of *kiššanu* ('bitter vetch'), half a litre of *pappasītu* (a mineral),

5 half a litre of *šammi ašî* ('*ašû* disease' plant), half a litre of *nīnû* ('mint'), half a litre of *zē summati* ('pigeon droppings'), a third of a litre of seed from *kamantu* (a plant), a third of a litre of *erišti eqli* ('sown in a field' plant),

443 For an extensive discussion of lines 1–13, see Heeßel 2016: 45–59. This first section of the text appears to be a diagnostic patch-test, in which blisters are induced, and the colour of the blister predicts the outcome of the illness. For a discussion of this rare diagnostic procedure, see also Ritter 1965: 304, Reiner 1995: 40–41 and Stol 2007: 23.

6 A$_{i\,6}$ 10 KISAL ILLU ^{šim}BULUḪ 10 KISAL KA A.AB.BA 1 SILA$_3$ ZI$_3$ GIB$_3$ 1 SILA$_3$ ZU$_2$.LUM.MA 1 SILA$_3$ ⸢DIDA⸣ SIG
10 KISAL ILLU ^{šim}BULUḪ 10 KISAL KA ⸢A⸣.A[B.BA . . .] (STO 2: 205)

7 A$_{i\,7}$ ⸢1⸣* SILA$_3$ ZI$_3$.KUM TEŠ$_2$.BI GAZ SIM *ina* KAŠ GIM *ra-bi-ki ta-rab-bak ina* TUG$_2$.ḪI.A SUR-*ri šu-lu-uš-ti* 9 ⸢UD-*me*⸣ LAL
[. . .] / 21 ⸢U$_2$.ḪI⸣.[A . . .] (STO 2: 205–206)

8 A$_{i\,8}$ *ina* 4 UD-*me* DU$_8$-*ma ta-mar šum$_2$-ma* U$_3$.BU$_2$.BU$_2$.UL BABBAR ŠA$_3$-*šu$_2$ i-pa-*⸢*šaḫ*⸣
[. . .] / ⸢*šum*⸣-*m*[*a* . . .] (STO 2: 206–207)

9 A$_{i\,9}$ *šum$_2$-ma* U$_3$.BU$_2$.BU$_2$.UL SA$_5$ ŠA$_3$-*šu$_2$* KUM$_2$ *u$_2$-kal šum$_2$-ma* U$_3$.BU$_2$.BU$_2$.UL SIG$_7$ UD.DA KUR-*id*
[. . .] / [. . .] (STO 2: 207–208)

10 A$_{i\,10}$ GUR.GUR-*šu šum$_2$-ma* U$_3$.BU$_2$.BU$_2$.UL GE$_6$ *u$_2$-šam-ra-su-ma* NU TI
[. . .] / [. . .] (STO 2: 208–209)

11 A$_{i\,11}$ *ana* U$_3$.BU$_2$.BU$_2$.UL *bu-le-e* ^{u2}LAG A.ŠA$_3$ IM.GU$_2$ *ša$_2$* UD.DA SA$_2$-*kat$_3$*
[. . . U]D.DA SA$_2$.SA$_2$ (STO 2: 209)

12 A$_{i\,12}$ GAZ SIM *ina* A GAZI^{sar} *ta-la-aš$_2$* LAL-*id* EGIR-*šu$_2$ saḫ-le$_2$-e ina* KAŠ NAG
GAZ SIM / [. . .] (STO 2: 209–210)

13 A$_{i\,13}$ UD-*ma* NAG-*u$_2$ ina* A ^{giš}*šu-nu* ^{giš}ŠINIG ^{u2}*ak-tam* ^{u2}IN$_6$.UŠ$_2$ *ir-ta-na-ḫaṣ*
[. . . ^{gi}]^{š}⸢*bi*⸣-*nu* ^{u2}IN$_6$.UŠ$_2$ RA-*ma* TI (STO 2: 210)

---

6 ten KISAL-measures of resin from *baluḫḫu* ('galbanum'), ten KISAL-measures of *imbū tâmti* ('algae'), one litre of flour from *kibtu* ('wheat'), one litre of *suluppū* ('dates'), one litre *billat našpi* (a kind of beerwort),

7 (and) one litre of *isqūqu* (a type of groats) together, you stir them as a paste in beer, you smear (*teṭerri*) (the mixture) on a piece of fabric, you bandage (*taṣammid*) him for one-third of nine days,

8 on the fourth day you remove (*tapaṭṭar-ma*) (the bandage), and you examine him. If the boil is white (*peṣiat*), his belly will calm down.

9 If the boil is red (*sāmat*), his belly will retain heat. If the boil is green-yellow (*arqat*), he will be overwhelmed by fever (*ṣēta kašid*),

10 (and) it will keep coming back to him (*uttanarrāšu*). If the boil is black (*ṣalmat*), it will make him sick, and he will not recover (*lā iballuṭ*).

11 In order to soothe the boil, you crush (and) sift *kirbān eqli* ('field clod' plant) (and) mud that . . . fever (*ṣēta* SA$_2$-*kat$_3$*),

12 you knead them in juice from *kasû* ('tamarind'), (and) you bandage (*taṣammid*) him. Afterwards, he drinks (*išatti*) *saḫlû* ('cress') in beer,

13 (and) while he drinks (*enūma išattû*) it, he keeps bathing in juice from *šunû* ('chaste tree'), *bīnu* ('tamarisk'), *aktam* (a plant) (and) *maštakal* ('soapwort').

---

14 A$_{i\,14}$ DIŠ NA ZE$_2$ GIG SUM^{sar} SUD$_2$ *ina* A NU *pa-tan* NAG
DIŠ KI MIN SUM^{sar} SUD$_2$ *ina* A NAG-*ma i-ar$_2$-ru$_3$* (STO 3: 140)
[x x x GI]G SUM^{sar} SUD$_2$ *ina* [. . .] (BAM 60: 1′)
[. . .] *ina* A.MEŠ NU *pa-tan* NAG (BAM 64 i$^!$ 9′)[444]

15 A$_{i\,15}$ A.GEŠTIN.NA KALAG.GA AL.US$_2$.SA GAZI^{sar} *kab-ru-ti* NAG
[x x x KAL]AG.GA AL.US$_2$.SA GAZI^{sar} *kab-*[*ru-ti* NAG] (BAM 60: 2′)
[. . .] *kab-ru-ti* [x] x (BAM 64 i$^!$ 10′)

16 A$_{i\,16}$ KAŠ.BIR$_8$ NAG *tu-ša$_2$-ʾ-raš-šu$_2$*
[. . .] *tu-ša$_2$-ʾ-r*[*aš-šu$_2$*] (BAM 64 i$^!$ 11′)

17 A$_{i\,17}$ GAZI^{sar} SUD$_2$ *ina* A NAG : MUN SUD$_2$ *ina* A NU *pa-tan* NAG : MUN SUD$_2$ *ina* KAŠ NU *pa-tan* NAG
[. . .] *ina* A.MEŠ NU *pa-ta*[*n* NAG] (BAM 64 i$^!$ 12′)

14 If someone suffers (*maruṣ*) from bile (*martu*): you pound (*tasâk*) *šūmū* ('garlic'), (and) he drinks (*išatti*) it in water on an empty stomach.

15 He drinks (*išatti*) strong vinegar, *šiqqu* ('garum') (and) thick[445] *kasû* ('tamarind').

16 He drinks (*išatti*) *ḫīqu* ('diluted beer'), (and) you make him vomit.

17 You pound (*tasâk*) *kasû* ('tamarind'), (and) he drinks (*išatti*) it in water. You pound salt, (and) he drinks it in water on an empty stomach. You pound salt, (and) he drinks it in beer on an empty stomach.

444 That BAM 64 i$^!$ 9′–13′ runs parallel with lines 14–18 of our text was first recognised by Scurlock (2014: 727), who also corrected Köcher's (1963) description of this fragment as coming from the reverse side of a tablet. The first column on the obverse of BAM 64 partially corresponds to our lines 14–18, and the second column corresponds to lines 156–164.

445 GUR$_4$ = Akk. *kabru* 'thick' normally qualifies meat or occasionally timber (CAD K 23) and is not otherwise used as a qualification of *kasû* ('tamarind'). It is, however, used as a qualification of *saḫlû* ('cress') in BAM 497 ii 17′ and parallels, with the spelling *saḫ-le$_2$-e kab-ra-ti* (Bácskay and Simkó 2017: 10). Moreover, the Old Babylonian culinary text YOS 11 27 obv. 10 has ^{u2}*ṣi-ib-bu-ra-tu ka-ba-ar-ta*.

18 A$_{i\,18}$ ILLU *a-bu-kat*$_3$ GAZ *ana* KAŠ$^!$.BIR$_8$[446] ŠUB-*di ina* MUL$_4$ *tuš-bat ina še-ri*$_3$ LAL$_3$ I$_3$ *ḫal-ṣa ana* ŠA$_3$ ŠUB NAG-*ma i-ar*$_2$*-ru*

ILLU LI.TAR [. . .] / [*ina* M]UL$_4$ *tuš-bat ina še-ri*$_3$ LAL$_3$ I$_3$ *ḫal-ṣi ana* Š[A$_3$ . . .] (BAM 60: 3′–4′)

[. . . NU *p*]*a-tan* ⸢NAG⸣ (BAM 64 i$^!$ 13′)

---

19 A$_{i\,19}$ NUMUN GI.ZU$_2$.LUM.MA SUD$_2$ *ina* KAŠ NAG : ^{u2}*nam-ruq-qa* SUD$_2$ *ina* KAŠ NAG

14 N[UMUN G]I.ZU$_2$.LUM.MA SUD$_2$ *ina* 5 GIN$_2$ ⸢I$_3$.GIŠ⸣ *u* KAŠ NAG-⸢*šu*$_2$⸣ / 21 ⸢^{u2}⸣[*na*]*b*-⸢*ruq*⸣-*qa ina* 10 GIN$_2$ I$_3$.GIŠ *u* KAŠ NAG-*šu*$_2$ (STO 3: 128–129)

[NUMUN G]I.ZU$_2$.LUM.MA SUD$_2$ *i*[*na* . . .] / [^{u2}*na*]*m-ru-qu* SUD$_2$ *ina* KAŠ SAG [. . .] (BAM 60: 5′–6′)

[DIŠ KI MIN] ^{u2}*nab-ru-qu* SUD$_2$ / [*ina* KA]Š ⸢NU *pa-tan* NAG⸣-*ma* / [. . .] (BAM 246: 11–13)

---

20 A$_{i\,20}$ U$_2$ DILI U$_2$ ZE$_2$ *ina* KAŠ NAG

21 A$_{i\,21}$ U$_2$ *me-er-gi-ra-nu* U$_2$ ZE$_2$ *ina* KAŠ ⸢NAG⸣* GAZI^{sar} U$_2$ ZE$_2$ *ina* KAŠ NAG

22 A$_{i\,22}$ U$_2$ ^{šim}LI U$_2$ ZE$_2$ *ina* KAŠ NAG U$_2$ NU.LUḪ.ḪA U$_2$ ZE$_2$ *ina* KAŠ NAG

☨

18 You crush (*taḫaššal*) resin from *abukkatu* (a tree), you put (*tanaddi*) it in *ḫīqu* ('diluted beer'), you leave (the mixture) out overnight under the stars, in the morning you put *dišpu* ('syrup') (and) pressed oil in it, he drinks (*išattī-ma*) it, and then he will vomit.

---

19 You pound (*tasâk*) seed from *kūru* (a plant),[447] (and) he drinks (*išatti*) it in beer. You pound *namruqqu* (a plant), (and) he drinks it in beer.

---

20 Drug:[448] *ēdu* ('lone' plant), a drug for bile, for drinking (*šatû*)[449] in beer.

21 Drug: *mergirānu* (a plant), a drug for bile, for drinking in beer. (Drug:) *kasû* ('tamarind'), a drug for bile, for drinking in beer.

22 Drug: *burāšu* (a kind of juniper), a drug for bile, for drinking in beer. Drug: *nuḫurtu* ('asafoetida'), a drug for bile, for drinking in beer.

---

446 The scribe seems to have written *ana* ŠA$_3$ SUD ŠUB-*di* initially and, after completing the line, he realised that he had omitted two of the signs from KAŠ.BIR$_8$ (= KAŠ.A.SUD), namely KAŠ and A, so he wrote KAŠ on top of the ŠA$_3$ sign and then squeezed in a small A sign between KAŠ and SUD. CAD M/1 325 cites our passage under *maslaḫtu* (DUG.A.SUD) 'a vessel for sprinkling', without recognising that KAŠ is inscribed over the ŠA$_3$ sign.

447 For a discussion of the different orthographies of *kūru*, namely GIŠ.GI.ZU$_2$.LUM.MA (used in STO 2) and GI.ZU$_2$.LUM.MA (used in STO 3 and 4), see STO 2: 15.

448 The assumption here is that in a list of drugs such as this, the determinative U$_2$ was read out aloud in Akkadian (presumably a form of *šammu*) before each item. For this usage, see Attia and Buisson 2012, Rumor 2017 and Geller 2020.

449 The logographically written verbs are almost certainly infinitives rather than finite verbs, as suggested by the syllabic orthography *sa*$_3$*-ku* for *sâku* 'to pound' or 'for pounding' in KADP 1 v 6–12. For the use of infinitives in medical texts, see Aro 1961: 28–29.

23 A$_{\text{i 23}}$ U$_2$ BAR ^{giš}*šu-ši* U$_2$ ZE$_2$ *ina* KAŠ NAG PA $^{\text{u2}}$*al-la-nu* U$_2$ ZE$_2$ *ina* KAŠ NAG

24 A$_{\text{i 24}}$ U$_2$ U$_5$ ARGAB^{mušen} U$_2$ ZE$_2$ *ina* KAŠ NAG U$_2$ LAG MUN U$_2$ ZE$_2$ *ina* KAŠ NAG

25 A$_{\text{i 25}}$ U$_2$ SUM^{sar} U$_2$ ZE$_2$ *ina* KAŠ NAG U$_2$ SUḪUŠ ^{giš}NAM.TAR NITA$_2$ U$_2$ ZE$_2$ SUD$_2$ *ina* KAŠ NAG

26 A$_{\text{i 26}}$ U$_2$ SUḪUŠ ^{giš}*šu-ši* U$_2$ ZE$_2$ (eras.) *ina* I$_3$ *u* KAŠ NAG U$_2$ *ṣi-ba-ru* U$_2$ ZE$_2$ SUD$_2$ *ina* A NAG
⸢$^{\text{u2}}$⸣*ṣi-bu-ru* // U$_2$ ZE$_2$ // SUD$_2$ *ina* KAŠ SAG NAG (BAM 1 i 30)

---

27 A$_{\text{i 27}}$ DIŠ NA NU *pa-tan* ŠA$_3$-*šu*$_2$ *ana pa-re-e e-te-ne*$_2$*-la-a* UḪ$_2$ *ma-gal* ŠUB.MEŠ A.MEŠ *ina* KA-*šu*$_2$ *mal-da-riš* DU-*ku*

28 A$_{\text{i 28}}$ *pa-nu-šu*$_2$ *iṣ-ṣa-nu-du* ŠA$_3$.MEŠ-*šu*$_2$ MU$_2$.MU$_2$-*ḫu* MURUB$_4$.MIN-*šu*$_2$ *kim-ṣa-šu*$_2$ TAG.GA.MEŠ-*šu*$_2$ KUM$_2$ SED ⸢IR⸣* TUKU.MEŠ-*ši*

†

23 Drug: bark from *šūšu* ('liquorice'), a drug for bile, for drinking in beer. (Drug:) leaves from *allānu* ('oak'), a drug for bile, for drinking in beer.

24 Drug: *rikibti arkabi* ('bat guano'), a drug for bile, for drinking in beer. Drug: lumps of salt, a drug for bile, for drinking in beer.

25 Drug: *šūmū* ('garlic'), a drug for bile, for drinking in beer. Drug: root from male *pillû* ('mandrake'), a drug for bile, for pounding (*sâku*) (and) drinking in beer.

26 Drug: root from *šūšu* ('liquorice'), a drug for bile, for drinking in oil and beer. Drug: *ṣibaru* ('aloe'), a drug for bile, for pounding (and) drinking in water.[450]

---

27 If someone has an empty stomach, (but) his belly continually heaves to vomit, he continually spits up (*ittanaddi*) a lot of phlegm (*rupuštu*), fluid regularly flows (*illakū*) from his mouth,[451]

28 he feels dizzy (lit. his face is spinning), his internal organs (*qerbū*) are swollen (*napḫū*), his hips (and) his shins keep bothering him (*iltanappatāšū-ma*), he gets hot (*immim*) (and then) gets cold (*ikaṣṣi*),[452] he is constantly sweating (*zūta irtanašši*),

450 There is a section of drugs for bile (*martu*) in the Therapeutic Vademecum BAM 1 i 30–34, but surprisingly these two lists have only one drug in common, namely *ṣibaru* ('aloe'). For further discussion, see Geller 2020, who rejects the idea that the two lists derive from the same source.

451 The contrast here is between *rupuštu* 'phlegm' and either 'liquid' or 'fluid' (A.MEŠ = Akk. *mû*), which probably corresponds to either *ru'tu* or *illatu*. Since the patient's stomach is empty, the term 'phlegm' probably refers to both bile and digestive enzymes from the stomach.

452 See CAD K 269, with the syllabic orthography *i-mi-im i-ka-aṣ-ṣi* (AMT 88/4 rev. 4', now as BAM 471 ii 26'). For further discussion of the finite form *immim*, see STO 5: 6.

29 A$_{\text{i}\,29}$ NINDA *u* KAŠ LAL A SED *ma-gal* NAG *i-par-ru ina* DUR$_2$-*šu*$_2$ GIŠ$_3$-*šu*$_2$ SIG$_7$ *u*$_2$-*tab-ba-kam* MUŠ$_2$.MEŠ-*šu*$_2$ *i-te-nen-nu-u*

30 A$_{\text{i}\,30}$ UZU.MEŠ-*šu tab-ku mim*$_3$-*ma* GU$_7$-*ma* UGU-*šu*$_2$ *ul* DU$_{10}$.GA NA BI ZE$_2$ *saḫ-pa-su ana* TI-*šu*$_2$ ^{šim}⸢GUR$_2$⸣.[GUR$_2$]

31 A$_{\text{i}\,31}$ ⸢^{šim}⸣LI ^{šim}GAM.MA 3 U$_2$.ḪI.A ŠEŠ SIG$_7$-*su*-⸢*nu*⸣* TI-*qe*$_2$ ḪAD$_2$.A SUD$_2$ *ina* GEŠTIN KALAG.GA NU *pa*-⸢*tan*⸣ N[AG*-*šu*$_2$]

32 A$_{\text{i}\,32}$ ⸢SI.SA$_2$-*ma* SAG ŠA$_3$⸣-*šu*$_2$ ŠA$_3$-*šu*$_2$ ⸢LAL-*id*⸣ *baḫ-ra* ⸢GU$_7$⸣* *b*[*aḫ**-*ra* NA]G ⸢UD*.3⸣*.KAM ⸢*tuš*⸣-*t*[*e-še-er-ma* TI]

---

33 A$_{\text{i}\,33}$ DIŠ KI MIN $^{\text{u2}}$*a-ra-ri-a-nu* SUD$_2$ *ina* KAŠ ⸢NU* *pa**-*tan*⸣* N[AG-*šu*$_2$ x x x]

$^{\text{u2}}$*a-ri-a-ni* SUD$_2$ *ina* KAŠ NU *pa-tan* NAG.MEŠ x [. . .] (BAM 558 i 21′)

---

†

29 he has a diminished appetite (*muṭṭu*) for bread and beer, he drinks (*išatti*) a lot of cold water, (and) he vomits, he discharges yellow effluvia (*arqūtu*)[453] through his anus (and) his penis, his looks (*zīmū*) constantly change,

30 his flesh is flabby (lit. poured out), (and) whatever he eats (*ikkalū-ma*) does him no good (*elīšu ul ṭāb*),[454] that man is 'overwhelmed by bile (*martu*)':[455] in order to heal him, *kukru* (an aromatic),

31 *burāšu* (a kind of juniper), (and) *ṣumlalû* (an aromatic)—you take (*teleqqe*) these three drugs when they are fresh (*arqūssunu*), you dry (*tubbal*) (and) pound (*tasâk*) them, you have him drink (*tašaqqīšu*)$^?$ them in strong wine on an empty stomach,

32 he will void (*ušeššer-ma*), and then you bandage (*taṣammid*) his epigastrium (*rēš libbi*) (and) his belly (*libbu*). He eats steaming hot (food), he drinks steaming hot (drinks) (and) on the third day, you purge$^?$ him; then he will recover (*iballuṭ*)$^?$.

---

33 If DITTO, you pound (*tasâk*) *arariānu* (a plant), you have him drink (*tašaqqīšu*) it in beer on an empty stomach . . .

---

453 The reading of SIG$_7$ is unknown, but it may be an abstract form of *arāqu* 'to be green-yellow', namely *arqūtu*, used here to describe the colour of the material being discharged from the body. The idiom is normally used in therapeutic texts to describe fresh ingredients, for which see SIG$_7$-*su-nu* in line 31 below. Interestingly, this would also be the form of a masculine plural adjective qualifying *mû* 'water' or 'liquid' as in 'he discharges yellow fluid (*mê arqūti*) through his anus (and) his penis'.

454 The same expression also occurs in the possible BRON text BAM 556 ii 70′.

455 Stol (2006: 107 with n. 26) understands *martu saḫpat* to mean the *martu* 'is flat' (*saḫpat*), citing Cadelli 2000: 389 n. 46 (see also Cadelli 2021: 19), which implies that *martu* is an organ, presumably the gallbladder. For a similar use of the verb *saḫāpu*, 'to lay flat (on its face)', said of the *riqītu* organ, see STO 1: 217. However, in STO *martu* always seems to refer to 'bile' rather than the 'gallbladder', as in line 1 above, where it is vomited up whenever the patient belches. For this use of *martu*, compare the Neo-Assyrian letters SAA 10 217 and SAA 10 326, where *martu* co-occurs with the verbs *gâ'u* 'to vomit, spew' and *ešēru* in the Š-stem, meaning 'to void, purge'.

34 A$_{i\,34}$ DIŠ KI MIN ^{u2}*saḫ-la-a-nu* SUD$_2$ *ina* GEŠTIN KALAG.GA NU *pa-tan* N[AG-*šu*$_2$ KI MIN][456]
ḪENBUR$_2$ ^{u2}UKUŠ$_2$.ḪAB ⸢^{u2}⸣*saḫ-la-na* SUD$_2$ *ina* GE[ŠTIN . . .] (STO 3: 76)

---

35 A$_{i\,35}$ DIŠ KI MIN ^{u2}*ṣi-bu-ru* SUD$_2$ *ina* GA KU$_7$.KU$_7$ ⸢NAG⸣-[*šu*$_2$ KI MIN]

---

36 A$_{i\,36}$ DIŠ KI MIN ḪENBUR$_2$ ^{u2}UKUŠ$_2$.ḪAB SUD$_2$ *ina* GEŠTIN LAL$_3$ *u* I$_3$ *ḫal-*⸢*ṣi*⸣* NAG-*šu*$_2$ K[I MIN][457]
ḪENBUR$_2$ ^{u2}UKUŠ$_2$.ḪAB ⸢^{u2}⸣*saḫ-la-na* SUD$_2$ *ina* GE[ŠTIN . . .] (STO 3: 76)

---

37 A$_{i\,37}$ DIŠ KI MIN ^{u2}SIG.MEŠ[458] *ša*$_2$ KUR-*e ina* GEŠTIN LAL$_3$ *u* I$_3$ ⸢*ḫal**-*ṣi*⸣* NAG-*šu*$_2$ ⸢KI⸣ [MIN]
KI MIN ^{u2}SIG *ša*$_2$ KUR-⸢*e*⸣ SUD$_2$ ⸢*ina*⸣ [. . .] (BAM 92 ii′ 33′)

---

34 If DITTO, you pound (*tasâk*) *saḫlânu* ('cress-like' plant), you have him drink (*tašaqqīšu*) it in strong wine on an empty stomach, DITTO.

---

35 If DITTO, you pound (*tasâk*) *ṣibaru* ('aloe'), you have him drink (*tašaqqīšu*) it in sweet milk, DITTO.

---

36 If DITTO, you pound (*tasâk*) shoots from *irrû* ('cucumber'), you have him drink (*tašaqqīšu*) it in wine, *dišpu* ('syrup'), and pressed oil, DITTO.

---

37 If DITTO, you have him drink (*tašaqqīšu*) *qatunu* ('thin' plant) from the mountains in wine, *dišpu* ('syrup'), and pressed oil, DITTO.

---

456 KI MIN at the end of lines 34–37 probably refers back to the instructions at the end of line 33, which are now missing. It is unlikely that they go back to the complex set of instructions in lines 30–32.

457 The horizontal ruling, which separates lines 36 and 37 from each other, was not copied by Köcher (1980).

458 Similar orthographies occur in our parallel (BAM 92 ii′ 33′), as well as in BAM 161 vii 23 and BAM 7 2 i 37. The Akkadian equivalent of ^{u2}SIG.MEŠ is probably *qatunu*, which is used as a plant name in BAM 254 rev. 7, viz. ^{u2}*qa-tu-nu ša* KUR-*e*, probably based on the adjective *qatnu* 'thin'. For the translation 'thin ones of the mountain'-plant, see Geller 2005: 47.

38 A$_{i\,38}$ DIŠ NA NINDA GU$_7$ KAŠ NAG-*ma u$_2$-nap-paq u* IGI.MEŠ-*šu$_2$* NIGIN.MEŠ-*du* NA BI GIG ⸢ZE$_2$⸣* GIG *ana* TI-*šu$_2$* ⸢^{u2}⸣[UKUŠ$_2$.ḪAB BI]L$_2$*[459]

[DIŠ NA NINDA G]U$_7$ KAŠ NAG-*ma u$_2$-nap-paq* IGI.MEŠ-*šu$_2$* NIGIN.MEŠ-*du* / [x x x x GI]G *ana* TI-*šu$_2$* ^{u2}UKUŠ$_2$.ḪAB BIL$_2$ (BAM 159 i 29–30)

[DIŠ NA NINDA GU$_7$ KA]Š NAG-*ma u$_2$-na-paq u* IGI.MEŠ-*šu$_2$* N[IGIN.MEŠ-*du*] / [x x x x GI]G *ana* TI-*šu$_2$* ^{u2}UKUŠ$_2$.ḪAB BIL$_2$ (BAM 60: 7′–8′)

39 A$_{i\,39}$ *ša$_2$* ^{im}SI.SA$_2$ *ina* A LUḪ-*si* ^{šim}BULUḪ *tu-sal-lat* ^{u2}NU.LUḪ.ḪA *te-⸢be$_2$⸣*-er* 3 U$_2$.⸢ḪI.A⸣ Š[EŠ *ina* KA]Š* SAG

[x x x x Z]I-*aḫ ina* A.MEŠ LUḪ-*si* / [x x x x x] ⸢^{u2}⸣NU.LUḪ.ḪA *te-be$_2$-er* / [. . . KAŠ] ⸢SAG⸣ (BAM 159 i 31–33)

⸢*ša*⸣ [x x x] / [x x x LUḪ-*s*]*i* ^{šim}BULUḪ *tu-sal-lat* ⸢^{u2}⸣[NU.LUḪ.ḪA x x x] / [. . .] x x 1/2 SILA$_3$ KAŠ (BAM 60: 8′–10′)

40 A$_{i\,40}$ *ki* (eras.)* *pi-i*[460] *mal-ma-liš tara-muk ana* IGI ^{mul}UZ$_3$ GAR-*an* GIŠ.ḪUR ⸢NIGIN⸣-*mi* ⸢*ina* A$_2$⸣.[GU$_2$.ZI.GA *ša-š*]*u$_2$*-⸢*nu*⸣[461] *ta-ša$_2$-ḫal*

ki pi-i / [. . . M]UL GE$_6$ GAR-*an* / GIŠ.ḪUR NIGIN-*mi ina* A$_2$.GU$_2$.ZI.[GA *ša-š*]*u$_2$*-⸢*nu*⸣ *ta-ša$_2$-ḫal* (BAM 159 i 33–35)

ki pi-[*i* . . .] / [. . . GI]Š.ḪUR NIGIN-*m*[*i* . . .] (BAM 60: 10′–11′)

38 If someone eats (*ikkal*) bread, drinks beer (*išattī-ma*), and then he becomes blocked up,[462] and he feels dizzy (lit. his face is spinning), that man suffers (*maruṣ*) from 'sickness of bile' (*muruṣ marti*): in order to heal him, you wash (*temessi*) roasted *irrû* ('cucumber'),

39 from the north side in water, you split up *baluḫḫu* ('ferula gummosa'), (and) you select (*tebêr*)[463] some *nuḫurtu* ('asafoetida'), (then) you soak these three drugs in high-quality beer

40 in proportion to equal amounts, you place (*tašakkan*) them under the Goat Star, you draw a circle around them (*uṣurta talammi*),[464] in the morning you filter those (ingredients),

459 For an edition of lines 38–41 and 50–52, as a parallel to BAM 159 i 29–42, see now Parys 2014: 14–15 and 29, who interprets the adjective following UKUŠ$_2$.ḪAB (in line with Cadelli 2000: 190) as GIBIL 'nouveau'.

460 As opposed to Köcher's (1980) copy, the MA sign in *ki-ma pi-i* seems to be partially erased, which brings the reading in line with the other duplicates and the expected form of the idiom *ki pi-i* for 'proportion' or 'ratio' (CAD P 467). The use of *kī pî*, here alongside *malmališ*, which normally occurs on its own, is probably made necessary by the different ways in which each ingredient has been prepared; it might suggest that the differently processed ingredients had divergent physical properties and the combination of *kī pî* with *malmališ* indicates that the three ingredients were quantified in a precise way (perhaps by weighing) before being combined.

461 The use of the demonstrative pronoun *šâšunu* to refer to ingredients normally only occurs following U$_2$.ḪI.A or U$_2$.MEŠ in the medical corpus, so we may have, instead, something like ŠEG$_6$-*šal ta-ša$_2$-ḫal* as in line 71 below, but the traces of signs after the break do not support such a reading.

462 The meaning of *nuppuqu*, viz. 'to be blocked up', is more general than *esēlu* 'to be constipated' and can be applied to other parts of the body such as the nose and throat (CAD N/1 277–278). The two terms co-occur in BAM 7 33: 13, which suggests that they cannot be identical in meaning. See also BAM 7 24 ii 8, where the verb, read as *u$_2$-na-⸢paq⸣*, is preceded by other gastrointestinal symptoms. For further discussion of *nuppuqu*, see Cadelli 2000: 359–360.

463 The other two ingredients here are processed before being added to the mixture, but *nuḫurtu* is simply 'picked out' (*tebêr*) in the form in which it was already available. For a similar use of the verb, see BM 78963 obv. 25 (Stadhouders and Johnson 2018: 572 ln. 25, and 592). Some texts actually suggest that a number of drugs were kept readily available by medical experts whre they practiced medicine; see generally Böck 2011: 700–702.

464 This circle was probably scratched on the ground rather than made with flour, as we usually find in magical contexts. It may have served to focus the stellar power of Gula's star on the ingredients in question, as suggested to us by I. Finkel (personal communication, February 2022).

41 A$_{i\,41}$ NU *pa-tan* NAG-*ma* ⸢*i-lap-pat-su-ma*⸣ *is-sal-la-’ la ta-na-k*[*ud*[465] T]I-⸢*uṭ*⸣* [*ina*] ⸢UD ŠE⸣.GA NAG-*šu*

NU *pa-tan* NAG *i-lap-pat-su-ma is-sa-la-’* / *la ta-na-kud* TI-*uṭ ina* UD ŠE.GA NAG-*šu*$_2$ (BAM 159 i 36–37)

[. . .] x x [. . .] (BAM 60: 12′)

---

42 A$_{i\,42}$ [x x] x x [x x] x ⸢IGI ta⸣ x [x x *u*]*r*$_2$-*ne*$_2$-*e* ^{šim}BAL $^{\text{u2}}$KUR.KUR ^{giš}GEŠTIN KA$_5$.A

43 A$_{i\,43}$ [x x] *ina* 3 SILA$_3$ ⸢KAŠ⸣ *ina* ⸢^{urudu}ŠEN⸣.[TUR ŠEG$_6$-*šal* E]N* ⸢*ana*⸣ 2 SILA$_3$ *i-tur-ru i-kaṣ*$_3$-*ṣa* <<*aṣ*>>[466]

44 A$_{i\,44}$ [x x *ana*] IGI ŠUB-*di pa-na* A GAZI^{sar} *i-š*[*aḫ*]-*ḫat*[467] EGIR-*šu*$_2$ *an-na-a ana* DUR$_2$-*šu*$_2$ DUB-*ak*

---

45 A$_{i\,45}$ [DIŠ] ⸢KI* MIN⸣ $^{\text{u2}}$UKUŠ$_2$.ḪAB ḪAD$_2$.A GAZ SIM KI ZI$_3$.KU[M Ḫ]I*.ḪI *ina* A GAZI^{sar} *tara-bak ina* KUŠ SUR LAL

---

41 he drinks (*išattī-ma*) them on an empty stomach, it (= the medicine) will then affect him, and consequently he will get worse, but you should not worry, he will recover (*iballuṭ*). You should have him drink (*tašaqqīšu*) it on a favourable day.

---

42 . . . *urnû* (a kind of mint), *ballukku* (an aromatic), *atā’išu* (a plant), *karān šēlebi* (‘fox-vine’),

43 . . . you bring them to a boil (*tušabšal*) in three litres of beer in a small copper pot until it turns (*iturru*)[468] into two litres (and) cools,

44 you add (*tanaddi*) . . ., (then) he rinses (himself) with juice from *kasû* (‘tamarind’) first, (and) afterwards you pour (*tašappak*) this (mixture) into his anus.

---

45 If DITTO, you dry (*tubbal*), crush (*taḫaššal*), (and) sift (*tanappi*) *irrû* (‘cucumber’), you mix (*tuballal*) it with *isqūqu* (a type of groats), you stir them into a paste in juice from *kasû* (‘tamarind’), you smear (*teṭerri*) it on a piece of leather, (and) you bandage (*taṣammid*) him.

---

465 For a similar use of *issalla’ lā tanakkud*, see BM 78963 obv. 3 (Stadhouders and Johnson 2018: 568–569 ln. 3, and 587). For an analysis of the verb *salā’u*, including its attestation in this passage, see Stol 2009c.

466 For a discussion of the reading *kasāsu* / *kaṣāṣu* ‘to chew’, see Cadelli 2019: 60, but this does not fit the context. In all likelihood the final AZ (= *aṣ*) sign was a gloss in the source text, as in *i-kaṣ*$_3^{\text{aṣ}}$-*ṣa*, which was accidentally moved to the end of the line.

467 For the same idiom used here to reconstruct the missing sign, see GAZI^{sar} *i-šaḫ-ḫat* in BAM 86 obv 7.

468 The verb *iturru* is a temporal (construct) relative going back to *adi*, which may explain why the order of *tušabšal* and *ana* (. . .) *iturru* varies considerably in their attestations. For this relatively rare instruction about cooking time, see Köcher 1978: 21–22 and Finkel 2000: 147.

46 A$_{i\,46}$ DIŠ NA *ina ti-bi-šu*$_2$ SAG.DU-*su ana* IGI-*šu*$_2$ *iš-ta-na-*⸢*da*⸣*-as-su* GU$_2$-*su* MURUB$_4$.MIN-*šu*$_2$ *kim-ṣa-šu*$_2$ GIR$_3$.MIN-*šu*$_2$ GU$_7$.MIN-*šu*$_2$

47 A$_{i\,47}$ ŠA$_3$-*šu*$_2$ *i*$^!$(IA)-*ʾ-aš*$_2$ ŠA$_3$-*šu*$_2$ *ana pa-re-e i-te-ne*$_2$*-*⸢*el-la*[469] IGI⸣.MEŠ-*šu*$_2$ *iṣ-ṣa-nu-du-šu*$_2$ NA BI ZE$_2$ DAB-*su ana* TI-*šu*$_2$[470]

48 A$_{i\,48}$ ^{giš}EREN ^{giš}ŠUR.MIN$_3$ ^{šim}GIR$_2$ GI DU$_{10}$ NAGA SI ^{šim}⸢IM⸣.[MAN.DU[471] MUN *e*]*me-sal-li*$_3$ *ina* KAŠ *tara-bak ina* NINDU UŠ$_2$-*er ana* DUR$_2$-*šu*$_2$ DUB-*ak*

---

49 A$_{i\,49}$ ^{u2}NU.LUḪ.ḪA ^{šim}LI NA$_4$ ZU$_2$.LUM.⸢MA *ina*⸣ [^{na4}*ur-ṣ*]*i*[472] ⸢DIŠ⸣-*niš* ARA$_3$.ARA$_3$ *ina* I$_3$.UDU ḪI.ḪI *alla-nu* DU$_3$-*uš* I$_3$.GIŠ SUD *ana* DUR$_2$-*šu*$_2$ GAR

---

46 If someone's head keeps pulling him forward when he gets up, his neck, his hips, his shins, (and) his feet cause him pain (*ikkalāšu*),

47 his belly (*libbu*) feels nauseated (*iʾʾaš*),[473] his belly continually heaves to vomit, (and) he feels dizzy (lit. his face is spinning), that man has been seized (*iṣbassu*) by bile (*martu*):[474] in order to heal him,

48 you stir into a paste *erēnu* ('cedar'), *šurmēnu* ('cypress'), *asu* ('myrtle'), *qanû ṭābu* ('sweet reed'), *uḫūlu qarnānû* ('horned alkali'), *suādu* (a kind of sedge), (and) *emesallu* salt in beer, you heat (*tesekker*) (the mixture) in an oven, (and) you pour (*tašappak*) it into his anus.

---

49 You grind (*teṭên*) *nuḫurtu* ('asafoetida'), *burāšu* (a kind of juniper), (and) *aban suluppi* ('date stone') together in a mortar, you mix (*tuballal*) them in fat, you make (*teppuš*) a suppository, you sprinkle (*tasallaḫ*) it with oil, (and) you place (*tašakkan*) it into his anus.

---

469 See the very similar entry ŠA$_3$-*šu*$_2$ *i-ta-na-*⸢*ša*$^?$⸣ : ŠA$_3$-*šu*$_2$ *ana* BURU$_8$ *e-te-ne*$_2$*-la-a* in STT 403 obv. 19, commenting on Sagig 3: 13 (Wee 2019, vol. 1: 17–18).

470 The beginning of lines 47–53 has been filled with the help of K 22008, which is a direct join to MS A. The join was made by Zs. Földi in 2022.

471 The reconstruction is based line 60 below.

472 The reconstruction of the missing passage is based on the relatively common instruction of having the specialist grind (ARA$_3$ = Akk. *ṭênu*) the ingredients in a mortar (^{na4}NA.ZA$_3$.ḪI.LI = Akk. *urṣu*): for this instruction, see NA$_4$.MEŠ *ina* ^{na4}NA.[ZA$_3$.ḪI.LI] / ARA$_3$-*en* in BAM 430 iii 38′–39′, as well as U$_2$.ḪI.A *ina* ⸢^{giš}⸣[. . .] x *ina* ^{na4}NA.ZA$_3$.ḪI.LI ARA$_3$-*en* in BAM 7 9 i 35.

473 The verb also occurs in slightly different orthographies, such as *i-ʾ-šam* in STT 262 obv. 3′ and *i-ʾ-šam-ma* in BAM 232 obv. 11.

474 The reference here is to various parts of the body, including the major joints like neck, hips, shins and feet. Here and later on we have other descriptions of symptoms affecting parts of the body that are not part of the gastrointestinal tract, yet they are explained as 'seizure by bile', suggesting that bile might have been conceived of as a somewhat abstract entity that could leave the gastrointestinal tract and move around within the body.

50 A$_{i\,50}$ DIŠ ⸢NA⸣ GABA-*su u ša*$_2$*-šal-la-šu*$_2$ KUM$_2$.MEŠ ZU$_2$.MEŠ-⸢*šu*$_2$⸣ [*i-ḫi-la*] ⸢*e*⸣*-peš* KA-*šu*$_2$ DUGUD NA BI ZE$_2$ GIG *ana* TI-*šu*$_2$

DIŠ NA GABA-*su u ša*$_2$*-šal-la-šu*$_2$ KUM$_2$.MEŠ ZU$_2$.MEŠ-*šu*$_2$ *i-ḫi-la* / *e-peš* KA-*šu*$_2$ DUGUD NA BI ZE$_2$ GIG *ana* TI-*šu*$_2$ (BAM 159 i 38–39)

51 A$_{i\,51}$ ^{š}[^{i}]^{m}GUR$_2$.GUR$_2$ ^{šim}LI ^{šim}GAM.MA MUN I[LLU LI.TA]R ^{u2}ḪA U$_2$ BABBAR ^{u2}ḪAB ^{u2}*ak-tam*

^{šim}GUR$_2$.GUR$_2$ ^{šim}LI ^{šim}GAM.MA MUN ILLU LI.TAR / ^{u2}ḪA U$_2$ BABBAR ^{u2}ḪAB ^{u2}*ak-tam* (BAM 159 i 40–41)

52 A$_{i\,52}$ ^{giš}Ḫ[AB] ⸢^{u2}⸣KUR.KUR U$_5$ ARGAB^{mušen} 12 ⸢U$_2$⸣.[ḪI.A ŠEŠ DIŠ]-⸢*niš*⸣ *ina* KAŠ *ba-lu pa-tan* NAG-*ma* BURU$_8$

^{giš}ḪAB ⸢^{u2}KUR.KUR⸣ U$_5$ ARGAB^{mušen} / [12 U$_2$.ḪI].⸢A⸣ ŠEŠ DIŠ-*niš* SUD$_2$ *ina* KAŠ NU *pa-tan* NAG-*ma i-ar*$_2$*-ru*$_3$ (BAM 159 i 41–42)

---

53 A$_{i\,53}$ x [x *sa*]*ḫ-le*$_2$*-e* ^{u2}KUR.RA *kam-mu* ILLU ⸢LI⸣.[TAR ^{š}]^{im}BULUḪ ⸢^{šim}⸣LI ^{šim}GUR$_2$.GUR$_2$ ILLU ^{šim}BULUḪ[475]

54 A$_{i\,54}$ [NUMUN] ⸢^{u2}⸣NU.LUḪ.ḪA ZI$_3$ ^{u2}NU.LUḪ.ḪA[476] [^{u2}*u*]*r*$_2$*-nu-u* TI-*su-nu ina* KAŠ ⸢NAG⸣-*ma* BURU$_8$

♆

50 If someone's chest and heel are warm (*emmā*), his gums (lit. teeth) exude (blood), (and) he has difficulty (*kabit*) speaking,[477] that man suffers (*maruṣ*) from bile (*martu*): in order to heal him,

51 *kukru* (an aromatic), *burāšu* (a kind of juniper), *ṣumlalû* (an aromatic), salt, resin from *abukkatu* (a tree), *urânu* ('anise'), *šammu peṣû* ('white plant'), *būšānu* ('smelly' plant), *aktam* (a plant),

52 *ḫûratu* ('madder'), *atā'išu* (a plant), (and) *rikibti arkabi* ('bat guano')—he drinks (*išattī-ma*) these twelve ingredients together on an empty stomach in beer, and then he will vomit (*i'arru*).[478]

---

53 . . . *saḫlû* ('cress'), *nīnû* ('mint'), *kammu* ('fungus'), resin from *abukkatu* (a tree), *baluḫḫu* ('ferula gummosa'), *burāšu* (a kind of juniper), *kukru* (an aromatic), resin from *baluḫḫu* ('galbanum'),

54 seed$^?$ from *nuḫurtu* ('asafoetida'), flour from *nuḫurtu* ('asafoetida'), (and) *urnû* (a kind of mint)—taken fresh (*balṭūssunu*),[479] he drinks (*išattī-ma*) them in beer, and then he will vomit (*i'arru*).

---

475 The gap in lines 53–57 has been filled with the help of AMT 5/4, which is a direct join to MS A. The join was made by K. Simkó in 2021.

476 Strictly speaking, ZI$_3$ ^{u2}NU.LUḪ.ḪA is flour made from *nuḫurtu* ('asafoetida'), which is not attested elsewhere, so the scribe may have misread the usual orthography for Akk. *tīyatu*, namely ^{u2}DUR$_2$.NU.LUḪ.ḪA, inverting the first two elements U$_2$ and KU (i.e., DUR$_2$ or ZI$_3$).

477 For a summary of different interpretations of this phrase, see Bácskay 2018: 96.

478 This is the first of ten sections in a row that all end with BURU$_8$ = Akk. *arû* 'to vomit', as the goal and conclusion of each prescription, with the exception of line 56, where KI MIN is used in place of BURU$_8$. Although similar sequences are known from BAM 193 ii 7′–iii 5, BAM 543 ii 15-18, 31, 33 and 35–38, and especially the opening section of BM 78963 (Stadhouders and Johnson 2018), which partially overlaps with STO 5, the largest set of short emetic prescriptions can be found here and lines 137–143 below.

479 Within the therapeutic corpus, the idiom TI-*su-nu* = Akk. *balṭūssunu* 'taken fresh' (with a play on the different meanings of TI such as Akk. *leqû* 'to take' and *balāṭu* 'to live') only seems to be used in STO 3: 54 and 91, as well as in CRAN 2: 120 (BAM 482+ ii 61). See also KUB 37 44: 9′, which has now been joined to a two-column tablet with a collection of prescriptions for undoing witchcraft (Abusch and Schwemer 2011: 27–39). For a broader discussion of 'leaf therapy', see Stadhouders 2017: 125, fn. 23.

55 A$_{i\,55}$ ⸢^{šim}⸣[x x x x] ⸢^{u2}⸣KUR.KUR ^{u2}NU.LUḪ.ḪA [^{u2}ḪAR].⸢ḪAR⸣ ^{šim}ŠEŠ ILLU LI.⸢DUR⸣ x x ⸢UḪ$_2$.^{d}ID$_2$⸣[480]

56 A$_{i\,56}$ ^{u2}x [x] ⸢U$_2$ NAM.TI.LA ^{u2}GAMUN ^{u2}⸣[x x] ⸢^{u2}KUR⸣.RA *saḫ-le$_2$-e* GAZI^{sar} 1[7 U$_2$.ḪI.A] ⸢ŠEŠ⸣ [KI MIN]

---

57 A$_{i\,57}$ ILLU $_{pa\ x}$ ⸢LI⸣.TAR U$_2$ BABBAR U$_5$ ARGAB^{mušen} ^{u2}*a*[*k-tam* x x x ^{ši}]^{m}⸢BULUḪ⸣ x x [*ina* KAŠ NA]G-*ma* BURU$_8$

---

58 A$_{i\,58}$ ^{u2}KUR.KUR ILLU LI.TAR U$_2$ BABBAR [........................ NAG-*m*]*a* BURU$_8$

---

59 A$_{i\,59}$ GI DU$_{10}$.GA ^{šim}MUG GAZI^{sar} U$_2$ BABBAR [.......................... *ina* IZ]I ŠEG$_6$-*šal* NAG-*ma* BURU$_8$
GI DU$_{10}$ ^{šim}MUG [. . .] (STO 5: 113′)

---

60 A$_{i\,60}$ ^{u2}⸢*ur$_2$*⸣-*nu-u* ^{u2}SUMUN.DAR ^{u2}*šib*-[*bu-ra-tu$_2$* x x x] ⸢^{u2}⸣KUR.RA ^{šim}IM.MAN.DU

55 . . . *atā'išu* (a plant), *nuḫurtu* ('asafoetida'), *ḫašû* ('thyme'), *murru* ('myrrh'), resin from *abukkatu* (a tree) . . . *ru'tītu* (a kind of sulphur),

56 . . . *šammi balāṭi* ('plant of life'), *kamūnu* ('cumin') . . . *nīnû* ('mint'), *saḫlû* ('cress'), (and) *kasû* ('tamarind')—these seventeen ingredients DITTO (= he drinks them in beer, and then he will vomit).

---

57 Resin (gloss: . . .)[481] from *abukkatu* (a tree), *šammu peṣû* ('white plant'), *rikibti arkabi* ('bat guano'), *aktam* (a plant) . . . *baluḫḫu* ('ferula gummosa') . . . he drinks (*išattī-ma*) in beer, and then he will vomit (*i'arru*).

---

58 *atā'išu* (a plant), resin from *abukkatu* (a tree), *šammu peṣû* ('white plant') . . . he drinks (*išattī-ma*) . . . and then he will vomit (*i'arru*).

---

59 You bring to a boil (*tušabšal*) *qanû ṭābu* ('sweet reed'), *ballukku* (an aromatic), *kasû* ('tamarind'), *šammu peṣû* ('white plant') . . . over fire, he drinks (*išattī-ma*) them, and then he will vomit (*i'arru*).

---

60 *urnû* (a kind of mint), *šumuttu* ('beetroot'), *šibburatu* ('rue')$^?$ . . . *nīnû* ('mint'), *suādu* (a kind of sedge),

---

480 The gap in lines 55–62 has partially been filled with the help of AMT 9/5 + AMT 17/7, which represents a direct join to MS A. AMT 17/7 was joined to MS A by K. Simkó in 2021, whereas the join between AMT 9/5 and AMT 17/7 was made by Zs. Földi in 2022.

481 The placement of the gloss beneath ILLU = Akk. *ḫīlu* 'resin' suggests that another part of the *abukkatu* plant is offered as an alternative, but the reading of the gloss is still unclear.

61 A$_{i\,61}$ GI [DU$_{10}$.G]A *an-daḫ-še na[b-ru-qu*[482] U$_2$.ḪI.A *an-nu-t]i ina* KAŠ NAG-*ma* BURU$_8$

---

62 A$_{i\,62}$ ⸢GI⸣ [DU$_{10}$.G]A ⸢PA ^{u2}⸣[............ ^{š}]^{im}BULUḪ U$_2$ NAM.TI.LA ZU$_2$.LUM.MA
63 A$_{i\,63}$ [.......................... *ina* MU]L$_4$ *tuš-bat ina še-ri*$_3$ NU *pa-tan* NAG-*ma* BURU$_8$

---

64 A$_{i\,64}$ [.........................] ⸢^{u2}⸣[x x x] x ⸢ILLU⸣ LI.TAR 7 U$_2$.ḪI.A ŠEŠ *ina* KAŠ NAG-*ma* BURU$_8$

---

65 A$_{i\,65}$ [................................] x ^{u2}⸢KUR⸣.K[UR ^{šim}GUR$_2$.GUR$_2$ NA]GA ⸢SI⸣* MUN ^{u2}IGI-*lim* ^{u2}IGI.NIŠ ^{u2}*tar-muš*
a-na ṣi-ri-iḫ-ti KUM$_2$ ⸢ŠA$_3$⸣ ZI-*ḫi* ⸢U$_2$⸣ [. . .] / ^{u2}KUR.RA ^{šim}GUR$_2$.GUR$_2$ ⸢NAGA⸣ SI MUN [. . .] (STO 5: 34–35)
[*a-na ṣi-r*]*i-iḫ-te* KUM$_2$ ŠA$_3$ ZI U$_2$ ⸢BABBAR⸣ [. . .] / [x x x NA]GA SI MUN ^{u2}IGI-*lim* ⸢^{u2}⸣[IGI.NIŠ . . .] (BAM 174 rev. 1–2)

☨

61 *qanû ṭābu* ('sweet reed'), *andaḫšu* ('lily'), (and) *namruqqu* (a plant)$^?$—he drinks (*išattī-ma*) these ingredients in beer, and then he will vomit (*i'arru*).

---

62 *qanû ṭābu* ('sweet reed')$^?$, leaves from . . . *baluḫḫu* ('ferula gummosa'), *šammi balāṭi* ('plant of life'), *suluppū* ('dates'),
63 . . . you leave them out overnight under the stars, in the morning he drinks (*išattī-ma*) them on an empty stomach, and then he will vomit (*i'arru*).

---

64 . . . (and) resin from *abukkatu* (a tree)—he drinks (*išattī-ma*) these seven ingredients in beer, and then he will vomit (*i'arru*).

---

65 *šammu peṣû* ('white plant')$^?$ . . . *atā'išu* (a plant), *kukru* (an aromatic)$^?$, *uḫūlu qarnānû* ('horned alkali'), salt, *imḫur-līm* ('faces a thousand' plant), *imḫur-ešrā* ('faces twenty' plant), *tarmuš* ('lupin'),

---

482 The determinative U$_2$ is omitted before both *andaḫšu* and *namruqqu*, which seems to occur here in its by-form *nabruqqu*. This plant is described as a drug for treating both *aḫḫāzu* (Uruanna II 42) and *amurriqānu* (BAM 1 ii 57), and these medical conditions are mentioned a few lines below in our text as well.

66 A$_{i 66}$ [............................ ^{u2}ḪA]R.ḪAR 14 ⸢U$_2$⸣*.[ḪI.A ŠE]Š DIŠ-*niš* SUD$_2$ *ina* KAŠ NAG-*ma* BURU$_8$
^{u2}KUR.⸢KUR NA$_4$ *ga-bi-i* ^{u2}*ak*⸣-*t*[*am* . . .] / ⸢TEŠ$_2$⸣.BI *ta-pa-aṣ ina* K[AŠ . . .] (STO 5: 36–37)
[. . .] / [NA$_4$ *ga-bi*]-*i* ^{u2}*ak-tam* ^{u2}ḪAR.ḪAR 14 U$_2$ *an-nu-*[*ti* . . .] (BAM 174 rev. 2–3)

---

67 A$_{i 67}$ [.......................... 10 GIN$_2$ ^{u2}*sa*]*ḫ*-⸢*la*⸣-*a*$^{!}$-*nu*$^{!}$[483] 10 GIN$_2$ AL.U[S$_2$*.S]A* ⸢10* GIN$_2$* A*.GEŠTIN⸣.NA KALAG.GA 10 GIN$_2$ KAŠ 10 GIN$_2$ *ut-ḫi-ra*

68 A$_{i 68}$ [......................... 10 GIN$_2$ ^{u2}ḪAR.Ḫ]AR 1 GIN$_2$ SUM^{sar} 1/2 GIN$_2$ M[UN 1/2 GIN$_2$ GA]ZI^{sar} *tuš-te-mid ina* MUL$_4$ *tuš-bat ina še-ri$_3$*

69 A$_{i 69}$ [......................... *ina* KA-*š*]*u$_2$ u* DUR$_2$-*šu$_2$* SI.SA$_2$-*ma* TI x [x] x A UZU *kab-ru-ti* NAG-*ma ina-eš*

---

66 *nīnû* ('mint')$^{?}$, *aban gabî* ('alum'), *aktam* (a plant), (and) *ḫašû* ('thyme')—you pound (*tasâk*) these fourteen[484] ingredients together, he drinks (*išattī-ma*) them in beer, and then he will vomit (*i'arru*).

---

67 . . . ten shekels of *saḫlânu* ('cress-like' plant), ten shekels of *šiqqu* ('garum'), ten shekels of strong vinegar, ten shekels of beer, ten shekels of *utḫiru* (a plant),[485]

68 . . . ten$^{?}$ shekels of *ḫašû* ('thyme'), one shekel of *šūmū* ('garlic'), half a shekel of salt, (and) half a shekel of *kasû* ('tamarind')—you mix them together, you leave them out overnight under the stars, in the morning

69 . . . (and) he will void (*ušeššer-ma*) from his mouth and from his anus; then he will recover (*iballuṭ*). He drinks (*išattī-ma*) . . . (and) broth from fatty meat; then he will get well.

---

483 The reading GIR$_2$-*nu*, instead of the much more conventional ^{u2}GIR$_2$-*a-nu* (Cadelli 2000: 192), is not impossible, but if so both the GIR$_2$ and the NU signs are malformed. In addition, the traces on the tablet indicate the presence of more than one sign before the malformed NU: these factors suggest our alternative rendering of the remaining traces as ^{u2}*saḫ-la-a-nu*. For this orthography, see also line 34 above.

484 There are probably three ingredients missing at the beginning of line 65. If the parallels with BAM 174 rev. 1–3 and STO 5: 34–37 hold, the first of these ingredients is *šammu peṣû* ('white plant'), but the identity of the other two ingredients is unclear. Our passage and STO 5: 37 have different verbs: *ta-sak$_3$* and *ta-pa-aṣ*, respectively, while the corresponding part in BAM 174 rev. 3 is missing. Moreover, the plants ^{u2}KUR.KUR = Akk. *atā'išu* and ^{u2}KUR.RA = Akk. *nīnû* seem to occur in a different order, with the parallels listing ^{u2}KUR.RA first and ^{u2}KUR.KUR second. The traces in line 65 support the reading ^{u2}KUR.K[UR], which thus presumably precedes ^{u2}KUR.RA in the list of ingredients in STO 3. ^{u2}KUR.RA might be one of the missing ingredients in the beginning of line 66, although there is probably not enough room in the break for three ingredients preceding ^{u2}ḪAR.ḪAR = Akk. *ḫašû*.

485 The rare ingredient *uthiru* (CAD U/W 334) is only attested a couple times in the medical literature, including the fragmentary passage in Uruanna II 134–136; in all of its other occurrences it is always preceded by ILLU = Akk. *ḫīlu* 'resin'.

70 A$_{\text{i 70}}$ [DIŠ NA *lu* ZE$_2$ *lu aḫ-ḫa*]-⸢*za lu*⸣ *a-mur-ri-qa-nu* ⸢DAB⸣-[*su* $^{\text{u2}}$*ur*$_2$]-⸢*ne*$_2$$^?$⸣-[*e*] ⸢$^{\text{u2}}$⸣KUR.KUR $^{\text{u2}}$GEŠTIN KA$_5$.A ^{šim}LI

[DIŠ N]A *lu-u*$_2$ ZE$_2$ *lu-u*$_2$ *aḫ-ḫa-za lu-u*$_2$ *a-mur-ri-qa* DAB-*su* $^{\text{u2}}$*ur*$_2$-[*nu*$_2$-*u*] / $^{\text{u2}}$KUR.KUR ^{giš}GEŠTIN KA$_5$.A ^{šim}LI (BAM 52 rev. 43–44)

[. . . *a-m*]*ur-ri-qa-nu* DAB-*su* $^{\text{u2}}$*ur*$_2$-*nu*-[*u*] / [. . .] (BAM 62 obv. 1–2)

71 A$_{\text{ii 1}}$ ^{šim}MUG 3 SILA$_3$ KAŠ *ina* ŠEN.TUR ŠEG$_6$-*šal ta-ša*$_2$-*ḫal* I$_3$.GIŠ *ana* I[GI ....][486]

^{šim}MUG *ina* 3 SILA$_3$ KAŠ *ina* ^{urudu}ŠE[N.TUR] / ŠEG$_6$-*šal ta-ša*$_2$-*ḫal* I$_3$.GIS *ana* IGI ŠUB-*di ina pa-ni* A GAZI^{sar} DUB-*ma* KI [x] x / ⸢NAG⸣ *ina* DUR$_2$-*šu*$_2$ SI.SA$_2$-*ma* TI-*u*[*ṭ*] (BAM 52 rev. 44–46)

[x x] ⸢3⸣ SILA$_3$ KAŠ *ina* ^{urudu}ŠEN.TUR / [. . . GA]ZI^{sar} DUB-*ma* / [. . . SI.SA$_2$-*m*]*a* TI (BAM 62 obv. 2–4)

---

72 A$_{\text{ii 2}}$ $^{\text{u2}}$GIR$_2$-*a-nu* $^{\text{u2}}$⸢MUR⸣.GABA.RI-*a-nu* $^{\text{u2}}$*a-ri-ḫu* ⸢$^{\text{u2}}$⸣[..]

73 A$_{\text{ii 3}}$ $^{\text{u2}}$*ṣa-ṣu-un-ta*$_5$ ⸢$^{\text{u2}}$⸣*si-si-ni* ŠA$_3$-*bi* $^{\text{u2}}$[..]

74 A$_{\text{ii 4}}$ $^{\text{u2}}$UKUŠ$_2$.ḪAB ⸢$^{\text{u2}}$ḪAB⸣ $_{\text{u2[x] ḪAB?}}$ $^{\text{u2}}$*tar-muš*$_8$ $^{\text{u2}}$N[U.LU]Ḫ.[ḪA ....]

☨

70 If someone has been seized (*iṣbassu*) by either bile (*martu*) or *aḫḫāzu*-jaundice or *amurriqānu*-jaundice: you bring to a boil (*tušabšal*) *urnû* (a kind of mint), *atā'išu* (a plant), *karān šēlebi* ('fox-vine'), *burāšu* (a kind of juniper),

71 (and) *ballukku* (an aromatic)[487] in three litres of beer in a small copper pot, you filter (the mixture), you add (*tanaddi*) oil, you pour (*tašappak-ma*) juice from *kasû* ('tamarind') on the surface,[488] and he drinks (*išatti*) it with . . . he will void (*ušeššer-ma*) from his anus; then he will recover (*iballuṭ*).

---

72 *patrānu* ('like a knife' plant), MUR.GABA.RI-*a-nu* (a plant),[489] *arīḫu* (a plant) . . .

73 *ṣaṣuntu* (a plant), *sissinni libbi* ('date spadix for the innards' plant) . . .[490]

74 *irrû* ('cucumber') (gloss: . . .), *būšānu* ('smelly' plant), *tarmuš* ('lupin'), *nuḫurtu* ('asafoetida') . . .

---

486 The gap in lines 71–80 has partially been filled with the help of AMT 58/8, which represents a direct join to MS A. The fragment was joined by K. Simkó in 2019.

487 The five ingredients in lines 70–71 are also included in two other more elaborate recipes: BAM 188 obv. 1–10 and BAM 186 obv. 1–11, each with 14 or 15 ingredients, for treating bile and both types of jaundice (in BAM 188), or only the two types of jaundice, without bile (in BAM 186).

488 For the same idiom, viz. *ina pa-ni* A GAZI^{sar} DUB, see STO 5: 54.

489 The identity of $^{\text{u2}}$MUR.GABA.RI-*a-nu* is unclear: given its context, it may represent a variant spelling for *mergirānu*, which is found between *patrānu* and *arariānu* in the Middle Babylonian letter PBS 1/2 72 rev. 10, edited by Parpola (1983b: 495–496) and discussed more recently by Sibbing-Plantholt (2014). The *mergirānu* plant is a rare medical ingredient, but it occurs two other times in our treatise, viz. STO 2: 145 and in line 136 below.

490 Although no clear parallel exists for this section, two of its ingredients, viz. *sissinni libbi* and *arīḫu*, appear in the pharmacological lists BAM 380 rev. 62–63 and BAM 381 iv 17–18; both ingredients are prescribed for the 'evacuation of the belly' (*šūšur libbi*). See also lines 131–136 below, together with the distant parallel in STO 2: 145–146.

75 A$_{\text{ii 5}}$ ḪENBUR$_2$ ^{u2}⸢EME⸣ UR.GI$_7$ $_{\text{ḪENBUR}_2\ ^{\text{šim}}\text{LI}}$ [ḪEN]BUR$_2$ ^{šim}GAM.ME *saḫ-le$_2$-⸢e⸣* [.................................]

---

76 A$_{\text{ii 6}}$ ḪENBUR$_2$ ^{u2}UKUŠ$_2$.ḪAB ⸢^{u2}⸣*saḫ-la-na* SUD$_2$ *ina* GE[ŠTIN ....]
DIŠ KI MIN ^{u2}*saḫ-la-a-nu* SUD$_2$ *ina* GEŠTIN KALAG.GA NU *pa-⸢tan⸣* N[AG-*šu$_2$* KI MIN] (STO 3: 34)
DIŠ KI MIN ḪENBUR$_2$ ^{u2}UKUŠ$_2$.ḪAB SUD$_2$ *ina* GEŠTIN LAL$_3$ *u* I$_3$ *ḫal-⸢ṣi⸣* NAG-*šu$_2$* K[I MIN] (STO 3: 36)
DIŠ KI MIN ḪENBUR$_2$ ^{u2}UKUŠ$_2$.⸢ḪAB⸣ [. . .] (AMT 69/1: 16′)

---

77 A$_{\text{ii 7}}$ DIŠ NA ZE$_2$ *qid-ḫa lu-ba-⸢ṭa⸣* GIG *ana* TI-*šu$_2$* ^{ši}[^{m} ....]
78 A$_{\text{ii 8}}$ ^{u2}*tar-muš* ^{u2}IGI-*lim* ⸢^{šim}⸣BULUḪ ^{u2}KUR.RA ILLU ^{ši}[^{m} ....]

---

79 A$_{\text{ii 9}}$ DIŠ NA *a-ša$_2$-a pa-šit-ta$_5$ u lu-⸢ba⸣-ṭi$_5$*[491] GIG ⸢^{u2}⸣[..................................]

75 shoots from *lišān kalbi* ('dog's tongue' plant) (gloss: shoots from *burāšu*), shoots from *ṣumlalû* (an aromatic), *saḫlû* ('cress') . . .

---

76 You pound (*tasâk*) shoots from *irrû* ('cucumber') (and) *saḫlânu* ('cress-like' plant), you have him drink (*tašaqqīšu*) them in strong wine on an empty stomach . . .[492]

---

77 If someone suffers (*maruṣ*) from bile (*martu*), *qidḫu* disease, (or) *lubāṭu* disease:[493] in order to heal him . . .
78 *tarmuš* ('lupin'), *imḫur-līm* ('faces a thousand' plant), *baluḫḫu* ('ferula gummosa'), *nīnû* ('mint'), resin from . . .

---

79 If someone suffers (*maruṣ*) from *ašû* disease, *pāšittu* disease,[494] or *lubāṭu* disease: . . .

491 The NE sign, read provisionally as *ṭi$_5$* via DE$_3$, may simply be a badly formed DA, meant to be read as *ṭa*.

492 The second half of the line is restored in the translation, based on line 34 above rather than line 36, where three different carrier substances are listed.

493 In line with Cadelli 2000: 229 n. 9 and 2021: 12, both *qidḫu* and *lubāṭu* are understood here as disease names. However, of these two terms, only *lubāṭu* is a clear designation of a disease (CAD L 231), while *qidḫu* may describe both a disease as in the Therapeutic Vademecum BAM 1 ii 41 with U$_2$ NA *ša$_2$ qid-ḫa* GIG, as well as a substance that is vomited up: see, for example, BAM 75 obv. 6, listing the symptom *qid-ḫa ip-te-ne$_2$-ru* 'he continuously vomits up *qidḫu*' in a gastric context. Samartian Aramaic has the root *l-b-ṭ* for 'affliction', but apparently not Syriac or Mandaic. In contrast, *qidḫu* is also found in Mandaic *qadhu* 'inflammation', from the root *q-d-h* 'to flare up'. See also CAD Q 251 for the alternative reading of the word as *saḫḫu* rather than *qidḫu*; Attia and Buisson (2012: 40) collect evidence in support of this reading from STT 92 ii 23 (with *sa-ḫi*) and AMT 51/2: 10 (with *sa-ḫa*).

494 For a discussion of *pāšittu* and its connection to *martu* here and in the Neo-Assyrian letter SAA 10 217, see Cadelli 2021: 22 with n. 608. The two terms, viz. *martu* and *pāšittu*, are equated in line 109 below.

80 A$_{ii\ 10}$ ^{u2}KUR.RA URUDU SUMUN 7 U$_2$.[ḪI].⸢A ŠEŠ DIŠ⸣-[*niš* ....]

---

81 A$_{ii\ 11}$ DIŠ NA ZE$_2$ DAB-*su* ^{u2}KUR.⸢RA NU⸣ *pa-tan a-ḫe-en-n*[*a-a* ....]

82 A$_{ii\ 12}$ *ina* KAŠ NAG-*ma* KAŠ SAL.LA ⸢NAG⸣ [..]

---

83 A$_{ii\ 13}$ *ana a-ša$_2$-a pa-šit-ta$_5$ u lu-ba-ṭi* ZI-*ḫi* U$_2$ BABBAR ILLU LI.T[AR ....]

[DIŠ N]A ⸢*a-ša$_2$-a*⸣ *pa-šit-ta$_5$ u lu-*⸢*ba*⸣*-ṭi* ⸢GIG⸣ / ⸢U$_2$⸣ BABBAR ILLU LI.DUR ^{u2}*ak-tam kam$_2$-mu* DIŠ-*niš* ḪI-*a*[*l*] / *ina* KAŠ NAG-*ma* TI-*u*[*ṭ*] (Labat and Tournay 1945–1946: 116 obv. 1–3)

---

84 A$_{ii\ 14}$ DIŠ NA *pa-šit-tu$_2$* DAB-*su* ^{šim}GUR$_2$.GUR$_2$ ^{u2}ḪAR.ḪAR ^{u2}KUR.KUR ^{u2}⸢KUR⸣.[RA ....] x

†

80 *nīnû* ('mint'), (and) old copper[495]—. . . these seven ingredients together . . .

---

81 If someone has been seized (*iṣbassu*) by bile (*martu*): . . . *nīnû* ('mint') separately on an empty stomach,

82 he drinks (*išattī-ma*) it in beer, and then he drinks (*išatti*) thin beer[496] . . .

---

83 In order to remove (*nasāḫi*) *ašû* disease, *pāšittu* disease, or *lubāṭu* disease:[497] you mix (*tuballal*) *šammu peṣû* ('white plant'), resin from *abukkatu* (a tree), *aktam* (a plant), (and) *kammu* ('fungus') together, he drinks (*išattī-ma*) them in beer; then he will recover (*iballuṭ*).

---

84 If someone has been seized (*iṣbassu*) by *pāšittu* disease: *kukru* (an aromatic), *ḫašû* ('thyme'), *atā'išu* (a plant), *nīnû* ('mint') . . .

---

495 See Uruanna III 476 for old copper, explained as 'soil that corrodes (lit. eats up) copper' (SAḪAR.URUDA.I$_3$.GU$_7$.E). The similarity between this logographic writing and the orthography for *pāšittu*, i.e. KA.MUŠ.I$_3$.GU$_7$.E, may have led to the inclusion of old copper here.

496 The qualification SAL in KAŠ SAL.LA probably corresponds to Akkadian *raqāqu* 'to be thin', which is also used to describe the appearance of oil in oil omens (CAD R 168). This unique designation should be contrasted with the much more common use of KAŠ.BIR$_8$ for Akkadian *ḫīqu* 'diluted beer' as in line 16 above.

497 Other than in STO 3: 79, 83 and 88, as well as the apparent parallel in Labat and Tournay 1945–1946: 116 obv. 1–3, the collocation of these three diseases is not known from other cuneiform medical texts.

85 A$_{ii\ 15}$ ILLU LI.TAR ^{u2}NU.LUḪ.ḪA *kam*$_2$*-mu ša*$_2$ ^{lu2}AŠGAB ^{u2}LAG A.⸢ŠA$_3$⸣ x [............................ *m*]*a** BURU$_8$*

---

86 A$_{ii\ 16}$ ^{u2}ḪAR.ḪAR ^{u2}NU.LUḪ.ḪA ILLU LI.TAR ^{šim}LI ^{šim}GUR$_2$.GUR$_2$ ⸢5* U$_2$⸣.[ḪI.A ....] x*
^{u2}ḪAR.Ḫ[AR . . .] / U$_2$.<ḪI>.⸢A⸣ [. . .] (STO 5: 114′–115′)

---

87 A$_{ii\ 17}$ ^{u2}*ak-tam* ^{u2}KUR.KUR NAGA SI ^{šim}GUR$_2$.GUR$_2$ ^{šim}LI ILLU LI.TAR MUN x* ⸢8* *šam*-me*$^{?}$* NAG⸣* [*i-ša*$_2$*-r*]*iš* IM[498]

---

88 A$_{ii\ 18}$ DIŠ NA SAG.KI.DAB.BA TUKU *a-ši-a pa-šit-tu*$_4$ *u lu-ba-ṭi* GIG *ana* TI-*šu*$_2$ 15 GIN$_2$ ^{šim}GUR$_2$.GUR$_2$ 15 GIN$_2$ ^{u2}*ur*$_2$*-nu-u*

†

85 resin from *abukkatu* (a tree), *nuḫurtu* ('asafoetida'), *kammu* ('fungus') from a leatherworker, *kirbān eqli* ('field clod' plant)[499] . . ., and then he will vomit (*i'arru*).

---

86 *ḫašû* ('thyme'), *nuḫurtu* ('asafoetida'), resin from *abukkatu* (a tree), *burāšu* (a kind of juniper), (and) *kukru* (an aromatic)[500]—. . . five ingredients . . .

---

87 *aktam* (a plant), *atā'išu* (a plant), *uḫūlu qarnānû* ('horned alkali'), *kukru* (an aromatic), *burāšu* (a kind of juniper), resin from *abukkatu* (a tree), salt, (and) . . .—he drinks (*išatti*) the eight ingredients . . .

---

88 If someone has (*irašši*) a headache (and) suffers (*maruṣ*) from *ašû* disease, *pāšittu* disease, or *lubāṭu* disease: in order to heal him, you crush (*taḫaššal*) (and) sift (*tanappi*) fifteen shekels of *kukru* (an aromatic), fifteen shekels of *urnû* (a kind of mint),

---

498 Cadelli's (2000: 196) reading of the traces of signs at the end of the line as SAG IM seems to be correct, and therefore the reading suggested earlier by Küchler (1904: 50–51), viz. SILIM-*im*, cannot be accepted. SAG may represent the ending of *išariš*, presumably an adverbial form of *ešēru*; for the use of this adverb in medical context, see BAM 248 iii 33, with parallels, as part of an incantation recited for easy childbirth.

499 The sequence of ingredients in lines 84–85 is not paralleled elsewhere, although the sequence *ḫašû, atā'išu, nīnû* reappears in BAM 158 ii 15, while the partially similar sequence *atā'išu*, resin from *abukkatu, nīnû, kasû* and *kammu* fungus from a leatherworker occurs in STO 5: 55, with parts of the line already lost in antiquity.

500 Lines 86–87 and 91 each include a sequence made up of resin from *abukkatu, burāšu* (and) *kukru* (line 86), or the same plants listed in reversed order (lines 87 and 91). Similar collocations appear in BAM 471 i 4′ as well as in Heeßel and Al-Rawi 2003: 231 iii 38.

89 A$_{\text{ii 19}}$ 15 GIN$_2$ ^{u2}KUR.KUR DIŠ-*niš* GAZ SIM *ina* I$_3$ KAŠ SAG *tu-ša$_2$-ḫa-an ana* DUR$_2$-*šu$_2$* DUB *ana še$_{20}$-bi* NAG-⸢*šu$_2$*⸣*

---

90 A$_{\text{ii 20}}$ DIŠ NA NU *pa-tan* SAG ŠA$_3$-*šu$_2$ i-kaṣ$_3$-ṣa-as-su* KUM$_2$ ŠA$_3$ TUKU.MEŠ *ina ge-ši-šu* ZE$_2$ *i-ar$_2$-ru$_3$* NA BI *pa-*⸢*šit***-ta$_5$*⸣*

91 A$_{\text{ii 21}}$ *tu-ga-na* GIG *ana* TI-*šu$_2$* ^{šim}GUR$_2$.GUR$_2$ ^{šim}LI ILLU LI.TAR ^{u2}*ak-tam* ^{u2}KUR.KUR MUN NAGA SI TI-*su-nu*

92 A$_{\text{ii 22}}$ *ina* KAŠ SAG *tara-muk ina* MUL$_4$ *tuš-bat ina še-ri$_3$* NU *pa-tan ta-ša$_2$-ḫal* NAG-*ma tu-ša$_2$-'-ra-šu-ma* TI

---

93 A$_{\text{ii 23}}$ ⸢DIŠ⸣ NA ZE$_2$ GIG x* [x x x x]

---

94 A$_{\text{ii 24}}$ ⸢EN$_2$⸣ ZE$_2$ *eṭ-li* ZE$_2$ ⸢*eṭ*⸣*-*li* : i x [...]

95 A$_{\text{ii 25}}$ ⸢*u$_2$*⸣-*ri eṭ-li e-il$_3$ ša li-li*[501] x [...]

89 (and) fifteen shekels of *atā'išu* (a plant) together, you heat them up in oil (and) high-quality beer, you pour (*tašappak*) (the mixture) into his anus, (and) you have him drink (*tašaqqīšu*) it until he can drink no more (lit. until he is satisfied).

---

90 If someone's epigastrium (*rēš libbi*) causes him a gnawing pain on an empty stomach, he continually has (*irtanaššī*) heat in the belly (*libbu*), (and) he vomits up bile whenever he belches,[502] that man suffers (*maruṣ*) from *pāšittu* disease

91 (and) *tuganû* disease: in order to heal him, you soak *kukru* (an aromatic), *burāšu* (a kind of juniper), resin from *abukkatu* (a tree), *aktam* (a plant), *atā'išu* (a plant), salt (and) *uḫūlu qarnānû* ('horned alkali'), taken fresh,

92 in high-quality beer, you leave (the mixture) out overnight under the stars, in the morning you filter it on an empty stomach, he drinks (*išattī-ma*) it, and you make him vomit;[503] then he will recover (*iballuṭ*).

---

93 If someone suffers (*maruṣ*) from bile (*martu*) . . .

---

94 Incantation: 'The bile of a young man,[504] the bile of a young man . . .

95 The loins of a young man are bound, . . . of Lilith . . .

---

501 It is unlikely that E belongs to the end of *eṭli*, since the orthography in the preceding line is consistently *eṭ-li*. The reading E DINGIR also makes little sense, so we take *e-il$_3$* here as a stative of the verb *e'ēlu*, as in '(the loins of the young man) are bound', followed by a reference to the demon Lilith.

502 The phrase *ina gešīšu* ('when he belches') recalls the incipit of the tablet and, thus, forms an *inclusio* before the start of the incantation section in line 94.

503 This is a literal translation of the word order in the line, but we would normally expect NU *pa-tan* to immediately precede NAG-*ma* in a context like this. Presumably it was not the physician who went without food, and the scribe has simply misplaced NU *pa-tan* along with *ina še-ri$_3$* before *ta-ša$_2$-ḫal*.

504 For a similar formulation in the context of eye diseases, see EYES 1: 159′ (BAM 10 p. 97): *i-ni* GURUŠ GIG-*at i-ni* ^{munus}KI.SIKIL GIG-*at* 'the eye of the lad is sick, the eye of the maiden is sick'.

96 A$_{ii\,26}$ [x] ti ma *ga-ra-aš-ga-ra-a*[*š*[505] ....]
97 A$_{ii\,27}$ [x] ⸢an⸣ ra ti *e-zib* ba ⸢mu⸣ x x [..]

---

98 A$_{ii\,28}$ [KA.INIM.M]A [..]

---

99 A$_{ii\,29}$ [EN$_2$ ze$_2$.am$_3$] ⸢u$_2$⸣* [..]

[EN$_2$ E$_2$].NU.RU / [ze$_2$.am$_3$] ⸢u$_2$⸣.šim.gen$_7$ / [ki] ⸢mu.un.dar⸣ (K 2841+ obv. 1–3)
EN$_2$ ⸢E$_2$⸣.NU.RU / ze$_2$.am$_3$ u$_2$.šim.gen$_7$ / ki mu.un.dar (Alster and van Dijk 1972: 357 Fig. 1 obv. 1–3)
⸢ze$_2$⸣.am$_3$ u$_2$.šim.⸢gen$_7$⸣ [ki mu.un.dar] (Alster and van Dijk 1972: 358 Fig. 2 obv. 1)
[ze$_2$.am$_3$ u$_2$.š]im$^?$.e ki m[u.un.dar] (Alster and van Dijk 1972: 358 Fig. 3 obv. 1′)
⸢ze$_2$.am$_3$ u$_2$⸣.šim.gen$_7$ ⸢ki mu.un⸣.d[ar] (CUSAS 32 7 iv 20′)
ze$_2$.a.am u$_2$.ši.im.ge.en ki mu.un.da.ar (Michalowski 1981: 14 obv. 1)

100 A$_{ii\,30}$ [..]

⸢ud$_5$⸣.da.⸢am$_3$⸣ [sag nam.i]l$_2$ / maš$_2$ ud$_5$.d[a.gen$_7$] / babbar$_2$ [nam.il$_2$] (K 2841+ obv. 4–6)
ud$_5$.da.am$_3$ sag nam.il$_2$ / maš$_2$ ud$_5$.da.gen$_7$ / babbar$_2$ nam.il$_2$ (Alster and van Dijk 1972: 357 Fig. 1 obv. 4–6)
ud$_5$.da.am$_3$ sa[g na]m.i[l$_2$] / maš$_2$ ud$_5$.da.gen$_7$ babb[ar$_2$ na]m.il$_2$ (Alster and van Dijk 1972: 358 Fig. 2 obv. 2–3)
[x x x] sag n[am.il$_2$] / [x x x] x en babbar$_2$ n[am.il$_2$] (Alster and van Dijk 1972: 358 Fig. 3 obv. 2′–3′)
u$_2$.da.⸢am sag nam.il$_2$⸣ / maš$_2$ u$_2$.da.⸢ke$_4$⸣ babbar nam.il$_2$ (CUSAS 32 7 iv 21′–22′)
ud.dam sag nam.il$_2$ / ma.aš$_2$ ud.da.⸢ge⸣.en ba.ba.ar il$_2$ (Michalowski 1981: 14 obv. 2–3)

96 . . . sexual intercourse . . .
97 . . . deserted . . .'

---

98 An invocation$^?$ for . . .

---

99 Incantation: 'It is bile that splits the ground like weeds,[506]
100 It is the nanny goat that raises its head, it is speckled (lit. carries) with white like the nanny goat's kid,[507]

505 CAD G 142 subsumes *ga-ra-aš-ga-ra-aš* under the lemma *guruš-garaš*, a term that occurs elsewhere in the medical literature, as in EYES 2: 27 (BAM 10 pp. 121 and 274), where 'vulva of a pig' appears as a medical ingredient, presumably a *Deckname*; see CT 41 45: 10′–11′, commenting on a passage in Uruanna III 603–604. In our text, however, in the context of an incantation with sexual connotations, it is probably related to the Akkadian verb *garāšu* 'to have sexual intercourse'. For this verb, see the commentary tablet TCL 6 17 rev. 29–30: GURUŠ : *ga-ra-šu*$_2$: *na-a-ku*, with the logogram GURUŠ = Akk. *eṭlu* 'young man' equated with Akk. *garāšu* 'to copulate' and *niāku* 'to have sexual intercourse' (Frazer 2016).
506 This is the well-known gall incantation which has been studied by Alster and van Dijk (1972), Michalowski (1981) and, more recently, Böck (2014a: 122–126; 2014b: 105–107), as well as George (2016: 6–7 and 123–125). The new join K 6941 allows for a more complete reconstruction of the passage. For this join, which could not be incorporated here, see the Addendum on page 38.
507 In line with standard translations, we do not take the prefix na- in lines 100–101 as negative modal but rather as non-negative reported speech marker; see Civil 2000: 37–38.

101 A$_{\text{ii 31}}$ [x x x] e[me* ....]

muš [a.gen$_7$] / ⸢eme$^!$(KA) na⸣.[na.ed$_3$.de$_3$] / muš ki b[il$_2$.la$_2$.a.gen$_7$] / ⸢ze$_2$ na⸣.n[a.dub$_2$.be$_2$] (K 2841+ obv. 7–10)

muš a.gen$_7$ / eme na.na.ed$_3$.de$_3$ / muš ki bil$_2$.la$_2$.a.gen$_7$ / ze$_2$ ⸢na⸣.na.dub$_2$.be$_2$ (Alster and van Dijk 1972: 357 Fig. 1 obv. 7–10)

muš a.a.gen$_7$ ⸢eme⸣ i$_3$.na.ed$_3$.de$_3$ / muš ki bil$_2$.la$_2$.gen$_7$ ze$_2$ na.na.⸢dub$_2^?$.be$_2^?$⸣ (Alster and van Dijk 1972: 358 Fig. 2 obv. 4–5)

[muš agrun.n]a.⸢ka ze$_2$⸣ s[ag nam.il$_2$] (Alster and van Dijk 1972: 358 Fig. 3 obv. 4′)

muš a.gen$_7$ eme ed$_3$.de$_3$ / muš agrun.na.ke$_4$ ze$_2$ sag$^!$(GUR.PA) nam.il$_2$ / muš.⸢gen$_7$⸣ BAD.ke$_4$ ze$_2$ na.an.ni.dub$_2$.be$_2$ (CUSAS 32 7 iv 23′–25′)

muš a.gen$_7$ e.⸢me⸣ na.e.de$_3$ / muš ki bi$_2$.il.⸢la$_2$⸣.gen$_7$ e.ne.par$_3$ i$_3$.si.⸢il.le⸣ (Michalowski 1981: 14 obv. 4–5)

102 A$_{\text{ii 32}}$ [ze$_2$ ni$_2$].⸢za⸣ mu.u[n.ši.du$_3$.a ....]

ze$_2$ ni$_2$.za / mu.e.ši.du$_3$.a / dug.gen$_7$ gaz.ba (Alster and van Dijk 1972: 357 Fig. 1 obv. 11–13)

za.e ni$_2$.za ⸢mu⸣.e.ši.⸢du⸣.a / ⸢dug⸣.gen$_7$ gaz.⸢ba⸣ (Alster and van Dijk 1972: 358 Fig. 2 obv. 6–7)

[ze$_2$ n]i$_2$.⸢zu⸣ mu.e.še$_3$.du.[a] / ⸢dug.gen$_7$⸣ gaz.b[a] (Alster and van Dijk 1972: 358 Fig. 3 obv. 5′–6′)

ze$_2$ ni.za.a mu.un.ši.du.un.⸢e⸣ / d[u.u]g.gen$_7$ ka.az.ba (CUSAS 32 7 iv 26′–27′)

ze$_2$.e ne.zu ⸢me⸣.ši.mi.na.ge.en / dug$_3$.ge.en ga.az.ba (Michalowski 1981: 14 obv. 6–7)

103 A$_{\text{ii 33}}$ ⸢izi.gen$_7$⸣ te.ni$^!$(ER).i[b$_2$* ....]

izi.gen$_7$ te.ni.ib / izi ^{u2}a.numun$_2$.gen$_7$ / ni$_2$.za te.bi$_2$.ib (Alster and van Dijk 1972: 357 Fig. 1 obv. 14–16)

⸢izi⸣.gen$_7$ ⸢te⸣.ni.[i]b / izi ^{u2}a.[num]un$_2$.gen$_7$ n[i$_2$.za t]e.ni.ib (Alster and van Dijk 1972: 358 Fig. 2 obv. 8–9)

⸢izi⸣.gen$_7$ te.ni.[ib] / izi ^{u2}numun$_2$.gen$_7$ ni$_2$.⸢zu⸣ [te.ni.ib] / izi ^{giš}gišimmar.gen$_7$ ni$_2$.z[u . . .] (Alster and van Dijk 1972: 358 Fig. 3 obv. 7′–9′)

izi.gen$_7$ ⸢te⸣.ni.ib / izi ^{u2}⸢numun$_2$.gen$_7$ ni$_2$.zu⸣ [te].ni.ib (CUSAS 32 7 iv 27′–28′)

i.zi.ge.en te.ni.ib / i.zi A.ME$_3$.⸢ŠA⸣.ge.en ne.za ⸢te.ni.ib⸣ / i.zi ^{giš}gišimmar.ge.e[n . . .] (Michalowski 1981: 14 obv. 7–9)

104 A$_{\text{ii 34}}$ tu$_6$.du$_{11}$.ga ^{d}ni[n.girim$_3$ ....]

tu$_6$.du$_{11}$.ga / ^{d}nin.girim$_3$ / nam.šub eridu^{ki}.ga (Alster and van Dijk 1972: 357 Fig. 1 obv. 17–19)

⸢tu$_6$⸣.d[u$_{11}$.g]a ⸢^{d}⸣n[in.gir]im$_3$ / ⸢nam⸣.[šub] eri[du^{k}]^{i}.ga (Alster and van Dijk 1972: 358 Fig. 2 obv. 10–11)

⸢nam⸣.šub eri[du^{ki}.ga] (Alster and van Dijk 1972: 358 Fig. 3 obv. 10′)

tu$_6$.dug$_4$.ga ⸢^{d}⸣nin.girim$_x$(ḪA.KUD.DU) mu.e / nam.giš.pa [erid]u^{ki}.ga (CUSAS 32 7 iv 29′–30′)

tu.du.ga ni.in.g[i.ri$^?$.im$^?$] / nam.šub eridu^{ki}.[ga] (Michalowski 1981: 14 obv. 10–11)

101 Like a water snake, it flicks its tongue, it spits bile like the snake from scorched ground,
102 O Bile, you who act on your own, be crushed like a pot,
103 Be extinguished like a fire, extinguish yourself like fire in the rushes!
104 The incantation spoken by Ningirima, the spell of Eridu,

105 A$_{ii\ 35}$ ^{d}en.ki.ke$_4$ d[ag ....]

^{d}en.ki.ke$_4$ / ⸢dag⸣ agrun.na.ka / ḫe$_2$.em.ma.an.du$_8$.du$_8$.e (Alster and van Dijk 1972: 357 Fig. 1 rev. 1–3)

[^{d}en.ki.ke$_4$ da]g ⸢agrun.na⸣.ke$_4$ / [ḫe$_2$].⸢em⸣.ma.an.du$_8$.du$_8$.e (Alster and van Dijk 1972: 358 Fig. 2 obv. 12–13)

⸢^{d}en.ki.ke$_4$ dag⸣ ag[run.na.ke$_4$] / [ḫe$_2$.em.m]a.an.d[u$_8$.du$_8$.e] (Alster and van Dijk 1972: 358 Fig. 3 obv. 11′–12′)

^{d}en.ki.k[e$_4$] d[ag ag]run.na.ke$_4$ ⸢im.ma⸣.ab.du$_8$.du$_8$.e (CUSAS 32 7 iv 31′)

^{d}en.ki.ke$_4$ dag agru[n.na.ke$_4$] ḫe$_2$.⸢em.ma.an⸣.[du$_8^?$.du$_8^?$.e$^?$] (Michalowski 1981: 14 obv. 12)

106 A$_{ii\ 36}$ lag mun šu u$_3$.[me.ti nam.šub eridu]⸢^{ki}*.ga⸣* [x x x x]

lag mun.na / ⸢šu⸣ u$_3$.me.ti / nam.šub u$_3$.me.si$_3$ (Alster and van Dijk 1972: 357 Fig. 1 rev. 4–6)

[lag mun.na] šu u$_3$.mu.e.[ti] / [. . .] (Alster and van Dijk 1972: 358 Fig. 2 obv. 14–rev. 1)

lag mun šu im.ma.an.ti / kaš sag 1 sila$_3$.ta.am$_3$ u$_3$.mu.e.⸢šub⸣ / [nam].⸢giš.pa⸣ u$_3$.me.ni.šub (CUSAS 32 7 v 3–5)

x x [. . .] / [. . .] (Michalowski 1981: 14 obv. 13–rev. 1′)

[. . . n]e$^?$.ke$_4$: u$_3$ ^{u2}ḫa.šu.u$_2$ šu u.me.ti / na[m.šub eridu^{ki}.ga u.m]e.ni.si$_3$ (STO 1: 128–129)

lag mun u$_3$ ḫa$^!$(GIR).še.na u$_3$.un.daḫ u$_3$.bi$_2$.i[n x (x)] / *ki-ir-ba-an ṭa-ab-ti u$_3$ ḫa-ši-i uṣ-ṣa-a[b$^?$* x x x] (CT 4 8 rev. 15–16)

[lag mun].na šu u$_4$.me.ti / [nam.šub er]idu^{ki}.ga u$_4$.me.si$_3$ (STVC 11 obv. 6′–7′)

107 A$_{ii\ 37}$ ka.ka.na$^!$(MA)[508] u$_3$.[me.ni.gar ....]

⸢ka⸣.ka.na u$_3$.me.gar / ⸢še$_{10}$⸣.gen$_7$ ḫe$_2$.dur$_2$.re / bu.lu.uḫ$_2$.gen$_7$ / ḫe$_2$.si.il.le (Alster and van Dijk 1972: 357 Fig. 1 rev. 7–10)

[. . .] / [še$_{10}$.gen$_7$] ⸢ḫe$_2$⸣.[dur$_2$.re] / [bu.lu.uḫ$_2$].⸢gen$_7$⸣ ḫe$_2$.si.⸢il.e⸣ (Alster and van Dijk 1972: 358 Fig. 2 rev. 2–4)

[lu$_2$.bi igi] ^{d}utu.še$_3$ u$_3$.mu.ni.nag / [še$_{10}$.gen$_7$ ḫe$_2$].⸢du.re⸣ / [. . .] (CUSAS 32 7 v 6–8)

[. . .] / ⸢še.ge.en ḫe$_2$⸣.d[u.re] / [bu].lu.uḫ$_2$.ge.e[n . . .] (Michalowski 1981: 14 rev. 2′–4′)

lu$_2$.u$_{18}$.lu dumu dingir.ra.na ka.bi.ta u.me.ni.gar / lu$_2$ du[mu dingir.ra.na še$_{10}$.gen$_7$ ḫe$_2$.du]r$_2$.re bu.luḫ.gen$_7$ «ri» ḫe$_2$.en.si.il.e (STO 1: 129–130)

še$_{10}$.<gen$_7$> ki.še$_3$ ḫe$_2$.si.il.le / *ki-ma ši-it-t[im li-id-di$^?$*]

bu.lu.uḫ.gen$_7$ ḫe$_2$.si.il.le / *ki-ma g[i-šu-tim li-ig-šu$^?$*] (CT 4 8 rev. 17–18)

[k]a.ka u$_3$.me.ni.gar (STVC 11 obv. 8′)

105 May Enki release it (= the bile) at the portico of (his) cella![509]
106 You should take a lump of salt, you should cast the spell of Eridu over it,[510]
107 You should put it in his mouth, so that it (= the bile) may come out like excrement,

508 Michalowski (1981: 16) reads the beginning of the line as ka.ka.še$_3$, but the last sign of this sequence is clearly MA, presumably a mistake or banalization based on the frequent invocation label KA.INIM.MA.

509 The subjunctive-optative ḫe$_2$- prefix in lines 105 and 107–108 originally had two separate uses: in line 105 the ḫe$_2$- prefix is deontic, whereas in lines 107–108 it is epistemic; see Civil 2000: 33 for the definition of these terms. In the first millennium, however, as shown by bilingual texts, these two uses were conflated and translated with the precative in Akkadian.

510 In CUSAS 32 7 there are a couple of additional instructions, namely kaš sag 1 sila$_3$.ta.am$_3$ u$_3$.mu.e.šub 'you put it in one litre of high-quality beer' (line 106) and [lu$_2$.bi igi] ^{d}utu.še$_3$ u$_3$.mu.ni.nag 'you should have that man drink it before sunrise' (line 107).

108 A$_{ii\ 38}$ im$^!$(AḪ).gen$_7$ gu.du.ni.ta ḫe$_2$.e[m.ma.ra].⸢e$_3$⸣ ⸢: bu⸣.lu.uḫ.⸢gen$_7$ ḫe$_2$⸣.[si.il.le]

⸢im⸣.gen$_7$ gu.du.ni.ta / ⸢ḫe$_2$⸣.em.ma.ra.du / ⸢ka⸣.inim.ma ze$_2$.kam (Alster and van Dijk 1972: 357 Fig. 1 rev. 11–13)

⸢im.gen$_7$⸣ gu$_3$.du$_{11}$.ni.ta ḫe$_2$.em.ma.ra.ed$_3$.de$_3$ / tu$_6$ en$_2$.ur$_5$.ru (Alster and van Dijk 1972: 358 Fig. 2 rev. 5–6)

⸢tu$_6^?$ en$^?$.nu⸣.[ru] (Alster and van Dijk 1972: 358 Fig. 3 rev. 1′)

[im.ge].⸢en gu.du⸣.n[i.ta . . .] ⸢ḫe$_2$⸣ x x [. . .] (Michalowski 1981: 14 rev. 5′)

im.ma gu.du.a.ni.ta ḫe$_2$.em.ma.ra.⸢e$_3$⸣ (STO 1: 130)

im.gen$_7$ gu$^!$(ŠE).du.še$_3$ e$_3$.ib$_2$.ta / *ki-ma š[a-ri-im li-še-ṣi$^?$*] (CT 4 8 rev. 19)

---

109 A$_{ii\ 39}$ EN$_2$ *mar-tu mar-tu mar-tu* ⸢*pa*⸣*-š[it-tu$_2$-ma]*[511]

110 A$_{ii\ 40}$ *mar-tu* GIM ⸢IGIRA$_2^{mušen}$⸣ SIG$_7$ *it-ta-na-al-lak* ⸢*a*⸣*-l[ak-ta]*[512]

111 A$_{ii\ 41}$ *it-ta-na-za-*⸢*az*⸣ *ina gi-sal-li ša* BAD$_3$

112 A$_{ii\ 42}$ *i-da-gal* ⸢*a-ki*⸣*-lum* ⸢*ak*⸣*-li i-da-gal ša$_2$-tu-u$_2$ ku-ru-un-ni*

113 A$_{ii\ 43}$ *ki-i tak-ka-la* ⸢*ak-la*⸣ *ki-i ta-ša-ta-a ku-ru-un-ni*

114 A$_{ii\ 44}$ *a-ma-qu$_2$-tak-ku-nu-šim-*⸢*ma*⸣ *tu-ga-ša-a ki-i* GUD TU$_6$ EN$_2$

---

115 A$_{ii\ 45}$ EN$_2$ UD$_5$ *ar-qa$_2$-at a-*⸢*ruq*⸣ DUMU-*ša a-ruq* ^{lu2}SIPA-*ša a-ruq na-qid-*⸢*sa*⸣[513]

✝

108 So that it may pass from his anus like wind, so that it may come up like a burp.'

---

109 Incantation: 'O Bile! O Bile! Bile is the *pāšittu* disease (viz., the one who obliterates),

110 Bile constantly travels the pathways$^?$ like a yellow heron,[514]

111 It constantly perches on the reed fence on top of the wall,

112 It looks at the one who is eating bread, it looks at the one who is drinking beer:

113 "When you all eat bread, when you all drink beer,

114 I will attack you, and then you will belch like an ox".' Incantation-formula.

---

115 Incantation: 'The nanny goat is yellow, her offspring is yellow, her shepherd is yellow, her overseer is yellow,

---

511 Lines 109–114 are edited by Collins (1999: 230–231) as Martu 1.

512 Collins (1999: 230) reads the final word in the line as ⸢*a-lak*$^?$⸣-[*ta*], hence the translation '*martu* keeps walking the pat[h$^?$]'. Alternatively, this fragmentary passage could perhaps be rendered *a-p*[*a-ra*] for *appāru* 'reed marsh' (Cadelli 2000: 198), although this is less likely since this word is usually spelled with the sign AP as the first element (CAD A/2 179–181).

513 Lines 115–119 are edited by Collins (1999: 231–232) as Martu 2. For an Old Assyrian version of this incantation, see Michel 2004 as well as Wasserman and Zomer 2022: 62–63.

514 It is difficult to establish a connection between bile and the yellow IGIRA$_2$ = Akk. *igirû* bird, normally equated with the heron: herons are usually white or grey but have yellow eyes (and beaks), which may have provided a link to patients suffering from medical conditions that are somehow related to bile, including the two types of jaundice, both of which are thematised in different parts of this tablet. The logographic sequence IGIRA$_2^{mušen}$ SIG$_7$ may have served, on a distinct orthographic level, as a pun for IGI RA SIG$_7$, meaning 'eyes struck with yellow'.

116 A$_{ii 46}$ *ina e-ki* SIG$_7$ U$_2$.MEŠ SIG$_7$.MEŠ ⸢*ik*⸣-*kal ina a-tap-pi a-ruq-ti* A.MEŠ SIG$_7$.MEŠ *i-šat-ti*
117 A$_{ii 47}$ *i-suk-ši* ^{giš}GIDRU *ul u$_2$-tir-*⸢*ra*⸣ *pa-ni-ša* : *i**-*suk**-*ši*[515] *kir-ba-na$_7$ ul u$_2$-šaq-qa-a re-ši-ša*
118 A$_{ii 48}$ ⸢*i*⸣*-*suk-ši bil$_2$-li*[516] ^{u2}ḪAR.⸢ḪAR⸣ *u* MUN : *mar-tu* GIM *im-ba-ri ana ša$_2$-ḫa-ḫi it-bi*
119 A$_{ii 49}$ ⸢EN$_2$ *ul*⸣ *ia-ut-tu* EN$_2$ ^{d}*e$_2$-*⸢*a*⸣ *u* ^{d}*asal-*⸢*lu$_2$-ḫi* EN$_2$ ^{d}*da*⸣-*mu u* ^{d}*gu-la* TU$_6$ EN$_2$[517]

---

120 A$_{ii 50}$ K[A.INIM.MA *š*]*a pa-šit-ti* ⸢DU$_3$⸣.D[U$_3$.B]I ^{u2}ḪAR.ḪAR ^{šim}LI MUN SUM^{sar} *pa-pi-ra* DIŠ-*niš* SIG$_3$-⸢*aṣ*⸣
121 A$_{ii 51}$ ⸢EN$_2$⸣ [x x] x [x x x] x ŠID-*nu la pa-tan* NAG-*ma* [x] x x ⸢TI-*uṭ*⸣

---

122 A$_{ii 52}$ EN$_2$ x [..............................] x ša e li *ša lib-*⸢*bi*⸣ [.................................] x ⸢ad$^?$⸣
123 A$_{ii 53}$ x [.................................. *lib-l*]*uṭ ina qi$_2$-bit* ^{d}*e$_2$-*⸢*a*⸣ [................ *l*]*ip-ṭur* ⸢EN$_2$⸣

☤

116 On a yellow canal bank, it eats yellow grass, it drinks yellow water from a yellow canal:
117 (Whenever) one throws a stick at it, it does not turn its face; (whenever) one throws a clod at it, it does not raise its head,
118 (But whenever) one throws a mixture of *ḫašû* ('thyme') and salt at it, the bile rises until it dissolves like a fog.
119 The incantation is not mine; it is the incantation of Ea and Asalluḫi; it is the incantation of Damu and Gula.' Incantation-formula.

---

120 An invocation for *pāšittu* disease. Its ritual: you stir (*tamaḫḫaṣ*) *ḫašû* 'thyme'), *burāšu* (a kind of juniper), salt, *šūmū* ('garlic'), (and) beer bread together,
121 you recite (*tamannu*) the incantation . . . he drinks (*išattī-ma*) it on an empty stomach, and then . . . he will recover (*iballuṭ*).

---

122 Incantation: '. . . of the belly . . .
123 . . . may he live, may Ea release . . .' Incantation.

---

515 The syllabic rendering *i-suk-ši* is nearly identical to NAG-*ši* in form. This similarity probably led Collins (1999: 232) to read, in line with Köcher's (1980) hand-copy, the second occurrence as NAG-*ši*, which he then emended to *i*$^!$-*suk*$^!$-*ši*. Collations of the tablet show that the signs in question are actually *i-suk-ši*.

516 For reading this form as a syllabic spelling of *billu* 'mixture', see already Cadelli 2000: 198 and 231. Collins (1999: 232) reads it as *pillû* 'mandrake'.

517 The gap in lines 119–125 has partially been filled with the help of K 13344 + K 17699, which is a direct joint to MS A. The join was found by Zs. Földi in 2023.

124 A$_{ii\ 54}$ [KID$_3$.KID$_3$.BI .... k]*ab-ru-ti u* ⸢MUN NU KU$_3$⸣*-ti* ŠUB-*di*
125 A$_{ii\ 55}$ [*ana* Š]A$_3$ ⸢EN$_2$⸣ Š[ID ....] *la pa-tan* NAG-*ma ina-eš*

---

126 A$_{ii\ 56}$ [5[518] K]A.INIM.MA ZE$_2$.A.KAM

---

127 A$_{ii\ 57}$ IG[I.4.G]AL$_2$.LA ILLU ⸢LI.TAR SUD$_2$⸣ *ina* A ⸢NAG⸣-*šu$_2$*
[I]GI.4.GAL$_2$.LA ILLU ⸢LI$^?$⸣.[TAR] / [. . .] (BAM 72: 2′–3′)

---

128 A$_{ii\ 58}$ 14 N[UMUN G]I.ZU$_2$.LUM.MA SUD$_2$ *ina* 5 GIN$_2$ ⸢I$_3$.GIŠ⸣ *u* KAŠ NAG-⸢*šu$_2$*⸣
NUMUN GI.ZU$_2$.LUM.MA SUD$_2$ *ina* KAŠ NAG (STO 3: 19)
[NUMUN G]I.ZU$_2$.LUM.MA SUD$_2$ *i*[*na* . . .] (BAM 60: 5′)

---

129 A$_{ii\ 59}$ 21 ⸢^{u2}⸣*[*na*]*b**-⸢*ruq*⸣*-*qa ina* 10 GIN$_2$ I$_3$.GIŠ *u* KAŠ NAG-*šu$_2$*
^{u2}*nam-ruq-qa* SUD$_2$ *ina* KAŠ NAG (STO 3: 19)
[^{u2}*na*]*m-ru-qu* SUD$_2$ *ina* KAŠ SAG [. . .] (BAM 60: 6′)
[DIŠ KI MIN] ^{u2}*nab-ru-qu* SUD$_2$ / [*ina* KA]Š ⸢NU *pa-tan* NAG⸣-*ma* / [. . .] (BAM 246: 11–13)

---

124 Its ritual: . . . you put (*tanaddi*) . . . thick . . . and impure salt,
125 you recite (*tamannu*)$^?$ the incantation over it . . . he drinks (*išattī-ma*) it on an empty stomach; then he will get well.

---

126 Five$^?$ invocations for bile.

---

127 You pound (*tasâk*) a fourth of a shekel of resin from *abukkatu* (a tree), (and) you have him drink (*tašaqqīšu*) it in water.

---

128 You pound (*tasâk*) fourteen seeds from *kūru* (a plant), (and) you have him drink (*tašaqqīšu*) it in five shekels of oil and beer.

---

129 You have him drink (*tašaqqīšu*) twenty-one (pieces of) *namruqqu* (a plant) in ten shekels of oil and beer.

---

518 Ritter (1965: 312) suggests reconstructing the number 5 before KA.INIM.MA, based on the number of incantations that precede this line, and there is room in the break for a numeral. It is unclear, however, whether the KA.INIM.MA statements in lines 98 and 120 are being counted as rubrics.

130 A$_{ii\ 60}$ 15 ŠE ⸢^{u2}⸣*[IG]I*-*lim ina* 1/2 SILA$_3$ I$_3$.GIŠ *u* KAŠ NAG-*šu*$_2$

---

131 A$_{ii\ 61}$ 90 ^{u2}[*sis-sin-n*]*i* ŠA$_3$-*bi ina* 10 GIN$_2$ A NAG-*šu*$_2$

90 ^{u2}*si-sin-ni* ŠA$_3$ *mal-ma-liš* SUD$_2$ *ina* KAŠ ^{lu2}KURUN$_2$.NA NU *pa-tan* NAG-*ma ina* ⸢DUR$_2$-*šu*$_2$⸣ SI.SA$_2$-*ma* ⸢TI⸣ (STO 2: 146)

⸢4$^?$⸣-*ut* ^{u2}*sis-sin-nu* ŠA$_3$-[*bi*] / [. . .] (BAM 72: 3′–4′)

---

132 A$_{ii\ 62}$ IGI.4.GAL$_2$.[LA] ⸢U$_2$⸣* *ma-at-qa ina* 10 GIN$_2$ A NAG-*šu*$_2$

ana ŠA$_3$ UTUL$_2$ ŠUB-*ma* ⸢IGI.4⸣.GAL$_2$.LA U$_2$ *mat-qa* IGI.4.GAL$_2$.LA U$_2$ TUR *mat*-⸢*qu*⸣ IGI.4.GAL$_2$.LA ^{u2}*a-ra-ri-ia*$_2$-⸢*nu*⸣ : ^{u2}*mer-gi-ra-a*-⸢*nu*⸣ (STO 2: 145)

---

133 A$_{ii\ 63}$ IGI.4.GAL$_2$.⸢LA U$_2$⸣ NAM.TI.LA *ina* 10 GIN$_2$ I$_3$.GIŠ NAG-*šu*$_2$

---

134 A$_{ii\ 64}$ 1/2 GIN$_2$ ^{u2}*a-ra-ri-a-nu ina* 10 GIN$_2$ A NAG-*šu*$_2$

ana ŠA$_3$ UTUL$_2$ ŠUB-*ma* ⸢IGI.4⸣.GAL$_2$.LA U$_2$ *mat-qa* IGI.4.GAL$_2$.LA U$_2$ TUR *mat*-⸢*qu*⸣ IGI.4.GAL$_2$.LA ^{u2}*a-ra-ri-ia*$_2$-⸢*nu*⸣ : ^{u2}*mer-gi-ra-a*-⸢*nu*⸣ (STO 2: 145)

[1/2 GI]N$_2$ ^{u2}*a*-⸢*ra*⸣-*ri-a-nu* / [. . .] (BAM 72: 8′–9′)

---

130 You have him drink (*tašaqqīšu*) fifteen grains of *imḫur-līm* ('faces a thousand' plant) in half a litre of oil and beer.

---

131 You have him drink (*tašaqqīšu*) ninety (grains)[519] of *sissinni libbi* ('date spadix for the innards' plant) in ten shekels of water.

---

132 You have him drink (*tašaqqīšu*) a fourth of a shekel of *šammu matqu* ('sweet plant') in ten shekels of water.

---

133 You have him drink (*tašaqqīšu*) a fourth of a shekel of *šammi balāṭi* ('plant of life') in ten shekels of oil.

---

134 You have him drink (*tašaqqīšu*) half a shekel of *arariānu* (a plant) in ten shekels of water.

---

519 For the 90 (grains of) *sissinni libbi*, see STO 2: 146.

135 A$_{ii\ 65}$ IGI.4.GAL$_2$.LA ^{u2}⸢IGI⸣.NIŠ *ina* 10 GIN$_2$ A NAG-*šu*$_2$

---

136 A$_{ii\ 66}$ IGI.4.GAL$_2$.LA ^{u2}*me-er-gi-ra-nu ina* 10 GIN$_2$ KAŠ [NAG-*šu*$_2$]
ana ŠA$_3$ UTUL$_2$ ŠUB-*ma* ⸢IGI.4⸣.GAL$_2$.LA U$_2$ *mat-qa* IGI.4.GAL$_2$.LA U$_2$ TUR *mat-*⸢*qu*⸣ IGI.4.GAL$_2$.LA ^{u2}*a-ra-ri-ia*$_2$-⸢*nu*⸣ : ^{u2}*mer-gi-ra-a-*⸢*nu*⸣ (STO 2: 145)

---

137 A$_{ii\ 67}$ DIŠ NA ZE$_2$ DAB-*su* GAZI^{sar} SUD$_2$ *ina* KAŠ NAG-*ma i-ar*$_2$-*ru*$_3$: DIŠ KI MIN *ḫi-qa* KAŠ NAG-⸢*ma i*⸣-*a*[*r*$_2$-*ru*$_3$]

---

138 A$_{ii\ 68}$ DIŠ KI MIN *ḫi-qa* A.GEŠTIN.NA KALAG.GA NAG-*ma i-ar*$_2$-*ru*$_3$: DIŠ KI MIN ^{šim}LI SUD$_2$ *ina* ⸢KAŠ⸣ NAG-⸢*ma*⸣ *i*-⸢*ar*$_2$⸣-*ru*$_3$

---

139 A$_{ii\ 69}$ DIŠ KI MIN ^{u2}*me-er-gi-ra-a-na* SUD$_2$ *ina* A NAG-*ma i-ar*$_2$-*ru*$_3$: DIŠ KI MIN ^{u2}IGI-*lim* SUD$_2$ *ina* KAŠ NAG-*ma i-ar*$_2$-*ru*$_3$

---

135 You have him drink (*tašaqqīšu*) a fourth of a shekel of *imḫur-ešrā* ('faces twenty' plant) in ten shekels of water.

---

136 You have him drink (*tašaqqīšu*) a fourth of a shekel of *mergirānu* (a plant) in ten shekels of beer.

---

137 If someone has been seized (*iṣbassu*) by bile (*martu*): you pound (*tasâk*) *kasû* ('tamarind'), he drinks (*išattī-ma*) it in beer, and then he will vomit. If DITTO, he drinks *ḫīqu* ('diluted beer') (and) beer, and then he will vomit.

---

138 If DITTO, he drinks (*išattī-ma*) *ḫīqu* ('diluted beer') (and) strong vinegar, and then he will vomit. If DITTO, you pound (*tasâk*) *burāšu* (a kind of juniper), he drinks it in beer, and then he will vomit.

---

139 If DITTO, you pound *(tasâk) mergirānu* (a plant), he drinks (*išattī-ma*) it in water, and then he will vomit. If DITTO, you pound *imḫur-līm* ('faces a thousand' plant), he drinks it in beer, and then he will vomit.

---

140 A$_{ii\ 70}$ DIŠ KI MIN MUN *lu ina* A *lu ina* KAŠ NAG-*ma i-ar*$_2$*-ru*$_3$: DIŠ KI MIN SUM^{sar} SUD$_2$ *ina* A NAG-*ma i-ar*$_2$*-ru*$_3$
DIŠ NA ZE$_2$ GIG SUM^{sar} SUD$_2$ *ina* A NU *pa-tan* NAG (STO 3: 14)
[x x x GI]G SUM^{sar} SUD$_2$ *ina* [. . .] (BAM 60: 1′)

---

141 A$_{iii\ 1}$ DIŠ KI MIN ILLU LI.TAR SUD$_2$ *ina* A ⸢NAG⸣*-*ma i-ar*$_2$*-ru*$_3$:[520] DIŠ KI MIN ILLU LI.TAR SUD$_2$ *ina* A *tara-muk ina* MUL$_4$ *tuš-bat* NAG-*ma i-ar*$_2$*-ru*$_3$

---

142 A$_{iii\ 2}$ DIŠ KI MIN ^{u2}UKUŠ$_2$.ḪAB ^{šim}BULUḪ ^{u2}ḪAR.ḪAR *ina* I$_3$ *ina* MUL$_4$ *tuš-bat* NAG-*ma i-ar*$_2$*-ru*$_3$
143 A$_{iii\ 3}$ DIŠ KI MIN ^{u2}⸢NU⸣.LUḪ.ḪA SUM^{sar} *a-ḫe-na-a* SUD$_2$ *ina* KAŠ NAG-*ma i-ar*$_2$*-ru*$_3$

---

†

140 If DITTO, he drinks (*išattī-ma*) salt in either water or beer, and then he will vomit. If DITTO, you pound (*tasâk*) *šūmū* ('garlic'),[521] he drinks it in water, and then he will vomit.

---

141 If DITTO, you pound (*tasâk*) resin from *abukkatu* (a tree), he drinks (*išattī-ma*) it in water, and then he will vomit. If DITTO, you pound resin from *abukkatu* (a tree), you soak it in water,[522] you leave it out overnight under the stars, he drinks it, and then he will vomit.

---

142 If DITTO, you leave *irrû* ('cucumber'), *baluḫḫu* ('ferula gummosa'), (and) *ḫašû* ('thyme')[523] in oil out overnight under the stars, he drinks (*išattī-ma*) them, and then he will vomit.
143 If DITTO, you pound (*tasâk*) *nuḫurtu* ('asafoetida') (and) *šūmū* ('garlic') separately, he drinks them in beer, and then he will vomit.

---

520 The scribe seems to have initially placed a *Glossenkeil* after *i*$_3$*-ar*$_2$ by mistake, which forced him to add the AŠ (= *ru*$_3$) on top of this first *Glossenkeil*, yielding *i*$_3$*-ar*$_2$*-ru*$_3$; he then had to write a second *Glossenkeil* after the complete form.
521 The last ingredient in the last line of the second column, namely SUM^{sar} = Akk. *šūmū* ('garlic'), harkens back to the list of simples against bile in lines 14–17 of the first column. The same list also occurs at the beginning of BAM 60.
522 At the beginning of the third column, the distinctive element for treating bile is soaking the resin from the *abukkatu* tree in water rather than beer. This element is also mentioned, in connection with bile, in BAM 429: 10′, which is usually thought to represent a manuscript of the Therapeutic Vademecum BAM 1. However, since the list of ingredients is missing from the passage mentioning bile in BAM 429: 6′–12′, we cannot be certain how much overlap there is between this passage and the corresponding part of the Therapeutic Vademecum BAM 1 i 30–34. For the section concerned with bile in BAM 1 i 30–34, see also the discussion in line 26 above.
523 The three ingredients *irrû*, *baluḫḫu* and *ḫašû* are found together in BAM 108 obv. 8–14 and BAM 168 rev. 21–24, both with the medical incipit: DIŠ NA ŠA$_3$-*šu*$_2$ KUM$_2$ TUKU-*ši* KUM$_2$ ŠA$_3$ *ša*$_2$*-ḫa-ṭi* 'if someone has heat in his belly: in order to remove the heat of the belly, (. . .)'. The fourth ingredient in both texts is *nuḫurtu*, which occurs here in the next line (143), as part of a separate prescription.

144 A$_{iii\ 4}$ DIŠ NA IGI.⸢SIG$_7$⸣.SIG$_7$ GIG-*ma* GIG-*su ana* ŠA$_3$ IGI.MIN-*šu*$_2$ E$_{11}$-*a* ŠA$_3$ IGI.MEŠ-*šu*$_2$ GU.MEŠ SIG$_7$.MEŠ *ud-du-ḫu*
DIŠ NA *aḫ-ḫa-zu ana* IGI.MIN-*šu*$_2$ E$_{11}$-*a-ma* IGI.MIN-*šu*$_2$ GU.MEŠ SIG$_7$.MEŠ ⸢*ud*⸣-*du-ḫa* (STO 3: 250)

145 A$_{iii\ 5}$ ŠA$_3$.MEŠ-⸢*šu*$_2$ *na*⸣-*šu-u* NINDA *u* KAŠ *u*$_2$-*tar-ra* NA BI IM DU$_3$.A.BI GIG *u*$_2$-*za-bal-ma* BA.UŠ$_2$
ŠA$_3$.MEŠ-*šu*$_2$ *na-šu-u*$_2$ NINDA *u* KAŠ *u*$_2$-*tar-ra* NA BI *u*$_2$-*za-bal-ma* [NU T]I ⸢UŠ$_2$⸣ (STO 3: 251)

---

146 A$_{iii\ 6}$ DIŠ ⸢NA* IGI⸣.SIG$_7$.SIG$_7$ ⸢GIG⸣*-*ma* SAG.DU-*su pa-nu-šu*$_2$ *ka-lu* ADDA-*šu*$_2$ SUḪUŠ EME-*šu*$_2$ *ṣa-bit ši-pir-šu*$_2$ SUMUN-*ma* BA.UŠ$_2$
DIŠ NA *aḫ-ḫa-zu* GIG SAG.DU-*su pa-nu-šu* SU-*šu*$_2$ *ka-la-šu*$_2$ *u*$_3$ SUḪUŠ E[ME-*šu*$_2$ DAB] / *ana* GIG *šu-a-tu* ^{lu2}A.ZU ŠU-*su* NU *ub-bal* NA BI UŠ$_2$ NU [TI] (STO 3: 252–253)

---

144 If someone suffers (*maruṣ-ma*) from *amurriqānu*-jaundice,[524] and then his illness goes up (*illâ*) into his eyes (and) yellow filaments cover the inside of his eyes,

145 his internal organs (*qerbū*) heave[525] (and) he regurgitates bread and beer, that man suffers (*maruṣ*) from every kind of wind, he will linger for a little while, and then he will die (*imât*).[526]

---

146 If someone suffers (*maruṣ-ma*) from *amurriqānu*-jaundice, and his head, his face, the entire trunk of his body (*pagru*),[527] (and) the root of his tongue are seized (*ṣabit*),[528] his affliction will last a long time (*ilabbir-ma*),[529] and then he will die (*imât*).

---

524 For a discussion of the type of jaundice called IGI.SIG$_7$.SIG$_7$ = Akk. *amurriqānu*, see Fincke 2000: 190–192 and Thavapalan 2020: 74–76.

525 For this symptom, see the discussion in Stol 2006: 108–109.

526 Here, in lines 144–146, as well as in lines 250–253 below, the text has negative diagnoses (*imât* 'he will die'), yet treatments for these seemingly untreatable conditions follow in lines 148–164; for an important discussion of diagnostic statements like these in therapeutic texts, see Stol 1991–1992. The use of a negative prognosis and certain turns of phrase might suggest that these lines come from the Diagnostic Handbook. If they derive from the Diagnostic Handbook, the negative prognoses could have resulted from copying the source text in a mechanical way (see Scheyhing 2007 for further discussion). Given the apparent competition between the disciplines of the physician and the exorcist (see Johnson 2018 and Geller 2018), however, it is more likely that the negative prognoses represent the standard view of the diagnostician (*āšipu*, or more specifically the KA.PIRIG), whereas the physician (*asû*) represented in these texts saw *amurriqānu* as treatable and offered treatments in lines 148–164. Still the inclusion of these diagnostic statements here makes clear that the physician saw this medical condition as more severe than the conditions earlier in the text. The further progression in the severity of the illnesses is apparent in lines 252–253 below, where the physician refuses to treat a patient with *aḫḫāzu* (*pace* Cadelli 2021: 20).

527 This translation attempts to bridge the term in the main text, viz. ADDA = Akk. *pagru*, and the different term in the parallel, viz. SU = Akk. *zumru*.

528 Presumably all the mentioned body parts 'are seized', but the list of body parts is followed by a syllabically written form of the stative in the singular, namely *ṣabit*. We might have expected a masculine plural form of the stative such as *ṣabtū*.

529 The same idiom is also found in EYES 2: 54 (BAM 10 p. 122). However, here we have a parallel between the temporal verbs referring to a relatively short period of time (*zabālu* in the D-stem) and a longer period (*labāru*), followed in both cases with the negative prognosis *imât* 'he will die'.

147 A$_{\text{iii 7}}$ DIŠ NA SU-*šu*$_2$ SIG$_7$ *pa-nu-šu*$_2$ SIG$_7$ *ši-ḫat* UZU TUKU (eras.)*[530] *a-mur-ri-qa-nu* MU.NI

[DIŠ SU-*šu*$_2$ SIG$_7$ IGI].MEŠ-*šu*$_2$ SIG$_7$ *šiḫ-ḫat* UZU TUKU.MEŠ *a-mur-*[*ri-q*]*a-nu* M[U.NI] (Sagig 33: 92)

[DIŠ IGI.MEŠ-*šu*$_2$ SI]G$_7$ ŠA$_3$ IGI.MIN-*šu*$_2$ SIG$_7$ *u* SUḪUŠ EME-*šu*$_2$ GE$_6$ [*a*]*ḫ-ḫ*[*a-zu* MU.NI] (Sagig 33: 93)

[DIŠ SU-*šu*$_2$ SI]G$_7$ IGI.MIN-*šu*$_2$ SIG$_7$.MEŠ *šiḫ-ḫat* UZU TUKU.MEŠ *a-mu-ri-qa-nu* (Sagig 18: 24)

DIŠ NA SU-*šu*$_2$ SIG$_7$ IGI-*šu*$_2$ SIG$_7$ *u* GE$_6$ SUḪUŠ EME-*šu*$_2$ GE$_6$ ⸢*aḫ*⸣-*ḫ*[*a-z*]*u* MU.NE (STO 3: 233)

---

148 A$_{\text{iii 8}}$ ^{šim}LI SUD$_2$ *ina* KAŠ NAG ^{šim}ŠE.LI SUD$_2$ *ina* KAŠ NAG ^{šim}ŠEŠ SUD$_2$ *ina* KAŠ NAG

149 A$_{\text{iii 9}}$ SUḪUŠ ^{giš}NAM.TAR NITA$_2$ *ša*$_2$ ^{im}SI.SA$_2$ *ša*$_2$ GURUN NU IL$_2$ SUD$_2$ *ina* KAŠ NAG $^{\text{u2}}$*mur-ra-an* KUR-*i* SUD$_2$ *ina* ⸢KAŠ* NAG⸣*

150 A$_{\text{iii 10}}$ $^{\text{u2}}$*kur-ka-na*$_7$ ⸢SUD$_2$⸣ *ina* KAŠ NAG $^{\text{u2}}$IGI-*lim* SUD$_2$ *ina* KAŠ NAG $^{\text{u2}}$*nam-ruq-qa* SUD$_2$ *ina* KAŠ ⸢NAG⸣

†

147 If someone's body is yellow (*aruq*), his face is yellow, (and) he has 'wasting away of the flesh' (*šiḫḫat šīri*), its name is *amurriqānu*-jaundice.[531]

---

148 You pound (*tasâk*) *burāšu* (a kind of juniper), (and) he drinks (*išatti*) it in beer. You pound *kikkirânu* ('juniper seed'), (and) he drinks it in beer. You pound *murru* ('myrrh'), (and) he drinks it in beer.[532]

149 You pound root from male *pillû* ('mandrake') from the north side that has not (yet) borne any fruit, (and) he drinks it in beer. You pound *murrānu* ('myrrh-like' plant)[533] of the mountains, (and) he drinks it in beer.

150 You pound *kurkanû* (a plant), (and) he drinks it in beer. You pound *imḫur-līm* ('faces a thousand' plant), (and) he drinks it in beer. You pound *namruqqu* (a plant),[534] (and) he drinks it in beer.

---

530 The sign indicated in Köcher's (1980) hand-copy as a small A written within the TUKU shows traces of intentional erasure.

531 This line, as well as line 233 below, both cite more or less verbatim two consecutive lines in the Diagnostic Handbook: our line here is an exact quote of Sagig 33: 92, whereas line 233 below seems to combine elements from Sagig 33: 92 and 93 (Labat 1951: 72–73; Heeßel 2000: 357). For further discussion, see STO 3: 233.

532 A number of the plants included in this long list of simples reappear in STT 92 ii 1–7, as a group of drugs for *amurriqānu*.

533 The logographic writing for *murrānu* is ^{giš}MA.NU.SIG$_7$.SIG$_7$ (CAD M/2 220), which is why this plant might be thought particularly appropriate for the treatment of *amurriqānu*-jaundice usually rendered with the logogram IGI.SIG$_7$.SIG$_7$.

534 Here again there seems to be a connection between the chosen ingredient, viz. *namruqqu*, and the medical condition *amurriqānu*: although *namruqqu* is actually a loanword into Akkadian, its phonetic make-up with the consonants *m-r-q* is extremely similar to *(w)arāqu*, the word for 'yellow' in Akkadian.

151 A$_{\text{iii 11}}$ $^{\text{u2}}$*nam-ruq-qa* SUD$_2$ *ina* A NAG IM.SAḪAR.NA$_4$.KUR.RA SUD$_2$ *ana* A.MEŠ ŠUB *tu*-ZAK NAG ^{šim}LI SUD$_2$ *ina* GA NAG

152 A$_{\text{iii 12}}$ ⸢^{šim}ŠE⸣.LI SUD$_2$ *ina* GA NAG ^{šim}ŠEŠ SUD$_2$ *ina* GA NAG $^{\text{u2}}$*nam-ruq-qa* SUD$_2$ *ina* GA NAG

153 A$_{\text{iii 13}}$ 5 ŠE EḪ$_3$ ⸢AN.ZAḪ⸣ *ina* KAŠ ŠUB *ina* MUL$_4$ *tuš-bat tu*-ZAK NAG ^{im}KAL.LA SUD$_2$ *ina* I$_3$ *e-re-ni u* KAŠ NAG

DIŠ NA MIN 15 ŠE.MEŠ AN.ZAḪ SUD$_2$ *ina* KAŠ *tara*-SUD *tu-zak-ka* I$_3$ *ḫal-ṣa ana* ŠA$_3$ ŠUB-*di* NU ⸢*pa*⸣-[*tan* NAG] / DIŠ NA MIN ^{im}KAL.LA SUD$_2$ *ina* I$_3$ *u* KAŠ NAG (STO 3: 246–247)

154 A$_{\text{iii 14}}$ NUMUN ^{giš}*bi-ni* ⸢$^{\text{u2}}$SUMUN⸣.DAR SUD$_2$ *ina* KAŠ NAG NUMUN ^{giš}*bi-ni* SUD$_2$ *ina* KAŠ NAG

NUMUN ^{giš}*bi-ni ina* KAŠ NAG NUMUN ^{giš}*bi-*⸢*ni*⸣ [x x x x] (STO 3: 247)

155 A$_{\text{iii 15}}$ NUMUN ^{giš}*bi-ni* SUD$_2$ *ina* ⸢I$_3$ *u* KAŠ NAG⸣ SUḪUŠ ^{giš}*šu-ši* SUD$_2$ MIN : $^{\text{u2}}$IGI.NIŠ SUD$_2$ *ina* KAŠ NAG[535]

NUMUN ^{giš}*bi-ni* SUD$_2$ *ina* I$_3$ *u* KAŠ NAG SUḪUŠ ^{giš}*šu-ši ina* I$_3$ *u* KAŠ NAG $^{\text{u2}}$IGI.NIŠ ⸢SUD$_2$⸣ *in*[*a* KAŠ NA]G.⸢MEŠ⸣ (STO 3: 248)

151 You pound *namruqqu* (a plant), (and) he drinks it in water. You pound *aban gabî* ('alum'), you put (*tanaddi*) it in water, you strain (*tuzakka*)[536] it, (and) he drinks it. You pound *burāšu* (a kind of juniper), (and) he drinks it in milk.

152 You pound *kikkirânu* ('juniper seed'), (and) he drinks it in milk. You pound *murru* ('myrrh'), (and) he drinks it in milk. You pound *namruqqu* (a plant), (and) he drinks it in milk.

153 You put five grains of powder from *anzaḫḫu* ('frit') in beer, you leave it out overnight under the stars, you strain it, (and) he drinks it. You pound *kalû* (a mineral), (and) he drinks it in oil from *erēnu* ('cedar') and beer.

154 You pound seed from *bīnu* ('tamarisk') (and) *šumuttu* ('beetroot'), (and) he drinks them in beer. You pound seed from *bīnu* ('tamarisk'), (and) he drinks it in beer.

155 You pound seed from *bīnu* ('tamarisk'), (and) he drinks it in oil and beer. You pound root from *šūšu* ('liquorice'), DITTO (= and he drinks it in oil and beer). You pound *imḫur-ešrā* ('faces twenty' plant), (and) he drinks it in beer.

---

535 The gap in lines 155–161 has been filled with the help of K 5762, which represents a direct join to MS A. The fragment was joined by Zs. Földi in 2019.

536 We take the form *tu*-ZAK as a D-stem of *zakû* 'to purify', perhaps with an overhanging /a/, to be read as *tu-zaka*(ZAK), hence *tuzakka* 'you strain', which could be analogous to orthographies like *tara*(TAR)-*bak* for *tarabbak* 'you stir into a paste'. For an explicit orthography of the verb, see *tu-zak-ka* in lines 245 and 246 below as well as *me-e-šu-nu u*$_2$*-za-ka-a* in the Old Babylonian therapeutic text CUSAS 32 73 obv 2–3. All recipes with *tuzakka* seem to involve purifying liquids by removing all non-liquid particulate matter, as in the perfume making recipes where it follows the verb *šaḫālu* 'to filter', perhaps describing a more fine-grained filtering process (Ebeling 1948: 312 ln. 4). The purified liquid is then consumed by the patient, so the removal of solid ingredients like *aban gabî* ('alum') or *anzaḫḫu* ('frit') must have played a central role in the procedure. For a survey of passages that use the D-stem of *zakû* meaning 'to strain', see Cadelli 2019: 60 and Stol 2020b: 568.

156 A$_{iii 16}$ SUḪUŠ ^{giš}MA.NU SUḪUŠ ^{giš}N[U.U]R$_{2}$.MA *ina* ⸢NINDU⸣ UŠ$_{2}$-*er* A.MEŠ *šu-nu-ti*$_{3}$ *tu*-ZAK *tu-kaṣ*$_{3}$*-ṣa* NAG-*ma ina-eš*

DIŠ MIN SUḪUŠ ^{giš}*šu-ši* SUḪUŠ ^{giš}NU.UR$_{2}$.MA *ana* A ŠUB *ina* NINDU UŠ$_{2}$-*er* E$_{11}$-*a ta-ša*$_{2}$*-ḫal* SED ⸢NU⸣ [*pa-tan*] ⸢NAG⸣.MEŠ (STO 3: 249)

[DIŠ KI MIN SUḪU]Š ^{giš}MA.NU SUḪUŠ ^{giš}⸢NU⸣.[UR$_{2}$.MA . . .] / [*tu*]-*sa*$_{3}$-*ak* [. . .] (BAM 64 ii$^{!}$ 2′–3′)

157 A$_{iii 17}$ ^{u2}*a-ṣu-ṣum-ta*$_{5}$ ^{u2}*a-nu-nu-ta*$_{5}$ *ina qut-rin-ni tu-qat-tar-šu*

DIŠ NA *aḫ-ḫa-za* DIRI ^{u2}*ṣu*$_{2}$*-ṣe-em-ta*$_{5}$ ^{u2}*a-nu-nu-ta*$_{5}$ *ina qut-ri-ni tu-qat-tar*-⸢*šu*$_{2}$⸣ (STO 3: 238)

DIŠ KI MIN ^{u2}*a-ṣu-ṣum-tu*$_{4}$ ⸢^{u2}⸣[*a-nu-nu-tu*$_{4}$ . . .] (BAM 64 ii$^{!}$ 4′)

158 A$_{iii 18}$ MUD$_{2}$ ^{d}NIN.KA$_{6}$.EDIN *ša ina* ^{u2}NINNI$_{5}$ GUB-*zu ta-maḫ-ḫar ina* I$_{3}$ EŠ.MEŠ

u MUD$_{2}$ KUN.⸢DAR.GURUN.NA⸣ ŠEŠ$_{2}$-*su-ma* ⸢*ina*⸣-[*eš*] (STO 3: 239)

MUD$_{2}$ ^{d}NIN.KA$_{6}$.EDIN ⸢*ša*⸣ [. . .] (BAM 64 ii$^{!}$ 5′)

159 A$_{iii 19}$ I$_{3}$.SUMUN *sip-pi*$_{2}$ ABUL *ki-lal-le-e* TI *ina* I$_{3}$ EŠ.MEŠ

⸢*ru-ša*⸣-*am ša si-ip-pi* ⸢ABUL *ki-lal-le*⸣-*en* TI-*qe*$_{2}$ *ana* I$_{3}$.GIŠ ŠUB-*di ta-ap-ta*-⸢*na*⸣-[*ša-aš*] (STO 3: 240)

ru-uš-ša ša sip-[*pi* x x x] (STO 3: 254)

ru-uš-ša ša ⸢*sip*$^{?}$*-pi*$^{?}$⸣ x x TI-⸢*qe*$_{2}$ KI⸣ [. . . ŠEŠ$_{2}$]-⸢*su-ma*⸣ TI (STO 4: 2)

DIŠ KI MIN I$_{3}$.SUMUN *ša sip-pi*$_{2}$ AB[UL . . .] (BAM 64 ii$^{!}$ 6′)

[. . .] / *ša* NA$_{4}$ ABUL TI-*qe*$_{2}$ ⸢KI I$_{3}$⸣ [. . .] (BAM 66 rev. 4′–5′)

156 You heat (*tesekker*) root from *ēru* (a tree) (and) root from *nurmû* ('pomegranate') in an oven, you strain this liquid, you let it cool, (and) he drinks it; then he will get well.

157 You fumigate him with *aṣuṣumtu* (a plant) (and) *anunūtu* (a plant) using a censer.

158 You collect the blood of an *ayāṣu* ('weasel') that was standing on rushes, (and) you keep anointing (*taptanaššaš*) him with it in oil.

159 You take (*teleqqe*) grease (*lušû*)[537] from both doorjambs of the city gate, you keep anointing him with it in oil,[538]

537 I$_{3}$.SUMUN = Akk. *lušû* 'old oil' is replaced by *rūšu* 'dirt' in line 240 below; both of these words also seem to pun on *russû* 'sullied' in the next line (cf. Scurlock 2014: 535 n. 47).

538 The translation of lines 159–160 partially reflects the placement of horizontal rulings and DIŠ KI MIN elements in the parallel text BAM 64 ii$^{!}$ 6′–7′, where these two lines are treated as a distinct unit. In the next line, which corresponds to line 161 of our text, BAM 64 returns to the *ina* KAŠ NAG pattern that was used earlier in the column.

160 A$_{\text{iii 20}}$ *ger$_3$-ra-am ru-⸢us⸣-sa$_3$-a*[539] *uš-te-eš-šir ti-tur-ra na-di-ta$_5$ e-ti-⸢iq⸣*

⸢*ge-er-ra ru*⸣*-us-sa$_3$-a-am* ⸢*uš-te-eš-še-er*⸣ *ti-tur-ra na-di-a-am* i x [x x] (STO 3: 241)

ger$_3$-ra-am ru-us-sa$_3$-a u[š-te-eš-šir . . .] (BAM 64 ii$^!$ 7′)

161 A$_{\text{iii 21}}$ ^{u2}NIG$_2$ GIDRU SA$_5$ SUD$_2$ *ina* ⸢KAŠ⸣ NAG ^{šim}GUR$_2$.GUR$_2$ SUD$_2$ *ina* KAŠ NAG GURUN ^{u2}*ka-zi-ri* SUD$_2$ *ina* K[AŠ NA]G*

DIŠ KI MIN ^{u2}NIG$_2$ GIDRU SA$_5$ SUD$_2$ *ina* KAŠ [. . .] / DIŠ KI MIN GURUN ^{u2}*ka-zi-ri* SU[D$_2$ . . .] (BAM 64 ii$^!$ 8′–9′)

DIŠ NA *a-mur-ri-qa-na* GIG ^{u2}NIG$_2$ GIDRU SUD$_2$ *ina* KAŠ [NAG] (Schmidtchen 2018: 464–465 obv. 12′)

DIŠ KI MIN ^{šim}KU$_7$.KU$_7$ *ina* KAŠ [NAG] / DIŠ KI MIN GURUN *ka-zi-ri ina* KAŠ [NAG] (Schmidtchen 2018: 464–465 obv. 14′–15′)

162 A$_{\text{iii 22}}$ ^{u2}ḪAR.ḪAR SUD$_2$ *ina* KAŠ NAG KUŠ[540] ^{giš}NU.UR$_2$.MA SUD$_2$ *ina* KAŠ ⸢NAG⸣ x x x x x [x x x]

[. . .] / DIŠ KI MIN SUḪUŠ ^{giš}NU.UR$_2$.MA SUD$_2$ [. . .] (BAM 64 ii$^!$ 9′–10′)

DIŠ KI MIN *ḫa-še-e in*[*a* KAŠ NAG] (Schmidtchen 2018: 464–465 rev. 1)

DIŠ KI.MIN 2 GIN$_2$ ^{giš}NU.UR$_2^!$.MA ⸢*ina*⸣ K[AŠ NAG] (Schmidtchen 2018: 464–465 rev. 3)

†

160 (and then) he / it goes straight out the sullied (*russû*) pathway, he / it marches through the abandoned causeway.[541]

161 You pound red *ḫaṭṭi rēʾi* ('shepherd's crook'), (and) he drinks it in beer. You pound *kukru* (an aromatic), (and) he drinks it in beer. You pound fruit from *kazīru* (a plant), (and) he drinks it in beer.

162 You pound *ḫašû* ('thyme'), (and) he drinks it in beer. You pound skin from *nurmû* ('pomegranate'), (and) he drinks it in beer . . .

---

539 For this reading, but understood differently as a by-form of *ruššû* 'to have a reddish sheen', see Scurlock 2014: 514 and 525. We take *ru-us-sa$_3$-a* as a D-stem verbal adjective from *russû* meaning 'sullied', parallel to the other verbal adjective later in the line, viz. *na-di-ta$_5$* 'abandoned'. Previous interpretations have read *ru-us-sa$_3$-a* as ŠUB *uṣ-ṣa-a*, with ŠUB as a logographic writing for the similar term *na-di-ta$_5$* later on in the same line (Cadelli 2000: 202 with n. 46). This is unlikely and interrupts the clear parallel between the two noun-adjective-verb sequences.

540 The logogram KUŠ, presumably for Akk. *mašku* 'skin', is not the standard orthography for the rind of a pomegranate, which is BAR, read as Akk. *qilpu*, as in *qilip nurmî*. This exceptional turn of phrase only occurs here and in AMT 73/1+ i 57 (Eypper 2016: 20–21 ln. 57). The two parallel texts have SUHUŠ and 2 GIN$_2$ in place of KUŠ, probably representing two different ways of correcting this anomalous phrase.

541 The gate with the old oil (i.e., grease), as well as the sullied and abandoned pathways in lines 159 and 160 seem to be a metaphorical representation of the patient's non-functioning orifices and gastrointestinal organs. The line clearly operates on two levels and can be translated accordingly: on the one level, it describes a patient looking for a deserted place to void his bowels, presumably after the action of walking has loosened them ('he goes straight out' and 'he marches through'), but it could also describe faecal matter passing through the rectum ('it goes straight out' and 'it marches through'), hence the reference to sullied pathways.

163 A$_{iii\ 23}$ SUḪUŠ ⸢^{u2}*EME⸣* UR.GI$_7$ SUD$_2$ *ina* KAŠ NAG IGI.6.GAL$_2$.⸢LA⸣ [..........]
DIŠ KI MIN SUḪUŠ ^{u2}EME UR.GI$_7$ SUD$_2$ [. . .] (BAM 64 ii$^!$ 11′)
DIŠ KI MIN IGI.6.GAL$_2$ ^{u2}*im-ḫur-lim i*[*na* KAŠ NAG] (Schmidtchen 2018: 464–465 rev. 2)
DIŠ KI MIN SUḪUŠ ^{u2}EME UR.GI$_7$ *ina* [KAŠ NAG] (Schmidtchen 2018: 464–465 rev. 4)

164 A$_{iii\ 24}$ ^{u2}IGI.NIŠ *qut-ri*$_3$ SUD$_2$ *ina* ⸢I$_3$⸣ *u* KAŠ NAG PA ^{giš}NU.U[R$_2$.MA ....]
DIŠ KI MIN ^{u2}IGI.NIŠ *qut-ri*$_3$ [. . .] / DIŠ KI MIN PA ^{giš}NU.UR$_2$.MA PA ^{giš}[. . .] (BAM 64 ii$^!$ 12′–13′)

---

165 A$_{iii\ 25}$ DIŠ NA IGI.SIG$_7$.SIG$_7$ DIRI ⸢SUḪUŠ⸣ ^{giš}*šu-ši* x x x [................................][542]
DIŠ KI MIN SUḪUŠ ^{giš}*šu-ši* ḪAD$_2$.DU SUD$_2$ *i*[*na* KAŠ NAG] / DIŠ KI MIN SUḪUŠ ^{giš}GI.ZU$_2$.LUM.MA *i*[*na* KAŠ NAG] (Schmidtchen 2018: 464–465 rev. 5–6)

166 A$_{iii\ 26}$ *ina* MUL$_4$ *tuš-bat* NAG *ḫu-*⸢*bi-bi-ta*$_5$⸣* [..]

---

167 A$_{iii\ 27}$ SUḪUŠ ^{giš}NU.UR$_2$.MA ⸢*ša*$_2$⸣* [^{im}SI].⸢SA$_2$⸣* [..]
168 A$_{iii\ 28}$ *šum-ma ina* x [..]

---

†

163 You pound root from *lišān kalbi* ('dog's tongue' plant), (and) he drinks it in beer. You pound a sixth of a shekel of *imḫur-līm* ('faces a thousand' plant), (and) he drinks it in beer.[543]

164 You pound *imḫur-ešrā* ('faces twenty' plant) (and) *qutru* (a plant), (and) he drinks it in oil and beer. You pound$^?$ leaves from *nurmû* ('pomegranate') (and) leaves from . . .

---

165 If someone is full (*mali*) of *amurriqānu*-jaundice: . . . root from *šūšu* ('liquorice') . . .

166 you leave it out overnight under the stars, (and) he drinks it. . . . *ḫumbabītu* (a kind of lizard)[544] . . .

---

167 Root from *nurmû* ('pomegranate') from the north side . . .

168 if . . . in . . .

---

542 Schmidtchen 2018: 465 rev. 5–6 is only a distant parallel, because the traces following SUḪUŠ ^{giš}*šu-ši* in STO do not seem to match up with either HAD$_2$.DU or SUD$_2$ in the suggested parallel. Therefore, we do not include it in our translation of the line.

543 The second half of the line has been restored using the parallel identified in Schmidtchen 2018: 465 rev. 2. While this parallel only instructs someone to drink the drugs in beer, earlier lines of STO 3 consistently include a reference to the pounding of the ingredients.

544 This rare term is listed under *humbabītu* in CAD H 234 and seems to refer to a type of lizard. The Principal Izbu Commentary describes it as *pizallur(t)u ša ṣēri* 'gecko from the steppe' (Leichty 1970: 213 ln. 43), while in Uruanna III 271 and 275 both *ḫu-bi-bi-it* A.ŠA$_3$ and *pi-za-lu-ur-tu* are equated with *iṣṣû rabītu* 'a large female gecko'. The *humbabītu* lizard is also mentioned as a medical ingredient in BAM 297 obv. 12′ (*ḫu-bi-bi-it* E$_2$), BAM 538+ ii 49′ (*ḫu-um-bi-bi-tu*$_2$) and CUSAS 32 73 obv. 7 (*li-pi-a-am ša ḫu-um-bi-bi-tim*).

169 $A_{\text{iii 29}}$ BAR ${}^{\text{giš}}$⸢NU.UR$_2$⸣.[MA ....]

170 $A_{\text{iii 30}}$ ⸢*saḫ-le$_2$*⸣*-[*e* ....]

ten missing lines

181 $A_{\text{iii 41'}}$ x x x x x [..........][545]

182 $A_{\text{iii 42'}}$ DIŠ NA IGI.SIG$_7$.SIG$_7$ DI[RI ....]
183 $A_{\text{iii 43'}}$ *ta-tab-bal* I$_3$.UDU U[KUŠ$_2$.ḪAB ....]

184 $A_{\text{iii 44'}}$ MUŠ.DIM$_2$.GURUN.⸢NA⸣ [..........]

185 $A_{\text{iii 45'}}$ x x x [..........]

twenty-two missing lines

†

169 Rind from *nurmû* ('pomegranate') . . .

170 *saḫlû* ('cress') . . .

ten missing lines

181 . . .

182 If someone is full (*mali*) of *amurriqānu*-jaundice . . .
183 you take away . . . pulp from *irrû* ('cucumber') . . .

184 *pizallur(t)u* ('gecko') . . .

185 . . .

twenty-two missing lines

545 The fragment AMT 9/6 was copied as an indirect join to MS A by Köcher (1980), but on closer examination in 2021, K. Simkó was able to join it directly to the main manuscript at this point.

208 A$_{iv\ 1}$ [DIŠ MIN x] x *ina* I$_3$.UDU UKUŠ$_2$.⸢ḪAB⸣ S[UD$_2$ *ina* KA]Š NAG : DIŠ MIN UZU GUD *kab-ra* GU$_7$.MEŠ ŠE$_{10}$ GE$_6$[546] NU IGI

---

209 A$_{iv\ 2}$ [DIŠ MIN ^{u2}]⸢NAM⸣.LU$_2$.U$_{18}$.LU[547] ^{šim}ŠEŠ *ina* ⸢I$_3$ *u*⸣ KAŠ NAG : DIŠ MIN AMA A.A ḪAD$_2$.DU SUD$_2$ *ina* I$_3$ *u* KAŠ ^{lu2}KURUN$_2$.NA NAG-*ma* BURU$_8$

---

210 A$_{iv\ 3}$ [DIŠ MI]N ^{u2}*ak-tam* ILLU LI.TAR U$_2$ BABBAR *ina* ⸢I$_3$⸣ *u* KAŠ NAG : DIŠ MIN I$_3$.UDU UKUŠ$_2$.ḪAB *ina* KAŠ NAG

---

211 A$_{iv\ 4}$ [DIŠ M]IN ^{šim}ŠEŠ NUMUN ^{šim}LI IM.SAḪAR.NA$_4$.KUR.RA SUD$_2$ *ina* I$_3$ *u* KAŠ NAG : DIŠ MIN ḪAR KUG.SIG$_{17}$ ḪUŠ.A *ina* ŠU-*šu*$_2$ GAR-*an*

---

208 If DITTO, you pound (*tasâk*) . . . in pulp from *irrû* ('cucumber'), (and) he drinks (*išatti*) it in beer. If DITTO, he keeps eating (*ītanakkal*) fatty beef, (and then) he will not have (lit. see) (*lā immar*) black faeces.

---

209 If DITTO, he drinks (*išatti*) *amīlānu* ('man-like' plant) (and) *murru* ('myrrh') in oil and beer. If DITTO, you dry (*tubbal*) (and) pound (*tasâk*) *ummi mê* ('mother of water' insect), he drinks (*išattī-ma*) it in oil and brewer's beer, and then he will vomit (*i'arru*).

---

210 If DITTO, he drinks (*išatti*) *aktam* (a plant), resin from *abukkatu* (a tree), (and) *šammu peṣû* ('white plant') in oil and beer. If DITTO, he drinks pulp from *irrû* ('cucumber') in beer.

---

211 If DITTO, you pound (*tasâk*) *murru* ('myrrh'), seed from *burāšu* (a kind of juniper), (and) *aban gabî* ('alum'), (and) he drinks them in oil and beer. If DITTO, you put a ring of red gold[548] on his hand.

---

546 Cadelli (2000: 204 and 236 n. 25) suggests reading ZI$_3$ GE$_6$ in reference to a specific kind of 'black flour' that the patient was not supposed to consume. The supporting lexical evidence, viz. AMT 91/4: 4', has since been reinterpreted as a reference to TUG$_2$ GE$_6$ 'black fabric' (Ambos 2004: 136–137). It is more likely that this statement, read as ŠE$_{10}$ GE$_6$ NU IGI, is a prognostic element meaning that the patient's faeces are no longer black, perhaps as a sign of improved health. Black faeces can be a sign of bleeding in the gastrointestinal tract.

547 See Scurlock 2014: 525 for the beginning of the line.

548 The use of a gold ring is unexpected, but it is known from at least one other therapeutic passage, namely BAM 494 iv 6: *ina an-ṣa-ab-ti* KUG.SIG$_{17}$ IGI GIG *ta-kaṣ*$_3$ 'you peel away the surface of the lesion with a golden ring'. KUG.SIG$_{17}$ ḪUŠ.A, literally 'red gold', is a designation for the highest quality or purity of gold (see Paoletti 2016); the purity of the gold may have played a role in its medicinal use.

212 A$_{iv\,5}$ [DIŠ N]A IGI.MIN-*šu*$_2$ IGI.SIG$_7$.SIG$_7$ <DIRI> PA ^{giš}NU.UR$_2$.MA SUD$_2$ *ina* ^{gi}SAG.KUD *ana* ŠA$_3$ IGI.MIN-*šu*$_2$ MU$_2$-*aḫ*
[DIŠ N]A IGI.MIN-*šu*$_2$ IGI.SIG$_7$.SIG$_7$ DIRI BAR ^{giš}NU.U[R$_2$.M]A SUD$_2$ *ina* ^{gi}SAG.KUD *ana* ŠA$_3$ IGI.MIN-*šu*$_2$ B[UN$_2^?$] (IGI 2: 115)

---

213 A$_{iv\,6}$ [DIŠ NA IGI.MIN-*š*]*u*$_2$ ⸢IGI⸣.SIG$_7$.SIG$_7$ <DIRI> IGI.MEŠ-*šu*$_2$ UZU.MEŠ-*šu*$_2$ DIRI 7 MUŠ.DIM$_2$.GURUN.NA *ri-it-ku-ba-ti*
214 A$_{iv\,7}$ [x x x x T]I-⸢*qe*$_2$ *tu-qal*⸣-*lap ina* ^{na4}NA.ZA$_3$.ḪI.LI SUD$_2$ *ina* DIDA ḪI.ḪI GU$_7$*.MEŠ-*ma ina-eš*

---

215 A$_{iv\,8}$ [..............................] x x x ⸢*saḫ*⸣-*le*$_2$-*e* (eras.)[549] ŠE.SA.A LAL-*su u* DIDA ḪI.ḪI GU$_7$*.MEŠ-*ma ina-eš*

---

212 If someone's eyes are full (*malâ*) of *amurriqānu*-jaundice: you pound (*tasâk*) leaves from *nurmû* ('pomegranate'), (and) you blow (*tanappaḫ*) it through a reed straw into his eyes.

---

213 If someone's eyes are full (*malâ*) of *amurriqānu*-jaundice, (and) his face (and) his flesh is (also) full (*malû*) of it (= *amurriqānu*): you take (*teleqqe*) seven (pairs of) copulating *pizallur(t)u* ('geckos')[550]
214 . . . you skin them, you pound (*tasâk*) them in a mortar, you mix (*tuballal*) them in *billatu* ('beerwort'), (and) he keeps eating them (*ītanakkal-ma*); then he will get well.

---

215 . . . (and) roasted *saḫlû* ('cress')—you bandage him (*taṣammissu*) with them, you mix (*tuballal*) them in *billatu* ('beerwort'), (and) he keeps eating them (*ītanakkal-ma*); then he will get well.

---

549 The sign between *saḫ-le*$_2$*-e* and ŠE.SA.A was copied as a damaged KU sign by Köcher (1980), which led to the reading ZI$_3$ ŠE.SA.A = Akk. *qēm labti* 'flour from roasted barley' in both Cadelli 2000: 205 and Scurlock 2014: 515. The KU was actually erased, partially, with parts of the following ŠE impressed over the second vertical of KU. The orthography ŠE.SA.A here probably stands for an adjectival form of the verb *qalû* 'to roast', as in *saḫlê qalûti* 'roasted cress'; the same orthography is found in AMT 82/2 iii 9 as well as NECK 5 (K 2418+) iii 155′. See also the instruction GAZI^{sar} *ki-ma* ŠE.SA.A *ta-qal*$_3$*-lu* 'you roast *kasû* ('tamarind') like *labtu* ('roasted barley')' in BAM 503+ iii 7. The scribe probably began to write the frequently occurring nominal phrase ZI$_3$ (= KU) ŠE.SA.A, but then realized that ŠE.SA.A is actually an adjective modifying *saḫlû*.
550 For the use of copulating geckos as a therapeutic ingredient, see also the Šaziga prescription KUB 4 48 ii 3-9, with further discussion in Biggs 1967: 59. For a more recent edition of the text, see Zisa 2021: 388–397 (as MS N).

216 A$_{\text{iv 9}}$ [...] x x x x *ina* I$_3$ *u* KAŠ NAG-*ma ina-eš*

217 A$_{\text{iv 10}}$ [.......................] x ḪU ⸢*ši-ši*⸣-[*ta*$_5$[551] ....] ⸢*ina** KAŠ⸣ NAG-*šu*$_2$

218 A$_{\text{iv 11}}$ [.............................] x *ta-qal-lap* x [...] ⸢NAG⸣-*šu*$_2$

219 A$_{\text{iv 12}}$ [DIŠ NA IGI.MIN-*šu*$_2$ IGI.SIG$_7$.SI]G$_7$ DIRI ^{u2}LAG A.ŠA$_3$ SUD$_2$ *ina* KAŠ NAG *an-*⸢*nu-ḫa*⸣*-r*[*a* SUD$_2$] ⸢*ina*⸣ KAŠ
220 A$_{\text{iv 13}}$ [x x x SU]D$_2$ *ina* KAŠ ŠIKA NUNUZ GA.⸢NU$_{11}$⸣^{mušen} SUD$_2$ *ina* KAŠ KUG.SIG$_{17}$ *ina* SIG$_2$ ⸢SA$_5$⸣ *ina* ŠU.MIN-*šu*$_2$ KEŠDA

221 A$_{\text{iv 14}}$ ⸢DIŠ* KI⸣* MIN ⸢^{u2}⸣[x] ⸢^{u2}⸣ŠAKIRA U$_2$ SA$_5$ ^{u2}LAL GAZ A.BI *ta-ṣa-ḫat ina* KAŠ NAG-*ma ina-eš*

216 . . . (and) he drinks (*išattī-ma*) it in oil and beer; then he will get well.

217 . . . membrane . . . (and) you have him drink (*tašaqqīšu*) it in beer.

218 . . . you skin it . . . (and) you have him drink (*tašaqqīšu*) it . . .

219 If someone's eyes are full (*malâ*) of *amurriqānu*-jaundice: you pound (*tasâk*) *kirbān eqli* ('field clod' plant), (and) he drinks (*išatti*) it in beer. You pound *alluḫaru* (a white mineral), (and he drinks it)[552] in beer.
220 You pound . . . (and he drinks it) in beer. You pound ostrich eggshell, (and he drinks it) in beer. You tie (*tarakkas*) gold in red wool[553] on both of his hands.

221 If DITTO, you crush (*taḫaššal*) . . . *šakirû* (a plant), *šammu sāmu* ('red plant'), (and) *ašqulālu* (a plant), you squeeze out their juice, he drinks (*išattī-ma*) it in beer; then he will get well.

551 The reading *ši-ši-*[*ta*$_5$] for Akkadian *šīštu* 'membrane, film' is more likely than IGI-*lim*, because the usual determinative for IGI-*lim* is missing, and the same word appears only five lines below in line 222.
552 This way of abbreviating, viz. the omission of NAG = Akk. *išatti*, is also found in STO 1: 68–69.
553 This statement harkens back to line 211, where a ring of pure red gold is placed on the patient's hand. Here we have gold used in combination with red wool, whereas in the next line (ln. 221) we have a red plant.

222 A$_{iv\ 15}$ DIŠ KI MIN G[AZI]^{sar} U$_5$ ARGAB^{mušen} U$_2$ BABBAR *ina* I$_3$.NUN SUD$_2$ IGI.MIN-*šu$_2$ te-te-ne$_2$-qi$_2$-ma ši-ši-⸢tu$_2$⸣* ZI-*aḫ*

---

223 A$_{iv\ 16}$ DIŠ NA ⸢SU⸣-*šu$_2$* SIG$_7$ 5 ŠE AN.ZAḪ SUD$_2$ *ina* I$_3$ *u* KAŠ NAG-*šu$_2$ tu-šam-ad-ma* BA.UŠ$_2$

---

224 A$_{iv\ 17}$ DIŠ NA ⸢IGI⸣.MIN-*šu$_2$ a-mur-ri-qa-nu* DIRI ^{u2}ḪAB SUD$_2$ *ina* KAŠ NAG-*ma ina-eš*

225 A$_{iv\ 18}$ DIŠ MIN SUḪUŠ ^{giš}*šu-ši tu-bal ta-sak$_3$ ina* KAŠ *tara$_3$-sa$_3$-an* IGI ^{d}UTU NAG-*ma ina-eš*

226 A$_{iv\ 19}$ DIŠ SUḪUŠ ^{u2}EME UR.GI$_7$ *tu-bal ta-sak$_3$ ina* KAŠ *tara$_3$-sa$_3$-an* NAG-*ma ina-eš*

227 A$_{iv\ 20}$ DIŠ ^{u2}*an-nu-ḫa-ra* SUD$_2$ *ina* KAŠ NAG-*ma ina-eš* : DIŠ NUNUZ GA$_2$.NU$_{11}$^{mušen} SUD$_2$ *ina* KAŠ NAG-*ma ina-eš*

228 A$_{iv\ 21}$ ⸢DIŠ SUḪUŠ⸣ ^{giš}NU.UR$_2$.MA SUD$_2$ *ina* KAŠ *ina* MUL *tuš-bat ina* A$_2$.GU$_2$.ZI.GA NAG-*šu$_2$*

222 If DITTO, you pound (*tasâk*) *kasû* ('tamarind'), *rikibti arkabi* ('bat guano'), (and) *šammu peṣû* ('white plant') in ghee, you keep daubing his eyes with it, and then the membrane can be removed (*innassaḫ*).[554]

---

223 If someone's body is yellow (*aruq*): you pound (*tasâk*) five grains of *anzaḫḫu* ('frit'),[555] you have him drink (*tašaqqīšu*) it in oil and beer; (if) you use too much, he will die (*imât*).

---

224 If someone's eyes are full (*malâ*) of *amurriqānu*-jaundice: you pound (*tasâk*) *būšānu* ('smelly' plant), (and) he drinks (*išattī-ma*) it in beer; then he will get well.

225 If DITTO, you dry (and) pound root from *šūšu* ('liquorice'), you steep it in beer, (and) he drinks it facing the sun; then he will get well.

226 If DITTO, you dry (and) pound root from *lišān kalbi* ('dog's tongue' plant), you steep it in beer, (and) he drinks it; then he will get well.

227 If DITTO, you pound (*tasâk*) *alluḫaru* (a white mineral), (and) he drinks it in beer; then he will get well. If DITTO, you pound ostrich eggshell, (and) he drinks it in beer; then he will get well.

228 If DITTO, you pound root from *nurmû* ('pomegranate'), you leave it out overnight under the stars in beer, (and) you have him drink (*tašaqqīšu*) it in the morning.

554 The word *šišītu* occurs in connection with the eyes: see EYES 2: 121′, 124′ and 139′ (BAM 10 pp. 136–137 and 139), as well as the discussion in Attia 2015: 66.

555 The warning attached to the use of the drug *anzaḫḫu* 'frit' is unique and is in line with other instances, where only small quantities are prescribed.

229 A$_{\text{iv 22}}$ ⸢DIŠ* NUMUN* GI*.ZU$_2$.LUM⸣.MA SUD$_2$ *ina* KAŠ *ina* MUL *tuš-bat ina* A$_2$.GU$_2$.ZI.GA NAG-*šu*$_2$

230 A$_{\text{iv 23}}$ DIŠ ^{giš}GEŠTIN KA$_5$.A SUD$_2$ *ina* ⸢KAŠ⸣ NAG-*šu*$_2$: DIŠ $^{\text{u2}}$NU.LUḪ.ḪA SUD$_2$ *ina* KAŠ NAG-*šu*$_2$

231 A$_{\text{iv 24}}$ DIŠ SUḪUŠ ^{giš}NAM.TAR SUD$_2$ *ina* KAŠ ⸢NAG-*šu*$_2$⸣ : DIŠ ILLU ⸢*a-bu*⸣*-ka-ti ta-sak*$_3$ *ina* KAŠ NAG-*šu*$_2$

232 A$_{\text{iv 25}}$ DIŠ $^{\text{u2}}$MUŠ.DIM$_2$.GURUN.NA GAL *ta-sak*$_3$ ⸢*ina*⸣ [KAŠ] ⸢*u*⸣ I$_3$ NAG-*šu*$_2$

---

233 A$_{\text{iv 26}}$ DIŠ NA SU-*šu*$_2$ SIG$_7$ IGI-*šu*$_2$[556] SIG$_7$ *u* GE$_6$ SUḪUŠ EME-*šu*$_2$ GE$_6$ ⸢*aḫ*⸣*-ḫ*[*a-z*]*u* MU.NE

[DIŠ SU-*šu*$_2$ SIG$_7$ IGI].MEŠ-*šu*$_2$ SIG$_7$ *šiḫ-ḫat* UZU TUKU.MEŠ *a-mur-*[*ri-q*]*a-nu* M[U.NI] (Sagig 33: 92)

[DIŠ IGI.MEŠ-*šu*$_2$ SI]G$_7$ ŠA$_3$ IGI.MIN-*šu*$_2$ SIG$_7$ *u* SUḪUŠ EME-*šu*$_2$ GE$_6$ [*a*]*ḫ-ḫ*[*a-zu* MU.NI] (Sagig 9: 13 and 33: 93)

DIŠ NA SU-*šu*$_2$ SIG$_7$ *pa-nu-šu*$_2$ SIG$_7$ *ši-ḫat* UZU TUKU (eras.) *a-mur-ri-qa-nu* MU.NI (STO 3: 147)

229 If DITTO, you pound seed from *kūru* (a plant), you leave it out overnight under the stars in beer, (and) you have him drink it in the morning.

230 If DITTO, you pound *karān šēlebi* ('fox-vine'), (and) you have him drink it in beer. If DITTO, you pound *nuḫurtu* ('asafoetida'), (and) you have him drink it in beer.

231 If DITTO, you pound root from *pillû* ('mandrake'), (and) you have him drink it in beer. If DITTO, you pound resin from *abukkatu* (a tree), (and) you have him drink it in beer.

232 If DITTO, you pound *pizallur(t)u rabû* ('big gecko' plant),[557] (and) you have him drink it in beer and oil.

---

233 If someone's body is yellow (*aruq*), his face is yellow and black (*ṣalim*) (and) the root of his tongue is black, its name is *aḫḫāzu*-jaundice:[558]

556 Although the orthography IGI-*šu*$_2$ is ambiguous, syllabic writings in lines 146, 147 and 252, with similar lists of symptoms, suggest that IGI represents Akk. *pānū* 'face' here. Both CAD A/1 185 and Cadelli (2000: 222) take IGI here as Akk. *īnu* 'eye', but the symptom descriptions in these four lines all refer to the patient's body and face, as well as the root of his tongue. Moreover, our line seems to combine elements from two consecutive lines of the Diagnostic Handbook, namely SU-*šu*$_2$ SIG$_7$ from Sagig 33: 92 with SUḪUŠ EME-*šu*$_2$ GE$_6$ *aḫ-ḫa-zu* MU.NI from Sagig 33: 93; both lines also include IGI.MEŠ for Akk. *pānū* (Labat 1951: 72–73; Heeßel 2000: 357).

557 There is a formal difference between the orthographies of the word 'gecko' at the end of the *amurriqānu* section in line 232 ($^{\text{u2}}$MUŠ.DIM$_2$.GURUN.NA GAL) and the beginning of the following *aḫḫāzu* section in line 234 (MUŠ.DIM$_2$.GURUN.NA GAL-*ta ša*$_2$ EDIN): in line 232 it is accompanied by the determinative for drugs, viz. U$_2$ = Akk. *šammu*, which is omitted in line 234. Following CAD P 452, we distinguish between *pizallūru* as a designation for a medicinal plant ($^{\text{u2}}$MUŠ.DIM$_2$.GURUN.NA) as opposed to its designation of an actual gecko (MUŠ.DIM$_2$.GURUN.NA). However, this may also be an arbitrary orthographic difference, since U$_2$ = Akk. *šammu* can designate all kinds of medicinal substances, not just plants (see CAD Š/1 319).

558 Our line here is a quotation from the Diagnostic Handbook and is analogous to line 147 above. However, the analogous line (147) occurs alongside other entries with negative prognoses (lines 144–146) as a block. Here a similar block of entries is split in two: line 233 corresponds to line 147, whereas lines 250–253, with the negative prognoses, correspond to lines 144–146 above. This was probably done to separate treatable forms of *aḫḫāzu* in lines 233–249 from the untreatable forms in lines 250–253, perhaps suggesting that some forms of *aḫḫāzu* were considered more serious than *amurriqānu* (see Adamson 1993: 157).

234 A$_{\text{iv }27}$ MUŠ.DIM$_2$.GURUN.NA GAL-*ta ša*$_2$ EDIN *ta-sak*$_3$ *ina* KAŠ NAG *aḫ-ḫa-zu* ⸢*ša*$_2$ ŠA$_3$-*šu*$_2$⸣ SI.SA$_2$-*am*

---

235 A$_{\text{iv }28}$ DIŠ NA *aḫ-ḫa-za* DIRI ^{šim}LI SUD$_2$ *ina* KAŠ NAG ^{šim}ŠE.LI BABBAR IM.SAḪAR.NA$_4$.KUR.RA SUD$_2$ *ina* I$_3$ *u* KAŠ ⸢NAG⸣-*ma ina-eš*

236 A$_{\text{iv }29}$ ^{šim}KU$_7$.KU$_7$ SUD$_2$ *ina* KAŠ NAG $^{\text{u2}}$*ḫa-še-e* SUD$_2$ *ina* KAŠ NAG SUḪUŠ GI.ZU$_2$.LUM.MA SUD$_2$ *ina* A NAG ^{šim}ŠEŠ SUD$_2$ *ina* GA NAG

---

237 A$_{\text{iv }30}$ DIŠ NA *aḫ-ḫa-za* DIRI SUḪUŠ ^{giš}*šu-še ta-sak*$_3$ *ina* KAŠ *tara-muk ina* MUL$_4$ *tuš-bat* NAG

---

238 A$_{\text{iv }31}$ DIŠ NA *aḫ-ḫa-za* DIRI $^{\text{u2}}$*ṣu*$_2$*-ṣe-em-ta*$_5$ $^{\text{u2}}$*a-nu-nu-ta*$_5$ *ina qut-ri-ni tu-qat-tar-*⸢*šu*$_2$⸣

$^{\text{u2}}$*a-ṣu-ṣum-ta*$_5$ $^{\text{u2}}$*a-nu-nu-ta*$_5$ *ina qut-rin-ni tu-qat-tar-šu* (STO 3: 157)

DIŠ KI MIN $^{\text{u2}}$*a-ṣu-ṣum-tu*$_4$ ⸢$^{\text{u2}}$⸣[*a-nu-nu-tu*$_4$ . . .] (BAM 64 ii$^!$ 4′)

†

234 you pound *pizallur(t)u rabītu* ('big gecko') from the steppe, he drinks (*išatti*) it in beer, (and then) the *aḫḫāzu*-jaundice in his belly will come straight out (*iššeram*).[559]

---

235 If someone is full (*mali*) of *aḫḫāzu*-jaundice: you pound (*tasâk*) *burāšu* (a kind of juniper), (and) he drinks (*išatti*) it in beer. You pound white *kikkirânu* ('juniper seeds') (and) *aban gabî* ('alum'), (and) he drinks (*išattī-ma*) it in oil and beer; then he will get well.[560]

236 You pound *kukru* (an aromatic) (and) he drinks it in beer. You pound *ḫašû* ('thyme'), (and) he drinks it in beer. You pound root from *kūru* (a plant), (and) he drinks it in water. You pound *murru* ('myrrh'), (and) he drinks it in milk.[561]

---

237 If someone is full (*mali*) of *aḫḫāzu*-jaundice: you pound root from *šūšu* ('liquorice'), you soak it in beer, you leave it out overnight under the stars, (and) he drinks it.

---

238 If someone is full (*mali*) of *aḫḫāzu*-jaundice: you fumigate him with *aṣuṣimtu* (a plant)[562] (and) *anunūtu* (a plant) using a censer,

---

559 Most translators have taken SI.SA$_2$-*am* as a description of a bowel movement (see CAD A/1 185 and Scurlock 2014: 526), but the use of the ventive suggests that SI.SA$_2$ corresponds to *ešēru* in the G-stem, meaning 'to go straight out', with the *ahhāzu*-jaundice as its subject.

560 The verb *ina-eš* 'he will improve' seems to be out of place here, since all other simples in lines 235 and 236 end with NAG alone.

561 Four of the ingredients in lines 235–236, namely *burāšu*, *kukru*, *ḫašû* and root from *kūru*, also appear in the treatments for *amurriqānu*-jaundice in Schmidtchen 2018: 464–465 obv. 12′–rev. 7, although not in the same sequence. For this passage see also lines 161–165 above.

562 For the *aṣuṣimtu* plant, cited as *ṣaṣuntu*, see Böck 2014a: 158–163.

239 $A_{\text{iv 32}}$ *u* MUD$_2$ KUN.⸢DAR⸣.GURUN.NA ŠEŠ$_2$-*su-ma ina-*[*eš*]
MUD$_2$ ^{d}NIN.KA$_6$.EDIN *ša ina* ^{u2}NINNI$_5$ GUB-*zu ta-maḫ-ḫar ina* I$_3$ EŠ.MEŠ (STO 3: 158)
MUD$_2$ ^{d}NIN.KA$_6$.EDIN ⸢*ša*⸣ [. . .] (BAM 64 ii$^{!}$ 5′)
[. . .] x MUD$_2$ *an-du-ḫal-la-ta$_5$ ina* I$_3$.GIŠ ḪI.ḪI ŠEŠ$_2$ (AMT 30/2: 7′)

---

240 $A_{\text{iv 33}}$ ⸢*ru-ša*⸣-*am ša si-ip-pi* ⸢ABUL *ki-lal-le*⸣-*en* TI-*qe$_2$ ana* I$_3$.GIŠ ŠUB-*di ta-ap-ta-*⸢*na*⸣-[*ša-aš*]
⸢I$_3$⸣ SUMUN *sip-pi$_2$* ABUL *ki-lal-le-e* TI *ina* I$_3$ EŠ.MEŠ (STO 3: 159)
DIŠ KI MIN I$_3$ SUMUN *ša sip-pi$_2$* AB[UL . . .] (BAM 64 ii$^{!}$ 6′)
ru-uš-šu ša ⸢*sip*$^{?}$-*pi*$^{?}$⸣ x x TI-⸢*qe$_2$* KI⸣ [. . . ŠEŠ$_2$]-⸢*su-ma*⸣ TI (STO 4: 2)

241 $A_{\text{iv 34}}$ ⸢*ge-er-ra ru*⸣-*us-sa$_3$-a-am* ⸢*uš-te-eš-še-er*⸣ *ti-tur-ra na-di-a-am* i x [x x]
ger$_3$-ra-am ru-⸢*us*⸣-*sa$_3$-a uš-te-eš-šir ti-tur-ra na-di-ta$_5$ e-ti-*⸢*iq*⸣ (STO 3: 160)
ger$_3$-ra-am ru-us-sa$_3$-a u[*š-te-eš-šir* . . .] (BAM 64 ii$^{!}$ 7′)

---

242 $A_{\text{iv 35}}$ DIŠ NA *aḫ-ḫa-za* DAB-*su* SUḪUŠ ^{giš}NAM.TAR NITA$_2$ *ša$_2$* IGI ^{im}⸢SI⸣*.SA$_2$ TI-*qe$_2$ ina* KAŠ NAG ^{u2}ḪAR.[ḪAR$^{?}$ x x x x]
243 $A_{\text{iv 36}}$ ^{u2}KUR.GI.RIN$_2$.NA SUD$_2$ *ina* KAŠ ^{šim}ŠE.LI BABBAR SUD$_2$ *ina* KAŠ NAG ^{u2}IGI-*lim* ^{u2}IGI.NIŠ *ina* KAŠ SUḪUŠ ⸢^{u2}⸣[. . .]

---

239 and you anoint him (*tapaššassū-ma*) with the blood of an *anduḫallatu* (a kind of lizard);[563] then he will get well.

---

240 You take (*teleqqe*) dirt from both doorjambs of the city gate, you put (*tanaddi*) it in oil, you keep anointing him with it,
241 (and then) he / it goes straight out the sullied (*russû*) pathway, he / it . . . the abandoned causeway.[564]

---

242 If someone is seized (*iṣbassu*) by *aḫḫāzu*-jaundice: you take (*teleqqe*) root from male *pillû* ('mandrake') from the north side, (and) he drinks (*išatti*) it in beer. . . . *ḫašû* ('thyme') . . .
243 You pound (*tasâk*) *kurkānû* (a plant), (and he drinks) it in beer. You pound white *kikkirânu* ('juniper seeds'), (and) he drinks it in beer. (He drinks) *imḫur-līm* ('faces a thousand' plant) (and) *imḫur-ešrā* ('faces twenty' plant) in beer. . . . root from. . .

---

563 The form KUN.DAR.GURUN.NA appears alongside a host of terms for gecko and lizard in Uruanna III 289, with the Akkadian equation *im-tu-ḫal-la-a-tu$_2$*, which is a slightly variant form of *anduḫallatu*. Two of the parallel texts replace the *anduḫallatu* lizard with ^{d}NIN.KA$_6$.EDIN (lit. 'mongoose of the steppe') = Akk. *ayāṣu*.

564 For the meaning of these two lines, see the discussions in lines 159 and 160 above.

244 A$_{iv\ 37}$ DIŠ ⸢NA⸣* MIN IGI.SIG$_7$.SIG$_7$ ^{šim}LI ^{šim}Š[EŠ SU]D$_2$ *ina* KAŠ ⸢NU⸣* [*pa-tan* NAG]

---

245 A$_{iv\ 38}$ DIŠ NA MIN IM.SAḪAR.NA$_4$.KUR.RA $_{IM.SAḪAR.BABBAR.KUR.RA}$ *[565] IM.SAḪAR.GE$_6$.KUR.RA DIŠ-*niš ina* KAŠ *tara*-SUD ⸢*tu-zak*⸣-*k*[*a* x x x x]

---

246 A$_{iv\ 39}$ DIŠ NA MIN 15 ŠE.MEŠ AN.ZAḪ SUD$_2$ *ina* KAŠ *tara*-SUD *tu-zak-ka* I$_3$ *ḫal-ṣa ana* ŠA$_3$ ŠUB-*di* NU ⸢*pa*⸣-[*tan* NAG]
5 ŠE EḪ$_3$ ⸢AN.ZAḪ⸣ *ina* KAŠ ŠUB *ina* MUL$_4$ *tuš-bat tu-sak*$_6$ NAG ^{im}KAL.LA SUD$_2$ *ina* I$_3$ *e-re-ni u* KAŠ NAG (STO 3: 153)

---

247 A$_{iv\ 40}$ DIŠ NA MIN ^{im}KAL.LA SUD$_2$ *ina* I$_3$ *u* KAŠ NAG NUMUN ^{giš}*bi-ni ina* KAŠ NAG NUMUN ^{giš}*bi*-⸢*ni*⸣ [x x x x]
^{im}KAL.LA SUD$_2$ *ina* I$_3$ *e-re-ni u* KAŠ NAG / NUMUN ^{giš}*bi-ni* ⸢^{u2}SUMUN⸣.DAR SUD$_2$ *ina* KAŠ NAG NUMUN ^{giš}*bi-ni* SUD$_2$ *ina* KAŠ NAG (STO 3: 153–154)

244 If someone DITTO (= is seized by *aḫḫāzu*-jaundice) (or) *amurriqānu*-jaundice:[566] you pound (*tasâk*) *burāšu* (a kind of juniper) (and) *murru* ('myrrh'), (and) he drinks (*išatti*)$^?$ them in beer on an empty stomach.

---

245 If someone DITTO (= is seized by *aḫḫāzu*-jaundice): you steep (*tarassan*)[567] *aban gabî* ('alum') (gloss: *alluḫaru*) (and) *qitmu* (a black mineral) together in beer, you strain them, (and then) . . .

---

246 If someone DITTO (= is seized by *aḫḫāzu*-jaundice): you pound (*tasâk*) fifteen grains of *anzaḫḫu* ('frit'), you steep (*tarassan*) it in beer, you strain it, you put (*tanaddi*) pressed oil in it, (and) he drinks (*išatti*) it on an empty stomach.

---

247 If someone DITTO (= is seized by *aḫḫāzu*-jaundice): you pound (*tasâk*) *kalû* ('yellow ochre'), (and) he drinks (*išatti*) it in oil and beer. He drinks seed from *bīnu* ('tamarisk') in beer. You pound seed from *bīnu* ('tamarisk') (and) he drinks it in beer.[568]

565 The gloss in this line is missing from both Küchler's (1904) and Köcher's (1980) hand-copies; it is also not included in Bácskay's (2021a) study of glosses in therapeutic texts.
566 For the same translation of this unusual expression, see Cadelli 2000: 238 and Scurlock 2014: 527. We take IGI.SIG$_7$.SIG$_7$ = Akk. *amurriqānu* as an embedded variant, although there is no *Glossenkeil* present.
567 The orthography *tara*-SUD is unclear: SUD normally corresponds to *salāḫu* 'to sprinkle', but here with *tara-* as its initial element, it presumably corresponds to either *tarammuk* 'you soak' or *tarassan* 'you steep'. CAD S 85 normalizes the form as *tarassan*, and we follow suit here.
568 The missing part of the line has been restored with the help of line 154 above, which seems to represent a distant parallel to this passage.

248 A$_{iv\ 41}$ NUMUN ^{giš}*bi-ni* SUD$_2$ *ina* I$_3$ *u* KAŠ NAG SUḪUŠ ^{giš}*šu-ši ina* I$_3$ *u* KAŠ NAG ^{u2}IGI.NIŠ $_{(eras.)}$ [569] ⸢SUD$_2$⸣ *in*[*a* KAŠ NA]G.⸢MEŠ⸣

NUMUN ^{giš}*bi-ni* SUD$_2$ *ina* ⸢I$_3$ *u* KAŠ NAG⸣ SUḪUŠ ^{giš}*šu-ši* SUD$_2$ MIN : ^{u2}IGI.NIŠ SUD$_2$ *ina* KAŠ NAG (STO 3: 155)

---

249 A$_{iv\ 42}$ DIŠ MIN SUḪUŠ ^{giš}*šu-ši* SUḪUŠ ^{giš}NU.UR$_2$.MA *ana* A ŠUB *ina* NINDU UŠ$_2$-*er* E$_{11}$-*a ta-ša$_2$-ḫal* SED ⸢NU⸣ [*pa-tan*] ⸢NAG⸣.MEŠ

SUḪUŠ ^{giš}MA.NU SUḪUŠ ^{giš}N[U.U]R$_2$.MA *ina* ⸢NINDU⸣ UŠ$_2$-*er* A.MEŠ-*šu-nu-ti$_3$ tu-sak$_6$ tu-kaṣ$_3$-ṣa* NAG-*ma ina-eš* (STO 3: 156)

[DIŠ KI MIN SUḪU]Š ^{giš}MA.NU SUḪUŠ ^{giš}⸢NU⸣.[UR$_2$.MA . . .] / [*tu*]-*sa$_3$-ak* [. . .] (BAM 64 ii$^!$ 2′–3′)

---

250 A$_{iv\ 43}$ DIŠ NA *aḫ-ḫa-zu ana** IGI.MIN-*šu$_2$* E$_{11}$-*a-ma* IGI.MIN-*šu$_2$* GU.MEŠ SIG$_7$.MEŠ ⸢*ud*⸣-*du-ḫa*

DIŠ NA IGI.⸢SIG$_7$⸣.SIG$_7$ GIG-*ma* GIG-*su ana* ŠA$_3$ IGI.MIN-*šu$_2$* E$_{11}$-*a* ŠA$_3$ IGI.MEŠ-*šu$_2$* GU.MEŠ SIG$_7$.MEŠ *ud-du-ḫu* (STO 3: 144)

251 A$_{iv\ 44}$ ŠA$_3$.MEŠ-*šu$_2$ na-šu-u$_2$* NINDA *u* KAŠ *u$_2$-tar-ra* NA BI *u$_2$-za-bal-ma* [NU T]I ⸢UŠ$_2$⸣

ŠA$_3$.MEŠ-⸢*šu$_2$ na*⸣-*šu-u* NINDA *u* KAŠ *u$_2$-tar-ra* NA BI IM DU$_3$.A.BI GIG *u$_2$-za-bal-ma* BA.UŠ$_2$ (STO 3: 145)

---

†

248 You pound seed from *bīnu* ('tamarisk') (and) he drinks it in oil and beer. He drinks root from *šūšu* ('liquorice') in oil and beer. You pound *imḫur-ešrā* ('faces twenty' plant), (and) he keeps drinking (*ištanatti*) it in beer.

---

249 If DITTO, you put (*tanaddi*) root from *šūšu* ('liquorice') (and) root from *nurmû* ('pomegranate') in water, you heat (*tesekker*) (the mixture) in an oven, (and when) you take it out (*tušellâ*), you filter it, you let it cool (*tukaṣṣa*), (and) he keeps drinking (*ištanatti*) it on an empty stomach.

---

250 If *aḫḫāzu*-jaundice goes up (*illâ-ma*) into someone's eyes, and then his eyes are covered by yellow filaments,

251 his internal organs (*qerbū*) heave, (and) he regurgitates bread and beer, that man will linger for a little while, but he will not recover (*lā iballuṭ*), he will die (*imât*).[570]

---

569 Faint traces of a gloss are still visible after ^{u2}IGI.NIŠ. The gloss shows signs of intentional erasure, but the remaining traces may still be rendered as ^{u2}IGI-*lim*, presumably given here as a variant ingredient used instead of ^{u2}IGI.NIŠ. For another erased gloss on ^{u2}IGI.NIŠ, see STO 1: 98.

570 The use of two antithetical verbs, viz *lā iballuṭ* and *imât*, the absence of any following treatment, and the reference to a physician withholding treatment in line 253 all suggest that physicians considered these two forms of *aḫḫāzu* to be untreatable. This is quite different from lines 144–146, where various treatments are offered in response to similarly negative diagnostic statements (see Scheyhing 2007 for a rather different account). Thus, the text seems to progress from relatively mild illnesses to severe illnesses that were sometimes considered untreatable: likewise in AMT 73/1+, the illness associated with the *kabbartu*-part of the foot seems to develop from a mild to a more severe form, with negative diagnoses occurring at the end of the section (see Eypper 2016: 5–7).

252 A$_{iv\ 45}$ DIŠ NA *aḫ-ḫa-zu* GIG SAG.DU-*su pa-nu-šu* SU-*šu*$_2$ *ka-la-šu*$_2$ *u*$_3$ SUḪUŠ E[ME-*šu*$_2$ DAB]
DIŠ ⸢NA IGI⸣.SIG$_7$.SIG$_7$ ⸢GIG⸣-*ma* SAG.DU-*su pa-nu-šu*$_2$ *ka-lu* ADDA-*šu*$_2$ SUḪUŠ EME-*šu*$_2$ *ṣa-bit* (STO 3: 146)

253 A$_{iv\ 46}$ *ana* GIG *šu-a-tu* ^{lu2}A.ZU ŠU-*su* NU *ub-bal* NA BI UŠ$_2$ NU [TI]
ši-pir-šu$_2$ SUMUN-*ma* BA.UŠ$_2$ (STO 3: 146)

---

254 A$_{iv\ 47}$ DIŠ NA UD.DA KUR-*id* ZI SAG.KI GIG *ina lam* DUGUD-*šu*$_2$ *ana* TI.BI *ru-uš-ša ša sip-*[*pi* x x x]
DIŠ NA UD.DA KUR-⸢*id* ZI SAG.KI⸣ G[IG . . .] (STO 4: 1)

255 A$_{iv\ 48}$ E$_2$.GAL ^{m}AN.ŠAR$_2$-DU$_3$-A MAN ŠU$_2$ MAN KUR AN.ŠAR$_2$^{ki} *ša* ^{d}AG *u* ^{d}*taš-me-tu*$_4$ GEŠTU.MIN *ra-pa-aš*$_2$*-tu*$_4$ *iš-*⸢*ru*⸣-[*ku-uš*]
256 A$_{iv\ 49}$ *e-ḫu-uz-zu* IGI.MIN *na-mir-tu*$_4$ *ni-siq ṭup-šar-*⸢*ru*⸣-[*ti*]
257 A$_{iv\ 50}$ *ša ina* LUGAL.MEŠ-*ni a-lik maḫ-ri-ia mam*$_2$*-ma šip-ru šu-a-tu la e-ḫu-*⸢*uz*⸣*-z*[*u*]*
258 A$_{iv\ 51}$ *bul-ṭi* TA *muḫ-ḫi* EN UMBIN *liq-ti* BAR.MEŠ *ta-ḫi-zu* [*nak-la*]
259 A$_{iv\ 52}$ *a-zu-gal-lu-ti* ^{d}*nin-urta u* ^{d}*gu-la ma-la ba-aš*$_2$*-m*[*u*]
260 A$_{iv\ 53}$ *ina ṭup-pa-a-ni aš*$_2$*-ṭur as-niq* IGI.KAR$_2$*-m*[*a*]*
261 A$_{iv\ 54}$ *a-na ta-mar-ti ši-ta-as-si-ia* ⸢*qe*$_2$*-reb*⸣ E$_2$.GAL-⸢*ia*⸣ *u*$_2$*-*⸢*kin*⸣

252 If someone suffers (*maruṣ)* from *aḫḫāzu*-jaundice, his head, his face, his whole body (*zumru*) and the root of his tongue are seized (*ṣabit*):[571]
253 the physician should not do anything (lit. should not bring his hand) for this illness, that man will die (*imât*), he will not recover (*lā iballuṭ*).

---

254 (Catchline:) 'If someone is overwhelmed by fever (*ṣēta kašid*) (and) suffers (*maruṣ*) from throbbing in (his) temple, before it gets worse for him: in order to heal him, dirt from the doorjamb . . .'
255 (Colophon:) Palace of Assurbanipal, ruler of everything, king of the land of Assur, on whom Nabû and Tašmētu have bestowed wisdom, lit. wide ears,
256 He acquired for himself shining eyes, the pinnacle of scholarship,
257 Of the kings who came before me, none were able to comprehend this task.
258 Prescriptions (organized) from head to foot, gleanings from extraneous materials, technical lore
259 (And) whatever pertains to the great medical expertise of Ninurta and Gula.
260 I have written on tablets, checked and double-checked, and
261 I deposited them in the middle of my palace for my reading and recitation.

571 For a discussion of the singular stative form *ṣabit* in combination with a list of body parts, see STO 3: 146.

Chapter 6
Edition of STO 4

Manuscript A = AMT 14/7
K 4114 + K 17800

Manuscript B = AMT 44/6 + AMT 45/1
K 11317 + Rm 250

Manuscript C = AMT 78/3 + AMT 45/6 + AMT 48/3 + AMT 48/1 + AMT 23/5
K 2386 + K 6779 + K 7258 + K 10247 + Sm 937

STO 4	Parallels		
	Publication number	**Museum number**	**Parallel passage**
1	AMC 30		
1–2	STO 3: 254		
1–2	BAM 66	VAT 9475 + VAT 10753 (+) VAT 9499	reverse, 4′–5′
2	STO 3: 159		
2	STO 3: 240		
2	BAM 64	A 207	column 2!, 6′
3–4	BAM 66	VAT 9475 + VAT 10753 (+) VAT 9499	reverse, 6′–7′
3–4	BAM 174	VAT 13761	obverse, 21′–22′
5–6	BAM 66	VAT 9475 + VAT 10753 (+) VAT 9499	reverse, 8′–9′
5–6	BAM 174	VAT 13761	obverse, 23′–24′
7–8	BAM 66	VAT 9475 + VAT 10753 (+) VAT 9499	reverse, 10′–11′
9–10	BAM 66	VAT 9475 + VAT 10753 (+) VAT 9499	reverse, 12′–13′
10	BAM 66	VAT 9475 + VAT 10753 (+) VAT 9499	obverse, 11–12
10	Sagig 31: 13–14		
11–12	BAM 66	VAT 9475 + VAT 10753 (+) VAT 9499	reverse, 14′–15′
13	BAM 66	VAT 9475 + VAT 10753 (+) VAT 9499	reverse, 16′
14	BAM 66	VAT 9475 + VAT 10753 (+) VAT 9499	reverse, 17′
15–18	BAM 66	VAT 9475 + VAT 10753 (+) VAT 9499	reverse, 18′–21′
19–20	BAM 66	VAT 9475 + VAT 10753 (+) VAT 9499	reverse, 22′–23′
21	BAM 66	VAT 9475 + VAT 10753 (+) VAT 9499	reverse, 24′
22	BAM 66	VAT 9475 + VAT 10753 (+) VAT 9499	reverse, 25′
49′–50′	BAM 174	VAT 13761	obverse, 25′–27′
a–o	BAM 174	VAT 13761	obverse, 28′–42′
e–h	BAM 52	VAT 13733 + VAT 13738	reverse, 18–22
i–n	BAM 175	VAT 11656	obverse, 1–8

https://doi.org/10.1515/9781501506574-006

1 A$_{i1}$ DIŠ NA UD.DA KUR-⸢*id* ZI SAG.KI⸣ G[IG ....]
B$_{i1}$ [..........] *ana* TI.BI
[DIŠ NA UD.DA KUR-*i*]*d* (AMC 30)
DIŠ NA UD.DA KUR-*id* ZI SAG.KI GIG *ina lam* DUGUD-*šu*$_2$ *ana* TI.BI (STO 3: 254)
DIŠ NA UD.DA KUR-*id* ZI SAG.KI [. . .] (BAM 66 rev. 4′)

2 A$_{i2}$ *ru-uš-šu ša* ⸢*sip*$^?$-*pi*$^?$⸣ x x TI-⸢*qe*$_2$ KI⸣ [..........]
B$_{i2}$ [.......... ŠEŠ$_2$]-⸢*su-ma*⸣ TI
ru-uš-ša ša sip-[*pi* x x x] (STO 3: 254)
[. . .] / *ša* NA$_4$ ABUL TI-*qe*$_2$ ⸢KI I$_3$⸣ [. . .] (BAM 66 rev. 4′–5′)
⸢I$_3$⸣.SUMUN *sip-pi*$_2$ ABUL *ki-lal-le-e* TI *ina* I$_3$ EŠ.MEŠ (STO 3: 159)
⸢*ru-ša*⸣-*am ša* ⸢*si-ip*⸣-*pi* ⸢ABUL *ki-lal-le*⸣-*en* TI-*qe*$_2$ *ana* I$_3$.GIŠ ŠUB-*di ta-ap-ta*-⸢*na*⸣-[*ša-aš*] (STO 3: 240)
DIŠ KI MIN I$_3$.SUMUN *ša sip-pi*$_2$ AB[UL . . .] (BAM 64 ii$^!$ 6′)

---

3 A$_{i3}$ DIŠ NA MIN KUM$_2$ ⸢TUKU⸣ *ana* ⸢TI.BI ^{u2}*ap*$_2^?$-*ru*$_3^?$-*šu*$_2^?$⸣ *ina* ⸢I$_3^?$⸣.[GIŠ ....]
B$_{i3}$ [..........] ⸢I$_3$.GIŠ⸣ ŠEŠ$_2$.MEŠ-*su* ^{u2}*an-ki-nu*-⸢*ti*⸣
DIŠ NA MIN KUM$_2$ TUKU *ana* TI.BI ^{u2}⸢*ap*⸣-*ru*$_3$-*ša*$_2$ [. . .] (BAM 66 rev. 6′)
DIŠ NA UD.DA KUR-*id* KUM$_2$ TUKU-*ši ana* TI-*šu*$_2$ ^{u2}*ap*$_2$-*ru-ša*$_2$ *ina* I$_3$.GIŠ ⸢ŠEŠ$_2$⸣ ^{u2}*an-ki-nu*-[*ti*] (BAM 174 obv. 21′)

1 If someone is overwhelmed by fever (*ṣēta kašid*) (and) suffers (*maruṣ*) from a throbbing temple, before it becomes severe for him (*ina lām kabātīšu*):[572] in order to heal him (*ana bulluṭīšu*),
2 you take (*teleqqe*) dirt from the doorjambs of the city gate, . . . with[573] oil, (and) you anoint him (*tapaššassū-ma*); then he will recover (*iballuṭ*).

---

3 If someone DITTO (= is overwhelmed by fever and suffers from a throbbing temple) (and continues to) have (*irašši*) a temperature:[574] in order to treat him, you keep anointing him (*taptanaššassu*) with *aprušu* (a plant) in oil.

572 The reading DIL-*lam* DUGUD-*šu*$_2$ = DIL-*lam ikabbissu* in Cadelli 2000: 207 and 224 seems to be wrong. Stol (2007: 31) renders the passage as 'it is difficult for him in . . . (LAM)', but the reference here is probably to a stage in the development of a condition, stressing that the treatment should take place before (*ina lām*) the illness becomes more severe for the patient (*kabātīšu*); see Scurlock 2014: 528 and Bácskay 2018: 215.
573 The use of the preposition KI = Akk. *itti* ('with') in our line suggests that there must have been a different verb in the break, perhaps *balālu* 'to mix' (Bácskay 2018: 215) rather than *nadû* 'to put' (ŠUB-*di*), which occurs in the parallels.
574 Stol (2007: 31) translates 'if a man, ditto, has fever'. The repeated reference to heat (viz. DITTO for *ṣēta kašid* and KUM$_2$ for Akk. *ummu*) and the expression *ina lām kabātīšu* ('before it becomes severe for him') in line 1 may suggest, however, that this incipit describes a further stage of the same condition mentioned in the previous prescription.

4 A$_{i4}$ *ta-sak*$_3$ *ina* KAŠ ⸢ŠEG$_6$-*šal* ŠEŠ$_2$-*su*⸣ [......................................]
B$_{i4}$ [..] ⸢*tu*⸣-*ta-na-ṣar*-BI-*ma* TI
ta-sak$_3$ *ina* KAŠ SAG *tu-šab-šal* ŠEŠ$_2$ [. . .] (BAM 66 rev. 7′)
SUD$_2$ *ina* KAŠ ŠEG$_6$-*šal* ŠEŠ$_2$ *tu-ta-*⸢*na-ṣa*?⸣-*raš*-⸢*šu*$_2$-*ma*⸣ TI-*uṭ* (BAM 174 obv. 22′)

---

5 A$_{i5}$ DIŠ NA ⸢MIN⸣ NINDA *u* KAŠ NU *i-*⸢*le*⸣-*em ana* T[I.BI ....]
B$_{i5}$ [... TI-*š*]*u*$_2$ I$_3$.GIŠ ^{šim}GUR$_2$.GUR$_2$ ŠEŠ$_2$-*su*
DIŠ NA MIN NINDA *u* KAŠ NU *i-le-em ana* TI.BI I$_3$ ^{š}[^{im}GUR$_2$.GUR$_2$ . .] (BAM 66 rev. 8′)
DIŠ NA UD.DA KUR-*id* NINDA *u* KAŠ *la i-ma-ḫar ana* T[I-*šu*$_2$ I$_3$.GI]Š ^{šim}GUR$_2$.GUR$_2$ ŠEŠ$_2$-*su* (BAM 174 obv. 23′)

6 A$_{i6}$ ILLU ⸢*a*⸣-*bu-kat*$_3$ ⸢KUR⸣-*i* ⸢*ta*⸣-*sak*$_3$ *ina ḫi-i*[*q* ....]
B$_{i6}$ [...] NAG-*šu*$_2$ *ina* A$_2$ *tu-šap-ra-šu*$_2$-*ma* TI
[. . .] / *ta-sak*$_3$ *ina ḫi-iq* KAŠ NAG-*šu*$_2$ *ina* A$_2$ *tu-ša*[*p-ra-šu*$_2$-*ma* TI] (BAM 66 rev. 8′–9′)
[ILLU L]I.TUR *ša*$_2$ KUR-*i* SUD$_2$ *ina ḫi-iq* KA[Š NAG]-*šu*$_2$ *ina* A$_2$ *tu*$_2$-*šap-raš-šum*-⸢*ma*⸣ [TI] (BAM 174 obv. 24′)

---

4 You pound *ankinūtu* (a plant), you bring it to a boil (*tušabšal*) in beer, you anoint him (*tapaššassu*), (and) you keep observing him (*tuttanaṣṣaršū-ma*);[575] then he will recover (*iballuṭ*).

---

5 If someone DITTO (= is overwhelmed by fever and suffers from a throbbing temple), (and) he cannot eat bread and beer: in order to heal him (*ana bulluṭīšu*), you anoint him (*tapaššassu*) with oil from *kukru* (an aromatic),

6 you pound resin from *abukkatu* (a tree) of the mountains, you have him drink (*tašaqqīšu*) it in diluted beer, (and) you make him throw up using a feather; then he will recover (*iballuṭ*).

---

575 We follow Maul's (2019: 301) recent edition of the parallel text BAM 174 obv. 22′, where he reads the verb as *tu-ta-*⸢*na-ṣa*⸣-*raš*-⸢*šu*$_2$-*ma*⸣. If so, then the only difference between this verbal form and the verb in our text, viz. *tu-ta-na-ṣar*-BI-*ma*, is the omission of the ventive. Moreover, as elsewhere in our text (lines 10 and 18, as well as STO 2: 165), BI stands for the object pronoun /*šu*/ in Akkadian, sometimes read as -*šu*$_{13}$. For this passage, see also Cadelli 2000: 241 n. 4 and Johnson 2014b: 29 n. 25.

7 A$_{i7}$ DIŠ NA MIN *ku-ṣu*$_2$ ⸢*ḫur-ba*⸣-*šu*$_2$ ŠUB.⸢ŠUB-*su ana* TI⸣-[*šu*$_2$ ....][576]

B$_{i7}$ [.. ŠUB.ŠUB-*s*]*u ana* TI-*šu*$_2$ I$_3$.GIŠ ^{u2}*ap-ru*$_3$*-ša*$_2$ ŠEŠ$_2$-*s*[*u*]

DIŠ NA MIN *ku-ṣu*$_2$ *ḫur-ba-šu* ŠUB.ŠUB-*su ana* TI.BI I$_3$ ⸢^{u2}⸣[*ap-ru*$_3$*-ša*$_2$ x x] (BAM 66 rev. 10′)

8 A$_{i8}$ *ana* UDUN ^{lu2}*se-*⸢*pi-i*⸣ SU$^!$(TU)-*šu*$_2$ ^{š}[$^{im?}$GUR$_2$.GUR$_2$ ....]

B$_{i8}$ [.. ^{š}]^{im}GUR$_2$.GUR$_2$ NAG.MEŠ-*ma* T[I]

ana UDUN ^{lu2}*se-pi-i* SU-*šu*$_2$ ^{šim}GUR$_2$.GUR$_2$ NAG.MEŠ-[*ma* TI] (BAM 66 rev. 11′)

---

9 A$_{i9}$ DIŠ NA MIN ⸢KUM$_2$ TUKU⸣ *ḫa-tu* ŠUB.ŠUB-*su ana* TI-*š*[*u*$_2$ ....]

B$_{i9}$ [.. *ana* T]I-*šu*$_2$ I$_3$.GIŠ ^{šim}GUR$_2$.GUR$_2$ I$_3$.GIŠ ^{šim}LI

DIŠ NA MIN KUM$_2$ TUKU *ḫa-tu* ŠUB.ŠUB-*su ana* TI.BI I$_3$ ^{šim}GUR$_2$.GUR$_2$ I$_3$ [x x] (BAM 66 rev. 12′)

7 If someone DITTO (= is overwhelmed by fever (and) suffers from a throbbing temple), (and) cold and chills keep afflicting him (*imtanaqqussu*): in order to heal him (*ana bulluṭīšu*), you anoint him (*tapaššassu*) with oil from *aprušu* (a plant),

8 you make him . . . to the oven of a knacker (*sēpû*),[577] (and) he keeps drinking (*ištanattī-ma*) *kukru* (an aromatic); then he will recover (*iballuṭ*).

---

9 If someone DITTO (= is overwhelmed by fever and suffers from a throbbing temple), he (continues to) have (*iraššī*) a temperature (and) terror keeps afflicting him (*imtanaqqassu*): in order to heal him (*ana bulluṭīšu*), you anoint him (*tapaššassu*) with oil from *kukru* (an aromatic) (and) oil from *burāšu* (a kind of juniper),

576 The gap in lines 7–12 has been partially filled with the help of K 17800, which is a direct join to MS A. The join was identified by K. Simkó in 2022.

577 Cadelli (2000: 242) emends the line by adding KUM$_2$ = Akk. *emēmu* after SU-*šu*$_2$, meaning that the patient heats his body at the oven of the tavern-keeper, but a rather different idiom seems to be at work here. We take ^{lu2}*se-pi-i* as Akkadian *sēpû* 'knacker', a profession that collected parts from dead animals in order to make glue and similar products; hence the connection to an oven (see Deller 1987: 63; Cancik-Kirschbaum 1999; Jakob 2003: 431–435). The parallel in BAM 66 clearly has SU-*šu*$_2$, as a possible verb, perhaps Akk. *riābu* 'to replace', but the new join to MS C seems to have the sign TU, perhaps to be read as KU$_4$ = Akk. *erēbu* 'to enter'. Earlier suggestions that SU-*šu*$_2$ should be rendered as KUŠ.BAR, as an abbreviation for KUŠ.BAR.RA = Akk. *maškaru*, are unlikely (Johnson 2014b: 30; Bácskay 2018: 214 and 216; Wee 2019, vol. 1: 300 and 442). Diagnostic Handbook Sagig 31: 4 has a similar instruction, with *sābû* (^{lu2}KURUN$_2$.NA) in place of *sēpû* (^{lu2}*se-pi-i*), but parts of the passage are similarly unclear: *ana* UDUN ^{lu2}KURUN$_2$.NA x ti ku GUB-*su-ma* 'you make him (= the patient) stand next to the oven of the inn-keeper . . .' (Heeßel 2000: 342).

10 A$_{i 10}$ ŠEŠ$_2$-⸢*su* IZI⸣ *ana* IGI-*šu ta-šar*$_2$*-rap* [...]

B$_{i 9-10}$ ŠEŠ$_2$-[*su*] / [...] ⸢*ina* TUG$_2$⸣ *tu-zar*-BI-*ma* [TI]

[x x] / IZI *ana* IGI-*šu ta-ša*$_2$*-rap šum*$_4$-⸢*ma*⸣ *ina* TUG$_2$ *tu-zar*-BI-*ma* [TI] (BAM 66 rev. 12′–13′)

ŠEŠ$_2$-*su* IZI *ana* IGI-*šu ta-ša*$_2$*-rap* / *ina* TUG$_2$ *tu*-[*zar*-BI-*ma* KUM$_2$-*ma* GU$_7$ KUM$_2$-*m*]*a* NAG 3 UD.MEŠ *tu-zar*-BI-*ma* TI (BAM 66 obv. 11–12)

ŠEŠ$_2$-*su* MU$_4$.MU$_4$-*su* IZI *ta-šar-rap-ma* / [KUM$_2$-*m*]*a* GU$_7$ KUM$_2$-*ma* NAG UD.3.KAM$_2$ *tuš-šar*$_2$*-šu-ma* TI-*uṭ* (Sagig 31: 13–14)[578]

---

11 A$_{i 11}$ DIŠ NA ⸢MIN⸣ [TAB-*iṭ*] ⸢UD.DA⸣ DU$_3$.A.BI-*ma* ^{u2}*a*[*p-ru*$_3$*-ša*$_2$ ....]

B$_{i 11}$ [...] ⸢^{u2}⸣*ap-ru*$_3$*-ša*$_2$ ^{u2}*il*$_3$*-kul*$_2$*-la ša*$_2$ ⸢PU$_2$⸣ [x x]

DIŠ NA MIN <<DIŠ>> (eras.)[579] TAB-*iṭ* UD.DA DU$_3$.A.BI-*ma* ^{u2}*ap-ru*$_3$*-ša*$_2$ ^{u2}*il*$_3$-⸢*kul*$_2$*-la*⸣ *ša*$_2$ PU$_2$ *ta-t*[*ab-bal*] (BAM 66 rev. 14′)

12 A$_{i 12}$ ⸢*ina* I$_3$ ^{šim}⸣[GUR$_2$.GUR$_2$] ⸢ḪI.ḪI⸣ Š[EŠ$_2$ ....]

B$_{i 12}$ [..] ŠEŠ$_2$-*su-m*[*a* TI]

ina I$_3$ ^{šim}GUR$_2$.GUR$_2$ ḪI.ḪI ŠEŠ$_2$.⸢MEŠ-*su*⸣-*ma* T[I] (BAM 66 rev. 15′)

---

10 you light a fire (*tašarrap*) in front of him, (and) you wrap him in cloth (*tuzāršū-ma*);[580] then he will recover (*iballuṭ*).

---

11 If someone DITTO (= is overwhelmed by fever and suffers from a throbbing temple) (and) any type of burning fever (*himiṭ ṣēti*): you take? *aprušu* (a plant) (and) *elkulla* (a plant) from the well, you mix (*tuballal*) *kukru* (an aromatic)

12 in oil, (and) you keep anointing him (*taptanaššassu-ma*); then he will recover (*iballuṭ*).

---

578 The standard version of Diagnostic Handbook Sagig 31:14 replaces 3 UD.MEŠ *tu-zar*-BI-*ma* 'you keep him wrapped for three days' in BAM 66 obv. 12 with UD.3.KAM$_2$ *tuš-šar*$_2$*-šu-ma* 'you release him on the third day' (Heeßel 2000: 342). Both turns of phrase specify a three-day period, however, during which the patient was to be kept warm.

579 The TAB seems to have been written over an erased UD sign which, as the first element of UD.DA, suggests that the scribe began to write *ṣēta*(UD.DA) *ḫamiṭ*(TAB), but then switched to the variant form *ḫimiṭ*(TAB) *ṣēti*(UD.DA). The significance of the DIŠ preceding TAB is unclear, but it may be related to this erasure.

580 The verb following *ina* TUG$_2$ is rendered here as *tu-zar*-BI-*ma*; von Soden reads this form as *tu-ṣar-raš*!(BI)-*ma* 'you continue the treatment' (AHw 1085), a reading that has been frequently adopted in the secondary literature (see, for example, Bácskay 2018: 214 and Wee 2019, vol 1: 300 and 442). Our reading of the passage as *ina* TUG$_2$ *tu-zar*-BI-*ma* 'you wrap him in cloth' is based on the parallel with MU$_4$.MU$_4$-*su* 'you dress him' in the related passage Sagig 31: 13–14 (Heeßel 2000: 342). In Sagig 31, the patient is first dressed and then a fire is built to warm him, but in the main parallel to our passage, viz. BAM 66 rev. 13′, the order seems to be reversed, with the surprising appearance of *šumma* 'if' between the building of the fire and the wrapping in cloth. The verb *tu-zar*-BI-*ma* derives from *zâru* 'to turn' in the D-stem with the patient as the direct object (with BI standing for /šu/), hence *tuzāršū-ma*.

13 B$_{i\,13}$ [...................................] ⸢*tu*⸣-*bal ta-sak*$_3$ *ina* I$_3$ ḪI.ḪI ŠEŠ$_2$.⸢MEŠ-*su*⸣-[*ma* TI]
DIŠ NA MIN ^{u2}*ḫa-am-ma ša*$_2$ A.⸢MEŠ *tu-bal*⸣ *t*[*a-sak*$_3$] *ina* I$_3$.GIŠ ḪI.ḪI ŠEŠ$_2$.MEŠ-*su-ma* MIN (BAM 66 rev. 16′)

---

14 B$_{i\,14}$ [... *t*]*u-bal ta-sak*$_3$ *ina* I$_3$ ḪI.ḪI ŠEŠ$_2$.MEŠ-*s*[*u-ma* TI]
⸢DIŠ NA MIN ^{u2}⸣x x x [. . . *ta-s*]*ak*$_3$ *ina* I$_3$.GIŠ ḪI.ḪI ŠEŠ$_2$.MEŠ-*su-ma* MIN (BAM 66 rev. 17′)

---

15 B$_{i\,15}$ [DIŠ NA ....] x MUR.MEŠ GIG-*ma* NA BI *ṣi-na-a*[*ḫ ti-ri*][581]
[. . .] GIG-*ma* NA *šu*$_2$ *ṣi-na-aḫ tu-ra* (BAM 66 rev. 18′)

16 B$_{i\,16}$ [... ^{šim}]⸢ŠEŠ⸣ 3 U$_2$.ḪI.A *ša*$_2$-*šu*$_2$-*nu* x [x x x]
[. . . SI]LA$_3$ ^{šim}ŠEŠ 3 U$_2$.MEŠ *ša*$_2$-*šu-nu* / [. . .] (BAM 66 rev. 19′–20′)

17 B$_{i\,17}$ [.. *t*]*a*-⸢*sak*$_3$ *ina* I$_3$⸣ x [x x x]
[. . . EME-*š*]*u* DAB-*bat ina* 2 UD-*me* U$_2$ BABBAR *ta-sak*$_3$ / [. . .] (BAM 66 rev. 20′–21′)

13 If someone DITTO (= is overwhelmed by fever, suffers from a throbbing temple, and any type of burning fever): you dry (and) pound *ḫammu* (an aquatic plant) from water,[582] you mix (*tuballal*) it in oil, (and) you keep anointing him (*taptanaššassu-ma*); then he will recover (*iballuṭ*).

---

14 If someone DITTO (= is overwhelmed by fever, suffers from a throbbing temple, and any type of burning fever): you dry (and) pound . . . you mix (*tuballal*) it in oil, (and) you keep anointing him (*taptanaššassū-ma*); then he will recover (*iballuṭ*).

---

15 If someone$^{?}$ . . . (and) he suffers (*maruṣ-ma*) from . . . of the lungs, that man has 'persistent diarrhoea' disease (*ṣinnaḫ tīri*):
16 . . . (and) . . . litres of *murru* ('myrrh')—. . . these three ingredients . . .
17 . . . you put (*tušaṣbat*) them on his tongue (lit. have his tongue seize them), . . . you pound *šammu peṣû* ('white plant') for two days . . . in oil . . .

581 We reconstruct the standard form of *ṣinnaḫ tīri* even though our parallel text has the apparently unique spelling *ṣi-na-aḫ tu-ra*, with *tu-ra* in place of *ti-ri*. This may be a playful variant that replaces *tīru* 'coil of the intestine' with TU.RA = Akk. *marāṣu* 'to be ill'.

582 For this reading, see Bácskay 2018: 215; this rare ingredient is equated with *alapû* 'algae' in Uruanna II 334 and III 351 (Kinnier Wilson 2005: 7–8). The plant *ḫammu* often occurs in connection with water, as in BAM 171 rev. 7, BAM 315 ii 2 and CTMMA 2 69: 9.

18 B$_{i\,18}$ [...]

[. . . *t*]*a-ša*$_2$*-ni-ma*[583] *ina* A$_2$ *tu-šap-ra*-BI-*ma* MIN (BAM 66 rev. 21′)

---

19 [...]

[. . . *in*]*a* I$_3$.GIŠ BARA$_2$ AK.A[584] *ba-lu pa-tan* (BAM 66 rev. 22′)

20 [...]

[. . .] TI (BAM 66 rev. 23′)

---

21 [...]

[. . . *ba-lu p*]*a-tan* NAG-*ma* TI (BAM 66 rev. 24′)

---

22 [...]

[. . .] x [. . . *ba-lu pa-ta*]*n* NAG-*ma* TI (BAM 66 rev. 25′)

---

approximately twelve missing lines

35′ C$_{i\,1'}$ [DIŠ NA x x] x ⸢*u*$_2$$^?$*-tan*$^?$*-ne*$_2$*-eḫ-šu*$_2$⸣[585] x [...]

†

18 . . . you make him throw up again using a feather; then DITTO (= he will recover).

---

19 . . . in pressed oil on an empty stomach . . .

20 . . . he will recover (*iballuṭ*).

---

21 . . . he drinks (*išattī-ma*) it on an empty stomach; then he will recover (*iballuṭ*).

---

22 . . . he drinks (*išattī-ma*) it on an empty stomach; then he will recover (*iballuṭ*).

---

approximately twelve missing lines

35′ If someone . . . it tires him out . . .

---

583 For the reading *ta-ša*$_2$*-ni-ma*, not recorded in Cadelli 2000: 243, see now Johnson 2014b: 31 with n. 29. The verb *ta-ša*$_2$*-ni-ma*, from Akk. *šanû* 'to do again', is probably in hendiadys with *tu-šap-ra*-BI-*ma*, meaning 'you make him throw up again'. This would mean that another instance of vomiting is lost in one of the breaks in line 17.

584 The signs read here as AK.A are crammed together, which makes our reading somewhat uncertain; however, the rare orthography ⸢i$_3$⸣.giš bara$_2$ ak.a = Akk. *šamnu ḫalṣu* appears in Ura 24: 14 (MSL 11 p. 79). For this orthography, see Waetzoldt 1985: 84.

585 For the reading *u*$_2$*-tan-ne*$_2$*-eḫ-šu*$_2$, from the verb *anāḫu* 'to be tired' in the Dt-stem, see Johnson 2014b: 16 with n. 12, but as emphasized there this verb is not otherwise attested in the Dt-stem and other possibilities should be considered.

36′ C$_{i\,2'}$ [^{u2}IG]I-*lim* ^{u2}IGI.⸢NIŠ⸣ [..]

37′ C$_{i\,3'}$ [DIŠ KI MIN] ⸢^{u2}⸣ḪAR.ḪAR ^{u2}*ur*$_2$-*ne*$_2$-*e* ^{ši}[^{m} ....]

38′ C$_{i\,4'}$ [DIŠ KI MIN] ⸢^{u2}⸣ḪAR.LUM.BA.ŠIR [..]

39′ C$_{i\,5'}$ [DIŠ N]A SAG ŠA$_3$-*šu*$_2$ *u*$_2$-*ṣar-rap-šu*$_2$ *na-piš* KIRI$_4$-*šu*$_2$ ⸢DUGUD NA⸣ B[I UD.DA SA$_2$.SA$_2$[586] ....]

40′ C$_{i\,6'}$ ⸢DIŠ⸣ NA SAG ŠA$_3$-*šu*$_2$ *i-ḫa-maṭ-su i-dak-ka-su* UḪ$_2$-*su* ⸢DU$^?$⸣ [.......................................]
41′ C$_{i\,7'}$ ⸢UD.DA⸣ SA$_2$.SA$_2$ I$_3$.GIŠ BARA$_2$.GA *ina* A NU *pa-tan* NAG.NAG-*šu*$_2$ [...........................]
42′ C$_{i\,8'}$ ⸢^{šim}⸣LI ^{šim}GUR$_2$.GUR$_2$ ILLU ^{šim}BULUḪ PA ^{giš}*bi-ni* PA ^{u2}IN$_6$.⸢UŠ$_2$⸣ [.....................................]

36′ *imḫur-līm* ('faces a thousand' plant), *imḫur-ešrā* ('faces twenty' plant) . . .

37′ If DITTO, *ḫašû* ('thyme'), *urnû* (a kind of mint) . . .

38′ If DITTO, *ḫarmunu* (a plant) . . .

39′ If someone's epigastrium (*rēš libbi*) burns him, (and) it is difficult (*kabit*) for him to breathe through his nose, that man is . . . by fever (*ṣēta* SA$_2$.SA$_2$) . . .

40′ If someone's epigastrium (*rēš libbi*) is inflamed, it causes him a pressing pain, his spittle (*ru'tu*) flows (*illak*)[587] . . . (and) . . .,
41′ he is . . . by fever (*ṣēta* SA$_2$.SA$_2$): you keep having him drink (*taštanaqqīšu*) pressed oil in water on an empty stomach,
42′ (then) . . . *burāšu* (a kind of juniper), *kukru* (an aromatic), resin from *baluḫḫu* ('galbanum'), leaves from *bīnu* ('tamarisk'), leaves from *maštakal* ('soapwort') . . .

586 For the suggested restoration of UD.DA SA$_2$.SA$_2$ in the break, see Bácskay 2018: 218.
587 The next to last sign in line 40′ is somewhat damaged, but the traces probably correspond to SU rather than ŠU. We would expect *illātu* here for UḪ$_2$, but the form of the possessive suffix (/su/ instead of /šu/) seems to suggest that it is *ru'tu*, hence *ru'ssu* 'his spittle'.

43′ C$_{i\,9′}$ ⸢DIŠ NA MURUB$_4$⸣ MAŠ.SILA$_3$.MIN-*šu$_2$* *u$_2$-ḫa-maṭ-su* KI UḪ$_2$-*šu$_2$* MUD$_2$ ŠUB.ŠUB *ana* UD.⸢DA⸣[588] [.................]

44′ C$_{i\,10′}$ ⸢^{šim}⸣LI ^{šim}GUR$_2$.GUR$_2$ ZA$_3$.ḪI.LI [...]

45′ C$_{i\,11′}$ ⸢PA GI⸣.ZU$_2$.LUM.MA IM.GU$_2$ EN.<NA> GAZ *ina* KAŠ SILA$_{11}$-*aš* x [......]

46′ C$_{i\,12′}$ ⸢DIŠ NA⸣ NINDA GU$_7$ KAŠ NAG-*ma* SAG ŠA$_3$-*šu$_2$* *i-kaṣ$_3$-ṣa-su* ŠA$_3$-*šu$_2$* MU$_2$.M[U$_2$ ....]

47′ C$_{i\,13′}$ [UD].⸢DA⸣ SA$_2$.SA$_2$ $^{\text{u2}}$*ak-tam* $^{\text{u2}}$IGI-*lim* $^{\text{u2}}$*tar-m*[*uš* ....]

48′ C$_{i\,14′}$ [DIŠ KI MIN] ⸢I$_3$⸣.GIŠ BARA$_2$.GA EME-*šu$_2$* DAB-*bat* [NAG *i-ar$_2$-ru$_3$*]

49′ C$_{i\,15′}$ [DIŠ NA *it-ta*]-⸢*na-ša-aš* *a-šu-uš-tu$_4$* ŠUB.ŠUB⸣-[*su* ....]

[DIŠ NA *i*]-⸢*ta*⸣-*na-ša-aš* *a-šu-uš-tu$_2$* ŠU[B.ŠUB]-*su* NUNDUM.MEŠ-*šu$_2$* *i-ta-n*[*a-ba-l*]*a* / ⸢A⸣.[MEŠ] ⸢*ma*⸣-*gal* NAG (BAM 174 obv. 25′–26′)

43′ If someone is entirely inflamed between his shoulders, he constantly spits up (*ittanaddi*) blood with his phlegm (*rupuštu*) (and) . . . into *ṣēta* . . .

44′ you crush (*taḫaššal*) *burāšu* (a kind of juniper), *kukru* (an aromatic), *saḫlû* ('cress') . . .

45′ leaves from *kūru* (a plant), (and) *qadūt šikāni* ('river mud'), you kneed (*talâš*) them in beer . . .

46′ If someone eats (*ikkal*) bread (and) drinks (*išatti*) beer, and subsequently, his epigastrium (*rēš libbi*) gnaws at him (*ikaṣṣassu*), his internal organs (*qerbū*) are swollen (*napḫū*) (and) . . .

47′ he is . . . by fever (*ṣēta* SA$_2$.SA$_2$): *aktam* (a plant), *imḫur-līm* ('faces a thousand' plant), *tarmuš* ('lupin') . . .

48′ If DITTO, you put (*tušaṣbat*) pressed oil on his tongue (lit. have his tongue seize it), he drinks (*išatti*) it, (and) he will vomit.

49′ If someone is always upset, (and) grief keeps afflicting him (*imtanaqqussu*), his lips keep getting dry (*ītanabbalā*),[589] (and) he drinks (*išatti*) a lot of water,

588 Based on the presence of the preposition *ana*, we expect a verb like GUR = Akk. *târu* in the break, indicating that the medical problem 'has turned' into some kind of feverish condition, perhaps even UD.DA SA$_2$.SA$_2$, given the fact that it is the main concern of our text at this point. For a similar reading, but without the preposition *ana*, see Bácskay 2018: 218.

589 The verb in the fragmentary parallel in BAM 174 obv. 25′ is probably *ītanabbalā*, the feminine plural form of *abālu* 'to be dry' in the Gtn-stem, with the feminine dual noun NUNDUM.MEŠ = Akk. *šaptā* 'lips' as its subject (Scurlock and Andersen 2005: 61, Bácskay 2018: 218). As a symptom, parched lips also feature in STO 1: 89, in an incantation recited against gastric constriction. The alternative reading that Maul (2019: 301) suggests for the fragmentary passage, viz. NUNDUM.MEŠ-*šu$_2$* *i-ta-na-*[*ša-k*]*a* 'he keeps biting his lips', does not occur elsewhere in our corpus but cannot be excluded.

50′ C$_{i\,16'}$ [UD.DA SA$_2$.S]A$_2$ ^{giš}GEŠTIN KA$_5$.A SUD$_2$ *ina* KAŠ NAG UZU ⸢GUR$_4$.RA GU$_7$⸣ ^{š}[^{im}LI ^{š}]^{im}⸢ḪAB *ina* KAŠ NAG *ina* KAŠ ŠEG$_6$-*šal ana* DUR$_2$⸣-[*šu*$_2$ DUB]

UD.DA SA$_2$.S[A$_2$ ^{gi}]^{š}GEŠTIN KA$_5$.A *ta-sak*$_3$ *ina* KAŠ ⸢NAG-*šu*$_2$⸣ UZU GUR$_4$ GU$_7$ / [^{ši}]^{m}LI ^{šim}ḪAB *ina* KAŠ ⸢NAG⸣ *ina* KAŠ ŠEG$_6$-*šal ana* DUR$_2$-*šu*$_2$ DUB-*ak* (BAM 174 obv. 26′–27′)

51′ C$_{i\,17'}$ [DIŠ KI MIN ^{giš}GE]ŠTIN KA$_5$.A SUD$_2$ *ina* KAŠ NAG IM.GU$_2$ EN.NA A.GAR.GAR MAŠ.DA$_3$ PA ⸢$^{giš.u2}$*ul*$_4$⸣-*ḫa-aḫ*[590] PA GI.ZU$_2$.LUM.M[A][591]

52′ C$_{i\,18'}$ [*g*]*u-ur* GI.ŠUL.ḪI ZI$_3$ GIB$_3$ DUḪ.ŠE.GIŠ.I$_3$ *ta-sak*$_3$ *ina* KAŠ *ta-la*$_3$-*aš ina* TUG$_2$ *te-ṭer*$_5$-*ri* L[AL]

53′ C$_{i\,19'}$ [DIŠ KI MI]N ^{u2}*ak-tam* SUD$_2$ *ina* KAŠ SAG ⸢NAG⸣

54′ C$_{i\,20'}$ [DIŠ NA *i*]*t-ta-na-ša-aš a-šu-uš-tu*$_4$ ŠUB.ŠUB-*su di-ik-ša* TAG.TAG-*su* UḪ$_2$-*šu*$_2$ *ma-a*-⸢*da*⸣

50′ he is . . . by fever (*ṣēta* SA$_2$.SA$_2$): you pound (*tasâk*) *karān šēlebi* ('fox-vine'), he drinks (*išatti*) it in beer, (and then) he eats (*ikkal*) fatty meat. He drinks *burāšu* (a kind of juniper) (and) *ṭūru* ('opopanax') in beer, (then) you bring (these ingredients) to a boil (*tušabšal*) in beer, (and) you pour (*tašappak*) them into his anus.

51′ If DITTO, you pound (*tasâk*) *karān šēlebi* ('fox-vine'), (and) he drinks (*išatti*) it in beer. You pound *qadūt šikāni* ('river mud'), gazelle droppings, leaves from *ulḫaḫ* (a kind of acacia), leaves from *kūru* (a plant),

52′ blades from *qan šalāli* (a kind of reed), *kibtu* ('wheat') flour, (and) *kupsu* ('sesame pomace'), you knead them in beer, you smear (the mixture) on a piece of fabric, (and) you bandage (*taṣammid*) him.

53′ If DITTO, you pound (*tasâk*) *aktam* (a plant), (and) he drinks (*išatti*) it in high-quality beer.

54′ If someone is always upset, grief keeps afflicting him (*imtanaqqussu*), pressing pain (*dikšu*)[592] repeatedly affects him (*iltanappassu*), (and) he keeps swallowing (*ištanatti*) (lit. drinking) a lot of his (own) phlegm (*rupuštu*),

---

590 Although the signs GIR$_2$ and UL$_4$ (= GIR$_2$*gunû*) are no longer distinguished in first-millennium Akkadian texts (Borger 2004: 247), this is presumably a form of *ulhah* as in Uruanna II 14–15, where it is syllabically written, viz. ^{u2}*ul-ḫa-aḫ*. The standard orthography is U$_2$.GIR$_2$-*ḫa-aḫ* (CAD P 515 and U/W 72), so the additional GIŠ determinative here in our line is unusual. Alternatively, one might consider rendering the word as ^{giš}KIŠI$_{16}$ = Akk. *ašāgu*, but this would not explain the -*ḫa-aḫ* at the end of the word. For a discussion of these different readings in earlier periods, see Biggs 1974: 70 and Hallo and van Dijk 1968: 75.

591 For the reading PA GI.ZU$_2$.LUM.MA, see line 45′ above.

592 The condition *dikšu* ('pressing pain') also occurs in STO 2: 200, accompanied by the same verb, viz. *itanappassu*. For the reading *di-ik-ša* in our line, see already Campbell Thompson 1929: 78 with n. 9 and more recently Stol 2018: 350.

55′ C$_{i\,21'}$ [NAG].NAG UD.DA SA$_2$.SA$_2$ ^{u2}IGI-*lim* ^{u2}*šiz-ba-na*$_7$ ^{šim}ŠE.LI BABBAR SUD$_2$ *ina* ⸢KAŠ⸣ N[AG]

56′ C$_{i\,22'}$ [DIŠ] ⸢NA NINDA GU$_7$⸣ KAŠ NAG-*ma* ŠA$_3$-*šu*$_2$ *in-nen-me-ru*$^!$(IR)[593] *nap-ḫu* A *ma-gal* NAG UD.DA SA$_2$.SA$_2$ ⸢^{u2}⸣[IGI-*lim*]

57′ C$_{i\,23'}$ [^{u2}]IGI.NIŠ ^{u2}*tar-muš* ^{šim}GAM.MA ^{u2}*ti-ia*$_2$-*ta*$_5$ ^{u2}ḪAR.ḪAR SUD$_2$ *ina* KAŠ NU *pa-t*[*an* NAG]

58′ C$_{i\,24'}$ [IM].⸢GU$_2$⸣ EN.NA A.GAR.GAR MAŠ.DA$_3$ ^{šim}LI ^{šim}GUR$_2$.GUR$_2$ ZA$_3$.ḪI.LI PA ^{gi}[^{š}GEŠ]TIN K[A$_5$.A x x x]

59′ C$_{i\,25'}$ [*g*]*u*-⸢*ur*⸣ ^{giš}GI.ŠUL.ḪI[594] ZI$_3$ GIB$_3$ DUḪ.ŠE.GIŠ.⸢I$_3$ SUD$_2$⸣ *ina* KAŠ SILA$_{11}$-⸢*aš*⸣ *i*[*na* TU]G$_2$ ⸢SUR⸣-*r*[*i* LAL-*su-ma* TI]

60′ C$_{i\,26'}$ [^{u2}*a*]*k-tam* SUD$_2$ *ina* KAŠ NAG UZU GUR$_4$.RA GU$_7$ ŠA$_3$-*šu*$_2$ *i*-⸢*ar*$_2$⸣-[*ru*$_3$ x x x SU]D$_2$ *ina* KAŠ NAG ⸢^{u2}IGI-*lim* SUD$_2$⸣

†

55′ he is . . . by fever (*ṣēta* SA$_2$.SA$_2$): you pound (*tasâk*) *imḫur-līm* ('faces a thousand' plant), *šizbānu* ('milkweed'), (and) white *kikkirânu* ('juniper seeds'), (and) he drinks (*išatti*) them in beer.

56′ If someone eats (*ikkal*) bread (and) drinks (*išattī-ma*) beer, and subsequently, his internal organs (*qerbū*) are bloated (and) swollen, (and) he drinks (*išatti*) a lot of water, he is . . . by fever (*ṣēta* SA$_2$.SA$_2$): you pound (*tasâk*) *imḫur-līm* ('faces a thousand' plant),

57′ *imḫur-ešrā* ('faces twenty' plant), *tarmuš* ('lupin'), *ṣumlalû* (an aromatic), *tīyatu* (a plant), (and) *ḫašû* ('thyme') (and) he drinks (*išatti*) them in beer on an empty stomach.

58′ You pound *qadūt šikāni* ('river mud'), gazelle droppings, *burāšu* (a kind of juniper), *kukru* (an aromatic), *saḫlû* ('cress'), leaves from *karān šēlebi* ('fox-vine') . . .

59′ blades from *qan šalāli* (a kind of reed), *kibtu* ('wheat') flour, (and) *kupsu* ('sesame pomace'), you kneed (*talâš*) them in beer, you smear (*teṭerri*) (the mixture) on a piece of fabric, (and) you bandage him (*taṣammissu*); then he will recover (*iballuṭ*).

60′ You pound (*tasâk*) *aktam* (a plant), he drinks (*išatti*) it in beer, (then) he eats (*ikkal*) fatty meat, (and) his belly (*libbu*) will (make him) vomit.[595] You pound . . . (and) he drinks it in beer. You pound *imḫur-līm* ('faces a thousand' plant),

---

593 In line with several neighbouring passages where the verb occurs in the plural, as in line 62′ *in-nem-me-ru*, we emend IR to RU and read this verb as plural in agreement with the following verb *naphū*.

594 Although *qan šalāli* is usually rendered without the GIŠ determinative, another example with this orthography, viz. ^{giš}GI.ŠUL.ḪI, is known from the Therapeutic Vademecum BAM 1 iv 1.

595 The verb *arû* usually has the patient and not the belly as its subject, which makes our wording here analogous to expressions like *libbašu ana parê ētenellâ* 'his belly continually heaves to vomit' (STO 3: 27 and 47), *libbašu ana parê ēteneppeš* 'his belly continually acts like it is going to vomit' (STO 2: 87) and *qerbūšu našû* 'his internal organs heave' (STO 3: 145 and 251). Unlike these expressions, however, 'his belly will (make him) vomit' in our line is not part of the symptomatology, but rather part of the therapeutic procedure.

61′ C$_{i\,27'}$ [*ina* I$_3$.GI]Š BARA$_2$.GA NAG IM.GU$_2$ EN.NA SUD$_2$ *ina* KAŠ N[AG ^{u2}*ti*]-⸢*ia*$_2$⸣-*ta*$_5$ SUD$_2$ *ina* KAŠ NAG

62′ C$_{i\,28'}$ [DIŠ] ⸢NA⸣ NINDA GU$_7$ KAŠ NAG-*ma* ŠA$_3$-*šu*$_2$ *in-nem-me-ru nap-ḫu* [A *ma-gal* NA]G UD.DA SA$_2$.SA$_2$
63′ C$_{i\,29'}$ ⸢GURUN⸣ UKUŠ$_2$.ḪAB EN *la uk-tap-pi-tu* ⸢ḪAD$_2$.DU⸣ [*ta-sa*]*k*$_3$ *ina* KAŠ NAG

64′ C$_{i\,30'}$ ⸢^{u2}⸣KUR.RA SUD$_2$ *ina* KAŠ NAG ^{u2}⸢ḪAR⸣.[LU]M.BA.ŠIR SUD$_2$ *ina* KAŠ NAG

65′ C$_{i\,31'}$ [DI]Š NA NINDA GU$_7$ KAŠ NAG-*ma* ŠA$_3$.⸢MEŠ-*šu*$_2$⸣ *in-nem-me-ru* KAŠ$_3$.⸢MEŠ⸣-*šu*$_2$ DAB.DAB-*at* UD.DA SA$_2$.SA$_2$

†

61′ (and) he drinks it in pressed oil. You pound *qadūt šikāni* ('river mud'), (and) he drinks it in beer. You pound *tīyatu* (a plant), (and) he drinks it in beer.

62′ If someone eats (*ikkal*) bread (and) drinks (*išattī-ma*) beer, and subsequently, his internal organs (*qerbū*) are bloated (and) swollen, (and) he drinks (*išatti*) a lot of water, he is . . . by fever (*ṣēta* SA$_2$.SA$_2$):
63′ you dry (*tubbal*) (and) pound fruit from *irrû* ('cucumber') before it shrinks (*uktappitu*),[596] (and) he drinks it in beer.

64′ You pound (*tasâk*) *nīnû* ('mint'), (and) he drinks (*išatti*) it in beer. You pound *ḫarmunu* (a plant), (and) he drinks it in beer.

65′ If someone eats (*ikkal*) bread (and) drinks (*išattī-ma*) beer, and subsequently, his internal organs (*qerbū*) are bloated, (and) he (unintentionally) holds back (*uṣabbat*) his urine,[597] he is . . . by fever (*ṣēta* SA$_2$.SA$_2$):

---

596 The verb *kupputu* occurs only here and in line 66′ below in connection with a medical ingredient. Other attestations of this verb suggest that it is used to describe the making of pill-shaped suppositories, with the possible meaning 'to roll (into a pill)' (Meier 1939a: 301–302 and Böck 2009: 124) or 'to form a pellet, pill, suppository' (CAD K 552–553). In our line *kupputu* describes the state of the fruit at the time of its use; either that (a) it was not allowed to ripen (Bácskay 2018: 222) or (b) that it was not allowed to dry and (hence) shrink (i.e., become more compact) after it had been picked. For an adjectival use of this word, specifying the shape of a stone, see Abusch, Schwemer, Luukko and Van Buylaere 2020: 51 ln. 2.

597 The same idiom also occurs in BAM 396 ii 19′, along with ŠE$_{10}$ = Akk. *zû* 'faeces': ŠE$_{10}$ *u*$_3$ KAŠ$_3$-*šu*$_2$ *u*$_2$-*ṣa-bat* with the patient as the subject of the verb. The idiom also seems to occur in the stative with the urine as the subject in Diagnostic Handbook Sagig 14: 136 (KAŠ$_3$.MEŠ-*šu*$_2$ DAB.DA[B-*ta*$_5^?$]; BAM 13 pp. 584–585) and BAM 7 2a: 14′ (KAŠ$_3$.MEŠ-*šu*$_2$ DAB.MEŠ-*t*[*a*]); however, in both cases the verb is partially restored, and the stative morphology is not preserved. Rather than an intentional action, this idiom probably refers to some kind of hindered urination, whether a reduction in urine volume, a feeling of incomplete emptying of the bladder, or the inability to produce urine altogether, even in those cases when the patient has consumed beer beforehand (Scurlock and Andersen 2005: 61).

66′ C$_{i\ 32′}$ [GU]RUN UKUŠ$_{2}$.ḪAB EN *la uk-tap-pi-tu* ḪAD$_{2}$.DU *ta-sak*$_{3}$ *ina* KAŠ NAG

67′ B$_{ii\ 1}$ DIŠ NA NINDA GU$_{7}$ KAŠ NAG-*ma* ŠA$_{3}$-*šu*$_{2}$ ⸢*in*⸣-*nem-me-ru in*-⸢*ne*$^{?}$⸣-[*bi-ṭu*$_{2}$ ....][598]
C$_{i\ 33′}$ [DIŠ N]A NINDA GU$_{7}$ KAŠ NAG-*ma* ŠA$_{3}$-*šu*$_{2}$ *in-nem-me-ru in*-⸢*ne*$_{2}$⸣-*bi-ṭu*$_{2}$ *ri-du-ut ir-ri* TUKU
68′ B$_{ii\ 2}$ ⸢UD.DA SA$_{2}$⸣.SA$_{2}$ NA$_{4}$ ZU$_{2}$.LUM.MA GAZ GIM UTUL$_{7}$.ZI$_{3}$.DA[599] *tara*-⸢*bak*⸣ [..............................]
C$_{i\ 33′}$ UD.DA SA$_{2}$.SA$_{2}$

69′ B$_{ii\ 3}$ [.. *ina*] ⸢^{dug}UTUL$_{7}$ ŠEG$_{6}$⸣-[*šal* ....]

approximately sixty-two missing lines

†

66′ you dry (*tubbal*) (and) pound fruit from *irrû* ('cucumber') before it shrinks, (and) he drinks (*išatti*) it in beer.

67′ If someone eats (*ikkal*) bread (and) drinks (*išattī-ma*) beer, and subsequently, his internal organs (*qerbū*) are bloated (and) have cramps, (and) he has (*iraššī*) diarrhoea,
68′ he is . . . by fever (*ṣēta* SA$_{2}$.SA$_{2}$): you crush (*taḫaššal*) *aban suluppi* ('date stone'), you stir them as a paste . . .

69′ . . . you bring it to a boil (*tušabšal*) in a pot . . .

approximately sixty-two missing lines

598 Manuscripts B and C seem to have been spaced differently, with the same piece of text (corresponding to our line 67′) occurring in different parts of the physical tablets: in Ms. B this is the incipit at the beginning of column 2, while in Ms. C the incipit occurs in the last line of column 1 and must have been continued into the first line of column 2, although we cannot entirely exclude the possibility that the two manuscripts in line 67′ present similar incipits and that other material may have intervened here. The symptom description in these two lines can be brought into alignment up to the verb *in-ne*$_{2}$*-bi-ṭu*$_{2}$, but if different material followed this verb in Ms. B, we would need to revisit the alignment of these two manuscripts.

599 The rare orthography UTUL$_{7}$.ZI$_{3}$.DA for Akk. *rabīku* 'paste' (German *Brei*) means literally 'a vessel (full) of flour'. See also the Old Babylonian form of the expression in YOS 11 28 obv. 5: *ki-ma* ZI$_{3}$.DA *ta-ra-ab-ba-ak-ma*.

a [...][600]
DIŠ NA ŠA$_{3}$-*šu*$_{2}$ NINDA *u* KAŠ *la i-ma-*⸢*ḫar*⸣ KI UḪ$_{2}$-*šu*$_{2}$ MUD$_{2}$ ŠUB.ŠUB-*a* NA BI UD.DA SA$_{2}$.SA$_{2}$ (BAM 174 obv. 28′)

b [...]
ana TI-*šu*$_{2}$ $^{\text{u2}}$GEŠTIN KA$_{5}$.⸢A⸣ [*ina* KA]Š NAG $^{\text{u2}}$*ap*$_{2}$*-ru-šum ina* I$_{3}$.GIŠ ŠEŠ$_{2}$ (BAM 174 obv. 29′)

c [...]
⸢^{šim}GUR$_{2}$⸣.GUR$_{2}$ ^{šim}⸢LI ^{šim}⸣MAN.DU NAGA SI *ina* ⸢A.GEŠTIN⸣.NA KAŠ SAG I$_{3}$ A GA[ZI^{sar}] (BAM 174 obv. 30′)

d [...]
⸢ŠEG$_{6}$.GA$_{2}$⸣ *ina* MU[L$_{4}$ *tuš-ba*]*t ina* A$_{2}$.GU$_{2}$.ZI.G[A x] x x x [x x] (BAM 174 obv. 31′)

---

e [...]
^{giš}LI ^{giš}[GUR$_{2}$.GUR$_{2}$ ^{š}]^{im}MAN.DU ^{šim}GAM.MA ^{šim}ŠEŠ $^{\text{u2}}$KUR.[KUR x x x x] (BAM 174 obv. 32′)
DIŠ NA ŠA$_{3}$.MEŠ-*šu*$_{2}$ *nik-mat* IM *u* UD.DA DIRI.ME ^{šim}GUR$_{2}$.GUR$_{2}$ ^{šim}LI ^{šim}M[AN.DU] / ^{šim}GAM.⸢MA⸣ ^{šim}ŠEŠ $^{\text{u2}}$KUR.KUR U$_{2}$ MAŠ.TAB.BA (BAM 52 rev. 18–19)

a If someone's stomach (*libbu*) does not accept bread and beer, (and) he constantly spits up (*ittanadâ*) blood with his phlegm (*rupuštu*), that man is ... by fever (*ṣēta* SA$_{2}$.SA$_{2}$):
b in order to heal him (*ana bulluṭīšu*), he drinks (*išatti*) *karān šēlebi* ('fox-vine') in beer, (and) you anoint (*tapaššaš*) him with *aprušu* (a plant) in oil.
c You bring to a boil (*tušabšal*) *kukru* (an aromatic), *burāšu* (a kind of juniper), *suādu* (a kind of sedge), (and) *uhūlu qarnānû* ('horned alkali') in vinegar, high-quality beer, oil, (and) juice from *kasû* ('tamarind'),
d you leave (the mixture) out overnight under the stars, in the morning ...

---

e *burāšu* (a kind of juniper), *kukru* (an aromatic), *suādu* (a kind of sedge), *ṣumlalû* (an aromatic), *murru* ('myrrh'), *atāʾišu* (a plant), *šammi ašî* ('*ašû* disease' plant),

600 The inclusion of BAM 174 obv. 28′–42′ at this point is warranted by the fact that it draws passages from various treatises, in the same sequence in which they occur in the Nineveh Medical Encyclopaedia: these excerpts are first taken from the fifth tablet of the fourth treatise (NECK 5), and then subsequently from BAM 558, which perhaps represents the sixth tablet of the seventh treatise (BRON 6). After these passages, the tablet turns to the eighth treatise (viz. the Stomach Treatise), with excerpts taken from the fourth and fifth tablets (STO 4 and 5). The last known parallel in BAM 174, namely lines obv. 25′–27′, corresponds to STO 4: 49′–50′, whereas the first excerpt from STO 5: 34–37 occurs in BAM 174 rev. 1–3: the lines in BAM 174 between these two sections, viz. obv. 28′–42′, presumably came from the missing part of STO 4, which we edit here as unplaced lines a–o. For a discussion of BAM 174, see Johnson 2014b: 34–35 as well as the new edition of the text available in Maul 2019: 300–309.

f [……………………………………………………………………………………………]

[x x ^{giš}]ŠUR.MIN$_3$ GI DU$_{10}$ ^{šim}BAL ^{giš}⸢EREN.SUMUN ŠIM⸣.[ŠAL x x x] (BAM 174 obv. 33′)

^{giš}EREN ^{šim}BULUḪ G[I DU$_{10}$.GA] / ^{šim}MUG ^{giš}EREN.SUMUN ŠIM.ŠAL ^{u2}ḪAR.ḪAR (BAM 52 rev. 19–20)

g [……………………………………………………………………………………………]

[x x x x] ^{u2}KUR.RA ^{u2}*ur*$_2$*-nu-u* GAZI⸢^{sar} ^{u2}ḪUR.SAG⸣ N[AGA SI x x] (BAM 174 obv. 34′)

^{u2}NU.LUḪ.ḪA ^{u2}KUR.[RA] / ^{u2}*ur*$_2$*-nu-u* GAZI^{sar} ^{u2}ḪUR.SAG NAGA SI LAGAB MUNU$_4$ (BAM 52 rev. 20–21)

h [……………………………………………………………………………………………]

[MU]N ZU$_2$.⸢LUM⸣.MA 23 U$_2$.ME *an-nu-ti ina* ⸢GEŠTIN ŠEG$_6$-*šal*⸣ I$_3$.GIŠ *ana* Š[A$_3$ . . .] (BAM 174 obv. 35′)

MUN ZU$_2$.L[UM.MA] / 23 U$_2$.ḪI.A *ina* KAŠ KALAG.GA ŠEG$_6$-*šal* I$_3$.GIŠ *ana* IGI ŠUB-*di ana* DUR$_2$-*šu*$_2$ DU[B-*ak*] (BAM 52 rev. 21–22)

---

i [……………………………………………………………………………………………]

[DIŠ N]A ŠA$_3$.MEŠ-*šu*$_2$ *na-šu-u* IGI.MIN.MEŠ-*šu*$_2$ *ur-ru-pa zi*-⸢*mu-u*$_2^?$-*šu*$_2^?$⸣[601] x x [. . .] (BAM 174 obv. 36′)

[. . . *na-šu*]-⸢*u*$_2$⸣ IGI.MIN-*šu*$_2$ *ur-ru-pa zi-mu* / [. . .] (BAM 175 obv. 1–2)

j [……………………………………………………………………………………………]

[NA B]I G[IG] ⸢*e*⸣-*sil-te* GIG *ana* GIG-*šu* ⸢*la* GID$_2$.DA⸣-*šu* G[IR$_2$.TAB . . .] (BAM 174 obv. 37′)

[N]A BI GIG *e-sil-te* GIG / [. . . *la* GID$_2$].⸢DA⸣-*šu* GIR$_2$.⸢TAB BABBAR⸣ ŠIKA NIG$_2$.⸢BUN.NA⸣ (BAM 175 obv. 2–3)

f *erēnu* ('cedar'), *šurmēnu* ('cypress'), *qanû ṭābu* ('sweet reed'), *ballukku* (an aromatic), *šupuḫru* ('old cedar'), *šimiššallû* ('box tree'), *ḫašû* ('thyme'),
g *nuḫurtu* ('asafoetida'), *nīnû* ('mint'), *urnû* (a kind of mint), *kasû* ('tamarind'), *azupīru* ('saffron'), *uḫūlu qarnānû* ('horned alkali'), *buqlu* ('malt') lumps
h salt, (and) *suluppū* ('dates')—you bring these twenty-three ingredients to a boil (*tušabšal*) in wine, you put (*tanaddi*) oil in (the mixture), and you pour (*tašappak*) it into his anus.

---

i If someone's internal organs (*qerbū*) heave, his eyes are darkened, his appearance . . .
j that man suffers (*maruṣ*) from 'constipation' (*muruṣ esilte*):[602] so that his disease would not be prolonged (*lā urrukīšu*), . . . white scorpion, turtle shell . . .

601 For the reading of the signs in this fragmentary passage, see Maul 2019: 302. The parallel in BAM 175 obv. 1 only has *zi-mu* without the third-person possessive suffix.

602 The precise meaning of *esiltu* is unclear, but some occurrences point to either 'constipation' or 'sphincter', both of which would derive from *esēlu* 'to be constipated'. The verb *esēlu* also occurs in STO 1: 83, STO 2: 136 and 138.

k [...]
[MUD$_2^?$ BURU$_5$].⸢ḪABRUD$^?$⸣.[DA]^{mušen} NITA[603] ⸢^{šim}⸣[x x] *saḫ-le$_2$-e* MUN *eme-sal-li$_3$* [. . .] (BAM 174 obv. 38′)
[. . . *saḫ-le$_2$*]-⸢*e*⸣ MUN *eme-sal-li$_3$* ^{šim}GUR$_2$.⸢GUR$_2$⸣ / [. . .] (BAM 175 obv. 4–5)

l [...]
[x x x x] ⸢^{u2}⸣KUR.RA ^{u2}*ṣa-ṣu-um-ta$_5$* ⸢5⸣ GIN$_2$.TA.AM$_3^!$(AN) x [. . .] (BAM 174 obv. 39′)
[. . . ^{u2}]*ṣa-ṣum-ta* 5 G[IN$_2$.TA.AM$_3$] / [. . .] *a-na* 1 SILA$_3$ A [x x x] (BAM 175 obv. 5–6)

m [...]
[*ina* A].⸢GEŠTIN.NA⸣ *u* KAŠ ŠUB-*ma* GIM ZI$_3$ ŠE.SA.A *ta-sak$_3$* x [. . .] (BAM 174 obv. 40′)
[. . .] ⸢ZI$_3$⸣ ŠE.SA.A *t*[*a-sak$_3$* x x] / [. . .] (BAM 175 obv. 7–8)

n [...]
[x x *l*]*a* ⸢*pa-tan*⸣ NAG-*šu$_2$-ma* SI.SA$_2$-*ma* ŠA$_3$.MEŠ-*šu$_2$* x [. . .] (BAM 174 obv. 41′)
[. . .] x x [. . .] (BAM 175 obv. 8)

o [...]
[. . .] ⸢*šiḫ*⸣-*ḫa-tu$_2$* [. . .] (BAM 174 obv. 42′)

132′ C$_{ii\ 1′}$ *ina* x [..]

133′ C$_{ii\ 2′}$ DIŠ ⸢NA⸣ [..]

†

k blood$^?$ from a male *iṣṣūr ḫurri* ('rock partridge')$^?$ . . . *saḫlû* ('cress'), *emesallu* salt, *kukru* (an aromatic) . . .
l . . . *nīnû* ('mint'), (and) *ṣaṣuntu* (a plant), five shekels each . . . to one litre of water . . .
m you put (*tanaddī-ma*) it in vinegar and beer, and then you pound it like *labtu* ('roasted barley') flour
n . . . you have him drink it (*tašaqqīšū-ma*) on an empty stomach, and then he will void (*ušeššer-ma*), and then his internal organs (*qerbū*) . . .
o . . . wasting away . . .

132′ . . . in . . .

133′ If someone . . .

603 The fragmentary passage at the beginning of the line might have contained a reference to the blood of *iṣṣūr ḫurri* ('rock partridge'), which however does not seem to be used as a medical ingredient elsewhere in our corpus. For this reading, see Maul 2019: 302 and 308.

134′ $C_{ii\ 3'}$ x [...]

approximately eighty-two missing lines

217′ $C_{iv\ 1'}$ [x] *šu*$_2$ i x [...]

218′ $C_{iv\ 2'}$ [DIŠ NA] mur ⸢ti⸣ [...]
219′ $C_{iv\ 3'}$ ⸢NA BI⸣ x x ⸢GIG⸣ [...]
220′ $C_{iv\ 4'}$ ^{u2}*ak-tam ina ḫi-*⸢*iq*⸣ K[AŠ ...]
221′ $C_{iv\ 5'}$ EGIR-*nu ḫi-iq* ⸢KAŠ⸣ x [...]

222′ $C_{iv\ 6'}$ DIŠ KI MIN *a-šu-uš-tu*$_2$ ŠUB.ŠUB-*s*[*u* ...]
223′ $C_{iv\ 7'}$ *ru-pu-uš-tu* NU TUKU.⸢TUKU⸣-*š*[*i* ...]
224′ $C_{iv\ 8'}$ NU ⸢GID$_2$.DA⸣ ^{u2}*ap*$_2$*-ru-ša*$_2$ x [...]
225′ $C_{iv\ 9'}$ ⸢DIŠ-*niš*⸣ [x x] x x [...]

226′ $C_{iv\ 10'}$ [DIŠ NA x x] ⸢*ma*⸣*-gal* TUKU.⸢TUKU⸣ [...]
227′ $C_{iv\ 11'}$ [...] x x x [...]

approximately thirty-two missing lines

†

134′ . . .

approximately eighty-two missing lines

217′ . . .

218′ If someone . . .
219′ that man suffers (*maruṣ*) from . . .
220′ *aktam* (a plant) in diluted beer . . .
221′ afterwards, . . . diluted beer . . .

222′ If DITTO, grief keeps afflicting him (*imtanaqqussu*) . . .
223′ he never has (*lā irtanašši*) phlegm (*rupuštu*) . . .
224′ so that it would not be prolonged (*lā urruki*): *aprušu* (a plant) . . .
225′ together . . .

226′ If someone continually has (*irtanašši*) a lot of . . .
227′ . . .

approximately thirty-two missing lines

260′ A$_{\text{iv 1′}}$ ⸢*ša*⸣ [*ina* LUGAL.MEŠ-*ni a-lik maḫ-ri-ia mam*$_{2}$*-ma šip-ru šu-a-tu la e-ḫu-uz-zu*][604]
261′ A$_{\text{iv 2′}}$ ⸢*bul-ṭi*⸣ T[A *muḫ-ḫi* EN UMBIN *liq-ti* BAR.MEŠ *ta-ḫi-zu nak-la*]
262′ A$_{\text{iv 3′}}$ ⸢*a-zu*⸣*-ga*[*l-lu-ut* ^{d}*nin-urta u* ^{d}*gu-la ma-la ba-aš*$_{2}$*-mu*]
263′ A$_{\text{iv 4′}}$ *ina ṭup-pa-a-n*[*i aš*$_{2}$*-ṭur as-niq* IGI.KAR$_{2}$*-ma*]
264′ A$_{\text{iv 5′}}$ *a-na ta-*⸢*mar-ti*⸣ [*ši-ta-as-si-ia qe*$_{2}$*-reb* E$_{2}$.GAL*-ia u*$_{2}$*-kin*]

260′ Of the kings who came before me, none were able to comprehend this task.
261′ Prescriptions (organized) from head to foot, gleanings from extraneous materials, technical lore
262′ (And) whatever pertains to the great medical expertise of Ninurta and Gula,
263′ I have written on tablets, checked and double-checked, and
264′ I deposited them in the middle of my palace for my reading and recitation.

604 Lines 260′–264′ are reconstructed according to the standard Assurbanipal q colophon (BAK 329), which almost always occurs in our treatise.

Chapter 7
Edition of STO 5

Manuscript A = BAM 579

K 5834 + K 6703 + K 7055 + K 8049 + K 8441 + K 8760 + K 9843 + K 10501 + K 13931 + K 18594 + Sm 1517 + 81–2–4, 195

STO 5	Parallels		
	Publication number	Museum number	Parallel passage
1	AMC 30		
1	CRAN 1: 121 (BAM 480+ ii 57)		
2	CRAN 1: 132 (BAM 480+ ii 68)		
4–5	STO 2: 101–102		
8	STO 2: 141		
34–37	STO 3: 65–66		
34–37	BAM 174	VAT 13761	reverse, 1–3
38	BAM 146	VAT 13793	reverse, 23–26
39	BAM 146	VAT 13793	reverse, 26
40–44	BAM 52	VAT 13733 + 13738	obverse, 39–44
40–44	BAM 67	VAT 13751	1′–9′
41–44	BAM 156	A 238 + VAT 13727 + 14208	obverse, 21–24
49–50	BAM 77	VAT 13737 + 13729$^{?}$ + 14300	obverse, 2′–4′
51–54	BAM 77	VAT 13737 + 13729$^{?}$ + 14300	obverse, 5′–9′
61–64	BAM 174	VAT 13761	reverse, 4–6
66–68	BAM 174	VAT 13761	reverse, 7–9
113′	STO 3: 59		
114′–115′	STO 3: 86		
119′–126′	BAM 168	VAT 9138	obverse, 18–28
119′–126′	BAM 68	A 258	obverse, 1–reverse, 2
119′–123′	BAM 69	A 242	1′–10′
119′–120′	BAM 226	A 224	reverse, 1′–6′
121′–126′	BAM 225	VAT 13845	obverse, 1′–13′
123′–126′	BAM 70	VAT 13907	reverse, 1′–7′
125′–126′	BAM 226	A 224	obverse, 1′–5′
127′–129′	BAM 168	VAT 9138	obverse, 28–32
127′–129′	BAM 68	A 258	reverse, 2–7
127′–128′	BAM 225	VAT 13845	obverse, 14′–16′
130′	BAM 68	A 258	reverse, 8
144′–148′	BAM 216	VAT 8911	obverse, 23′–28′
149′–153′	BAM 7 50	K 3550	reverse, 22′–25′
193′–203′	BAM 159	A 198	column 5, 37–46
204′–215′	BAM 54	VAT 8027	4–12
225′–234′	BAM 49	VAT 7822	reverse, 9–21
225′–234′	BAM 50	VAT 14082	reverse, 7–21
235′	BAM 49	VAT 7822	reverse, 22–23
235′	BAM 50	VAT 14082	reverse, 22–23
236′	AMT 43/6	81–7–27, 57	column 1, 1

https://doi.org/10.1515/9781501506574-007

1 A$_{i\,1}$ DIŠ NA ŠA$_3$-*šu*$_2$ KUM$_2$ DAB PA ^{giš}*šu-še* ZI$_3$.KUM ḪI.ḪI *ina* A GAZI⸢^{sar}⸣ [SILA$_{11}$-*a*]*š* LAL$_2$-*du*
DIŠ NA ŠA$_3$-*šu*$_2$ KUM$_2$ DAB-*it* (AMC 30)
DIŠ K[I MIN . . . Z]I$_3$.KUM ḪI.ḪI *ina* A GAZI^{sar} SILA$_{11}$-*aš* ⸢LAL-*id*⸣ (CRAN 1: 121 = BAM 480+ ii 57)

---

2 A$_{i\,2}$ ^{u2}GEŠTIN KA$_5$.A ḪAD$_2$.DU GAZ SIM (eras.)[605] *ina* A GAZI⸢^{sar}⸣ [SILA$_{11}$-*a*]*š* ⸢LAL$_2$⸣-*du*
[DIŠ KI MIN ^{u2}GEŠTIN] ⸢KA$_5$⸣.A ḪAD$_2$.A SUD$_2$ *ina* A GAZI^{sar} SILA$_{11}$-*aš* LAL (CRAN 1: 132 = BAM 480+ ii 68)

---

3 A$_{i\,3}$ NUMUN ^{u2}*qut-ra-te* GAZ *ina* A GAZI^{sar} *ta-la*$_3$-*aš* LAL *ina* A GAZI⸢^{sar}⸣ x [x] x ⸢LAL$_2$⸣

---

4 A$_{i\,4}$ DIŠ NA SAG ŠA$_3$-*šu*$_2$ KUM$_2$ ŠA$_3$-*šu*$_2$ MU$_2$.MU$_2$ *ana* TI-*šu* 1/2* SILA$_3$ ⸢^{šim}⸣ḪAB *ina* *š*[*ur-šu*]*m-me* KAŠ
DIŠ NA SAG ŠA$_3$-*šu*$_2$ KUM$_2$ ⸢ŠA$_3$⸣-*š*[*u*$_2$ M]U$_2$.MU$_2$-*ḫu* 1/2 SILA$_3$ ^{šim}ḪAB *ina šur-šum-me* KAŠ (STO 2: 101)

†

1 If someone's belly (*libbu*) has been seized (*ṣabit*) by heat: you mix (*tuballal*) leaves from *šūšu* ('liquorice') (and) *isqūqu* (a type of groats), (and) you knead (*talâš*) them in juice from *kasû* ('tamarind'); to be used as a bandage (*ṣamādu*).[606]

---

2 You dry (*tubbal*), crush (*taḫaššal*) (and) sift (*tanappi*) *karān šēlebi* ('fox-vine'), (and) you knead (*talâš*) it in juice from *kasû* ('tamarind'); to be used as a bandage (*ṣamādu*).

---

3 You crush (*taḫaššal*) seed from *qutrātu* ('smoke' plant), you knead it in juice from *kasû* ('tamarind'), (and) you bandage (*taṣammid*) him. . . . in juice from *kasû* ('tamarind'), (and) you bandage him.

---

4 If someone's epigastrium (*rēš libbi*) is hot (*ēm*) (and) his internal organs (*qerbū*) are swollen (*napḫū*): in order to heal him (*ana bulluṭīšu*), you stir into a paste a third of a litre of *ṭūru* ('opopanax') in beer dregs,

---

605 It seems that the scribe first wrote the instruction *ina* A GAZI^{sar} immediately after SIM, but he then erased this instruction and placed it further to the right, so that it would be in the same position as the same instruction one line above.

606 Due to the phonetic complement *-du*, the verb here and in line 2 may be understood as an infinitive (Cadelli 2000: 270 n. 1), used in a similar way as in STO 3: 20–26 and other pharmacological lists, to express that the medicine is 'for bandaging'. See Aro 1961: 28–29 for the use of infinitives in medical texts.

5 A$_{i\,5}$ *tara-bak ina* TUG$_2$ SUR-*ri* GAZI^{sar} ^{šim}BULUḪ SUD$_2$ *ana* IGI SUR *ta-*⸢*za*⸣*-ru$_3$** ⸢IGI⸣ *u* MAŠ.SILA$_3$ LA[L-*m*]*a** *ina-*⸢*eš*⸣

ta-r[*ab-bak*] / *ina* TUG$_2$ *te-*<(*ṭer-ri*)> LAL-*id ana* ⸢*na*⸣-[*aṣ*]-*ma-ti* GAZI^{sar} ŠIM.ŠAL *ta-*⸢*za-ru$_3$* IGI *u* MAŠ.SILA$_3$⸣ [LAL] (STO 2: 101–102)

---

6 A$_{i\,6}$ DIŠ NA ŠA$_3$-*šu$_2$* KUM$_2$-*im* PA ^{giš}ŠE.ḪAR PA ^{giš}*šu-še* 10 ⸢KISAL⸣ MUN *ana* ŠA$_3$ KA[Š ŠU]B-⸢*di*⸣

7 A$_{i\,7}$ *ina* MUL$_4$ *tuš-bat ina še-ri$_3$* NU *pa-tan* NAG-[*ma*] ⸢TI*⸣

---

8 A$_{i\,8}$ DIŠ NA ŠA$_3$-*šu$_2$* KUM$_2$ *u$_2$-kal* NINDA *u* A *la i-maḫ-ḫar* NUMUN ^{giš}ŠINIG SUD$_2$ *ina* LAL$_3$ *u* [.....................]

DIŠ NA ŠA$_3$-*šu$_2$* NINDA *la i-maḫ-*⸢*ḫar*⸣ NUMUN ^{giš}ŠINIG SUD$_2$ *ina* LAL$_3$ *u* I$_3$.NUN ḪI.ḪI *ba-lu pa-tan* N[AG-*šu$_2$-ma* TI] (STO 2: 141)

---

9 A$_{i\,9}$ DIŠ KI MIN 1/3 SILA$_3$ A ZU$_2$.LUM.MA 1/3 SILA$_3$ A ⸢GAZI⸣^{sar} 1/3 SILA$_3$ [................]

DIŠ NA ŠA$_3$-*šu$_2$* NINDA *u* KAŠ *la i-*⸢*maḫ*⸣*-ḫar* 1/3 SILA$_3$ A ZU$_2$.⸢LUM.MA 1/3 SILA$_3$⸣ [A] ⸢GAZI^{sar}⸣ [x x x x x x] (STO 2: 139)

⚚

5 you smear (*teṭerri*) (the mixture) on a piece of fabric, you pound (*tasâk*) *kasû* ('tamarind') (and) *baluḫḫu* ('ferula gummosa'), you scatter them over what you smeared on (SUR),[607] (and) you bandage (*taṣammid-ma*) him front and back (lit. shoulder blades); then he will get well.

---

6 If someone's belly (*libbu*) gets hot (*immim*): you put (*tanaddi*) leaves from ŠE.ḪAR (a tree),[608] leaves from *šūšu* ('liquorice'), (and) ten KISAL measures of salt in beer,

7 you leave them out overnight under the stars, (and) in the morning he drinks (*išattī-ma*) them on an empty stomach; then he will recover (*iballuṭ*).

---

8 If someone's belly (*libbu*) retains heat (and) does not accept bread and water: you pound (*tasâk*) seed from *bīnu* ('tamarisk'), you mix (*tuballal*) it in *dišpu* ('syrup') and ghee (and), you have him drink (*tašaqqīšū-ma*)$^?$ it on an empty stomach; then he will recover (*iballuṭ*).

---

9 If DITTO, he drinks (*išatti*) a third of a litre of juice from *suluppū* ('dates'), a third of a litre of juice from *kasû* ('tamarind'), (and) a third of a litre . . .

---

607 In line with Cadelli 2000: 270 n. 2, SUR can be related to the verb *ṭerû*, which is mentioned earlier in the line: SUR presumably indicates a nominal form from the same verb root, used here to refer to the part of the fabric that was coated in the mixture. For the same expression, viz. *ana* IGI SUR *ta-za-ru$_3$*, see BAM 571 ii 24′, in a collection of therapeutic instructions for the respiratory tract.

608 For a discussion of the ŠE.ḪAR tree, see STO 1: 24.

10 A$_{i\,10}$ NU *pa-tan* 1-*šu*$_2$ 2-*šu*$_2$ 3-*šu*$_2$ NAG AL.US$_2$.SA ⸢A⸣.GEŠTIN.NA NAG *ana* DUR$_2$-[*šu*$_2$ DUB-*ak-ma* TI][609]
EGIR-*šu*$_2$ AL.US$_2$.SA A.GEŠTIN.NA NAG-*ma* KUM$_2$ *ša*$_2$ ŠA$_3$-*šu*$_2$ *i-ša*$_2$*-ḫaṭ*^{aṭ} *im-me-*⸢*si*⸣ [x x x x] (STO 2: 140)

---

11 A$_{i\,11}$ *a-na* KUM$_2$ ŠA$_3$ *šu-li-i* I$_3$.UDU ⸢UKUŠ$_2$⸣.Ḫ[AB ^{š}]^{im}ḪAB[610] ⸢^{u2}⸣[..................]
12 A$_{i\,12}$ *ana* A ŠUB-*di ina* MUL$_4$ *tuš-bat* NU *p*[*a-tan* NA]G [................................]

---

13 A$_{i\,13}$ DIŠ NA ŠA$_3$-*šu*$_2$ KUM$_2$.KUM$_2$ ^{šim}GU[R$_2$.GUR$_2$] ⸢^{šim}⸣[....................................]
14 A$_{i\,14}$ *tuš-bat ina še-ri*$_3$ SUD$_2$ *ana* ŠA$_3$ KAŠ ŠUB [..]

---

15 A$_{i\,15}$ DIŠ NA ŠA$_3$-*šu*$_2$ KUM$_2$-*im* ⸢*la*⸣ x [...]
16 A$_{i\,16}$ *ana* A ŠUB-⸢*di*⸣ *ina* NIN[DU UŠ$_2$-*er* ....]
17 A$_{i\,17}$ ⸢^{u2}*ur*$_2$⸣-[*ne*$_2$*-e* ....] ⸢^{šim}LI⸣ ^{š}[^{im}x x x]

☨

10 once, twice, three times on an empty stomach, (and then) he drinks *šiqqu* ('garum') (and) vinegar, you pour (*tašappak-ma*) them into his anus; then he will recover (*iballuṭ*).

---

11 In order to remove the heat from the belly (*libbu*), . . . pulp from *irrû* ('cucumber'), *ṭūru* ('opopanax') . . .
12 you put (*tanaddi*) them in water, you leave (the mixture) out overnight under the stars, he drinks (*išatti*) it on an empty stomach . . .

---

13 If someone's belly (*libbu*) is constantly hot (*ītenemmim*): *kukru* (an aromatic) . . .
14 you leave it out overnight, in the morning you pound (*tasâk*) it, you put (*tanaddi*) it in beer . . .

---

15 If someone's belly (*libbu*) gets hot (*immim*) (and) does not . . .
16 you put (*tanaddi*) it in water, you heat (*tesekker*) it in an oven . . .
17 you pound (*tasâk*) *urnû* (a kind of mint) . . . *burāšu* (a kind of juniper) (and) . . .

---

609 Based on the expression that directly precedes the break, viz. *ana* DUR$_2$-*šu*$_2$, this seems to be a likely restoration, suggested here in line with Cadelli 2000: 253.

610 The amount of room in the break preceding ^{šim}ḪAB could have accommodated the name of another ingredient, if it consisted of no more than two signs, such as ^{šim}LI. However, the spacing of the line, with empty room left between entries, suggests instead that there was no other ingredient written between I$_3$.UDU UKUŠ$_2$.ḪAB and ^{šim}ḪAB.

18 A$_{i\,18}$ TEŠ$_2$.BI SUD$_2$ ⸢*ina** A⸣*.[GEŠTIN.NA NAG ....] ⸢*ina*⸣ I$_3$.UDU ḪI.ḪI *ina* KUŠ SUR ⸢ŠA$_3$⸣*-*š*[*u*$_2$* LAL-*ma* TI]

---

19 A$_{i\,19}$ NUMUN ^{giš}ŠINIG ^{u2}x* [..................................] x KI MIN *ina* I$_3$.⸢GIŠ⸣ x [x x]

---

20 A$_{i\,20}$ DIŠ NA SAG ŠA$_3$-*šu*$_2$ *um-m*[*a-am* TUKU-*ši*[611] .... KI MI]N ⸢*ina*⸣ x [x x x]

---

21 A$_{i\,21}$ DIŠ KI MIN ⸢DIDA$_2$ *ba*⸣-*l*[*u pa-ta*]*n* [NAG]

---

22 A$_{i\,22}$ DIŠ NA SAG ŠA$_3$-*šu*$_2$ *um-ma-am* TUKU-*ši a-na* KUM$_2$ *ša*$_2$ S[AG* Š]A$_3$-*šu*$_2$ *ša*$_2$-*ḫa-ṭi* [......................]
23 A$_{i\,23}$ I$_3$.GIŠ BARA$_2$.GA *lu* A UZU ŠAḪ *kab-ra* NA[G.NA]G-⸢*ma*⸣ *um-mu š*[*a*$_2$* SAG ŠA$_3$-*šu*$_2$]
24 A$_{i\,24}$ *iš-ša*$_2$-*ḫa-aṭ im-me-*⸢*es*⸣-[*si* x] x ib x [x x x]

---

25 A$_{i\,25}$ DIŠ NA SAG ŠA$_3$-*šu*$_2$ KUM$_2$ *u*$_2$-*ka-al-ma* NINDA *u* ⸢A⸣* [NU IGI ....]

✝

18 together (and) he drinks (*išatti*)$^?$ them in vinegar$^?$ . . . you mix (*tuballal*) it in fat, you smear (*teṭerri*) (the mixture) on a piece of leather, (and) you bandage (*taṣammid-ma*) his belly; then he will recover (*iballuṭ*).

---

19 Seed from *bīnu* ('tamarisk') . . . DITTO in oil . . .

---

20 If someone has (*iraššši*) heat in his epigastrium (*rēš libbi*): . . . DITTO in . . .

---

21 If DITTO, he drinks (*išatti*) *billatu* ('beerwort') on an empty stomach.

---

22 If someone has (*irašši*) heat in his epigastrium (*rēš libbi*): in order to drain the heat from his epigastrium, . . .
23 he keeps drinking (*ištanattī-ma*) either pressed oil or broth from fatty pork, and then the heat in his epigastrium
24 will be drained (and) washed off[612] . . .

---

25 If someone's epigastrium (*rēš libbi*) retains heat and, subsequently, does not accept bread and water: you pulverize (*tapâṣ*)[613] . . .

---

611 The reconstruction is based on line 22 below.

612 For the same formulation, written as *i-ša*$_2$*-ḫaṭ*^{at} *im-me-si*, see STO 2: 140.

613 The verb *pa'āṣu*, which is rendered with the same logogram as *ḫašālu* (viz. GAZ), is another way to describe that the ingredients need to be crushed during the preparation of medications (Herrero 1984: 63). Within the Stomach Treatise, this verb only seems to occur here in STO 5, but it is attested in other therapeutic texts. For *pa'āṣu*, see now Stol 2020a: 107.

26 A$_{i\,26}$ *ta-pa-aṣ lu ana* 1/2 SILA$_3$ KAŠ SAG *lu ana* ⸢1/2⸣ [SILA$_3$ ....]

---

27 A$_{i\,27}$ DIŠ NA SAG ŠA$_3$-*šu*$_2$ *um-ma-am ṣe*-⸢*e*⸣-*en ana u*[*m-mi* SAG ŠA$_3$-*šu*$_2$ *ša*$_2$-*ḫa-ṭi* ....]
28 A$_{i\,28}$ ZA$_3$.ḪI.LI *ṭe*$_4$-*ne*$_2$-*ti* KI NINDA[614] x [x] x *ina* x [..]
29 A$_{i\,29}$ KUM$_2$ *ša*$_2$ SAG ŠA$_3$-*šu*$_2$ *iš*-⸢*ša*$_2$-*ḫa-aṭ*⸣ [..]

---

30 A$_{i\,30}$ DIŠ NA KUM$_2$ ŠA$_3$ TUKU.TUKU-*ši* UD.DA SA$_2$.SA$_2$ x* [..]
31 A$_{i\,31}$ ^{u2}KUR.RA GAZI^{sar} ^{u2}*ak-tam* U$_2$ BABBAR ^{š}[^{im} ....]
32 A$_{i\,32}$ ^{u2}IGI-*lim* ^{u2}IGI.NIŠ 14 U$_2$.[ḪI.A ....]
33 A$_{i\,33}$ SUD$_2$ *ina* ZA$_3$.ḪI.LI *si-ka-a-ti* [..]

---

34 A$_{i\,34}$ *a-na ṣi-ri-iḫ-ti* KUM$_2$ ŠA$_3$ ZI-*ḫi* ⸢U$_2$⸣ [...]
[. . .] x (STO 3: 65)
[*a-na ṣi-r*]*i-iḫ-te* KUM$_2$ ŠA$_3$ ZI U$_2$ ⸢BABBAR⸣ [. . .] (BAM 174 rev. 1)

✝

26 . . . it in either half a litre of high-quality beer or half a litre of . . .

---

27 If someone's epigastrium (*rēš libbi*) is loaded (*ṣēn*)[615] with heat: in order to drain the heat from his epigastrium, . . .
28 . . . ground *saḫlû* ('cress') with bread . . . in . . .
29 the heat in his epigastrium will be drained . . .

---

30 If someone continually has (*irtanašši*) heat in the belly (*libbu*), he is . . . by fever (*ṣēta* SA$_2$.SA$_2$): in order to heal him (*ana bulluṭīšu*), . . .
31 *nīnû* ('mint'), *kasû* ('tamarind'), *aktam* (a plant), *šammu peṣû* ('white plant') . . .
32 *imḫur-līm* ('faces a thousand' plant), (and) *imḫur-ešrā* ('faces twenty' plant)— . . . fourteen ingredients . . .
33 you pound (*tasâk*) them, . . . in powdered *saḫlû* ('cress') . . .

---

34 In order to remove (*nasāḫi*) burning heat from the belly (*libbu*), *šammu peṣû* ('white plant') . . .

614 As Cadelli (2000: 254 n. 7) notes, the sign GAR could also be used here to denote a measurement as in 4-*ut* for Akk. *rebūt* 'a fourth of a shekel'; for GAR as a measurement in Late Babylonian texts, see also Finkel 2000: 147. Its co-occurrence with ground *saḫlû* ('cress') reminds us, however, of CRAN 1: 10–12 (BAM 480+ i 10–12), where the same material needs to be skimmed off from the mouth of a mortar using a piece of bread. For a discussion of this passage, see also STO 1: 85.

615 The imagery here is probably based on loading cargo onto a boat or coals into a brazier (CAD Ṣ 132). For the same verb describing a belly loaded with wind (i.e., flatulence), see STO 2: 124.

35 A$_{i\,35}$ ^{u2}KUR.RA ^{šim}GUR$_2$.GUR$_2$ NAGA SI MUN [..........]
^{u2}⸢KUR⸣.K[UR ^{šim}GUR$_2$.GUR$_2$ NA]GA ⸢SI⸣ MUN ^{u2}IGI-*lim* ^{u2}IGI.NIŠ ^{u2}*tar-muš* (STO 3: 65)
[. . .] / [x x x NA]GA SI MUN ^{u2}IGI-*lim* ⸢^{u2}⸣[IGI.NIŠ . . .] (BAM 174 rev. 1–2)

36 A$_{i\,36}$ ^{u2}KUR.KUR ⸢NA$_4$ *ga-bi-i* ^{u2}*ak*⸣-*t*[*am* ....]
[. . . ^{u2}ḪA]R.ḪAR 14 ⸢U$_2$⸣.[ḪI.A ŠE]Š (STO 3: 66)
[. . .] / [NA$_4$ *ga-bi*]-*i* ^{u2}*ak-tam* ^{u2}ḪAR.ḪAR 14 U$_2$ *an-nu-*[*ti*] (BAM 174 rev. 2–3)

37 A$_{i\,37}$ TEŠ$_2$.BI *ta-pa-aṣ ina* K[AŠ ....]
DIŠ-*niš* SUD$_2$ *ina* KAŠ NAG-*ma* BURU$_8$ (STO 3: 66)
[. . .] (BAM 174 rev. 3)

---

38 A$_{i\,38}$ U$_2$ *a-re-e* GA[ZI^{sar} ....]
U$_2$ *a-re-e* ^{u2}x [. . .] / ZA$_3$.ḪI.LI⸢^{sar}⸣ [x x] ⸢^{šim}⸣x [. . .] / ^{u2}IGI-⸢*lim*⸣ [^{u2}I]GI.NIŠ ^{u2}*t*[*ar*$^{?}$-*muš*$_8$ . . .] / NA$_4$ *ga-bi*-⸢*i*⸣ ^{u2}*ak-tam* (BAM 146 rev. 23–26)

---

39 A$_{i\,39}$ PAP *an-nu-tu*$_4$ *bul-ṭu* D[U$_8$[616] ....]
PAP [x] U$_2$.⸢ḪI.A⸣ *an-nu-ti* (BAM 146 rev. 26)

---

†

35 *nīnû* ('mint'), *kukru* (an aromatic), *uḫūlu qarnānû* ('horned alkali'), salt, *imḫur-līm* ('faces a thousand' plant), *imḫur-ešrā* ('faces twenty' plant), *tarmuš* ('lupin'),
36 *atā'išu* (a plant), *aban gabî* ('alum'), *aktam* (a plant), (and) *ḫašû* ('thyme')—you pulverize these fourteen ingredients
37 together, he drinks (*išattī-ma*) them in beer, and then he will vomit (*i'arru*).

---

38 Drugs to induce vomiting: *kasû* ('tamarind')[617] . . .

---

39 All these are remedies to release . . .[618]

---

616 Cadelli (2000: 254) correctly, in our view, reads DU$_8$, which corresponds to Akkadian *paṭāru* 'to release'. This is a rarely used verb in our text but occurs elsewhere in the Diagnostic Handbook, as in Sagig 17: 5–6, to describe 'releasing' symptoms, including heat (*ummu*), from a patient (Heeßel 2000: 195 and 206).

617 The structure of the thematic units in lines 38–39 is unusual: the two headers in these lines (U$_2$ *a-re-e* and PAP *an-nu-tu*$_4$ *bul-ṭu* D[U$_8$]) sit in between two recipes for *ṣiriḫti (ummi) libbi* and probably refer to the recipes for emetics that follow in lines 40–55. For similar headers, see BAM 146 rev. 23–26, included here as a distant parallel without any attempt at a more complete reconstruction of our passage in lines 38–39.

618 The rubrics in line 38 and 39 seem to mark a division between the first section of the text, concerned with heat in the belly, and the following section, where heat-related conditions are treated with the help of various emetics. Rubrics like this were sometimes deleted in different stages of the editorial work: see, for example, the discussion in STO 1: 131a.

40 A$_{i\,40}$ DIŠ NA *ṣi-ri-iḫ-ti* ŠA$_3$ TUKU-*ma* ŠA$_3$-*šu*$_2$ KUM$_2$ ⸢*u*$_2$⸣-[*ka-al mi-n*]*a*-⸢*tu-šu*$_2$⸣* D[UB.DUB]
DIŠ NA *ṣi-ri-iḫ-ti* ŠA$_3$-*bi* TUKU-*ma* ŠA$_3$-*šu*$_2$ KUM$_2$ *u*$_2$-*kal mi-na-tu*-⸢*šu*$_2$⸣ [DUB.DUB] (BAM 52 obv. 39)
[. . .] x x ⸢ŠA$_3$⸣ [. . .] / [. . .] ⸢*mi*⸣-[*na-t*]*u-šu*$_2$ DUB.D[UB] (BAM 67: 1′–2′)

41 A$_{i\,41}$ GABA-*su i-ka-sa-su* LU$_2$ BI UD.DA *ḫa-miṭ* [*ana*] ⸢TI⸣-*šu*$_2$[619] ^{šim}GUR$_2$.GUR$_2$ ^{ši}[^{m}LI]
GABA-*su i-ka-sa-su* NA BI UD.DA *ḫa-miṭ ana* ⸢TI-*šu*$_2$ ^{šim}GUR$_2$⸣.GUR$_2$ ^{ši}[^{m}LI] (BAM 52 obv. 40)
[GABA-*s*]*u u*$_2$-*kas*$_3$-<*sa*>-*su* UD.DA *ḫ*[*a-miṭ*] / ⸢*ana* TI-*šu*$_2$⸣ ^{giš}GUR$_2$.GUR$_2$ ^{giš}⸢LI⸣ (BAM 67: 3′–4′)
^{šim}GUR$_2$.GUR$_2$ ^{šim}LI (BAM 156 obv. 21)

42 A$_{i\,42}$ ^{u2}KUR.KUR ^{u2}*tar-muš* ^{u2}IGI-*lim* ^{u2}⸢IGI*.NIŠ⸣ ^{šim}ŠEŠ NA$_4$ *ga-bi*-⸢*i*⸣
^{u2}KUR.KUR ^{u2}*tar-muš* ^{u2}IGI-*lim* ^{u2}IGI.NIŠ ^{š}[^{im}ŠEŠ x x x x] (BAM 52 obv. 41)
^{u2}KUR.KUR ^{u2}⸢*tar*⸣-[*muš*] / ^{u2}IGI-⸢*lim* ^{u2}⸣IGI.NIŠ ^{šim}ŠE[Š] / NA$_4$ *ga*-⸢*bi*⸣-*i* (BAM 67: 4′–6′)
^{u2}KUR.KUR ^{u2}*tar-muš*$_8$ ^{u2}IGI-*lim* ^{u2}IGI.NIŠ / ^{šim}ŠEŠ NA$_4$ *gab-i* (BAM 156 obv. 21–22)

43 A$_{i\,43}$ ILLU LI.TAR ^{u2}ḪAB ^{u2}*ak-tam saḫ-lu-u* GA[ZI^{sar}] ⸢^{u2}⸣KUR.RA 14 U$_2$.ḪI.A ŠEŠ
ILLU LI.DUR ^{u2}ḪAB ^{u2}*ak-tam saḫ-lu-u* [x x x x x] / 14 U$_2$.ḪI.A *an-nu-ti* (BAM 52 obv. 42–43)
ILLU LI.DUR ⸢^{u2}⸣[ḪAB] / ^{u2}*ak-tam* [*sa*]*ḫ-li*$_2$-*i* GAZI^{sar} ⸢^{u2}⸣[KUR.RA] / [14] ⸢U$_2$⸣.MEŠ ⸢ŠEŠ⸣ (BAM 67: 6′–8′)
ILLU LI.TAR ^{u2}ḪAB ^{u2}*ak-tam* / *saḫ-li*$_2$-*i ni-nu-u*$_2$ GAZI^{sar} 14 U$_2$.ḪI.A ŠEŠ (BAM 156 obv. 22–23)

40 If someone has (*iraššī-ma*) a burning sensation in the belly (*libbu*), and subsequently, his belly retains heat, his limbs are flaccid (*tabkā*)[620]

41 (and) his chest gnaws at him, that man is burning with fever (*ṣēta ḫamiṭ*): in order to heal him (*ana bulluṭīšu*), *kukru* (an aromatic), *burāšu* (a kind of juniper),

42 *atā'išu* (a plant), *tarmuš* ('lupin'), *imḫur-līm* ('faces a thousand' plant), *imḫur-ešrā* ('faces twenty' plant), *murru* ('myrrh'), *aban gabî* ('alum'),

43 resin from *abukkatu* (a tree), *būšānu* ('smelly' plant), *aktam* (a plant), *saḫlû* ('cress'), *kasû* ('tamarind') (and) *nīnû* ('mint')—you pulverize these fourteen ingredients

619 A similar symptom description is found in BAM 145 obv. 16–17, with *ṣiriḫtu* and *ummu* combined into a single statement: [*ṣi-ri-iḫ*]-⸢*ti*⸣ KUM$_2$ ŠA$_3$ TUKU.MEŠ / [NA BI UD.DA TAB.BA *ana* TI-*šu*$_2$]. See also BM 78963, which begins in lines 1–2 with the same symptom description as in STO 5: 40–41, but the prescription itself is different (Stadhouders and Johnson 2018: 568 ll. 1–2, and 585).

620 For the straightforward syllabic spelling *tab-ka* of the verb *tabāku* 'to pour out', used here in the sense of 'limp, flaccid' (CAD T 27–28), see CRAN 1: 234 (BAM 480+ iv 33) and parallels.

44 A$_{\text{i}\,44}$ DIŠ-*niš ta-pa-aṣ ina* KAŠ NU *pa-tan* NAG-*ma* BURU$_8$ [*maš-qit* NAM.E]RIM$_2$.BUR$_2$.RU.DA.KE$_4$

DIŠ-*niš ta-pa-aṣ ina* K[AŠ x x x x x] / BURU$_8$ *maš-qit* NAM.ERIM$_2$ (BAM 52 obv. 43–44)

DIŠ-*niš* SUD$_2$ NU *pa-tan ina* ⸢KAŠ⸣ [NAG] / [*i-a*]*r*$_2$-*ru*$_3$ *maš-qit* NAM.RIM.BUR$_2$.RU.D[A] (BAM 67: 8′–9′)

DIŠ-*niš* SUD$_2$ / *ina* KAŠ *ba-lu pa-tan* NAG.MEŠ-*ma ina-eš maš-qit* NAM.RIM (BAM 156 obv. 23–24)

---

45 A$_{\text{i}\,45}$ DIŠ KI MIN ^{u2}*saḫ-le*$_2$-*e* ⸢SUD$_2$⸣ *b*[*a-l*]*u p*[*a-tan ina* K]AŠ NAG-*ma* (eras.)[621] BURU$_8$

---

46 A$_{\text{i}\,46}$ DIŠ NA KUM$_2$ ŠA$_3$ TUKU *saḫ-le*$_2$-*e* ⸢^{u2}⸣[KU]R.RA ^{u2}KUR.KUR

47 A$_{\text{i}\,47}$ ^{u2}*ur*$_2$-*nu-u* ^{u2}*ak-tam* NA$_4$ *ga-*⸢*bi*⸣-*i* ^{u2}ḪAR.⸢ḪAR⸣ *ina* KAŠ NAG-*ma* BURU$_8$

---

48 A$_{\text{i}\,48}$ DIŠ KI MIN NAGA SI ILLU LI.⸢DUR ^{u2}⸣ḪAR.ḪAR ^{u2}*ti-ia-*⸢*ta*$_5$⸣ *ina* KAŠ NAG-*ma* BURU$_8$

---

49 A$_{\text{i}\,49}$ DIŠ KI MIN ^{u2}ḪAR.ḪAR ^{u2}KUR.⸢KUR⸣ NAGA SI GI DU$_{10}$.GA ^{u2}ḪA ⸢U$_2$⸣ BABBAR ^{u2}⸢*ak*⸣*-*tam*

[. . . ^{u2}]ḪAR.ḪAR ^{u2}KUR.KUR NAGA ⸢SI⸣ [. . .] / [. . . ^{u2}*ak*]-*tam* (BAM 77 obv. 2′–3′)

†

44 together, he drinks (*išattī-ma*) them in beer on an empty stomach, and then he will vomit (*i'arru*); a potion for relieving (broken) oaths.

---

45 If DITTO, you pound (*tasâk*) *saḫlû* ('cress'), he drinks (*išattī-ma*) it in beer on an empty stomach, and then he will vomit (*i'arru*).

---

46 If someone has (*iraššī*) heat in the belly (*libbu*): he drinks (*išattī-ma*) *saḫlû* ('cress'), *nīnû* ('mint'), *atā'išu* (a plant),

47 *urnû* (a kind of mint), *aktam* (a plant), *aban gabî* ('alum'), (and) *ḫašû* ('thyme') in beer, and then he will vomit (*i'arru*).

---

48 If DITTO, he drinks (*išattī-ma*) *uḫūlu qarnānû* ('horned alkali'), resin from *abukkatu* (a tree), *ḫašû* ('thyme'), (and) *tīyatu* (a plant) in beer, and then he will vomit (*i'arru*).

---

49 If DITTO, he drinks (*išattī-ma*) *ḫašû* ('thyme'), *atā'išu* (a plant), *uḫūlu qarnānû* ('horned alkali'), *qanû ṭābu* ('sweet reed'), *urânu* ('anise'), *šammu peṣû* ('white plant'), *aktam* (a plant),

---

621 There seem to be traces of the syllabic orthography *i-ar*$_2$*-ru* that were erased at some point and replaced with the logographic rendering of the verb, viz. BURU$_8$.

50 A$_{i\,50}$ $^{ḫe\text{-}pi_2}$ ILLU LI.TAR MUN ⸢*eme*⸣-*sal-li*$_3$ ^{šim}GUR$_2$.GUR$_2$ ⸢*ina*⸣ KAŠ NAG-*ma* BURU$_8$
$^{he\text{-}pi_2}$ ILLU LI.TAR MUN ⸢*eme*⸣-[*sal-li*$_3$ . . .] / [. . . *i*]-*na* KAŠ NAG-*ma* [. . .] (BAM 77 obv. 3′–4′)

---

51 A$_{i\,51}$ *ana* KUM$_2$ ŠA$_3$ ZI-*ḫi* ^{ši}[^{m}BA]L ^{šim}IM.MAN.DU GI DU$_{10}$.⸢GA⸣ ^{u2}⸢ḪAR.ḪAR⸣
[. . .] ⸢^{šim}⸣MUG ^{šim}IM.MAN.DU [. . .] (BAM 77 obv. 5′)

52 A$_{i\,52}$ $^{ḫe\text{-}pi_2}$ ^{u2}NU.LUḪ.ḪA [Z]U$_2$.LUM.MA ^{šim}GUR$_2$.GUR$_2$ 7 U$_2$.ḪI.A *an-nu-ti* DIŠ-*niš* ⸢GAZ⸣ SIM
[. . .] ⸢^{u2}⸣NU.LUḪ.ḪA ZU$_2$.L[UM.MA . . .] / [. . . DIŠ]- ⸢*niš*⸣ GAZ SIM (BAM 77 obv. 6′–7′)

53 A$_{i\,53}$ *ina* KAŠ *tara-muk ina* NINDU UŠ$_2$-*er* ⸢E$_{11}$-*ma*⸣ *ta-ša*$_2$-*ḫal* SED LAGAB MUNU$_6$ *ana* ⸢ŠA$_3$⸣ ŠUB-*di* GAR-*an*
ina KA[Š . . .] / [. . .] ⸢*ta*⸣-*ša*$_2$-*ḫal* S[ED . . .] (BAM 77 obv. 7′–8′)

54 A$_{i\,54}$ *ina pa-ni* A GAZI^{sar} D[UB] ⸢U$_2$$^{?}$⸣[622] *an-na-a ana* DUR$_2$-*šu*$_2$ D[UB*-*a*]*k-ma* TI-*uṭ*
[. . .] ⸢DUB$^{?}$⸣ [. . .] (BAM 77 obv. 9′)

---

50 ^{broken} resin from *abukkatu* (a tree), *emesallu* salt, (and) *kukru* (an aromatic) in beer, and then he will vomit (*i'arru*).

---

51 In order to remove (*nasāḫi*) heat from the belly (*libbu*), *ballukku* (an aromatic), *suādu* (a kind of sedge), *qanû ṭābu* ('sweet reed'), *ḫašû* ('thyme'),

52 ^{broken} *nuḫurtu* ('asafoetida'), *suluppū* ('dates'), (and) *kukru* (an aromatic)— you crush (*taḫaššal*) (and) sift (*tanappi*) these seven ingredients together,

53 you soak them in beer, you heat (*tesekker*) (the mixture) in an oven, you take it out (*tušellâ-ma*), and then you filter it, you let it cool (*tukaṣṣa*), you put (*tanaddi*) *buqlu* ('malt') lumps in it, (and) you let it stand (*tašakkan*),[623]

54 (then) you pour (*tašappak*) juice from *kasû* ('tamarind') on the surface, (and) you pour (*tašappak-ma*) this medication$^{?}$ into his anus; then he will recover (*iballuṭ*).

---

622 The wedges after the break may either represent the right side of DI, as in Š[UB-*d*]*i* (Böck 2009: 121 with n. 72), or the last two horizontals of U$_2$ = Akk. *šammu*, presumably used here to describe the whole mixture as a single medication (CAD Š/1 318–320). However, the traces before the break do not seem to correspond to ŠUB, perhaps representing DUB instead. Our reading here is in line with the same idiom, namely *ina pa-ni* A GAZI^{sar} DUB, found in STO 3: 71.

623 The use of GAR-*an* = Akk. *tašakkan* 'you let it stand' may be largely temporal, meaning you let the mixture sit for a period of time, until the malt forms a layer on the surface. The *kasû* juice is then poured on top of this layer of malt (in the next line).

55 A$_{i\,55}$ DIŠ $^{ḫe\text{-}pi_2}$ ^{u2}KUR.KUR ILL[U LI.TAR] ⸢^{u2}KUR⸣.RA GAZI^{sar} $^{ḫe\text{-}pi_2*}$ *kam-mi* ^{lu2}[AŠGAB *ina* KAŠ NA]G-*ma i-ar$_2$-ru*

---

56 A$_{i\,56}$ DIŠ $^{ḫe\text{-}pi_2}$ ^{u2}KUR.RA ^{šim}L[I ^{ši}]^{m}MUG $^{ḫe\text{-}pi_2}$ ^{šim}GIG ^{š}[^{im}x x ^{šim}ŠE.L]I ⸢BABBAR⸣ LAGAB MUNU$_6$

57 A$_{i\,57}$ $^{ḫe\text{-}pi_2}$ DIDA$_2$ PAP 14 ⸢U$_2$⸣.[ḪI.A *a*]*n-nu-ti* $^{ḫe\text{-}pi_2}$ *ina* ^{urudu}ŠEN*.T[UR* ŠEG$_6$-*šal šum$_4$-ma* E]N.TE.NA

58 A$_{i\,58}$ $^{ḫe\text{-}pi_2}$ *tu-kaṣ$_3$-ṣa*[624] I$_3$.GIŠ *ana* I[GI ŠUB]-*di ana* DUR$_2$-*šu$_2$* DUB-*a*[*k* .... SI.SA$_2$-*a*]*m*[625] *ina-eš*

---

59 A$_{i\,59}$ *ana* KUM$_2$ ŠA$_3$ *šu-ṣi$_2$-i* ⸢^{šim}⸣[BULU]Ḫ x [x x x^{u2}Ḫ]AR.ḪAR

☨

55 If ^{broken}: he drinks (*išattī-ma*) *atā'išu* (a plant), resin from *abukkatu* (a tree), *nīnû* ('mint'), *kasû* ('tamarind'), ^{broken} (and) *kammu* ('fungus') from a leather worker in beer, and then he will vomit.

---

56 If ^{broken}: *nīnû* ('mint'), *burāšu* (a kind of juniper), *ballukku* (an aromatic) ^{broken} *kanaktu* (an aromatic) . . . white *kikkirânu* ('juniper seeds'), *buqlu* ('malt') lumps,

57 ^{broken} (and) *billatu* ('beerwort')—altogether, these fourteen ingredients ^{broken} you bring them to a boil (*tušabšal*) in a small copper pot, if it is winter

58 ^{broken} you let it cool, you add (*tanaddi*) oil, you pour (*tašappak*) (the mixture) into his anus (and) . . . will come straight out (*iššeram*)$^{?}$; (then) he will get well.

---

59 In order to drive the heat from the belly (*libbu*): you soak *baluḫḫu* ('ferula gummosa')$^{?}$ . . . *ḫašû* ('thyme'),

---

624 The frequency of the *ḫepi* glosses in this part of the text shows that the tablet used by the scribe to produce his copy was in a fragmentary state of preservation in antiquity. AMT 98/3: 4′–5′ could give us some idea about the instructions that might have been included at this point: *šum$_4$-ma* EN.TE.NA *ba-aḫ-ru-us-su šum$_4$-ma* AMA.MEŠ *tu-kaṣ$_3$-ṣa* 'if it is winter, (you use the medicine) while it is steaming hot, (and) if it is summer, you let (the medicine) cool'. For a discussion of seasonal treatments, see Stadhouders and Johnson 2018: 597–598.

625 For the orthography SI.SA$_2$-*am*, which is otherwise rare in our corpus, see STO 3: 234 where it is said that the therapy will result in the *aḫḫāzu*-jaundice 'coming straight out' from the patient's belly (*aḫ-ḫa-zu ša$_2$* ŠA$_3$-*šu$_2$* SI.SA$_2$-*am*). Our prognosis here differs only in the ailment that is coming out of the patient's body: presumably 'heat' (Akk. *ummu*) instead of the *aḫḫāzu*-jaundice.

60 A$_{i\,60}$ ^{u2}NU.LUḪ.ḪA *ina* KAŠ *tara-muk ina* x [..................] *ta-ḫaṭ*[626]

---

61 A$_{i\,61}$ *ana* KUM$_2$ ŠA$_3$ ZI-*ḫi* 1 SILA$_3$ LAGAB MUNU$_6$ *ina* KA[Š *tara-muk ina* ^{na4}NA.ZA$_3$.ḪI.L]I SUD$_2$
[x x x x Z]I 1 SILA$_3$ LAGAB MUNU$_6$ <*ina*> KAŠ *tara-muk* <*ina*> ^{na4}NA.Z[A$_3$.ḪI.LI . . .] (BAM 174 rev. 4)

62 A$_{i\,62}$ 1 GIN$_2$ ^{šim}LI 1 GIN$_2$ ŠIM.ŠAL 15 GIN$_2$ [NUMUN GADA ŠE]Š
[. . .] / [1 GIN$_2$ ŠIM].ŠAL 15 GIN$_2$ NUMUN GADA *an-na-a* (BAM 174 rev. 4–5)

63 A$_{i\,63}$ *ina* ^{na4}NA.ZA$_3$.ḪI.LI SUD$_2$ *ina* 1 SILA$_3$ KAŠ *dan-na ta-ḫaṭ ina* ⸢*še*⸣-*r*[*i*$_3$ *ina* NINDU UŠ$_2$-*er*] *tu-kaṣ*$_3$-*ṣa*
ina ^{na4}NA.ZA$_3$.Ḫ[I.LI . . .] / [x x x x Š]EG$_6$-*šal* E$_{11}$-*ma tu-kaṣ*$_3$-*ṣa* (BAM 174 rev. 5–6)

64 A$_{i\,64}$ *ta-ḫaṭ ta-ḫi-it-tu*$_4$ *an-ni-tu*$_4$ *ina* ITI 5-*šu*$_2$ 3 5/6$^!$(UR) GIN$_2$ *ša*$_2$ *t*[*a*$^?$-*ḫi-it-ti* x x x] ⸢^{u2}⸣KUR.RA
ta-ḫaṭ ta-ḫi-i[*t-tu*$_4$ . . .] (BAM 174 rev. 6)

60 (and) *nuḫurtu* ('asafoetida') in beer, . . . in . . . (and) you measure out (the doses) (*taḫâṭ*).[627]

---

61 In order to remove (*nasāḫi*) the heat from the belly (*libbu*), you soak one litre
of *buqlu* ('malt') lumps in beer (and) you pound (*tasâk*) it in a mortar,
62 (then) you pound (*tasâk*) one shekel of *burāšu* (a kind of juniper), one shekel
of *šimišallû* ('box tree'), fifteen shekels of seed from *kitû* ('flax'), (and)
the aforementioned (mixture of malt and beer)
63 in the mortar, you measure (this mixture) into one litre of strong beer, in the
morning you heat (*tesekker*) it in an oven, (and) you let it cool,
64 (then) you measure it (again) (and) . . . this batch within a month, up to five
times, three and five-sixths shekels of the batch$^?$ (each time),

---

626 The verb at the end of this line is most likely *ḫâṭu*, not *sâku*, which often occurs in the syllabic form *ta-sak*$_3$, but the occurrence of *ta-sak*$_3$ at the end of a prescription would make little sense. The verb *ḫâṭu* and its nominalised form *taḫittu* (see CAD T 50) occur several times in the next prescription, and in this prescription *sâku* is always rendered with SUD$_2$. Elsewhere in the medical texts *sâku* is never the final verb in a recipe.

627 There is no lexical evidence that would imply that *ḫâṭu* (CAD H 162) can describe the administration of a drug. This seems to be in agreement with the different discourse pattern here and in the following prescription: a purpose clause (the preposition *ana* followed by an infinitive) is used to specify the goal of the procedure, no patient is mentioned, and the usual concluding formula (*inêš* or *iballuṭ*) is omitted. The prescriptions here and in lines 61–65 were clearly meant to describe the preparation of medicines in advance, without any particular patient in mind. For a somewhat different interpretation, see Chalender 2020: 66–68.

65 A$_{i\,65}$ *ina* 5 SILA$_3$ GA *ta-ḫi-it-tu$_4$ an-ni-tu$_2$* [(...)] ⸢*ta*⸣-*ḫaṭ*

---

66 A$_{ii\,1}$ ⸢DIŠ NA KUM$_2$⸣ ŠA$_3$ TUKU.MEŠ ^{u2}ḪAR.ḪAR ⸢^{u2}⸣[NU.LUḪ.ḪA ....]

[DIŠ NA KU]M$_2$ ŠA$_3$ TUKU.MEŠ-*ši* ^{u2}ḪAR.ḪAR ^{u2}NU.[LUḪ.ḪA . . .] / [^{u2}ḪUR].SAG (BAM 174 rev. 7–8)

67 A$_{ii\,2}$ ^{u2}KUR.RA GAZI^{sar} ^{šim}LI ^{ši}[^{m} ....]

^{u2}KUR.RA GAZI^{sar} ^{šim}LI [. . .] / [NAG]A SI (BAM 174 rev. 8–9)

68 A$_{ii\,3}$ *saḫ-le$_2$-e* 13 U$_2$.ḪI.A *ina* KAŠ *ina* A.GEŠTIN.N[A ....]

saḫ-lu-u 13 U$_2$ *an-nu-ti$_3$ ina* ⸢NINDU⸣ UŠ$_2$-[*er* . . .] (BAM 174 rev. 9)

---

69 A$_{ii\,4}$ DIŠ KI MIN *saḫ-le$_2$-e* ARA$_3$-*ti$_3$ ina* ⸢A⸣.[GEŠTIN.NA ....]

---

70 A$_{ii\,5}$ DIŠ KI MIN 10 GIN$_2$ ^{giš}*e-re-nu* 10 GIN$_2$ ^{g}[^{iš}* ....]

71 A$_{ii\,6}$ 10 GIN$_2$ ^{šim}⸢BAL⸣ 10 G[IN$_2$ ....]

approximately thirty-eight missing lines

†

65 you measure this batch into five litres of milk together with *nīnû* ('mint').[628]

---

66 If someone continually has (*irtanašši*) heat in the belly (*libbu*): *ḫašû* ('thyme'), *nuḫurtu* ('asafoetida') . . . *azupīru* ('saffron'),[629]

67 *nīnû* ('mint'), *kasû* ('tamarind'), *būrāšu* (a kind of juniper) . . . *uḫūlu qarnānû* ('horned alkali'),

68 (and) *saḫlû* ('cress')—. . . the thirteen ingredients in beer (and) in vinegar . . .

---

69 If DITTO, . . . ground *saḫlû* ('cress') in vinegar$^?$ . . .

---

70 If DITTO, ten shekels of *erēnu* ('cedar'), ten shekels . . .

71 ten shekels of *ballukku* (an aromatic), ten shekels . . .

approximately thirty-eight missing lines

---

628 This elaborate procedure seems to include several steps, with the mixture measured at the end of each step. The first two steps in lines 61–63 involve the combination of two sets of ingredients, which are then measured (the first occurrence of *taḫâṭ*) into beer. The second occurrence of *taḫâṭ* in line 64 takes place after the mixture has been placed in an oven and presumably cooked down to a dry substance. The second measurement served as the basis for the calculation of the amounts of dosages that follow; this specific amount seems to be listed in line 64: the mixture could then be used for up to a month, presumably in five equal doses, each of which was specified as three and five-sixths shekels. Each of these doses was presumably combined with one litre of fresh milk, but our text summarises this by saying that the entire batch was measured into—third occurrence of *taḫâṭ*—five litres of milk. Interestingly, the fourth column of our text also contains many different notations for fractions of shekels and ends with an analogous use of *ḫâṭu*.

629 The lexical lists equate ^{u2}ḪUR.SAG^{sar} with *azupīru* (CAD A/2 530), whereas Uruanna I 607 has clear equations between ^{u2} ḪUR.SAG^{sar} and *azupīrānu*.

110′ A$_{ii\ 45'}$ x [..]

111′ A$_{ii\ 46'}$ ^{u2}*tar-m*[*uš* ....]
112′ A$_{ii\ 47'}$ ša šap x [..]

113′ A$_{ii\ 48'}$ GI DU$_{10}$ ^{šim}MUG [..]
[GI D]U$_{10}$.GA ^{šim}MUG GAZI^{sar} U$_2$ BABBAR x [. . . *ina* IZ]I ŠEG$_6$-*šal* NAG-*ma* BURU$_8$ (STO 3: 59)

114′ A$_{ii\ 49'}$ ^{u2}ḪAR.Ḫ[AR ....]
^{u2}ḪAR.ḪAR ^{u2}NU.LUḪ.ḪA ILLU LI.TAR ^{šim}LI ^{šim}GUR$_2$.GUR$_2$ (STO 3: 86)

115′ A$_{ii\ 50'}$ 5 U$_2$.<ḪI>.⸢A⸣ [..]
⸢5 U$_2$⸣.[ḪI.A . . .] x (STO 3: 86)

116′ A$_{ii\ 51'}$ ^{u2}*a*[*k-tam* ....]
117′ A$_{ii\ 52'}$ ⸢PAP 4 U$_2$⸣*.[ḪI.A ....]

---

†

110′ . . .

111′ *tarmuš* ('lupin') . . .
112′ . . .

113′ *qanû ṭābu* ('sweet reed'), *ballukku* (an aromatic), *kasû* ('tamarind'), *šammu peṣû* ('white plant') . . . you bring them to a boil (*tušabšal*) over fire, he drinks (*išattī-ma*) them, and then he will vomit (*i'arru*).

114′ *ḫašû* ('thyme'), *nuḫurtu* ('asafoetida'), resin from *abukkatu* (a tree), *burāšu* (a kind of juniper), (and) *kukru* (an aromatic)—

115′ . . . five ingredients . . .

116′ *aktam* (a plant) . . .
117′ altogether four ingredients . . .

118′ A$_{ii\ 53'}$ ^{u2}*ak-tam* ^{šim}⸢BULUḪ⸣* [...]

119′ A$_{ii\ 54'}$ DIŠ NA *ši-biṭ* IM *ḫi-miṭ* UD.⸢DA⸣ [...][630]

DIŠ NA TAB UD.DA *ši-biṭ* IM *šim-ma-tu$_2$ ri-mu-tu$_2$ ša$_2$-aš$_2$-ša$_2$-ṭu* / ŠU.GIDIM$_7$.MA (BAM 168 obv. 18–19)

DIŠ NA *ši-biṭ* IM *ḫi-miṭ* [UD].DA *šim-ma-tu$_2$ r*[*i-mu-tu$_2$*] / *ša$_2$-aš$_2$-ša$_2$-ṭu* ŠU.GID[IM].MA (BAM 68 obv. 1–2)

[DIŠ NA] *ši-biṭ* ⸢IM⸣ *ḫi-*[*miṭ* UD.DA x x x] / *ri-mu-tu$_2$ ša$_2$-aš$_2$-ša$_2$-ṭu* ŠU.[GIDIM.MA] (BAM 69: 1′–2′)

PAP 28 U$_2$.MEŠ *mar-ḫa-ṣi ḫi-miṭ* UD.DA / *ši-pit* IM *šim-mat* / *ri-mu-tu$_2$ ša$_2$-aš$_2$-ša$_2$-ṭu* (BAM 226 rev. 1′–4′)

120′ A$_{ii\ 55'}$ ŠU.NAM.ERIM$_2$ DUR$_2$.GIG *u* [...]

ŠU.NAM.ERIM$_2$ DUR$_2$.GIG DU$_3$ GIG *ana* TI-*šu$_2$* / 10 GIN$_2$ U$_2$ NAM.TI.LA (BAM 168 obv. 19–20)

ŠU.NAM.ERIM$_2$.M[A DUR$_2$.GIG] / *u ka-la* GIG *an*[*a* T]I-*šu$_2$* 10 GIN$_2$ U$_2$ NA[M.TI.LA] (BAM 68 obv. 2–3)

ŠU.NAM.ERIM$_2$.MA DUR$_2$.GIG [x x] / *ana* TI-*šu$_2$* 10 GIN$_2$ U$_2$ NAM.TI.LA (BAM 69: 3′–4′)

ŠU.GIDIM$_7$.MA ŠU.NAM.RIM / DUR$_2$.GIG *u* DU$_3$ GIG *an-*[*ni-ti*] (BAM 226 rev. 5′–6′)

118′ *aktam* (a plant), *baluḫḫu* (‘ferula gummosa’) . . .

119′ If someone has ‘blast of wind’ disease (*šibiṭ šāri*), burning fever (*ḫimiṭ ṣēti*), paralysis (*šimmatu*), numbness (*rimûtu*), stiffness (*šaššaṭu*), hand-of ghost (*šugidimmakku*),[631]

120′ hand-of-oath (*šunamerimmakku*), rectal disease (*durgiqqu*), or all (other) diseases: in order to heal him (*ana bulluṭīšu*), ten shekels of *šammi balāṭi* (‘plant of life’),

630 For lines 119′–129′, see Cadelli 2000: 257 with n. 14, who includes BAM 189 i 6′–12′, BAM 228 obv. 14–16, BAM 216 obv. 26′–28′, BAM 52 obv. 35–37, BAM 229 obv. 9′–11′ and BAM 409 rev. 23–24 as additional parallels, even though these texts only present the same symptom description, with different therapeutic procedures. Most of the texts that Cadelli treats as distant parallels have recently been re-published by Maul (2019: 284–287), who edits our passage in STO 5: 119′– 129′ as his ‘Rezeptsammlung 2’, based on the three Assur tablets BAM 68, BAM 69 and BAM 168.

631 For the rendering of ŠU.GIDIM.MA as *šugidimmakku* (a calque of the Sumerian logogram into Akkadian) rather than *qāt eṭemmi* (a translation of the logogram into Akkadian), especially in therapeutic context, see Heeßel 2007 and 2018b.

121′ A$_{ii\ 56'}$ 10 GIN$_2$ ^{u2}*ti-ia-tu* 10 GIN$_2$ ⸢^{u2}⸣[KUR.KUR ....]

10 GIN$_2$ ^{u2}*ti-ia$_2$-tu$_2$* 10 GIN$_2$ ^{u2}KUR.KUR / 10 GIN$_2$ ^{u2}ḪAR.ḪAR 10 GIN$_2$ ^{u2}NU.LUḪ.ḪA (BAM 168 obv. 20–21)

10 GIN$_2$ ^{u2}*ti-ia$_2$-tu$_2$* 10 GIN$_2$ ^{u2}KUR.KUR 10 GIN$_2$ ^{u2}[ḪAR.ḪAR] / 10 GIN$_2$ ^{u2}NU.LUḪ.ḪA (BAM 68 obv. 4–5)

10 [GIN$_2$] / ^{u2}*ti-ia$_2$-tu$_2$* 10 GIN$_2$ ^{u2}KUR.KUR 10 GIN$_2$ ^{u2}[ḪAR.ḪAR] / 10 GIN$_2$ ^{u2}NU.LUḪ.ḪA (BAM 69: 4′–6′)

[10 GIN$_2$ ^{u2}DUR$_2$.NU.L]UḪ.ḪA / 10 GIN$_2$ ⸢^{u2}⸣[KUR.KUR] / [10 GIN$_2$ ^{u2}]⸢ḪAR⸣.ḪAR 10 GIN$_2$ ^{u2}NU.[LUḪ.ḪA] (BAM 225 obv. 1′–2′)

122′ A$_{ii\ 57'}$ 10 GIN$_2$ ^{u2}KUR.RA 10 GIN$_2$ ^{u2}*u[r$_2$-nu-u* ....]

10 GIN$_2$ ^{u2}KUR.RA / 10 GIN$_2$ ^{u2}*ur$_2$-nu-u* 10 GIN$_2$ MUN *ku$_3$-pad* 10 GIN$_2$ ^{u2}ḪUR.SAG (BAM 168 obv. 21–22)

10 GIN$_2$ ^{u2}KUR.RA 10 GIN$_2$ ^{u2}*u[r$_2$-nu-u]* / 10 GIN$_2$ MUN *ku$_3$-bad* 10 GIN$_2$ ^{u2}ḪUR.SAG (BAM 68 obv. 5–6)

10 GIN$_2$ ^{u2}KUR.RA / 10 GIN$_2$ ^{u2}*ur$_2$-nu-u* 10 GIN$_2$ MUN *ku$_3$-b[ad]* / 10 GIN$_2$ ^{u2}ḪUR.SAG (BAM 69: 6′–8′)

[10 GIN$_2$] ⸢^{u2}⸣KUR.RA 10 GIN$_2$ ^{u2}*ur$_2$-[nu-u]* / [10 GIN$_2$] MUN *ku$_3$-pad* 10 GIN$_2$ ^{u2}ḪUR.[SAG] (BAM 225 obv. 3′–4′)

123′ A$_{ii\ 58'}$ 10 GIN$_2$ ^{u2}*šib-bur-ra-tu$_4$* [..]

10 GIN$_2$ ^{u2}LUḪ.MAR.TU$_2$ 10 GIN$_2$ U$_2$ BABBAR 10 GIN$_2$ NA$_4$ *ga-bi-i* / 10 GIN$_2$ ^{giš}LI (BAM 168 obv. 23–24)

10 GIN$_2$ ^{u2}*šib-bur-rat* / 10 GIN$_2$ U$_2$ BABBAR 10 ⸢GIN$_2$⸣ NA$_4$ *ga-be$_2$-e* 10 GIN$_2$ ^{šim}LI (BAM 68 obv. 6–7)

10 GIN$_2$ ^{u2}*si-bur-[rat]* / [10 GI]N$_2$ U$_2$ BABBAR 10 GIN$_2$ NA$_4$ *ga-[bi-i]* / [. . .] (BAM 69: 8′–10′)

[10 GIN$_2$] *saḫ-le$_2$-e* 10 GIN$_2$ ^{u2}SUMUN.[DAR] / [10 G]IN$_2$ ^{u2}*si-bir-ru* 10 GIN$_2$ NUMUN [x x] / [10] GIN$_2$ ^{šim}LI (BAM 225 obv. 5′–7′)

[. . .] x x x / [. . . 1]0 GIN$_2$ ^{giš}LI (BAM 70 rev. 1′–2′)

121′ ten shekels of *tīyatu* (a plant), ten shekels of *atā'išu* (a plant), ten shekels of *ḫašû* ('thyme'), ten shekels of *nuḫurtu* ('asafoetida'),

122′ ten shekels of *nīnû* ('mint'), ten shekels of *urnû* (a kind of mint), ten shekels of *kupad*[632] salt, ten shekels of *azupīru* ('saffron'),

123′ ten shekels of *šibburatu* ('rue'), ten shekels of *šammu peṣû* ('white plant'), ten shekels of *aban gabî* ('alum'), ten shekels of *burāšu* (a kind of juniper),

632 For the reading of this form, based on the syllabic orthography *ṭa$_3$-ab-ti ku-pa-ad* in the Old Babylonian medical text BAM 393 obv. 1, see now Maul 2019: 286.

124′ A$_{ii\,59′}$ 10 GIN$_2$ ⸢^{šim}GUR$_2$⸣.G[UR$_2$* ....]

10 GIN$_2$ ^{giš}GUR$_2$.GUR$_2$ 10 GIN$_2$ *ak-tam* 10 GIN$_2$ MUN / 10 GIN$_2$ NUMUN ^{giš}ḪAB 10 GIN$_2$ ^{šim}GAM.MA (BAM 168 obv. 24–25)

10 GIN$_2$ ^{šim}GUR$_2$.GUR$_2$ 10 GIN$_2$ ^{u2}*ak-tam* 10 GIN$_2$ NUMUN ^{giš}ḪAB / 10 GIN$_2$ ^{šim}GAM.⸢MA⸣ (BAM 68 obv. 8–9)

10 GIN$_2$ ^{šim}GUR$_2$.[GUR$_2$] / [10] GIN$_2$ ^{šim}GAM.MA (BAM 225 obv. 7′–8′)

10 GIN$_2$ ⸢^{giš}⸣[GUR$_2$.GUR$_2$] / [. . .] x 10 GIN$_2$ NUMUN ^{giš}ḪAB / [. . .] (BAM 70 rev. 2′–4′)

125′ A$_{ii\,60′}$ 10 GIN$_2$ ^{šim}MAN.DU 10 GIN$_2$ ^{š}[^{im}BULUḪ ....]

10 GIN$_2$ ^{šim}MAN.DU / 10 GIN$_2$ ^{šim}BULUḪ 10 GIN$_2$ ^{giš}EREN 10 GIN$_2$ ^{šim}ŠEŠ (BAM 168 obv. 25–26)

10 GIN$_2$ ^{šim}MAN.DU 10 GIN$_2$ ^{šim}[BULUḪ] / 10 GIN$_2$ ^{giš}EREN 10 GIN$_2$ [^{šim}ŠE]Š (BAM 68 obv. 9–10)

10 GIN$_2$ ^{šim}MAN.D[U] / [10 GIN$_2$] ^{šim}BULUḪ 10 GIN$_2$ ^{giš}EREN / [10 GIN$_2$] ^{šim}ŠEŠ (BAM 225 obv. 8′–10′)

[. . .] ^{šim}ŠEŠ (BAM 226 obv. 1′)

[10 G]IN$_2$ ^{šim}MAN.DU / [. . .] ^{giš}EREN 10 GIN$_2$ ^{šim}⸢ŠEŠ⸣ (BAM 70 rev. 4′–5′)

126′ A$_{ii\,61′}$ 10 GIN$_2$ GI DU$_{10}$ 5 GIN$_2$ ^{giš}*si-ḫu* [..]

10 GIN$_2$ GI DU$_{10}$ 5 GIN$_2$ ^{giš}*si-ḫu* 5 GIN$_2$ ^{giš}*ar$_2$-gan-nu* / 5 GIN$_2$ LUM.ḪA 5 GIN$_2$ U$_2$ ^{d}UTU (BAM 168 obv. 27–28)

10 GIN$_2$ GI DU$_{10}$ / 5 GIN$_2$ ^{giš}*si-ḫu* 5 GIN$_2$ ^{giš}*[a]r-ga-nu* / 5 GIN$_2$ ^{giš}*ba-⸢ri⸣-rat* 5 GIN$_2$ U$_2$ ⸢^{d}UTU⸣ (BAM 68 obv. 10–rev. 2)

10 GIN$_2$ GI DU$_{10}$.GA / [10 GI]N$_2$ ^{u2}*si-ḫa* [10] GIN$_2$ ^{u2}*ar$_2$-ga[n-nu]* / ⸢10⸣ GIN$_2$ ^{u2}*ba-ri-ra-[ta$_5$]* / [10] GIN$_2$ ^{u2}*ka-ši-ru*[633] (BAM 225 obv. 10′–13′)

GI DU$_{10}$.GA / ^{giš}*si-ḫu* / ^{giš}*ar$_2$-ga$_2$-nu* / ^{giš}LUM.ḪA / U$_2$ ^{d}UTU (BAM 226 obv. 1′–5′)

[. . . ^{gi}]^{š}⸢*si*⸣*-ḫa* 5 GIN$_2$ ⸢*ar$_2$*⸣*-g[a-nu]*[634] / [. . .] (BAM 70 rev. 6′–7′)

124′ ten shekels of *kukru* (an aromatic), ten shekels of *aktam* (a plant), ten shekels of salt, ten shekels of seed from *ḫûratu* ('madder'), ten shekels of *ṣumlalû* (an aromatic),

125′ ten shekels of *suādu* (a kind of sedge), ten shekels of *baluḫḫu* ('ferula gummosa'), ten shekels of *erēnu* ('cedar'), ten shekels of *murru* ('myrrh'),

126′ ten shekels of *qanû ṭābu* ('sweet reed'), five shekels of *sīḫu* ('wormwood'), five shekels of *argannu* (a conifer), five shekels of *barīrātu* ('sagapenum'), (and) five shekels of *šammi Šamaš* ('plant of Šamaš').

---

633 The *kašīrû* plant, cross-referenced to *šakirû* in CAD K 289 (not listed in AHw), is probably a variant form of the *šakirû* plant, with the same syllable structure but /k/ and /š/ in an inverted order. ^{u2}ŠAKIRA = Akk. *šakirû*, in turn, is equated with U$_2$ ^{d}UTU = Akk. *šammi Šamaš* in Uruanna I 27; the parallels in our line 126′ seem to support this link, since 5 GIN$_2$ U$_2$ ^{d}UTU in a number of these texts is aligned with BAM 225 obv 13′, which has [10] GIN$_2$ ^{u2}*ka-ši-ru*.

634 According to Maul (2019: 286), the hand-copy of BAM 70 is unreliable at this point: the passage clearly has ⸢*ar$_2$*⸣*-g[a-nu]*.

127′ A$_{\text{ii 62′}}$ 25[635] U$_2$.ḪI.A ŠIM.ḪI.A ŠEŠ DIŠ-*niš* G[AZ ....]

25 U$_2$.ḪI.A.MEŠ / *u* ŠIM.ḪI.A ŠEŠ DIŠ-*niš* GAZ SIM KAŠ SAG A GAZI^{sar} (BAM 168 obv. 28–29)

26 U$_2$.[ḪI.A.MEŠ] / *an-nu-ti-ma* GAZ SIM *ina* KAŠ SAG A GAZI^{sar} ŠEG$_6$-*šal* (BAM 68 rev. 2–3)

⸢28⸣ U$_2$.ḪI.A [ŠE]Š DIŠ-*niš* GAZ SI[M . . .] / [A GA]ZI^{sar} BIL-*ti* (BAM 225 obv. 14′–15′)

128′ A$_{\text{ii 63′}}$ *u* A.GEŠTIN.NA *dan-na-ti* TI-*qe*$_2$ ⸢ZI$_3$⸣ [...]

u A.GEŠTIN.NA KALAG.GA TI-*qe*$_2$ ZI$_3$.DA.MEŠ *an-nu-ti ana* ŠA$_3^{!}$ ŠUB-*di* / *ina* NINDU UŠ$_2$-*er* (BAM 168 obv. 30–31)

u A.GEŠTIN.NA *dan*-⸢*na*⸣-*ti* TI-*qe*$_2$ ZI$_3$.DA.MEŠ *an-nu-ti* / *ana* ŠA$_3$ ŠUB-*di ina* ⸢NINDU⸣ UŠ$_2$-*er* (BAM 68 rev. 4–5)

u A.GEŠTIN.NA [. . .] / [. . . *an-nu*]-⸢*ti*$^{?}$ *ana*⸣ [. . .] (BAM 225 obv. 15′–16′)

129′ A$_{\text{ii 64′}}$ *ina še-ri*$_3$ E$_{11}$-*ma* SED *ta-ša*$_2$-*ḫal* I$_3$ *ḫal*-[*ṣa* ....]

ina še-ri$_3$ E$_{11}$ SED LAL$_3$ *u* I$_3$ *ḫal-ṣa ana* IGI ŠUB-*di* / 1-*šu*$_2$ 2-*šu*$_2$ ⸢3-*šu*$_2$⸣ *ana* DUR$_2$-*šu*$_2$ DUB-*ak* (BAM 168 obv. 31–32)

ina še-ri$_3$ E$_{11}$-*ma tu-kaṣ*$_3$-*ṣa* / *ta-ša*$_2$-*ḫal* I$_3$.GIŠ BARA$_2$.GA *ana* IGI ŠUB-[*di*] / ⸢1⸣-*šu*$_2$ 2-*šu*$_2$ 3-*šu*$_2$ *ana* DUR$_2$-*šu*$_2$ DUB-*ak-m*[*a* TI] (BAM 68 rev. 5–7)

130′ A$_{\text{iii 1}}$ 10 GIN$_2$ $^{\text{u2}}$NU.LUḪ.ḪA 10 G[IN$_2$ ....]

[10] GIN$_2$ $^{\text{u2}}$NU.LUḪ.ḪA 10 GIN$_2$ $^{\text{u2}}$*am-ḫ*[*a-ra* . . .] (BAM 68 rev. 8)[636]

131′ A$_{\text{iii 2}}$ 10 GIN$_2$ $^{\text{u2}}$ḪUR.SAG^{sar} 10 ⸢GIN$_2$* $^{\text{u2}}$⸣[..]

†

127′ You crush (*taḫaššal*) (and) sift (*tanappi*) these twenty-five plants (and) aromatics together, you take (*teleqqe*) high-quality beer, juice from *kasû* ('tamarind')

128′ and strong vinegar, you put (*tanaddi*) these powdered substances in (the mixture), you heat (*tesekker*) it in an oven,

129′ in the morning you take it out (*tušellâ-ma*), and then you let it cool (*tukaṣṣa*), you filter it, you add pressed oil, (and) you pour (*tašappak*) it into his anus once, twice, three times.

130′ Ten shekels of *nuḫurtu* ('asafoetida'), ten shekels of *amḫaru* (a plant) . . .

131′ ten shekels of *azupīru* ('saffron'), ten shekels . . .

635 If our reconstruction is correct, there are 27 ingredients mentioned in the preceding drug list. The number given here may thus be a mistake, as in our first parallel BAM 168 obv. 28 (Maul 2019: 286), where the number of listed ingredients ('27') differs from what is given as the total number of drugs in the summary section of the prescription ('25').

636 As Maul (2019: 287) points out, the sequence of prescriptions is the same in BAM 68 and STO 5. The first prescription in BAM 68 obv. 1–rev. 7 runs parallel with STO 5: 119′–129′, whereas the catchline in BAM 68 rev. 8 refers to the prescription that starts in STO 5: 130′.

132′ A$_{iii\,3}$ 10 GIN$_2$ MUN 10 GIN$_2$ ^{u2}x [...]
133′ A$_{iii\,4}$ 10 GIN$_2$ ^{šim}MAN.DU [...]
134′ A$_{iii\,5}$ 10 GIN$_2$ ^{šim}BULUḪ [...]
135′ A$_{iii\,6}$ 10 GIN$_2$ ^{giš}*si-ḫu* [...]
136′ A$_{iii\,7}$ 10 GIN$_2$ GI DU$_{10}$.GA [...]
137′ A$_{iii\,8}$ 10 GIN$_2$ ⸢^{šim}⸣*BAL [...]
138′ A$_{iii\,9}$ 10 G[IN$_2$] ⸢^{šim}⸣x [...]
139′ A$_{iii\,10}$ 10 [GIN$_2$ ....]
140′ A$_{iii\,11}$ [...]
141′ A$_{iii\,12}$ [x x x x] 10 ⸢GIN$_2$⸣ [...]
142′ A$_{iii\,13}$ [x x x] x[637] 10 GIN$_2$ ^{giš}ER[EN ....]
143′ A$_{iii\,14}$ ⸢^{giš}*si-ḫu*⸣ ^{giš}*ar$_2$-ga-nu* ⸢^{u2}⸣*b[a-ri-ra-tu$_2$* ....]
144′ A$_{iii\,15}$ ^{u2}KUR.RA ^{u2}KI.^{d}IŠKUR DIŠ-*n[iš* ....][638]

LAGAB MUNU$_6$ ^{u2}KI.^{d}IŠKUR DIŠ-*niš* GAZ SI[M] / *ina* A.GEŠTIN.NA KALAG.GA (BAM 216 obv. 23′–24′)

145′ A$_{iii\,16}$ KAŠ SAG *u* ⸢A⸣ GAZI^{sar} ŠEG$_6$-*šal* ZI$_3$.M[EŠ ....][639]

u A GAZI^{sar} *ina* IZI ŠEG$_6$-⸢*šal*⸣ / ZI$_3$.ḪI.A *an-nu-tu$_2$ ana* ŠA$_3$ ŠUB-*di* (BAM 216 obv. 24′–25′)

132′ ten shekels of salt, ten shekels . . .
133′ ten shekels of *suādu* (a kind of sedge) . . .
134′ ten shekels of *baluḫḫu* ('ferula gummosa') . . .
135′ ten shekels of *sīḫu* ('wormwood') . . .
136′ ten shekels of *qanû ṭābu* ('sweet reed') . . .
137′ ten shekels of *ballukku* (an aromatic) . . .
138′ ten shekels . . .
139′ ten shekels . . .
140′ . . .
141′ . . . ten shekels . . .
142′ . . . ten shekels of *erēnu* ('cedar') . . .
143′ (then) you crush (*taḫaššal*) (and) sift (*tanappi*) *sīḫu* ('wormwood'),[640] *argannu* (a conifer), *barīrātu* ('sagapenum') . . .
144′ *nīnû* ('mint') (and) *qutru* (a plant) together, you bring to a boil (*tušabšal*) strong vinegar,
145′ high-quality beer and juice from *kasû* ('tamarind'), you put (*tanaddi*) these powdered substances in (the mixture),

637 Cadelli (2000: 263) read this fragmentary passage as [^{giš}ER]EN, but the traces do not support this reading.

638 BAM 216 obv. 23′–28′ contains a procedure that is similar to our lines 143′–148′, so we have used it here to reconstruct some missing words in our passage. This applies, however, only to the preparation of the medicine. The list of ingredients is quite different in BAM 216, but it also uses the same measurement (ten shekels) up until the last two entries.

639 The gap in lines 145′–153′ has been partially filled with the help of K 18594, which is a direct join to MS A. The join was identified by Zs. Földi in 2022.

640 The repetition of ^{giš}*si-ḫu* in lines 135′ and 143′ strongly suggests that the ingredients up to line 142′, all of which include 10 GIN$_2$ as a place-holder measurement, were manipulated in some way in line 142′ and that the ^{giš}*si-ḫu* that follows in line 143′ belongs to a different stage in the recipe.

146′ A$_{iii 17}$ *u* I$_{3}$.GIŠ BARA$_{2}$.GA *ana* IGI ⸢ŠUB-*di*⸣-*ma* 1-[*šu*$_{2}$ ....]

u$_{3}$ I$_{3}$.GIŠ *ḫal-ṣa ana* I[GI x x x] / 1-*šu*$_{2}$ 2-*šu*$_{2}$ 3-*šu*$_{2}$ *ana* DUR$_{2}$-*šu*$_{2}$ DUB-*ma* (BAM 216 obv. 25′–26′)

147′ A$_{iii 18}$ *ana ši-biṭ* IM *u ḫi-miṭ* U[D.DA ....]

a-na ši-bi[*ṭ* IM] / *ḫi-miṭ* UD.DA *šim-ma-tu*$_{4}$ *ša-aš*$_{2}$*-ša*$_{2}$*-ṭu r*[*i-mu-tu*$_{4}$] (BAM 216 obv. 26′–27′)

148′ A$_{iii 19}$ ŠU.GIDIM.MA ŠU.[NAM.ERIM$_{2}$ ....]

[ŠU.GIDIM.MA] / ^{d}NAM.ERIM$_{2}$ *u*$_{3}$ *kal* GIG x [x x x] (BAM 216 obv. 27′–28′)

149′ A$_{iii 20}$ DIŠ NA IR-*šu* na di x [...]

[. . . ^{gi}]^{š}⸢ŠA$_{3}$⸣.GI ^{šim}GUR$_{2}$.GUR$_{2}$ ^{šim}LI (BAM 7 50 rev. 22′)

150′ A$_{iii 21}$ GAZI^{sar} *saḫ-le*$_{2}$*-e* ⸢^{u2}⸣ [...]

⸢GAZI⸣^{sar} *saḫ-lu-u* / [. . . ^{u2}]ḪAR.ḪAR (BAM 7 50 rev. 22′–23′)

151′ A$_{iii 22}$ ^{u2}*ur*$_{2}$*-nu-u* ⸢^{u2}⸣[KUR.RA ....]

^{u2}*ur*$_{2}$*-ne*$_{2}$*-e* ^{u2}KUR.RA ^{u2}ḪUR.SAG / [. . .] (BAM 7 50 rev. 23′–24′)

152′ A$_{iii 23}$ U$_{2}$ MAŠ.TAB.BA x [..]

[. . .] x x 14 U$_{2}$.MEŠ (BAM 7 50 rev. 24′)

153′ A$_{iii 24}$ *ina* KAŠ A NIG$_{2}$.⸢AR$_{3}$.RA⸣ [...]

ina KAŠ A NIG$_{2}$.AR$_{3}$.RA / [. . . *ina* DUR$_{2}$-*šu*$_{2}$] DUB-*ak* (BAM 7 50 rev. 24′–25′)

154′ A$_{iii 25}$ ^{šim}GUR$_{2}$.GUR$_{2}$ ^{š}[^{im} ....]

ϯ

146′ and you add pressed oil, then you pour (*tašappak-ma*) it into his anus once, twice, three times,

147′ so that ‘blast of wind’ disease (*šibiṭ šāri*), burning fever (*himiṭ ṣēti*), paralysis (*šimmatu*), stiffness (*šaššaṭu*), numbness (*rimûtu*),

148′ hand-of-ghost (*šugidimmakku*), hand-of-oath (*šunamerimmakku*), or all (other) diseases . . .

149′ If someone . . . *ḫandû* (‘reed pulp’), *kukru* (an aromatic), *burāšu* (a kind of juniper),

150′ *kasû* (‘tamarind’), *saḫlû* (‘cress’) . . . *ḫašû* (‘thyme’),

151′ *urnû* (a kind of mint), *nīnû* (‘mint’), *azupīru* (‘saffron’) . . .

152′ *šammi ašî* (‘*ašû* disease’ plant) . . .—. . . fourteen ingredients

153′ in beer, juice from *mundu* (‘groats’) . . . (and) you pour (*tašappak*) it into his anus.

154′ *kukru* (an aromatic) . . .

155′ $A_{iii\ 26}$ ŠIM.ŠAL [..]

156′ $A_{iii\ 27}$ ^{u2}*ur_2-n[u-u* ....]

157′ $A_{iii\ 28}$ ^{u2}KUR.[KUR ....]

158′ $A_{iii\ 29}$ [..]

159′ $A_{iii\ 30}$ x [..]

160′ $A_{iii\ 31}$ ⸢^{šim}⸣[..]

161′ $A_{iii\ 32}$ ^{šim}[..]

162′ $A_{iii\ 33}$ ⸢^{u2}⸣[..]

163′ $A_{iii\ 34}$ x [..]

164′ $A_{iii\ 35}$ [..]

165′ $A_{iii\ 36}$ [..]

166′ $A_{iii\ 37}$ x [..]

approximately twenty-six missing lines

193′ $A_{iv\ 1}$ ^{giš}*e-re-nu* ^{giš}ŠUR.MIN_3 ^{giš}*dap_2-ra-nu* ^{giš}*a-sa* ŠIM.ŠAL GI DU_{10}.GA
^{giš}*e-re-nu* ^{giš}ŠUR.MIN_3 ^{giš}*dap_2-ra-nu* ^{šim}GIR_2 ŠIM.ŠAL / GI DU_{10}.GA (BAM 159 v 37–38)

194′ $A_{iv\ 2}$ ^{šim}BAL $^{šim.d}$MAŠ ^{šim}EN.DI ^{šim}GUR_2.GUR_2 ^{šim}LI ^{šim}GAM.⸢MA⸣
^{šim}BAL $^{šim.d}$MAŠ ^{šim}MAN.DU ^{u2}KUR.KUR / ^{šim}GUR_2.GUR_2 ^{šim}LI ^{šim}ŠE.LI BABBAR ^{šim}GAM.MA (BAM 159 v 38–39)

195′ $A_{iv\ 3}$ ^{u2}KUR.KUR ^{šim}ŠE.LI BABBAR ^{u2}ḪAR.ḪAR ^{giš}*si-ḫa* ^{giš}LUM.ḪA NAG[A S]I
^{u2}ḪAR.ḪAR ^{u2}*si-ḫu* ^{giš}*ar_2-gan_2-nu* ^{giš}LUM.ḪA NAGA SI (BAM 159 v 40)

☩

155′ *šimišallû* ('box tree') . . .

156′ *urnû* (a kind of mint) . . .

157′ *atā'išu* (a plant)$^?$ . . .

158′ . . .

159′ . . .

160′ . . .

161′ . . .

162′ . . .

163′ . . .

164′ . . .

165′ . . .

166′ . . .

approximately twenty-six missing lines

193′ *erēnu* ('cedar'), *šurmēnu* ('cypress'), *daprānu* (a kind of juniper), *asu* ('myrtle'), *šimišallû* ('box tree'), *qanû ṭābu* ('sweet reed'),

194′ *ballukku* (an aromatic), *nikiptu* ('spurge'), *suādu* (a kind of sedge), *kukru* (an aromatic), *burāšu* (a kind of juniper), *ṣumlalû* (an aromatic),

195′ *atā'išu* (a plant), white *kikkirânu* ('juniper seeds'), *ḫašû* ('thyme'), *sīḫu* 'wormwood'), *barīrātu* ('sagapenum'), *uḫūlu qarnānû* ('horned alkali'),

196′ A$_{iv\ 4}$ ^{u2}NU.⸢LUḪ.ḪA⸣ [19] ⸢U$_2$.ḪI⸣.A ŠEŠ *mal-la ṣi-bu-te-ka*[641] T[I-*q*]*e*$_2$
  ^{u2}NU.LUḪ.ḪA MUN *saḫ-le*$_2$*-e* GAZI^{sar} 23 U$_2$.ḪI.A ŠEŠ / 1/3 SILA$_3$.TA.AM$_3$ TI-*qe*$_2$ (BAM 159 v 41–42)

197′ A$_{iv\ 5}$ *ina* ⸢KAŠ⸣ [*tu-la-bak in*]*a* GE$_6$ *ana* IGI ^{mul}UZ$_3$ *t*[*uš-ba*]*t*
  ina KAŠ *tu-*^{la}*lab-bak ina* GE$_6$ / *ana* IGI ^{mul}UZ$_3$ *tuš-bat* (BAM 159 v 42–43)

198′ A$_{iv\ 6}$ *ina š*[*e**-*ri*$_3$] ŠEG$_6$-*šal ta-š*[*a*$_2$*-*ḫ*]*al*
  ina še-ri$_3$ ŠEG$_6$-*šal ta-ša*$_2$*-ḫal* (BAM 159 v 43)

199′ A$_{iv\ 7}$ *ir-r*[*i* x x x] x U$_2$.ḪI.A *u* I$_3$.GIŠ ^{šim}EN.DI *t*[*a-qal*$_3$]*-lu*
  ḪENBUR$_2$ ^{u2}UKUŠ$_2$.ḪAB ⸢U$_2$⸣.[ḪI].⸢A⸣.MEŠ SUD$_2$ (BAM 159 v 44)

200′ A$_{iv\ 8}$ *ma-l*[*a ṣi-bu-ti-ka* TI]-*qe*$_2$* *ina* KAŠ *ša* ŠIM.ḪI.A ⸢*ina* IZI$^?$⸣ ŠEG$_6$.GA$_2$

201′ A$_{iv\ 9}$ *ma-l*[*a ṣi-bu-ti-ka t*]*u-maḫ-ḫa-aḫ* 10 GIN$_2$ LAL$_3$ 1/3 SILA$_3$ I$_3$ *ḫal-ṣa ana* ŠA$_3$ GAZ
  KI 1 SILA$_3$ LAL$_3$ / 11 SILA$_3$ I$_3$.GIŠ ⸢GAZ⸣ (BAM 159 v 44–45)

202′ A$_{iv\ 10}$ *ana* KU[Š *maš-qi*$_2$*-te*] *te-si-ip*
  ana KUŠ *maš-qi*$_2$*-te te-sip* (BAM 159 v 45)

203′ A$_{iv\ 11}$ *ana* DUR$_2$*-š*[*u*$_2$ DUB-*a*]*k* SI.SA$_2$*-ma* TI
  ana DUR$_2$*-šu*$_2$ DUB-*ak maš-qi*$_2$*-tu ša* ANŠE.KUR.RA (BAM 159 v 46)

196′ (and) *nuḫurtu* ('asafoetida')—you take (*teleqqe*) as much as you need of these nineteen ingredients,
197′ you soften them in beer, you leave them out for the night under the Goat Star,
198′ in the morning you bring them to a boil (*tušabšal*), you filter them,
199′ (and then) you roast *irrû* ('cucumber')$^?$ . . . (these) ingredients and oil from *suādu* (a kind of sedge),
200′ you take as much as you need of them, (and) you bring them to a boil (*tušabšal*) in aromatic beer over fire$^?$,
201′ you soften as much as you need (of the mixture), you crush (*taḫaššal*) ten shekels of *dišpu* ('syrup') (and) a third of a litre of pressed oil in it,
202′ (and) you skim it off into a leather (bag) for potions,[642]
203′ you pour (*tašappak*) it into his anus, (and) he will void (*ušeššer-ma*); then he will recover (*iballuṭ*).

---

641 There are four Assyrianisms previously recognised in our text by Meier (1939b: 215 with n. 3): *nakuāri* (lines 228′ and 229′), *taḫiaq* (line 229′), *ḫadiāta* (line 232′) and *ṭabiūni* (line 233′). Our phrase here, viz. *mal-la ṣi-bu-te-ka*, also seems to be an Assyrian formulation, with the *e*-colouring of the genitive ending in *ṣi-bu-te-ka* and the spelling of the adverb *mala* as *malla*. For the latter, see De Ridder 2018: 340, who includes a reference to Middle Assyrian *ma-al-la* in MARV 1 14 obv. 4.

642 For the same procedure, see STO 1: 85 with further discussion.

204′ A$_{\text{iv 12}}$ 1 GIN$_2$ ^{giš}*e-⸢re-nu* 1⸣ 1/2 GIN$_2$ ^{giš}ŠUR.MIN$_3$ 1 GIN$_2$ ^{giš}*dap$_2$-ra-nu* 1 GIN$_2$ ^{šim}GIR$_2$
DIŠ KI MIN 1 GIN$_2$ ^{giš}*eri-nu* 1 1/2 GIN$_2$ ^{giš}ŠUR.MIN$_3$ 1 GIN$_2$ ^{giš}*dap$_2$-ra-nu* 1 GIN$_2$ ^{šim}GIR$_2$ (BAM 54: 4)

205′ A$_{\text{iv 13}}$ 1 GIN$_2$ ŠIM.ŠAL 2 GIN$_2$ GI DU$_{10}$.GA 2 GIN$_2$ ^{šim}BAL
2 GIN$_2$ ŠIM.ŠAL / 2 GIN$_2$ GI DU$_{10}$.GA 2 GIN$_2$ ^{šim}BAL (BAM 54: 4–5)

206′ A$_{\text{iv 14}}$ 1/2 GIN$_2$ $^{\text{šim.d}}$MAŠ 1 GIN$_2$ ^{šim}EN.DI 1/2 GIN$_2$ ^{šim}GUR$_2$.GUR$_2$ 1/2 GIN$_2$ ^{šim}⸢LI⸣
1/2 GIN$_2$ $^{\text{giš.d}}$MAŠ 1 GIN$_2$ ^{giš}EN.DI 1/2 GIN$_2$ ^{giš}GUR$_2$.GUR$_2$ / 1/2 GIN$_2$ ^{giš}LI (BAM 54: 5–6)

207′ A$_{\text{iv 15}}$ LUM[643] GIN$_2$ ^{šim}GAM.MA 1/2 GIN$_2$ $^{\text{u2}}$KUR.KUR 3 GIN$_2$ ^{šim}ŠE.LI $_{\text{: 2 GIN}_2\ ^{\text{u2}}\text{ḪAR.ḪAR}}$ 2 GIN$_2$ ^{šim}GIG
LIMMU$_2$ GIN$_2$ ^{šim}GAM.MA 1/2 GIN$_2$ $^{\text{u2}}$KUR.KUR 2 GIN$_2$ ^{šim}ŠE.LI 2 GIN$_2$ $^{\text{u2}}$ḪAR.ḪAR / ⸢2⸣ GIN$_2$ ^{šim}GIG (BAM 54: 6–7)

208′ A$_{\text{iv 16}}$ *bit-qu* ^{giš}*si-ḫu bit-qu* ^{giš}LUM.ḪA 1/2 *bit-qi$_2$* ^{šim}ŠEŠ
bit-qu ^{giš}*si-ḫu bit-qu* ^{giš}*ar$_2$-gan$_2$-nu* 1/2 *bit-qu* ^{šim}ŠEŠ (BAM 54: 7)

204′ One shekel of *erēnu* (‘cedar’), half a shekel of *šurmēnu* (‘cypress’), one shekel of *daprānu* (a kind of juniper), one shekel of *asu* (‘myrtle’),
205′ one shekel of *šimišallû* (‘box tree’), two shekels of *qanû ṭābu* (‘sweet reed’), two shekels of *ballukku* (an aromatic),
206′ half a shekel of *nikiptu* (‘spurge’), one shekel of *suādu* (a kind of sedge), half a shekel of *kukru* (an aromatic), half a shekel of *burāšu* (a kind of juniper),
207′ a fourth of a shekel of *ṣumlalû* (an aromatic), half a shekel of *atā’išu* (a plant), three shekels of *kikkirânu* (‘juniper seeds’) (gloss: two shekels of *ḫašû*), two shekels of *kanaktu* (an aromatic),
208′ an eighth of a shekel of *sīḫu* (‘wormwood’), an eighth of a shekel of *barīrātu* (‘sagapenum’), a sixteenth of a shekel of *murru* (‘myrrh’),

643 In the partially parallel BAM 54, the corresponding sign is LIMMU$_2$ (two sets of two horizontal wedges). Given the use of one-half and one-eighth elsewhere in the same recipe, we should probably infer that both LUM and LIMMU$_2$ are partially distorted writings of the Old Assyrian sign for ‘one-fourth’. As emphasized by Powell (1979: 96–97) and more recently Michel (2020: 403), the sign for ‘one-fourth’ (two stacked occurrences of an oblique and a horizontal) is only used in the Old Assyrian documents. LUM can then be described as a misunderstanding of either LIMMU$_2$ (with the four horizontals that occur in LUM) or the Old Assyrian sign for ‘one-fourth’ (with two obliques that occur on the left side of LUM). LUM also appears in BAM 42 obv. 28, where it is parallel with four other manuscripts that use the notations 4-*ut* and IGI.4.GAL$_2$.LA for ‘one-fourth (of a shekel)’. See Stadhouders and Johnson 2018: 573 and Bácskay 2021b: 163, but now with the emended reading IGI.4.GAL$_2$.LA in BAM 44 rev. 36′: Köcher’s (1980) hand-copy mistakenly shows IGI.5.GAL$_2$.LA.

209′ A$_{\text{iv 17}}$ 1/2 *bit-qi*$_2$ ^{šim}ḪAB 1/2 *bit-qi*$_2$ ^{šim}BULUḪ.ḪI.A[644] 1 GIN$_2$ GAZI^{sar}
1/2 *bit-qu* ^{šim}ḪAB 1/2 *bit-qu* ^{šim}BULUḪ.ḪI.A 1 GIN$_2$ GAZI^{sar} (BAM 54: 8)

210′ A$_{\text{iv 18}}$ 1 GIN$_2$ NAGA 1 GIN$_2$ $^{\text{u2}}$DUR$_2$.NU.LUḪ.ḪA 24 U$_2$.ḪI.A ŠIM.ḪI.A ŠEŠ
1 GIN$_2$ NAGA SI / 1 GIN$_2$ $^{\text{u2}}$NU.LUḪ.ḪA 24 U$_2$.MEŠ ŠEŠ (BAM 54: 8–9)

211′ A$_{\text{iv 19}}$ *ta-ka-sim ina* ^{giš}*zi-ba-ni-ti ta-ša*$_2$*-qal*$_3$ *ana* IGI ^{mul}UZ$_3$ GIN-*an*
ta-ka-sim ina ^{giš}ERIN$_2$ LA$_2$-*al* / ⸢*ana* IGI⸣ ^{mul}UZ$_3$ GIN-*an* (BAM 54: 9–10)

212′ A$_{\text{iv 20}}$ *ina* KAŠ *tu-la-bak* 1/2 SILA$_3$ *mi-ḫat* $^{\text{lu2}}$KURUN$_2$.NA *ša*$_2$ *ina* ⸢NINDU NU UŠ$_2$⸣-*er* NU ŠUB-*u*
ina KAŠ *tu-lab-bak* 1 SILA$_3$ *mi-ḫat* $^{\text{lu2}}$KURUN$_2$.NA / [*ša*$_2$] *ina* NINDU NU ŠUB-*u* (BAM 54: 10–11)

213′ A$_{\text{iv 21}}$ 1/3 SILA$_3$ A.GEŠTIN.NA *ana* ŠA$_3$ DUB *ina šer*$_3$*-ti* ⸢ŠEG$_6$-*šal*⸣ *ta-ša*$_2$*-ḫal*
5/6 SILA$_3$ A.⸢GEŠTIN⸣.NA *ana* ŠA$_3$ DUB-*ak ina šer*$_3$*-ti* ŠEG$_6$-*šal* (BAM 54: 11)

214′ A$_{\text{iv 22}}$ 1/3 SILA$_3$ LAL$_3$ 1/2 SILA$_3$ I$_3$ *ḫal-ṣa ana* ŠA$_3$ ŠUB-*di*
5/6 SILA$_3$ LAL$_3$ 1/2 SILA$_3$ I$_3$.GIŠ *ḫal-ṣa ana* ŠA$_3$ ŠUB-*di* (BAM 54: 12)

215′ A$_{\text{iv 23}}$ *baḫ-ru-su ana* DUR$_2$-*šu*$_2$ DUB-*ak* SI.SA$_2$-*ma* TI-*uṭ*
baḫ-ru-su ana DUR$_2$-*šu*$_2$ DUB-*ak* S[I.SA$_2$] (BAM 54: 12)

---

†

209′ a sixteenth of a shekel of *ṭūru* ('opopanax'), a sixteenth of a shekel of *baluḫḫu* ('ferula gummosa'), one shekel of *kasû* ('tamarind'),

210′ one shekel of *uḫūlu* ('alkali'), (and) one shekel of *tīyatu* (a plant)—you chop up these twenty-four drugs (and) aromatics,

211′ you weigh them in a balance, you set them out (*tukān*) before the Goat Star,

212′ you soften them in beer, (and then) you pour (*tašappak*) half a litre of *miḫḫatu* (a kind of beer) from an innkeeper, which was not heated (*lā seker*) (or) put (*lā nadû*) in an oven,

213′ (and) a third of a litre of vinegar in (the mixture), in the morning you bring it to a boil (*tušabšal*), you filter it,

214′ you put (*tanaddi*) a third of a litre of *dišpu* ('syrup') (and) half a litre of pressed oil in it,

215′ you pour it into his anus while it is steaming hot, (and) he will void (*ušeššer-ma*); then he will recover (*iballuṭ*).

---

644 The orthography ^{šim}BULUḪ.ḪI.A is unusual but not without other occurrences in the therapeutic corpus: see, for instance, BM 78963 obv. 28 in Stadhouders and Johnson 2018: 573 ln. 28 and n. 25. The form is also attested in EYES 1: 79′; here however, it does not feature as a medical ingredient but is used in a metaphorical sense, presumably to describe some kind of sticky discharge from the eyes that resembled the resin of the *baluḫḫu* aromatic, namely 'galbanum' (BAM 10 pp. 79 and 259–260). For a discussion of ^{šim}BULUḪ.ḪI.A, see also Attia 2015: 32–35, Panayotov 2017: 238 and Bácskay 2021b: 163 n. 15.

216′ A$_{\text{iv 24}}$ 1 ŠU$_2$[645] ^{šim}⸢ŠEŠ 1⸣ ŠU$_2$ ^{šim}ḪAB 1 ŠU$_2$ ILLU ^{šim}BULUḪ 1 ŠU$_2$ ILLU LI.TUR

217′ A$_{\text{iv 25}}$ 1 ŠU$_2$ ^{giš}SU.⸢ḪU.RA⸣ 1 ŠU$_2$ ^{giš}⸢EN.DI⸣ 1 ŠU$_2$ ^{šim}GUR$_2$.GUR$_2$ 1 ŠU$_2$ NUMUN $^{\text{u2}}$DILI

218′ A$_{\text{iv 26}}$ 1 ŠU$_2$ U$_2$ BABBAR 1 ŠU$_2$ $^{\text{u2}}$*tar-⸢muš⸣* 1 ŠU$_2$ $^{\text{u2}}$*ak-tam ta-qal$_3$-lu*

219′ A$_{\text{iv 27}}$ 1 ŠU$_2$ NUMUN ^{giš}ŠE.NU$_2$.A 1 ŠU$_2$ ŠUḪUŠ $^{\text{u2}}$ḪUR.SAG^{sar} 1/2 ŠU$_2$ KUŠ *a-ia-ri* DINGIR

220′ A$_{\text{iv 28}}$ 1/2 ŠU$_2$ $^{\text{u2}}$*kal-la-ṣu-di* 1/2 ŠU$_2$ ZE$_2$ *ša* ^{gud}AB$_2$ 1/2 ŠU$_2$ ZE$_2$ *ša* KU$_6$

216′ A sixth of a shekel of *murru* ('myrrh'), a sixth of a shekel of *ṭūru* ('opopanax'), a sixth of a shekel of resin from *baluḫḫu* ('galbanum'), a sixth of a shekel of resin from *abukkatu* (a tree),

217′ a sixth of a shekel of SU.ḪU.RA[646] (a tree), a sixth of a shekel of *suādu* (a kind of sedge), a sixth of a shekel of *kukru* (an aromatic), a sixth of a shekel of seed from *ēdu* ('lone' plant),

218′ a sixth of a shekel of *šammu peṣû* ('white plant'), a sixth of a shekel of *tarmuš* ('lupin'), a sixth of a shekel of *aktam* (a plant)—you roast (these / it)[647]—

219′ a sixth of a shekel of seed from *šunû* ('chaste tree'), a sixth of a shekel of root from *azupīru* ('saffron'), a twelfth of a shekel of skin from *ayyar ili* ('chameleon'),

220′ a twelfth of a shekel of *kallaṣūdu* (a plant), a twelfth of a shekel of bile from a cow, a twelfth of a shekel of bile from a fish,

---

645 ŠU$_2$ is treated here as a pseudo-logogram for 'one-sixth', although its linguistic and orthographic form need to be dealt with separately. Powell (1971: 84–116) devotes an entire chapter to the question, but ŠU$_2$ almost certainly derives from the Akkadian word *šuššu* 'one-sixth', which becomes *šuduš* in the construct state (see, in particular, Powell 1979: 101 and 1987–1990: 512). Alternative readings like DIŠ-*šu*$_2$, where DIŠ stands for 'sixty' and -*šu*$_2$ is a phonetic, viz. *šuššu* 'one-sixth', seem to be challenged by the occurrence of 1/2 ŠU$_2$ later in our recipe. Our text consistently writes 1 ŠU$_2$ for 'one-sixth (of a shekel)' (equivalent to 1 *suddû* in the late texts) or 1/2 ŠU$_2$ for 'one-twelfth' (equivalent to 2 *girû* in the late texts). For the measurement ŠU$_2$, see the recent discussion in Chalendar 2020: 61–63, who connects the usage of ŠU$_2$ in our passage to BAM 78 rev. 1–6, where 1 ŠU$_2$ or 2 ŠU$_2$ occurs after the names of each ingredient. In our view, however, orthographies like 1 ŠU$_2$ or 2 ŠU$_2$ in BAM 78 are probably multiplicative forms, namely *ištīššu* ('one time') and *šinīšu* ('two times'); this would also explain the use of ŠU, instead of ŠU$_2$, in the parallel recipe AMT 55/4: 6–8.

646 The form ^{giš}SU.ḪU.RA is a hapax that might be rendered as ^{giš}SU.BAḪ.RA, perhaps as a kind of pseudo-logographic writing of *šupuhru* ('old cedar'), which is normally written with the logogram ^{giš}ERIN.SUMUN. For a similar pseudo-logographic writing, compare the form $^{\text{u2}}$ZA.BA.LAM for Akk. *supālu* (a kind of juniper).

647 The verb *taqallu* 'you roast' is placed, rather unusually, in the middle of the drug list: it is preceded by eleven ingredients and followed by another seven, after which the prescription gives the total number of all listed drugs. The occurrence of the verb *taqallu* in such a position may suggest that the action described by it, viz. 'roasting', only applied to the first eleven ingredients (or some subset thereof), whereas the other seven were used in an unroasted state.

221′ A$_{iv 29}$ 1/2 ŠU$_2$ ŠIR *ša$_2$ ga-ri-di* 18 U$_2$.ḪI.A ŠIM.ḪI.A ⸢ŠEŠ⸣
222′ A$_{iv 30}$ KI *sa-ḫu-ni u* I$_3$ ^{giš}EN.DI *tu-sa-ḫap* SAG-*ka* ⸢*u$_2$*⸣*-*q*[*a-a*]
223′ A$_{iv 31}$ U$_2$.ḪI.A ŠEŠ *ni-ṣir-ti* LUGAL-*t*[*i*]

224′ A$_{iv 32}$ 3 *maš-qi-a-ti ša qer-be$_2$-na$_7$* GIG *ni-ṣir-ti* LUGAL-⸢*ti*⸣

225′ A$_{iv 33}$ DIŠ NA SAG ŠA$_3$-*šu$_2$* GIM *ša* NAM.ERIM$_2$ *i-ka-su-šu$_2$ ana*[648] GIG-*šu$_2$* GUR.⸢GUR⸣
[DIŠ NA S]AG ŠA$_3$-*šu$_2$* GIM *ša* ^{d}NAM.ERIM$_2$ *i-ka-su-šu$_2$* / *ana* GIG-*šu$_2$* GUR.GUR (BAM 49 rev. 9–10)
DIŠ NA S[AG . . .] / [. . .] (BAM 50 rev. 7–8)

221′ (and) a twelfth of a shekel of castoreum (lit. testicle from a beaver)[649]—you cover (*tusaḫḫap*)[650] these eighteen drugs (and) aromatics
222′ with *saḫunu* (a foodstuff)[651] and oil from *suādu* (a kind of sedge), (and then) it will be at your disposal.
223′ These ingredients are a royal secret.

224′ Three potions for those who suffer (*maruṣ*) internally. Royal secret.

225′ If someone's epigastrium (*rēš libbi*) binds him like in the case of a (broken) oath, (and) he continually has reoccurrences (*ittanâr*) of his disease,

648 As suggested by Maul (2019: 283), the reading of the single vertical wedge here is much more likely *ana* than DIŠ, as in *ana* GIG-*šu$_2$* GUR.GUR. This idiom, which literally means 'he keeps coming back to his disease', probably describes a patient that has relapsed (see Cadelli 2000: 279 n. 14 and CAD T 255).

649 For this rare medical ingredient, see the Syriac 'šky brd' in Gignoux 2011: 29, as well as Butz 1977: 285 and Stol 2012: 628.

650 The action applied to all eighteen ingredients follows the summary section and is expressed with the rarely used verb *saḫāpu* in the D-stem, meaning 'to cover' or 'to lay flat' (hence our translation 'you cover', as opposed to 'you sprinkle' in CAD S 35), but never with the preposition KI = Akk. *itti*. The occurrence of this rare verb in our corpus may have been influenced by the use of ŠU$_2$, the Sumerian equivalent of *saḫāpu*, as a unit of measure in the same recipe.

651 The word *saḫunu* is found a couple of times in the medical literature: see, for example, BAM 556 ii 69 // BAM 42 obv. 11–12, BAM 555 ii 14–15, as well as BAM 42 obv. 41 and rev. 6, in connection with the respiratory tract. In BAM 556 ii 69 and its parallel, *saḫunu* co-occurs with the idiom *rēška uqa''a* ('it is at your disposal') and the secrecy label *niṣirti šarrūti*. It is used there, however, as the designation of a certain type of medicine (see CAD S 67, Haussperger 1999: 179 and Scurlock 2014: 240). What sets our passage apart from these texts is that *saḫunu* here cannot designate a medicine; instead, it is most likely the name of an ingredient (CAD S 67) that is used alongside *suādu* oil.

226′ A$_{iv\ 34}$ IM *ina* ŠA$_3$-*šu*$_2$ GIM *ša* DUR$_2$.GIG *uš-tar-ʾ-ab* DU$_3$ UZU.MEŠ-*šu*$_2$ *ša*$_2$-*ḫu*$^!$(SIG)[652]
IM *ina* ŠA$_3$-*šu*$_2$ GIM *ša* DUR$_2$.GIG *uš-tar-ʾ-ab* / DU$_3$ UZU.MEŠ-*šu*$_2$ *šaḫ-ḫu* (BAM 49 rev. 10–11)
⸢IM⸣ *ina* ŠA$_3$-⸢*šu*$_2$⸣ [x x x x] / *uš-tar-*⸢*ʾ-ab*⸣ [DU$_3$] UZU.MEŠ-[*šu*$_2$ x x] (BAM 50 rev. 8–9)

227′ A$_{iv\ 35}$ ŠA$_3$-*šu*$_2$ *ru-uq-šu*$_2$ *ana* TI-*šu*$_2$ ^{u2}*ḫa-ša*$_2$-*na* ^{šim}GUR$_2$.GUR$_2$
ŠA$_3$-*šu*$_2$ *ru-uq-šu*$_2$ *ana* TI-*šu*$_2$ / ^{u2}*ḫa-ša*$_2$-*nu* ^{šim}GUR$_2$.GUR$_2$ (BAM 49 rev. 11–12)
ŠA$_3$-*šu*$_2$ *ru-uq-šu*$_2$ *ana* TI-*šu*$_2$ ^{u2}[. . .] (BAM 50 rev. 10)

228′ A$_{iv\ 36}$ *ina a-bat-ti tu-daq-qaq ina na-ku-a-ri ša* A.⸢MEŠ⸣
ina a-bat-te tu-daq$_3$*-qaq* / [*ina na-ku-a-r*]*i ša* A.MEŠ (BAM 49 rev. 12–13)
ina a-bat-[*te*] ⸢*tu*⸣-[*daq*$_3$*-qaq*] / *ina na-ku-*[*a-ri* . . .] (BAM 50 rev. 11–12)

229′ A$_{iv\ 37}$ *tu-la-bak šum*$_4$*-ma na-ku-a-ri ḫa-mar* A.MEŠ *ana* ŠA$_3$ *ta-ḫi-*⸢*aq*⸣
tu-lab-bak šum$_4$*-ma na-ku-a-ru* / [. . .] *ta-ḫi-aq* (BAM 49 rev. 13–14)
[. . .] / *šum*$_4$*-ma na-ku-a-*[*ri* . . .] / *ta-ḫi-aq* (BAM 50 rev. 12–14)

230′ A$_{iv\ 38}$ *ana* IGI ^{mul}UZ$_3$ TUR$_3$ ^{d}*gu-la tuš-bat ina šer*$_3$*-ti* ŠEG$_6$*-šal*
ana IGI ^{mul}UZ$_3$ / [. . . ^{d}*gu-l*]*a tuš-bat ina še-ri*$_3$ ŠEG$_6$*-šal* (BAM 49 rev. 14–15)
ana IGI ^{mul}UZ$_3$ [. . .] / *ana* IGI ^{d}*gu-la tuš-bat ina š*[*e-ri*$_3$ x x] (BAM 50 rev. 14–15)

†

226′ flatus (lit. wind) churns in his belly (*libbu*) like in the case of rectal disease (*durgiqqu*), all his flesh is wasting away,
227′ (and) his belly is distant (*rūqšu*)[653] from him: in order to heal him (*ana bulluṭīšu*), you crush minutely *ḫašânu* ('thyme-like' plant) (and) *kukru* (an aromatic)
228′ using a pestle, you dissolve them in a *nakmaru*[654] jug,
229′ if the *nakmaru* jug becomes dry, you mix water into it,
230′ you leave (the mixture) out overnight under the Goat Star, the cattle pen (*tarbaṣu*) of Gula, (and) in the morning you bring it to a boil (*tušabšal*),

652 The emendation here (*pace* Maul 2019: 283) is required by the context as well as the parallel passage in BAM 49 rev. 11, which has *šaḫ-ḫu*. The signs SIG and ḪU are similar in form, differing only in the rotation of the first wedge (see also Cadelli 2019: 58). For the medical condition *šiḫḫat šīri* 'wasting away of the flesh', see STO 3: 147. The reading *ša-pik* (CAD Š/1 419 and Cadelli 2000: 267) is less likely and does not take into account the plural subject of the verb, viz. UZU.MEŠ-*šu*$_2$.

653 The meaning of the idiom *libbašu rūqšu*, viz. impenetrable or unfathomable (of the mind), is clearly transferred here to the gastrointestinal system, describing a belly that feels distant or strange (Cadelli 2000: 288 n. 9). In the therapeutic corpus, this idiom only occurs here and in BAM 87 obv. 2, as part of a longer symptom description mentioning a throbbing and hurting belly as well as flaccid limbs. Following CAD R 425, Maul (2019: 281) takes this literally as a description of the loss of mental coherence, namely 'er nicht mehr ganz bei Sinnen ist'.

654 For *nakmuru*, see Gaspa 2014: 255 and 409–410.

231′ A$_{iv\ 39}$ U$_2$ *an-nu-ti$_3$-ma ana mar-kas$_3$-te ana* ŠA$_3$ *ṭe$_4$-ḫi*[655] *ša$_2$* UTUL$_2$ ŠUB
[. . . *mar-kas$_3$-t*]*i ana* ŠA$_3$ *ṭe$_4$-ḫi ša* UTUL$_2$ ŠUB-*di* (BAM 49 rev. 16)
U$_2$.ḪI.A ŠEŠ *ana mar-kas$_3$-ti* [x x x x] / *ša* UTUL$_2$ ŠUB-*di* (BAM 50 rev. 16–17)

232′ A$_{iv\ 40}$ *šum$_4$-ma ḫa-di-a-ta a-na* 1-*et qa-ti* ^{u2}*bu-uṭ-na-nu tu-qar-rab*
[. . . *a-n*]*a* 1-*et qa-ti* / [. . . *tu-qa*]*r-rab* (BAM 49 rev. 17–18)
šum$_4$-ma ḫa-⌜*di*⌝-[*a-ta*] / *a-na* 1-*et qa-ti* ^{u2}*bu-uṭ-na-nu* ⌜*tu*⌝-[*qar-rab*] (BAM 50 rev. 17–18)

233′ A$_{iv\ 41}$ *a-bat-ta-te* DIDLI-*ta$_5$ ta*$^!$(TAB)-*pa-aṣ$_2$*[656] *ša ṭa-bi-u$_2$-ni*[657] *qa-a-ta tu-šal-pat*
a-bat-ta-te / [. . . *ṭ*]*a-bi-u$_2$-ni* / [. . .] (BAM 49 rev. 18–20)
a-bat-ta-te DIDLI-*ta$_5$ ta-pa-aṣ$_2$* / *ša$_2$ ṭa-bi-u$_2$-ni qa-a-ta tu-ša*[*l-pat*] (BAM 50 rev. 19–20)

231′ (then) you put (*tanaddi*) these ingredients for a compress in . . . from the bowl,
232′ if you wish, you can serve it (*tuqarrab*)[658] with *buṭnānu* ('terebinth-like' plant) for each portion,[659]
233′ crushing the individual seeds (and) setting (*tušalpat*)[660] them next to the portion, as (you think) best,

655 The difficult form *ṭe$_4$-ḫi* may be related to Akk. *ṭaḫû* / *ṭeḫû*, which describes a culinary practice involving a fatty substance smeared or glazed on bread (Waerzeggers 2010: 231; see also CDA 414). The term also appears in the ritual text Thureau-Dangin 1921: 77 ln. 46, which seems to have the nominal form *ṭa-ḫu-u$_2$ ša im-mi-e-ti*, as in our line, presumably referring to the material used as well as the act of glazing.
656 The first half of line 233′ has long been a puzzle. While CAD A/1 40 and P 268 read it as *abatta* TE AŠ AŠ without any translation, von Soden (1966: 359) takes AŠ AŠ as DIL.DIL (i.e., DIDLI) for the Akkadian adverb *aḫennâ*. In line with Maul 2019: 283, DIDLI here probably stands for Akk. (*w*)*ēdû*, as an adjectival modifier of *abattāte*. We differ only in the reading of the following UD sign, which we take as a phonetic complement indicating the feminine plural DIDLI-*ta$_5$*. Maul (2019: 280–281) interprets this sign as part of the following verb, yielding *a-bat-ta-te* DIDLI *tu$_2$-ta-pa-aš$_2$*, a verb that he sees as a D-stem form of *tapāšu* meaning '(Einzelne Steinchen (??)) nimmst du an dich (?)' (AHw 1320 and CAD T 476). Following AHw 846, we take this as the verb *pa'āṣu* 'to crush', which occurs elsewhere in the therapeutic corpus with orthographies like *tu-pa-aṣ$_2$* (AMT 14/5 obv.$^!$ 10) and *ta-pa-aṣ* (BAM 494 ii 40 with parallels in Bácskay and Simkó 2017: 13).
657 The verb here is most likely *ṭâbu* 'to be good', with the Assyrian subjunctive ending, yielding *ša ṭābiāni*, which lines up nicely with *šumma ḫadiāta* 'if you wish' in line 232′. Maul (2019: 281 and 283), however, derives this form from *ṭebû* 'to sink' and translates 'Das, was (in der Flüssigkeit) nach unten gesunken ist'.
658 The D-stem of *qerēbu* normally means 'to bring near' or 'to present' but is also used in the sense of 'to serve (a meal to a god or king)' (CAD Q 236). Here, the meaning seems to be extended slightly to describe the use of *buṭnānu* as a kind of garnish. This usage is explained in more detail in line 233′, where the crushed seeds of the *buṭnānu* plant are set next to the mixture. Both CAD B 358 and Q 194–195 as well as Maul 2019: 281 ln. 40 take this verb to mean roughly 'to add'.
659 For a recent discussion of *qātu* in this passage, see Chalendar 2020: 66 with earlier literature.
660 The meaning of the verb *lapātu* in the Š-stem is somewhat unclear but may further specify the way in which the *buṭnānu* plant comes into contact with the mixture, as described in the preceding line. Both here and in CRAN 1: 11 (BAM 480+ i 11), the suggested translation of the verb as 'to sprinkle' (CAD L 93) does not seem to be justified.

234′ A$_{iv\ 42}$ MU ^{d}*gu-la u* ^{d}*nin-maḫ ta-zak-kar ta-ḫi-as-su*
[. . .] ^{d}*gu-la u* ^{d}MAḪ / [. . . *ta-ḫi*]*-as-su* (BAM 49 rev. 20–21)
MU ^{d}*gu-la u* ^{d}MAḪ MU-*ar*$_2$ *ta-ḫi-a*[*s-su*] (BAM 50 rev. 21)

235′ A$_{iv\ 43}$ *maš-qi-tu an-ni-tu* URU$_3$*-ti* LUGAL*-ti šaq-lu-tu*
[. . . *an-n*]*a-*⸢*ti*⸣ / [. . . LUGAL*-t*]*i šaq-*[*lu-tu*] (BAM 49 rev. 22–23)
maš-qi-a-ti an-na-a-t[*i*] / *ni-ṣir-ti* LUGAL*-u-*⸢*ti*⸣ [x x x] (BAM 50 rev. 22–23)

236′ A$_{iv\ 44}$ DIŠ ⸢NA SAG ŠA$_3$*-šu*$_2$ *na*⸣*-ši* MURUB$_4$.MEŠ*-šu*$_2$ *mi-na-tu-šu*$_2$ GU$_7$.MEŠ*-šu*$_2$
[DIŠ NA] ⸢SAG⸣ ŠA$_3$*-šu*$_2$ *na-ši* MURUB$_4$.MEŠ*-šu*$_2$ *mi-na-*⸢*tu-šu*$_2$⸣ GU$_7$.MEŠ*-šu*$_2$ NA ⸢BI⸣ [x x] (AMT 43/6 i 1)
237′ A$_{iv\ 45}$ ⸢DUB.5⸣*.[KAM$_2$ DIŠ NA *su-a-la*]*m* GIG *ana ki-is* ŠA$_3$ GUR*-šu*
238′ A$_{iv\ 46}$ E$_2$.[GAL ^{m}AN.ŠAR$_2$-DU$_3$-A MAN ŠU$_2$ MAN KUR AN.ŠAR$_2$^{ki}] ⸢*ša*⸣ ^{d}AG *u* ⸢^{d}⸣[*taš*]-⸢*me*⸣*-tu*$_4$ GEŠTU.MIN *ra-pa-aš*$_2$*-tu*$_4$ *iš-ru-ku-u*[*š*]
239′ A$_{iv\ 47}$ ⸢*e*⸣-[*ḫu-uz-zu* IGI.MIN *na-m*]*ir-tu*$_4$ *ni-siq ṭup***-šar-ru-t*[*i*]
240′ A$_{iv\ 48}$ [*ša ina* LUGAL.MEŠ*-ni a-lik maḫ-r*]*i-ia mam*$_2$*-ma šip-ru šu-a-tu la e-ḫu-uz-z*[*u*]

234′ you invoke the name of Gula and Ninmaḫ, (and) you measure out (the doses) for him.

235′ This potion,[661] a royal secret, (with) weighed (ingredients).[662]

236′ (Catchline:) 'If someone's epigastrium (*rēš libbi*) heaves, his hips, (and) his limbs constantly cause him pain (*ītanakkalšu*)'.
237′ (Tablet designation:) Fifth tablet of 'If someone suffers (*maruṣ*) from phlegm (*suālu*), which has turned into (*itūršu*) gastric constriction (*kīs libbi*)'.
238′ (Colophon:) Palace of Assurbanipal, ruler of everything, king of the land of Assur, on whom Nabû and Tašmētu have bestowed wisdom (lit. wide ears),
239′ He acquired for himself shining eyes, the pinnacle of scholarship,
240′ Of the kings who came before me, none were able to comprehend this task.

---

661 The label clearly defines this medicine as a healing potion, viz. *mašqītu* (plural *mašqiātu* in the parallel); however, a few lines earlier the drugs are summarised as a *markastu* (line 231′). This hapax derives from the verb *rakāsu* and presumably describes a kind of bandage (AHw 612, CAD M/1 282 and Maul 2019: 283).

662 Weighing is a central theme in this text, as shown by the exact measurements and complex recipes that involve the verb *ḫiāṭu* 'to measure' (see line 59–65 and 225′–234′). The masculine plural adjective *šaqlūtu* 'weighed' does not modify any of the nouns in this line, so we assume with CAD Š/2 15 and Maul 2019: 281 that it agrees with the measured ingredients earlier in the prescription, summarised in line 231′ with the masculine plural noun *šammū* 'ingredients'.

241′ A$_{\text{iv 49}}$ *b[ul-ṭi* TA *muḫ-ḫi* EN UMBIN *liq]**-⸢*ti*⸣* BAR.MEŠ *ta-ḫi-zu nak-l[a]*
242′ A$_{\text{iv 50}}$ *a-zu-gal-lu-ut* [d]⸢*nin-urta u* [d]*gu-la*⸣ *ma-la ba-a[š$_2$-mu]*
243′ A$_{\text{iv 51}}$ *ina ṭup-pa-a-ni aš$_2$-ṭur as-niq* IGI.KAR$_2$-*m[a]*
244′ A$_{\text{iv 52}}$ *a-na ta-mar-ti ši-ta-as-si-ia qe$_2$-reb* E$_2$.GAL-*ia u$_2$-[kin]*

†

241′ Prescriptions (organized) from head to foot, gleanings from extraneous materials, technical lore
242′ (And) whatever pertains to the great medical expertise of Ninurta and Gula,
243′ I have written on tablets, checked and double-checked, and
244′ I deposited them in the middle of my palace for my reading and recitation.

Bibliography

Abusch 2016 = Tz. Abusch, *The Magical Ceremony Maqlû: A Critical Edition*, Ancient Magic and Divination 10, Leiden / Boston: Brill.

Abusch and Schwemer 2009 = Tz. Abusch and D. Schwemer, 'The Chicago Maqlû Fragment (A 7876)', *Iraq* 71, 53–87.

Abusch and Schwemer 2011 = Tz. Abusch and D. Schwemer, *Corpus of Mesopotamian Anti-Witchcraft Rituals*, Vol. 1, Ancient Magic and Divination 8/1, Leiden / Boston: Brill.

Abusch and Schwemer 2016 = Tz. Abusch and D. Schwemer, *Corpus of Mesopotamian Anti-Witchcraft Rituals*, Vol. 2, Ancient Magic and Divination 8/2, Leiden / Boston: Brill.

Abusch, Schwemer, Luukko and Van Buylaere 2020 = Tz. Abusch, D. Schwemer, M. Luukko and G. Van Buylaere, *Corpus of Mesopotamian Anti-Witchcraft Rituals*, Vol. 3, Ancient Magic and Divination 8/3, Leiden / Boston: Brill.

Adamson 1993 = P.B. Adamson, 'An Assessment of Some Akkadian Medical Terms', *Revue d'Assyriologie et d'archéologie orientale* 87, 153–159.

Algaze 2018 = G. Algaze, 'Entropic Cities: The Paradox of Urbanism in Ancient Mesopotamia', *Current Anthropology* 59, 23–54.

Alster and van Dijk 1972 = B. Alster and J.J.A. van Dijk, 'A Sumerian Incantation against Gall', *Orientalia* Nova Series 41, 349–358.

Ambos 2004 = C. Ambos, *Mesopotamische Baurituale aus dem 1. Jahrtausend v. Chr.*, Dresden: Islet.

Annus 2016 = A. Annus, *The Overturned Boat: Intertextuality of the Adapa Myth and Exorcist Literature*, State Archives of Assyria Studies 24, Helsinki: The Neo-Assyrian Text Corpus Project.

Arnaud 1987 = D. Arnaud, *Recherches au pays d'Aštata, Emar VI/4, Textes de la bibliothèque: transcriptions et traductions*, Paris: Éditions Recherche sur les Civilisations.

Aro 1961 = J. Aro, *Die akkadischen Infinitivkonstruktionen*, Studia Orientalia 26, Helsinki: Suomalaisen Kirjallisuuden Kirjapaino.

Attia 2015 = A. Attia, 'Traduction et commentaires des trois premières tablettes de la série IGI', *Le Journal des Médecines Cunéiformes* 25, 1–120.

Attia and Buisson 2012 = A. Attia and G. Buisson, 'BAM 1 et consorts en transcription', *Le Journal des Médecines Cunéiformes* 19, 22–50.

Attinger 2021 = P. Attinger, *Glossaire sumérien-français: principalement des textes littéraires paléobabyloniens*, Wiesbaden: Harrassowitz.

Bácskay 2015 = A. Bácskay, 'Magical-medical prescriptions against fever: an edition of BM 42272', *Le Journal des Médecines Cunéiformes* 26, 1–32.

Bácskay 2018 = A. Bácskay, *Therapeutic Prescriptions against Fever in Ancient Mesopotamia*, Alter Orient und Altes Testament 447, Münster: Ugarit-Verlag.

Bácskay 2021a = A. Bácskay, *Glosses and Embedded Variants in Mesopotamian Therapeutic Texts*, Dubsar 22, Münster: Zaphon.

Bácskay 2021b = A. Bácskay, 'Medical Treatments against Respiratory Diseases, Ear Complaints and Migraine: An Edition of a Late Babylonian Medical Compendium, BM 32277+', *Revue d'Assyriologie et d'archéologie orientale* 115, 159–174.

Bácskay and Niederreiter 2021 = A. Bácskay and Z. Niederreiter, 'Two New Fragments Belonging to the 16th Tablet of the Omen Series *Šumma Ālu*', *Bibliotheca Orientalis* 78, 39–48.

Bácskay and Simkó 2017 = A. Bácskay and K. Simkó, 'Edition of BAM 494: The fifth tablet of UGU or a compilation of recipes against the skin diseases of the head', *Le Journal des Médecines Cunéiformes* 30, 1–71.

Balke 2015 = T. Balke, 'Die Zeichensequenz /ÁB.ŠÀ.GI/ in den altsumerischen Inscriften aus Ĝirsu/Lagas: Ein Fall orthographischer Verkomplizierung?', *Studia Mesopotamica: Jahrbuch für altorientalische Geschichte und Kultur* 2, 1–15.

Barrett and Armelagos 2013 = R. Barrett and G.J. Armelagos, *An Unnatural History of Emerging Infections*, Oxford: Oxford University Press.

Barjamovic 2015 = G. Barjamovic, 'Contextualizing Tradition: Magic, Literacy and Domestic Life in Old Assyrian Kanesh', in: *Texts and Contexts: Approaches to Textual Transmission in the Cuneiform World*, Studies in Ancient Near Eastern Records 9, ed. P. Delnero and J. Lauinger, Berlin / Boston: Walter de Gruyter, 48–86.

Beckman and Foster 1988 = G. Beckman and B.R. Foster, 'Assyrian Scholarly Texts in the Yale Babylonian Collection', in: *A Scientific Humanist: Studies in Memory of Abraham Sachs*, Occasional Publications of the Samuel Noah Kramer Fund 9, Philadelphia: The University Museum, 1–26.

Biggs 1967 = R.D. Biggs, *ŠÀ.ZI.GA: Ancient Mesopotamian Potency Incantations*, Texts from Cuneiform Sources 2, New York: J.J. Augustin Publisher.

Biggs 1974 = R.D. Biggs, *Inscriptions from Tell Abū Ṣalābīkh*, Oriental Institute Publications 99, Chicago / London: The University of Chicago Press.

Böck 2000 = B. Böck, *Die babylonisch-assyrische Morphoskopie*, Archiv für Orientforschung Beiheft 27, Wien: Institut für Orientalistik der Universität Wien.

Böck 2003 = B. Böck, 'Hauterscheinungen in altmesopotamischer Divination und Medizin, Teil 1: Das *kurāru*-Mal', *Aula Orientalis* 21, 161–184.

Böck 2007 = B. Böck, *Das Handbuch Muššu'u "Einreibung". Eine Serie sumerischer und akkadischer Beschwörungen aus dem 1. Jt. vor Chr.*, Biblioteca del Próximo Oriente Antiguo 3, Madrid: Consejo Superior de Investigaciones Científicas.

Böck 2009 = B. Böck, 'On Medical Technology in Ancient Mesopotamia', in: *Advances in Mesopotamian Medicine from Hammurabi to Hippocrates: Proceedings of the International Conference "Oeil malade et mauvais oeil," Collège de France, Paris, 23rd June 2006*, Cuneiform Monographs 37, Leiden / Boston: Brill, 105–128.

Böck 2011 = B. Böck, 'Sourcing, Organizing, and Administering Medical Ingredients', in: *The Oxford Handbook of Cuneiform Culture*, ed. K. Radner and E. Robson, Oxford: Oxford University Press, 690–705.

Böck 2014a = B. Böck, *The Healing Goddess Gula: Towards an Understanding of Ancient Babylonian Medicine*, Culture and History of the Ancient Near East 67, Leiden / Boston: Brill.

Böck 2014b = B. Böck, 'Die Hymne *Ninisina A* Z. 30–42 mit einem Exkurs über $\check{s}a_3$ ‚Bauch, Magen-Darm-Trakt' als Sitz der Gefühle', in: *Studies in Sumerian Language and Literature: Festschrift für Joachim Krecher*, Babel und Bibel 8, ed. N. Koslova, E. Vizirova and G. Zólyomi, Winona Lake, Indiana: Eisenbrauns, 101–121.

Borger 1969 = R. Borger, 'Die erste Tafel der zi-pà Beschwörung (ASKT 11)', in: *Lišān mitḫurti: Festschrift Wolfram Freiherr von Soden zum 19. VI. 1968 gewidmet von Schülern und Mitarbeitern*, Alter Orient und Altes Testament 1, ed. W. Röllig, Kevelaer / Neukirchen-Vluyn: Verlag Butzon & Bercker / Neukirchener Verlag, 1–22.

https://doi.org/10.1515/9781501506574-008

Borger 2004 = R. Borger, *Mesopotamisches Zeichenlexikon*, Alter Orient und Altes Testament 305, Münster: Ugarit-Verlag.

Bottéro 1995 = J. Bottéro, *Textes culinaires Mésopotamiens*, Mesopotamian Civilisations 6, Winona Lake, Indiana: Eisenbrauns.

Buisson 2009 = G. Buisson, 'Chroniques bibliographiques 13. Moyens médico-magiques pour contrer les fantômes', *Revue d'Assyriologie et d'archéologie orientale* 103, 149–158.

Burde 1974 = C. Burde, *Hethitische medizinische Texte*, Studien zu den Boğazköy-Texten 19, Wiesbaden: Harrassowitz.

Butz 1977 = K. Butz, 'Bemerkungen zu Jagdtieren in Mesopotamien', *Bibliotheca Orientalis* 34, 282–290.

Cadelli 2000 = D.S. Cadelli, *Recherche sur la médecine Mésopotamienne: la série šumma amêlu suâlam maruṣ*, Doctorat de l'Université de Paris I Panthéon Sorbonne.

Cadelli 2019 = D.S. Cadelli, 2019, 'Symptomatologie dans Suâlam (première partie)', *Le Journal des Médecines Cunéiformes* 34, 4–68.

Cadelli 2021 = D.S. Cadelli, 'Symptomatologie dans Suâlam (seconde partie)', *Le Journal des Médecines Cunéiformes* 37, 9–30.

Campbell Thompson 1923 = R. Campbell Thompson, *Assyrian Medical Texts from the Originals in the British Museum*, London: Humphrey Milford.

Campbell Thompson 1926 = R. Campbell Thompson, 'Assyrian Medical Texts', *Proceedings of the Royal Society of Medicine* 19, 29–78.

Campbell Thompson 1929 = R. Campbell Thompson, 'Assyrian Medical Prescriptions for Diseases of the Stomach', *Revue d'Assyriologie et d'archéologie orientale* 26, 47–92.

Campbell Thompson 1949 = R. Campbell Thompson, *A Dictionary of Assyrian Botany*, London: The British Academy.

Cancik-Kirschbaum 1999 = E. Cancik-Kirschbaum, '^{lú}*sāpi'u/sēpû*: Eine akkadische Berufsbezeichnung aus dem Bereich der Textilherstellung', in: *Munuscula Mesopotamica. Festschrift für Johannes Renger*, Alter Orient und Altes Testament 267, ed. B. Böck, E. Cancik-Kirschbaum and T. Richter, Münster: Ugarit-Verlag, 79–93.

Cavigneaux and Al-Rawi 1993 = A. Cavigneaux and F. Al-Rawi, 'New Sumerian Literary Texts from Tell Haddad (Ancient Meturan): A First Survey', *Iraq* 55, 91–105.

Cavigneaux 2014 = A. Cavigneaux, 'Une version sumérienne de la légende d'Adapa (Textes de Tell Haddad X)', *Zeitschrift für Assyriologie und Vorderasiatische Archäologie* 104, 1–41.

Chalendar 2020 = V. Chalendar, 'Le dosage des ingrédients dans les prescriptions thérapeutiques Mésopotamiennes: Quelques observations à partir du texte BAM 579', *Histoire & mesure* 35, 55–76.

Civil 1960 = M. Civil, 'Prescriptions médicales sumériennes', *Revue d'Assyriologie et d'archéologie orientale* 54, 57–72.

Civil 1961 = M. Civil, 'Une nouvelle prescription médicale sumérienne', *Revue d'Assyriologie et d'archéologie orientale* 55, 91–94.

Civil 1982 = M. Civil, 'Studies on Early Dynastic Lexicography, I', *Oriens Antiquus* 21, 1–26.

Civil 1983 = M. Civil, 'The Sign LAK 384', *Orientalia* Nova Series 52, 233–240.

Civil 2000 = M. Civil, 'Modal Prefixes', *Acta Sumerologica* 22, 29–42.

Cohen 1976 = S. Cohen, 'Studies in Sumerian Lexicography I', in: *Kramer Anniversary Volume: Cuneiform Studies in Honor of Samuel Noah Kramer*, Alter Orient und Altes Testament 25, ed. B.L. Eichler, Kevelaer / Neukirchen-Vluyn: Verlag Butzon & Bercker / Neukirchener Verlag, 97–110.

Cohen 2015 = E. Cohen, 'Circumstantial Clause Combining in Old Babylonian Akkadian', in: *Clause Combining in Semitic: The Circumstantial Clause and Beyond*, Abhandlungen für die Kunde des Morgenlandes 96, ed. B. Isaksson and M. Persson, Wiesbaden: Harrassowitz, 365–406.

Collard and Samama 2021 = F. Collard and E. Samama (eds.), *Histoire du ventre: Entrailles, tripes et boyaux. Antiquité, Moyen Age, Époque moderne*, Paris: L'Harmattan.

Collins 1999 = T.J. Collins, *Natural Illness in Babylonian Medical Incantations*, PhD Dissertation, University of Chicago.

Corcoran-Todd, Price and Caramanica 2022 = N. Corcoran-Todd, M. Price and A. Caramanica, 'The Political Economy of Livestock in Early States', *Cambridge Archaeological Journal* First View, 1–18 (accessed on the 12th of November 2022).

Couto-Ferreira 2009 = M.E. Couto-Ferreira, *Etnoanatomía y partonomía del cuerpo humano en sumerio y acadio. El léxico Ugu-mu*, PhD Dissertation, Universitat Pompeu Fabra.

Cunningham 1997 = G. Cunningham, *'Deliver Me from Evil': Mesopotamian Incantations 2500–1500 BC*, Studia Pohl: Series Maior 17, Roma: Editrice Pontificio Istituto Biblico.

Curtis 1984 = R.I. Curtis, 'Salted Fish Products in Ancient Medicine', *Journal of the History of Medicine and Allied Sciences* 39, 430–445.

Deller 1987 = K. Deller, Review of H. Freydank, *Mittelassyrische Rechtsurkunden und Verwaltungstexte II* (1982), *Archiv für Orientforschung* 34, 58 –66.

Devecchi and Sibbing-Plantholt 2020 = E. Devecchi and I. Sibbing-Plantholt, '"See Ḫattuša and Die": A New Reconstruction of the Journeys of the Babylonian Physician Rabâ-ša-Marduk', *Journal of Near Eastern Studies* 79, 305–322.

Drower and Macuch 1963 = E.S. Drower and R Macuch, *A Mandaic Dictionary*, Oxford: Clarendon Press.

Ebeling 1922–1923 = E. Ebeling, *Keilschrifttexte medicinischen Inhalts*, Berliner Beiträge zur Keilschriftkunde Beiheft 1–2, Berlin: Selbstverlag.

Ebeling 1931 = E. Ebeling, *Tod und Leben nach den Vorstellungen der Babylonier. I. Teil: Texte*, Berlin / Leipzig: Walter de Gruyter.

Ebeling 1948 = E. Ebeling, 'Mittelassyrische Rezepte zur Herstellung von wohlriechenden Salben (Fortsetzung)', *Orientalia* Nova Series 17, 299–313.

Ebeling 1949 = E. Ebeling, 'Mittelassyrische Rezepte zur Herstellung von wohlriechenden Salben (Fortsetzung)', *Orientalia* Nova Series 18, 404–418.

Enders 2015 = G. Enders, *Gut: The Inside Story of Our Body's Most Underrated Organ*, Vancouver: Greystone Books Ltd.

Eypper 2016 = S.Ch. Eypper, 'Diseases of the Feet in Babylonian-Assyrian Medicine: A Study of Text K.67+', *Le Journal des Médecines Cunéiformes* 27, 1–58.

Eypper 2019 = S.Ch. Eypper, '*kasû* (^{u2}GAZI^{sar}) Revisited', *Le Journal des Médecines Cunéiformes* 33, 35–49.

Falkenstein 1931 = A. Falkenstein, *Die Haupttypen der sumerischen Beschwörung*, Leipziger Semitische Studien Neue Folge 1, Leipzig: J. C. Hinrichs'sche Buchhandlung.

Farber 1984 = W. Farber, 'Early Akkadian Incantations: Addenda et Subtrahenda', *Journal of Near Eastern Studies* 43, 69–71.

Farber 1987 = W. Farber, 'Ein Abschnitt aus einem jungbabylonischen medizinischen Traktat gegen Leibschmerzen', in: *Religiöse Texte*, Texte aus der Umwelt des Alten Testaments II/2, ed. W. Farber, H.M. Kümmel and W.H.Ph. Römer, Gütersloh: Gütersloher Verlagshaus, 272.

Farber 1990 = W. Farber, 'Mannam lušpur ana Enkidu: Some New Thoughts about an Old Motif', *Journal of Near Eastern Studies* 49, 299–321.

Farber 1993 = W. Farber, 'Myrrhe. B. Philologisch', *Reallexikon der Assyriologie* 8: 536–537.

Farber 2014 = W. Farber, *Lamaštu: An Edition of the Canonical Series of Lamaštu Incantations and Rituals and Related Texts from the Second and First Millennia B.C.*, Mesopotamian Civilisations 17, Winona Lake, Indiana: Eisenbrauns.

Fincke 2000 = J.C. Fincke, *Augenleiden nach keilschriftlichen Quellen: Untersuchungen zur altorientalischen Medizin*, Würzburger medizinhistorische Forschungen 70, Würzburg: Königshausen & Neumann.

Finkel 1994 = I. L. Finkel, 'On TDP Tablets XXIX and XXXI, and the Nature of SA.GIG', *Journal of Cuneiform Studies* 46, 87–88.

Finkel 1999 = I.L. Finkel, 'On Some Dog, Snake and Scorpion Incantations', in: *Mesopotamian Magic: Textual, Historical, and Interpretative Perspectives* (Ancient Magic and Divination 1), ed. Tz. Abusch and K. van der Toorn, Groningen: Styx, 213–250.

Finkel 2000 = I.L. Finkel, 'On Late Babylonian Medical Training', in: *Wisdom, Gods and Literature: Studies in Assyriology in Honour of W. G. Lambert*, ed. A.R. George and I.L. Finkel, Winona Lake, Indiana: Eisenbrauns, 137–223.

Foster [2]1996 = B.R. Foster, *Before the Muses: An Anthology of Akkadian Literature*, Vol. 1: *Archaic, Classical, Mature*, 2nd ed., Bethesda, Maryland: CDL Press.

Foster [3]2005 = B.R. Foster, *Before the Muses: An Anthology of Akkadian Literature*, 3rd ed., Bethesda, Maryland: CDL Press.

Frahm 2010 = 'Kommentar zum 10. Abschnitt der therapeutischen Serie', in: *Texte zur Heilkunde*, Texte aus der Umwelt des Alten Testaments, Neue Folge 5, ed. B. Janowski and D. Schwemer, Gütersloh: Gütersloher Verlagshaus, 172–173.

Frahm 2015 = E. Frahm, 'Commentary on Therapeutic (*CCP* 4.2.D)', *Cuneiform Commentaries Project* (E. Frahm, E. Jiménez, M. Frazer, and K. Wagensonner), 2013–2022; accessed October 10, 2022, at https://ccp.yale.edu/P348468.

Frahm 2018 = E. Frahm, 'The Exorcist's Manual: Structure, Language, *Sitz im Leben*', in: *Sources of Evil: Studies in Mesopotamian Exorcistic Lore*, Ancient Magic and Divination 15, ed. G. Van Buylaere, M. Luukko, D. Schwemer and A. Mertens-Wagschal, Leiden / Boston: Brill, 9–47.

Frazer 2016 = M. Frazer, 'Commentary on Enūma Anu Enlil 8 (*CCP* 3.1.8.A.a)', *Cuneiform Commentaries Project* (E. Frahm, E. Jiménez, M. Frazer, and K. Wagensonner), 2013–2022; accessed October 11, 2022, at https://ccp.yale.edu/P363690.

Frazer 2017 = M. Frazer, 'Commentary on Therapeutic (Qutāru) (*CCP* 4.2.M.a)', *Cuneiform Commentaries Project* (E. Frahm, E. Jiménez, M. Frazer, and K. Wagensonner), 2013–2022; accessed October 11, 2022, at https://ccp.yale.edu/P296515.

Fronzaroli 1998 = P. Fronzaroli, 'A Pharmaceutical Text at Ebla (TM.75.G.1623)', *Zeitschrift für Assyriologie und Vorderasiatische Archäologie* 88, 225–239.

Gabbay 2016 = U. Gabbay, *The Exegetical Terminology of Akkadian Commentaries*, Culture and History of the Ancient Near East 82, Leiden / Boston: Brill.

Gadotti 2014 = A. Gadotti, *'Gilgamesh, Enkidu, and the Netherworld' and the Sumerian Gilgamesh Cycle*, Untersuchungen zur Assyriologie und Vorderasiatischen Archäologie 10, Boston / Berlin: Walter de Gruyter.

Gaspa 2014 = S. Gaspa, *Contenitori neoassiri: Studi per un repertorio lessicale*, Philippika 67, Wiesbaden: Harrassowitz.

Geller 1984 = M.J. Geller, Review of F. Köcher, *Die assyrisch-babylonische Medizin in Texten und Untersuchungen Vol. V–VI* (1980), *Zeitschrift für Assyriologie und Vorderasiatische Archäologie* 74, 292–297.

Geller 1991 = M.J. Geller, 'Akkadian Medicine in the Babylonian Talmud', in *A Traditional Quest: Essays in Honour of Louis Jacobs*, Journal for the Study of the Old Testament Supplement 114, ed. D. Cohn-Sherbok, Sheffield: JSOT Press, 102–112.

Geller 2004 = M.J. Geller, 'Diet and Regimen in the Babylonian Talmud', in: *Food and Identity in the Ancient World*, History of the Ancient Near East Studies 9, ed. C. Grottanelli and L. Milano, Padua: S.A.R.G.O.N, 217–242.

Geller 2005 = M.J. Geller, *Renal and Rectal Disease Texts*, Die babylonisch-assyrische Medizin in Texten und Untersuchungen 7, Berlin / New York, Walter de Gruyter.

Geller 2006 = M.J. Geller, 'Les maladies et leurs causes, selon un texte médical paléobabylonien', *Le Journal des Médecines Cunéiformes* 8, 7–12.

Geller 2010 = M.J. Geller, *Ancient Babylonian Medicine: Theory and Practice*, Chichester, West Sussex: Wiley-Blackwell.

Geller 2018 = M.J. Geller, 'Babylonian Medicine as a Discipline', in: *The Cambridge History of Science*, Vol. 1: *Ancient Science*, ed. A. Jones and L. Taub, Cambridge: Cambridge University Press, 29–57.

Geller 2020 = M.J. Geller, 'An Apothecary's Handbook', *Le Journal des Médecines Cunéiformes* 35, 1–33.

George 2015 = A.R. George, 'On Babylonian Lavatories and Sewers' *Iraq* 77, 75–106.

George 2016 = A.R. George, *Mesopotamian Incantations and Related Texts in the Schøyen Collection*, Cornell University Studies in Assyriology and Sumerology 32, Bethesda, Maryland: CDL Press.

Gignoux 2011 = P. Gignoux, *Lexique des termes de la pharmacopée syriaque*, Cahiers de Studia Iranica 47, Chrétiens en terre d'Iran vol. V, Leuven: Peeters.

Goetze 1955 = A. Goetze, 'An Incantation against Diseases', *Journal of Cuneiform Studies* 9, 8–18.

Hallo and van Dijk 1968 = W.W. Hallo and J.J.A. van Dijk, *The Exaltation of Inanna*, Yale Near Eastern Researches 3, New Haven / London: Yale University Press.

Hankinson 1990 = R.J. Hankinson, 'Saying the Phenomena', *Phronesis* 35, 194–215.

Haussperger 1997 = M. Haussperger, 'Ein kleines medizinisches Kompendium aus altbabylonischer Zeit', *Würzburger medizinhistorische Mitteilungen* 16, 131–149.

Haussperger 2009 = M. Haussperger, 'Das „Fachbuch" der Erkrankungen der Atmungsorgane', *Zeitschrift für Assyriologie und Vorderasiatische Archäologie* 89, 165–200.

Heeßel 2000 = N.P. Heeßel, *Babylonisch-assyrische Diagnostik*, Alter Orient und Altes Testament 43, Münster: Ugarit-Verlag.

Heeßel 2002 = N.P. Heeßel, 'Ein neubabylonisches Rezept zur Berauschung und Ausnüchterung', in: *Mining the Archives: Festschrift for Christopher Walker on the Occasion of His 60th Birthday, 4 October 2002*, ed. C. Wunsch, Dresden: Islet, 99–106.

Heeßel 2007 = N.P. Heeßel, 'The Hands of the Gods: Disease Names and Divine Anger', in: *Disease in Babylonia*, Cuneiform Monographs 36, ed. I.L. Finkel and M.J. Geller, Leiden / Boston: Brill, 120–130.

Heeßel 2009 = N.P. Heeßel, 'The Babylonian Physician Rabâ-ša-Marduk. Another Look at Physicians and Exorcists in the Ancient Near East', in: *Advances in Mesopotamian Medicine from Hammurabi to Hippocrates: Proceedings of the International Conference "Oeil malade et mauvais oeil," Collège de France, Paris, 23rd June 2006*, Cuneiform Monographs 37, Leiden / Boston: Brill, 13–28.

Heeßel 2016 = N.P. Heeßel, 'Medizinische Texte aus dem Alten Mesopotamien', in: *Translating Writings of Early Scholars in the Ancient Near East, Egypt, Greece and Rome. Methodological Aspects with Examples*, Beiträge zur Altertumskunde 344, ed. A. Imhausen and T. Pommerening, Berlin / Boston: De Gruyter, 17–73.

Heeßel 2018a = N.P. Heeßel, 'A New Medical Therapeutic Text on Rectal Disease', in: *Mesopotamian Medicine and Magic: Studies in Honor of Markham J. Geller*, Ancient Magic and Divination 14, Leiden / Boston: Brill, 310–342.

Heeßel 2018b = N.P. Heeßel, 'Identifying Divine Agency: The Hands of the Gods in Context', in: G. van Buylaere et al., eds., Sources of Evil: Studies in Mesopotamian Exorcistic Lore, Ancient Magic and Divination 15, Leiden / Boston: Brill, 135–149.

Heeßel and al-Rawi 2003 = N.P. Heeßel and F.N.H. Al-Rawi, 'Tablets from the Sippar Library XII. A Medical Therapeutic Text', *Iraq* 65, 221–239.

Heimpel 2011 = W. Heimpel, 'Twenty-Eight Trees Growing in Sumer', in: *Garšana Studies*, Cornell University Studies in Assyriology in Sumerology 6, ed. D. Owen, Bethesda, Maryland: CDL Press, 75–152.

Herrero 1984 = P. Herrero 1984, *La thérapeutique mésopotamienne*, Paris: Editions Recherche sur les civilisations.

Hrůša 2010 = I. Hrůša, *Die akkadische Synonymenliste malku = šarru. Eine Textedition mit Übersetzung und Kommentar*, Alter Orient und Altes Testament 50, Münster: Ugarit-Verlag.

Jakob 2003 = S. Jakob, *Mittelassyrische Verwaltung und Sozialstruktur. Untersuchungen*, Cuneiform Monographs 29, Leiden / Boston: Brill / Styx.

Johnson 2014a = J.C. Johnson, 'The Origins of Scholastic Commentary in Mesopotamia: Second-order Schemata in the Early Dynastic Exegetical Imagination', in: *Visualizing Knowledge and Creating Meaning in Ancient Writing Systems*, Berliner Beiträge zum Vorderen Orient 23, ed. S. Gordin, Berlin: PeWe Verlag, 11–55.

Johnson 2014b = J.C. Johnson, 'Towards a reconstruction of SUALU IV: Can we localize K 2386+ in the therapeutic corpus?', *Le Journal des Médecines Cunéiformes* 24, 11–38.

Johnson 2015 = J.C. Johnson, 'Depersonalized Case Histories in the Babylonian Therapeutic Compendia', in: *In the Wake of the Compendia: Infrastructural Contexts and the Licensing of Empiricism in Ancient and Medieval Mesopotamia*, Science, Technology, and Medicine in Ancient Cultures 3, ed. J.C. Johnson, Boston / Berlin: Walter de Gruyter, 289–316.

Johnson 2018 = J.C. Johnson, 'Towards a New Perspective on Babylonian Medicine: The Continuum of Allegoresis and the Emergence of Secular Models in Mesopotamian Scientific Thought', in: *Assyrian and Babylonian Scholarly Text Catalogues: Medicine, Magic and Divination*, Die babylonisch-assyrische Medizin in Texten und Untersuchungen 9, ed. U. Steinert, Boston / Berlin: Walter de Gruyter, 55–88.

Jursa 2003–2005 = M. Jursa, 'Parfüm(rezepte). A. In Mesopotamien', *Reallexikon der Assyriologie* 10: 335–336.

Keetman 2021 = J. Keetman, 'Die Zeichenkombination ÁB.ŠÀ.GE und das Wort für „Galle", *Nouvelles Assyriologiques Brèves et Utilitaires* 2021/1, 5–8.

Kienast 1961 = B. Kienast, 'Weiteres zum R-Stamm des Akkadischen', *Journal of Cuneiform Studies* 15, 59–61.

Kinnier Wilson 1968 = J.V. Kinnier Wilson, 'Gleanings from the Iraq Medical Journals', *Journal of Near Eastern Studies* 27, 243–247.

Kinnier Wilson 2005 = J.V. Kinnier Wilson, 'On the Cryptograms in the lexical and related texts', *Le Journal des Médecines Cunéiformes* 6, 1–21.

Kinnier Wilson 2011 = J.V. Kinnier Wilson, 'A Journey through the Prescriptions', *Le Journal des Médecines Cunéiformes* 17, 1–24.

Kinnier Wilson and Reynolds 2007 = J.V. Kinnier Wilson and E.H. Reynolds, 'On Stroke and Facial Palsy in Babylonian Texts', in: *Disease in Babylonian* (Cuneiform Monographs 36), ed. I.L. Finkel and M.J. Geller, Leiden / Boston: Brill, 67–99.

Klinger 2010 = J. Klinger, 'Hethitische Texte zur Medizin – Einleitung', in: *Texte zur Heilkunde*, Texte aus der Umwelt des Alten Testaments, Neue Folge 5, ed. B. Janowski and D. Schwemer, Gütersloh: Gütersloher Verlagshaus, 177–188.

Köcher 1963 = F. Köcher, *Die babylonisch-assyrische Medizin in Texten und Untersuchungen*, Vol. 1: *Keilschrifttexte aus Assur 1*, Berlin: Walter de Gruyter.

Köcher 1971 = F. Köcher, *Die babylonisch-assyrische Medizin in Texten und Untersuchungen*, Vol. 4: *Keilschrifttexte aus Assur 4, Babylon, Nippur, Sippar, Uruk und unbekannter Herkunft*, Berlin: Walter de Gruyter.

Köcher 1978 = F. Köcher, 'Spätbabylonische medizinische Texte aus Uruk', in: *Medizinische Diagnostik in Geschichte und Gegenwart. Festschrift für Heinz Goerke zum sechzigsten Geburtstag*, ed. Ch. Habrich, F. Marguth and J.H. Wolf, München: Werner Fritsch, 17–39.

Köcher 1980 = F. Köcher, *Die babylonisch-assyrische Medizin in Texten und Untersuchungen*, Vol. 5–6: *Keilschrifttexte aus Ninive 1–2*, Berlin: Walter de Gruyter.

Krebernik 1984 = M. Krebernik, *Die Beschwörungen aus Fara und Ebla. Untersuchungen zur ältesten keilschriftlichen Beschwörungsliteratur*, Texte und Studien zur Orientalistik 2, Hildesheim / Zürich / New York: Georg Olms Verlag.

Küchler 1904 = F. Küchler, *Beiträge zur Kenntnis der Assyrisch-Babylonischen Medizin, Texte mit Umschrift, Übersetzung und Kommentar*, Leipzig: J. C. Hinrichs'sche Buchhandlung.

Labat 1951 = R. Labat, *Traité akkadien de diagnostics et pronostics médicaux*, Leiden: Brill.

Labat and Tournay 1945–1946 = R. Labat and J. Tournay, 'Un texte médical inédit', *Revue d'Assyriologie et d'archéologie orientale* 40, 113–122.

Lambert 1969 = W.G. Lambert, 'A Middle Assyrian Medical Text', *Iraq* 31, 28–39.

Lambert 1970 = W.G. Lambert, 'Fire Incantations', *Archiv für Orientforschung* 23, 39–45.

Lambert 1974 = W.G. Lambert, 'Dingir.šà.dib.ba Incantations', *Journal of Near Eastern Studies* 33, 267–270 + 272–322.

Lambert 1989 = W.G. Lambert, 'A Late Babylonian Copy of an Expository Text', *Journal of Near Eastern Studies* 48, 215–221.

Landsberger 1966 = B. Landsberger, 'Einige unerkannt gebliebene oder verkannte Nomina des Akkadischen', *Die Welt des Orients* 3, 246–268.

Landsberger 1967 = B. Landsberger, *The Date Palm and its By-products according to the Cuneiform Sources*, Archiv für Orientforschung Beiheft 17, Graz: Selbstverlag des Herausgebers.

Landsberger and Gurney 1957–1958 = B. Landsberger and O.R. Gurney, 'Practical Vocabulary of Assur', *Archiv für Orientforschung* 18, 328–341.

Landsberger and Jacobsen 1955 = B. Landsberger and Th. Jacobsen, 'An Old Babylonian Charm against Merḫu', *Journal of Near Eastern Studies* 14, 14–21.

Lassen, Frahm and Wagensonner 2019 = A.W. Lassen, E. Frahm and K. Wagensonner, *Ancient Mesopotamia Speaks: Highlights of the Yale Babylonian Collection*, New Haven: Yale University Press.

Leichty 1970 = E. Leichty, *The Omen Series Šumma Izbu*, Texts from Cuneiform Sources 4, Locust Valley, New York: J.J. Augustin Publisher.

Leichty 2011 = E. Leichty, *The Royal Inscriptions of Esarhaddon, King of Assyria (680–669 BC)*, The Royal Inscriptions of the Neo-Assyrian Period 4, Winona Lake, Indiana: Eisenbrauns.

Lenzi 2008 = A. Lenzi, *Secrecy and the Gods: Secret Knowledge in Ancient Mesopotamia and Biblical Israel*, State Archives of Assyria Studies 19, Helsinki: The Neo-Assyrian Text Corpus Project.

Livingstone 2007 = A. Livingstone, 'Ashurbanipal: literate or not?', *Zeitschrift für Assyriologie und Vorderasiatische Archäologie* 97, 98–118.

Livingstone 2014 = A. Livingstone, *Hemerologies of Assyrian and Babylonian Scholars*, Cornell University Studies in Assyriology and Sumerology 25, Bethesda, Maryland: CDL Press.

Loretz 2011 = O. Loretz, *Hippologia Ugaritica: Das Pferd in Kultur, Wirtschaft, Kriegführung und Hippiatrie Ugarits – Pferd, Esel und Kamel in biblischen Texten – Mit einem Beitrag von M. Stol über Pferde, Pferdekrankheiten und Pferdemedizin in altbabylonischer Zeit*, Alter Orient und Altes Testament 386, Münster: Ugarit-Verlag.

Löw 1924 = I. Löw, *Die Flora der Juden*, Band 3: *Pedaliaceae – Zygophyllaceae*, Wien: R. Loewit.

Marchesi 2013 = G. Marchesi, 'Of Plants and Trees: Crops and Vegetable Resources at Ebla', in: *Ebla and its Landscape: Early State Formation in the Ancient Near East*, ed. P. Matthiae and N. Marchetti, California: Left Coast Press, 274–292.

Maul 1994 = S.M. Maul, *Zukunftsbewältigung. Eine Untersuchung altorientalischen Denkens anhand der babylonisch-assyrischen Löserituale (Namburbi)*, Baghdader Forschungen 18, Mainz am Rhein: Verlag Philipp von Zabern.

Maul 2019 = S.M. Maul, *Bannlösung (nam-érim-búr-ru-da). Die Therapie eines auf eidliche Falschaussage zurückgeführten Leidens*, Teil 1: *Einleitung, Katalog und Textbearbeitungen*, Teil 2: *Verzeichnisse, Keilschriftautographien und Photographien*, Keilschrifttexte aus Assur literarischen Inhalts 10, Wiesbaden: Harrassowitz.

Mayer 2009 = W.R. Mayer, 'Akkadische Lexikographie: CAD T unt Ṭ'. *Orientalia* Nova Series 78, 423–439.

Meier 1939a = G. Meier, 'Lexikalische Bemerkungen', *Orientalia* Nova Series 8, 301–305.

Meier 1939b = G. Meier, 'Ein akkadisches Heilungsritual aus Boğazköy', *Zeitschrift für Assyriologie und Vorderasiatische Archäologie* 45, 195–215.

Michalowski 1981 = P. Michalowski, 'Carminative Magic: Towards an Understanding of Sumerian Poetics', *Zeitschrift für Assyriologie und Vorderasiatische Archäologie* 71, 1–18.

Michalowski 1992 = P. Michalowski, 'The Early Mesopotamian Incantation Tradition', in: *Literature and Literary Language at Ebla* (Quaderni di Semitistica 18), ed. P. Fronzaroli, Firenze: Dipartimento di linguistica, Università di Firenze, 305–326.

Michel 2004 = C. Michel, 'Deux incantations paléo-assyriennes. Une nouvelle incantation pour accompagner la naissance', in: *Assyria and Beyond: Studies Presented to Mogens Trolle Larsen* (Publications de l'Institut historique et archéologique néerlandais de Stamboul 100), ed. J.G. Dercksen, Leiden: Nederlands Instituut voor het Nabije Oosten, 395–420.

Michel 2020 = C. Michel, 'Computation Practices of the Assyrian Merchants During the Nineteenth Century BCE', in: *Mathematics, Administrative and Economic Activities in the Ancient Worlds*, Why the Sciences of the Ancient World Matter 5, ed. C. Michel and K. Chemla, Cham, Switzerland: Springer.

Nougayrol 1979 = J. Nougayrol, 'Tablettes diverses du Musée du Louvre', *Revue d'Assyriologie et d'archéologie orientale* 73, 63–80.

Oefele 1902 = F. von Oefele, *Keilschriftmedicin: Einleitendes zur Medicin der Kouyunjik-Collection*, Abhandlungen zur Geschichte der Medicin 111, Breslau: J.U. Kern's Verlag.

Oefele ²1904 = F. von Oefele, *Keilschriftmedizin in Parallelen mit der Wiedergabe einer medizinischen Keilschrifttafel*, Der Alte Orient 2, 2nd ed., Leipzig: J.C. Hinrichs'sche Buchhandlung.

Panayotov 2013 = S.V. Panayotov, 'A Copper Bell to Expel Demons in Berlin', *Nouvelles Assyriologiques Brèves et Utilitaires* 2013/3 , 80–87.

Panayotov 2017 = S.V. Panayotov, 'Eye Metaphors, Analogies and Similes within Mesopotamian Magico-Medical Texts', in: *The Comparable Body: Analogy and Metaphor in Ancient Mesopotamian, Egyptian, and Greco-Roman Medicine*, Studies in Ancient Medicine 49, ed. J.Z. Wee, Leiden / Boston: Brill, 204–246.

Panayotov 2018 = S.V. Panayotov, 'Notes on the Assur Medical Catalogue with Comparison to the Nineveh Medical Encyclopaedia', in: *Assyrian and Babylonian Scholarly Text Catalogues: Medicine, Magic and Divination*, Die babylonisch-assyrische Medizin in Texten und Untersuchungen 9, ed. U. Steinert, Boston / Berlin: Walter de Gruyter, 89–120.

Paoletti 2016 = P. Paoletti, '„Raffiniertes" Gold? Gold und seine Qualität(sbezeichnung)en in den altbabylonischen Quellen aus Mesopotamien im 20.–18. Jahrhundert v. Chr.', in: *Bernstorf. Archäologisch-naturwissenschaftliche Analysen der Gold- und Bernsteinfunde vom Bernstorfer Berg bei Kranzberg, Oberbayern*, ed. R. Gebhard and R. Krause, München: Archäologische Staatssammlung.

Parpola 1983a = S. Parpola, 'Assyrian Library Records', *Journal of Near Eastern Studies* 42, 1–29.

Parpola 1983b = S. Parpola, *Letters from Assyrian Scholars to the Kings Esarhaddon and Assurbanipal*. Part II: *Commentary and Appendices*, Alter Orient und Altes Testament 5/2, Kevelaer / Neukirchen-Vluyn: Verlag Butzon & Bercker / Neukirchener Verlag.

Parpola 1988 = S. Parpola, 'The Neo-Assyrian Word for "Queen"', *State Archives of Assyria Bulletin* 2, 73–76.

Parys 2014 = M. Parys, 'Édition d'un texte médical thérapeutique retrouvé à Assur (BAM 159)', *Le Journal des Médecines Cunéiformes* 23, 1–88.

Paulette 2016 = T. Paulette, 'Grain, Storage, and State Making in Mesopotamia (3200–2000 BC)', in: *Storage in Ancient Complex Societies: Administration, Organisation, and Control*, ed. L.R. Manzanilla and M.S. Rothman, New York / London: Routledge, 85–109.

Peterson 2013 = J. Peterson, 'A Catalogue of Old Babylonian Sumerian Incantations and Rituals from Nippur in the University Museum, Philadelphia', *Nouvelles Assyriologiques Brèves et Utilitaires* 2013/1, 1–2.

Peterson 2019 = J. Peterson, 'A Brief OB Incantation Against Stomach Ailments from Nippur, Area TA, House F', *Nouvelles Assyriologiques Brèves et Utilitaires* 2019/4, 172.

Picchioni 1981 = S.A. Picchioni, *Il poemetto di Adapa*, Assyriologia 6, Budapest: Eötvös Loránd Tudományegyetem.

Pietrobelli 2021 = A. Pietrobelli, 'Théories et imaginaire de la digestion dans l'Antiquité', in: *Histoire du ventre: Entrailles, tripes et boyaux. Antiquité, Moyen Age, Époque moderne*, ed. F. Collard and E. Samama, Paris: L'Harmattan, 31–43.

Postgate 1987 = J.N. Postgate, 'Some Vegetables in the Assyrian Sources', *Bulletin on Sumerian Agriculture* 3, 93–100.

Powell 1971 = M.A. Powell, *Sumerian Numeration and Metrology*, PhD Dissertation, University of Minnesota.

Powell 1979 = M.A. Powell, 'Ancient Mesopotamian Weight Metrology: Methods, Problems and Perspectives', in: *Studies in Honor of Tom B. Jones* (Alter Orient und Altes Testament 203), ed. R.H. Sack, Kevelaer / Neukirchen-Vluyn: Verlag Butzon & Bercker / Neukirchener Verlag, 71–110.

Powell 1984 = M.A. Powell, 'Sumerian Cereal Crops', *Bulletin on Sumerian Agriculture* 1, 48–72.

Powell 1987–1990 = M.A. Powell, 'Masse und Gewichte', *Reallexikon der Assyriologie und Vorderasiatischen Archäologie* 7, 457–517.

Powell 1994 = M.A. Powell, 'Metron Ariston: Measure as a Tool for Studying Beer in Ancient Mesopotamia', in: *Drinking in Ancient Societies*, History of the Ancient Near East, Studies 6, ed. L. Milano, Padova: Sargon srl, 90–119.

Reade 1998–2000 = J.E. Reade, 'Nineve (Nineveh)', *Reallexikon der Assyriologie und Vorderasiatischen Archäologie* 9, 388–433.

Reiner 1958 = E. Reiner, *Šurpu: A Collection of Sumerian and Akkadian Incantations*, Archiv für Orientforschung Beiheft 11, Osnabrück: Biblio Verlag.

Reiner 1963 = E. Reiner, 'Deux cryptogrammes akkadiens', *Revue d'Assyriologie et d'archéologie orientale* 63, 170–171.

Reiner 1985 = E. Reiner, *Your Thwarts in Pieces, Your Mooring Rope Cut: Poetry from Babylonia and Assyria*, Michigan Studies in the Humanities 5, Ann Arbor: Horace H. Rackham School of Graduate Studies at the University of Michigan.

Reiner 1995 = E. Reiner, *Astral Magic in Babylonia*, Transactions of the American Philosophical Society 85/4, Philadelphia: The American Philosophical Society.

de Ridder 2018 = J.J. De Ridder, *Descriptive Grammar of Middle Assyrian*, Leipziger Altorientalische Studien 8, Wiesbaden: Harrassowitz.

Ritter 1965 = E.K. Ritter, 'Magical-Expert (= *Āšipu*) and Physician (= *Asû*): Notes on Two Complementary Professions in Babylonian Medicine', in: *Studies in Honor of Benno Landsberger on His Seventy-Fifth Birthday, April 21, 1965*, Assyriological Studies 16, ed. H.G. Güterbock and T. Jacobsen, Chicago: The University of Chicago Press, 299–322.

Rudik 2011 = N. Rudik, *Die Entwicklung der keilschriftlichen sumerischen Beschwörungsliteratur von den Anfängen bis zur Ur III-Zeit*, PhD Dissertation, Friedrich-Schiller Universität Jena.

Rumor 2017 = M. Rumor, 'The 'AŠ section' of Uruanna III in Partitur', *Le Journal des Médecines Cunéiformes* 29, 1–34.

Rumor 2021 = M. Rumor, 'Babylonian Astro-medicine, Quadruplicities and Pliny the Elder', *Zeitschrift für Assyriologie und Vorderasiatische Archäologie* 111, 47–76.

Rutz 2011 = M.T. Rutz, 'Threads of Esagil-kīn-apli: The Medical Diagnostic-Prognostic Series in Middle Babylonian Nippur', *Zeitschrift für Assyriologie und Vorderasiatische Archäologie* 101, 294–308.

Sayce 1885 = A.H. Sayce, 'An ancient Babylonian Work on Medicine', *Zeitschrift für Keilschriftforschung und verwandte Gebiete* 2, 1–14.

Scheyhing 2007 = H. Scheyhing, 'Der Patient wird sterben! Tod in den medizinisch-therapeutischen Texten des Alten Orients', *Die Welt des Orients* 37, 112–134.

Schmidtchen 2018 = E. Schmidtchen, 'Simplicia and Unpublished Fragments of *Alamdimmû* from the British Museum', in: *Mesopotamian Medicine and Magic: Studies in Honor of Markham J. Geller*, Ancient Magic and Divination 14, Leiden / Boston: Brill, 462–500.

Schmidtchen 2021 = E. Schmidtchen, *Mesopotamische Diagnostik. Untersuchungen zu Rekonstruktion, Terminologie und Systematik des babylonisch-assyrischen Diagnosehandbuches und eine Neubearbeitung der Tafeln 3–14*, Die babylonisch-assyrische Medizin in Texten und Untersuchungen 13, Berlin / Boston: Walter de Gruyter.

Schuster-Brandis 2008 = A. Schuster-Brandis, *Steine als Schutz- und Heilmittel. Untersuchung zu ihrer Verwendung in der Beschwörungskunst Mesopotamiens im 1. Jt. v. Chr.*, Alter Orient und Altes Testament 46, Münster: Ugarit-Verlag.

Schwemer 1998 = D. Schwemer, *Akkadische Rituale aus Ḫattuša: Die Sammeltafel KBo XXXVI 29 und verwandte Fragmente*, Texte der Hethiter 23, Heidelberg: Winter.

Schwemer 2004 = D. Schwemer, 'Ein akkadischer Liebeszauber aus Ḫattuša', *Zeitschrift für Assyriologie und Vorderasiatische Archäologie* 94, 59–79.

Schwemer 2007 = D. Schwemer, *Abwehrzauber und Behexung: Studien zum Schadenzauberglauben im alten Mesopotamien.* Wiesbaden: Harrassowitz.

Schwemer 2010 = D. Schwemer, 'Eine Rezeptsammlung aus Ur', in: *Texte zur Heilkunde*, Texte aus der Umwelt des Alten Testaments, Neue Folge 5, ed. B. Janowski and D. Schwemer, Gütersloh: Gütersloher Verlagshaus, 36.

Schwemer 2021 = D. Schwemer, 'KU.KU = *supantu, supandu*', *Nouvelles Assyriologiques Brèves et Utilitaires* 2021/2 , 117.

Scott 2017 = J.C. Scott, *Against the Grain: A Deep History of the Earliest States*, New Haven: Yale University Press.

Scurlock 2006 = J.A. Scurlock, *Magico-Medical Means of Treating Ghost-Induced Illnesses in Ancient Mesopotamia*, Ancient Magic and Divination 3, Leiden / Boston: Brill / Styx Publications.

Scurlock 2014 = J.A. Scurlock, *Sourcebook for Ancient Mesopotamian Medicine*, Writings from the Ancient World 36, Atlanta, Georgia: SBL Press.

Scurlock and Andersen 2005 = J.A. Scurlock and B.R. Andersen, *Diagnoses in Assyrian and Babylonian Medicine: Ancient Sources, Translations, and Modern Medical Analyses*, Urbana / Chicago: University of Illinois Press.

Sibbing-Plantholt 2014 = I. Sibbing-Plantholt, 'A New Look at the Kassite Medical Letters, and an Edition of Šumu-libši Letter N 969', *Zeitschrift für Assyriologie und Vorderasiatische Archäologie* 104, 171–181.

Sibbing-Plantholt 2022 = I. Sibbing-Plantholt, *The Image of Mesopotamian Divine Healers: Healing Goddesses and the Legitimization of Professional* asûs *in the Mesopotamian Medical Marketplace*, Cuneiform Monographs 53, Leiden / Boston: Brill.

Simkó 2018 = K. Simkó, 'BAM 7 44: Suppositories for Rectal and Gastro-Intestinal Diseases', in: *Mesopotamian Medicine and Magic: Studies in Honor of Markham J. Geller*, Ancient Magic and Divination 14, Leiden / Boston: Brill, 537–555.

von Soden 1947 = W. von Soden, 'Zum akkadischen Wörterbuch. 6–14', *Orientalia* Nova Series 16, 66–84.

von Soden 1966 = W. von Soden, Review of CAD Vol. 1: A Part 1, *Orientalistische Literaturzeitung* 61, 356–360.

von Soden 1968 = W. von Soden, 'Aramäische Wörter in neuassyrischen und neu- und spätbabylonischen Texten. Ein Vorbericht. II (n-z und Nachträge)', *Orientalia* Nova Series 37, 261–271.

von Soden 1977 = W. von Soden, 'Aramäische Wörter in neuassyrischen und neu- und spätbabylonischen Texten. Ein Vorbericht. III', *Orientalia* Nova Series 46, 183–197.

Sokoloff 2002 = M. Sokoloff, *A Dictionary of Jewish Babylonian Aramaic of the Talmudic and Geonic Periods*, Dictionaries of Talmud, Midrash and Targum 3, Ramat-Gan: Bar Ilan University Press.

Sokoloff 2009 = M. Sokoloff, *A Syriac Lexicon: A Translation from the Latin, Correction, Expansion, and Update of C. Brockelmann's Lexicon Syriacum*, Winona Lake, Indiana: Eisenbrauns.

von Staden 1989 = H. von Staden, *Herophilus: The Art of Medicine in Early Alexandria: Edition, Translation and Essays*, Cambridge: Cambridge University Press.

Stadhouders 2011 = H. Stadhouders, 'The Pharmacopoeial Handbook *Šammu šikinšu* – An Edition', *Le Journal des Médecines Cunéiformes* 18, 3–51.

Stadhouders 2018 = H. Stadhouders, 'The *mirišmarû*-Plant: Orthographic Novelties and a Consecratory Spell', *Die Welt des Orients* 48, 116–127.

Stadhouders and Johnson 2018 = H. Stadhouders and C.J. Johnson, 'A Time to Extract and a Time to Compile: The Therapeutic Compendium Tablet BM 78963', in: *Mesopotamian Medicine and Magic: Studies in Honor of Markham J. Geller*, Ancient Magic and Divination 14, Leiden / Boston: Brill, 556–622.

Steinert 2012 = U. Steinert, *Aspekte des Menschseins im Alten Mesopotamien: Eine Studie zu Person und Identität im 2. und 1. Jt. v. Chr.*, Cuneiform Monographs 44, Leiden / Boston: Brill.

Steinert 2013 = U. Steinert, 'Fluids, Rivers and Vessels: Metaphors and Body Concepts in Mesopotamian Gynaecological Texts', *Le Journal des Médecines Cuneiformes* 22, 1–23.

Steinert 2018a = U. Steinert, 'The Assur Medical Catalogue (AMC)', in: *Assyrian and Babylonian Scholarly Text Catalogues: Medicine, Magic and Divination*, Die babylonisch-assyrische Medizin in Texten und Untersuchungen 9, ed. U. Steinert, Boston / Berlin: Walter de Gruyter, 203–291.

Steinert 2018b = U. Steinert, 'Catalogues, Texts and Specialists: Some Thoughts on the Assur Medical Catalogue, Mesopotamian Medical Texts and Healing Professions', in: *Assyrian and Babylonian Scholarly Text Catalogues: Medicine, Magic and Divination*, Die babylonisch-assyrische Medizin in Texten und Untersuchungen 9, ed. U. Steinert, Boston / Berlin: Walter de Gruyter, 158–200.

Steinert and Vacín 2018 = U. Steinert and L. Vacín, 'BM 92518 and Old Babylonian Incantations for the "Belly"', in: *Mesopotamian Medicine and Magic: Studies in Honor of Markham J. Geller*, Ancient Magic and Divination 14, ed. S.V. Panayotov and L. Vacín, Leiden / Boston: Brill, 698–744.

Stol 1985a = M. Stol, 'Remarks on the Cultivation of Sesame and the Extraction of its Oil', *Bulletin on Sumerian Agriculture* 2, 119–126.

Stol 1985b = M. Stol, 'Beans, Peas, Lentils and Vetches in Akkadian Texts', *Bulletin on Sumerian Agriculture* 2, 127–139.

Stol 1985c = M. Stol; 'Felix von Oefele and Babylonian Medicine', *Janus* 72, 7–16.

Stol 1987 = M. Stol, 'The Cucurbitaceae in the Cuneiform Texts', *Bulletin on Sumerian Agriculture* 3, 81–92.

Stol 1991–1992 = M. Stol, 'Diagnosis and Therapy in Babylonian Medicine', *Jaarbericht van het Vooraziatisch-Egyptisch Genootschap "Ex Oriente" Lux* 32, 42–65.

Stol 1993 = M. Stol, *Epilepsy in Babylonia and the Bible*, Cuneiform Monographs 2, Groningen: Styx.

Stol 1994 = M. Stol, 'Beer in Neo-Babylonian Times', in: *Drinking in Ancient Societies*, History of the Ancient Near East, Studies 6, ed. L. Milano, Padova: Sargon srl, 155–183.

Stol 1998 = M. Stol, 'Einige kurze Wortstudien', in: *Festschrift für Rykle Borger zu seinem 65. Geburtstag am 24. Mai 1994. tikip santakki mala bašmu . . .*, Cuneiform Monographs 10, ed. S.M. Maul, Groningen: Styx, 343–352.

Stol 2004 = M. Stol, 'An Assyriologist Reads Hippocrates', in: *Magic and Rationality in Ancient Near Eastern and Graeco-Roman Medicine* (Studies in Ancient Medicine 27), ed. H.F.J. Horstmanshoff and M. Stol, Leiden / Boston: Brill, 63–78.

Stol 2006 = M. Stol, 'The Digestion of Food According to Babylonian Sources', in: *Médecine et médecins au Proche-Orient ancien. Actes du Colloque International organisé à Lyon les 8 et 9 novembre 2002, Maison de l'Orient et de la Mediterranée* (BAR International Series 1528), ed. L. Battini and P. Villard, Oxford: Archaeopress, 103–119.

Stol 2007 = M. Stol, 'Fevers in Babylonia', in: *Disease in Babylonian*, Cuneiform Monographs 36, ed. I.L. Finkel and M.J. Geller, Leiden / Boston: Brill, 1–39.

Stol 2009a: M. Stol, 'Sesame', *Reallexikon der Assyriologie und Vorderasiatischen Archäologie* 12, 400–404.

Stol 2009b = M. Stol, 'Insanity in Babylonian Sources', *Le Journal des Médecines Cunéiformes* 13, 1–12.

Stol 2009c = M. Stol, '"To be ill" in Akkadian: The Verb *Salā'u* and the Substantive *Sili'tu*', in: *Advances in Mesopotamian Medicine from Hammurabi to Hippocrates: Proceedings of the International Conference "Oeil malade et mauvais oeil," Collège de France, Paris, 23rd June 2006*, Cuneiform Monographs 37, Leiden / Boston: Brill, 29–46.

Stol 2012 = M. Stol, Review of P. Gignoux, *Lexique des termes de la pharmacopée syriaque* (2011), *Bibliotheca Orientalis* 69, 627–628.

Stol 2013 = M. Stol, Review of Tz. Abusch and D. Schwemer, *Corpus of Mesopotamian Anti-Witchcraft Rituals* Vol. 1 (2011), *Bibliotheca Orientalis* 70, 125–130.

Stol 2018 = M. Stol, Review of A. Bácskay, *Therapeutic Prescriptions against Fever in Ancient Mesopotamia* (2018), *Bibliotheca Orientalis* 75, 344–351.

Stol 2020a = M. Stol, Review of SAD Vol. 1: B, P, *Bibliotheca Orientalis* 77, 101–110.

Stol 2020b = M. Stol, Review of Tz. Abusch, D. Schwemer, M. Luukko and G. Van Buylaere, *Corpus of Mesopotamian Anti-Witchcraft Rituals* Vol. 3–4 (2020), *Bibliotheca Orientalis* 77, 567–573.

Stol 2021 = M. Stol, Review of SAD Vol. 2: D, T, Ṭ, *Bibliotheca Orientalis* 78, 431–458.

Sullivan 1980 = B.B. Sullivan, *Sumerian and Akkadian Sentence Structure in Old Babylonian Literary Bilingual Texts*, PhD Dissertation, Hebrew Union College.

Thavapalan 2020 = S. Thavapalan, *The Meaning of Color in Ancient Mesopotamia*, Culture and History of the Ancient Near East 104, Leiden / Boston: Brill.

Thureau-Dangin 1921 = F. Thureau-Dangin, *Rituels accadiens*, Paris: Éditions Ernest Leroux.

van der Toorn 1985 = K. van der Toorn, *Sin and Sanction in Israel and Mesopotamia: A Comparative Study*, Studia Semitica Neerlandica 22, Assen / Maastrich: Van Gorcum.

Tsukimoto 1999 = A. Tsukimoto, '"By the Hand of Madi-Dagan, the Scribe and *Apkallu*-Priest": A Medical Text from the Middle Euphrates Region', in: *Priests and Officials in the Ancient Near East: Papers of the Second Colloquium on the Ancient Near East – The City and its Life, held at the Middle Eastern Culture Center in Japan (Mitaka, Tokyo) March 22–24, 1996*, ed. K. Watanabe, Heidelberg: Universitätsverlag C. Winter, 187–200.

Turner 2021 = G. Turner, *The British Museum's Excavations at Nineveh, 1846–1855*, Culture and History of the Ancient Near East 115, Leiden / Boston: Brill.

Veldhuis 1990 = N.C. Veldhuis, 'The Heart Grass and Related Matters', *Orientalia Lovaniensia Periodica* 21, 27–44.

Veldhuis 1993 = N.C. Veldhuis, 'The Fly, the Worm, and the Chain: Old Babylonian Chain Incantations', *Orientalia Lovaniensia Periodica* 24, 41–64.

Waetzoldt 1985 = H. Waetzoldt, 'Ölpflanzen und Pflanzenöle im 3. Jahrtausend', *Bulletin on Sumerian Agriculture* 2, 77–96.

Waerzeggers 2010 = C. Waerzeggers, *The Ezida Temple of Borsippa: Priesthood, Cult, Archives*, Achaemenid History 15, Leiden: Nederlands Instituut voor het Nabije Oosten.

Wasserman 2003 = N. Wasserman, *Style and Form in Old Babylonian Literary Texts*, Cuneiform Monographs 27, Leiden / Boston: Brill / Styx.

Wasserman 2012 = N. Wasserman, *Most Probably: Epistemic Modality in Old Babylonian*, Languages of the Ancient Near East 3, Winona Lake, Indiana: Eisenbrauns.

Wasserman and Zomer 2022 = N. Wasserman and E. Zomer, *Akkadian Magic Literature, Old Babylonian and Old Assyrian Incantations: Corpus – Context – Praxis*, Leipziger Altorientalische Studien 12, Wiesbaden: Harrassowitz.

Wee 2017 = J.Z. Wee (ed.), *The Comparable Body: Analogy and Metaphor in Ancient Mesopotamian, Egyptian and Greco-Roman Medicine*, Studies in Ancient Medicine 49, Leiden / Boston: Brill.

Wee 2019 = J.Z. Wee, *Knowledge and Rhetoric in Medical Commentary: Ancient Mesopotamian Commentaries on a Handbook of Medical Diagnosis (Sa-gig)*, Cuneiform Monographs 49/1, Leiden / Boston: Brill.

Wilcke 1985 = C. Wilcke, 'Liebesbeschwörung aus Isin', *Zeitschrift für Assyriologie und Vorderasiatische Archäologie* 75, 188–209.

Whiting 1985 = R.M. Whiting, 'An Old Babylonian Incantation from Tell Asmar', *Zeitschrift für Assyriologie und Vorderasiatische Archäologie* 75, 179–187.

Worthington 2006 = M. Worthington, 'Edition of BAM 3', *Le Journal des Médecines Cunéiformes* 7, 18–48.

Zilberg and Horowitz 2016 = P. Zilberg and W. Horowitz, 'A Medico-Magical Text from the Otago Tablets, Dunedin New Zealand', *Zeitschrift für Assyriologie und Vorderasiatische Archäologie* 106, 175–184.

Zimmern 1917[2] = H. Zimmern, *Akkadische Fremdwörter als Beweis für babylonischen Kultureinfluss*, Leipzig: J.C. Hinrichs'sche Buchhandlung.

Zisa 2021 = G. Zisa, *The Loss of Male Sexual Desire in Ancient Mesopotamia: ›Nīš Libbi‹ Therapies*, Medical Traditions 5, Berlin / Boston: Walter de Gruyter.

Zomer 2018 = E. Zomer, *Corpus of Middle Babylonian and Middle Assyrian Incantations*, Leipziger Altorientalische Studien 9, Wiesbaden: Harrassowitz.

Index

All Akkadian words in the currently reconstructed form of the Stomach Treatise are indexed here. Adjectives and participial forms are listed under the corresponding verbal infinitive unless there is a specific lexical nuance that needs to be highlighted, viz. *aḫḫāzu* is listed separately from *aḫāzu* ('to take') because it distinctly refers to a type of jaundice. Bipartite phrases in which neither term occurs separately (or where the meaning of the phrase as a whole is distinct from its components) are listed as a single unit and alphabetised under the first term: *aban gabî, ana libbi, ana maḫri, ana muḫḫi, ana pāni, ayyar ili, balu patān, billat našpi, biṣṣūr atāni, bišīt libbi, bīt zumbi labbini, erišti eqli, ḫaṭṭi rē'î, ḫimiṭ ṣēti, ḫīq šikari, imbu' tâmti, ina libbi, ina maḫri, ina muḫḫi, ina pāni, iṣ pišri, išku ša gāridi, ištēt qati, karān šēlebi, kī pî, kirbān eqli, kīs libbi, kiṣir libbi, kiṣirti libbi, lā patān, liblibbi gišimmari, lišān kalbi, naptan šēri, pappāsi buqli, pizalluru rabû, qadūt šikāni, qān šalāli, qanû ṭābu, qāt ṣēri, rēš libbi, ridût irrī, rikibti arkabi, sebet ūmī, sissinni libbi, ṣēta ḫamiṭ, ṣēta kašid, ṣinnaḫ tīri, šalāšat ūmī, šammi ašî, šammi balāṭi, šammu peṣû, šibiṭ šāri, šiḫḫat šīri, šikar sābî, šikaru rēštû, šinā ūmī, tē šipti, ṭābat amāni, ṭābat emesalli, ubānu rabītu, uḫūlu qarnānu, ummi mê, zē summati,* and *zīr karši*. Logograms for which the correct Akkadian reading is unclear, such as MIN or KI MIN, are listed under the logographic form; numerals are generally listed under the masculine singular absolute form; and complex prepositions are listed separately. Entirely Sumerian phrases, which seem to have been read in Sumerian, including STO 1: 5–7a and the monolingual Sumerian incantation in STO 3: 99–108, have not been included in the index. Occurrences of the logogram PA, which can correspond to a number of Akkadian words, are somewhat artificially collected under Akk. *artu*, while occurrences of PA.MEŠ are collected under Akk. *ḫasḫalātu*

Only one occurrence is listed if the same word occurs more than once in a line. Where multiple manuscripts are in play, only distinct orthographies or orthographies that are damaged in a different way are listed separately. Parallels are not included in any way.

Entries are listed in terms of orthographic completeness and complexity, with fully preserved forms of the standard logogram coming first, then increasingly damaged versions of the same orthography, and then syllabic and unusual orthographies at the end.

Words

https://doi.org/10.1515/9781501506574-009

Divine Names

Personal Names

Geographical Names

www.ingramcontent.com/pod-product-compliance
Lightning Source LLC
LaVergne TN
LVHW081347011026
849161LV00013BB/3021